Handbook of Gastroenterology and Hepatology

Handbook of Gastroenterology and Hepatology

Handbook of Gastroenterology and Hepatology

Editor: Jonas Dexter

FOSTER ACADEMICS

www.fosteracademics.com

www.fosteracademics.com

FOSTER ACADEMICS

Cataloging-in-Publication Data

Handbook of gastroenterology and hepatology / edited by Jonas Dexter.
p. cm.
Includes bibliographical references and index.
ISBN 978-1-63242-934-6
1. Gastroenterology. 2. Hepatology. 3. Digestive organs--Diseases. 4. Internal medicine. I. Dexter, Jonas.
RC801 .H36 2020
616.33--dc23

Foster Academics,
118-35 Queens Blvd., Suite 400,
Forest Hills, NY 11375, USA

ISBN 978-1-63242-934-6 (Hardback)

Contents

Preface

Gastroenterology is a branch of medicine that is concerned with the treatment of the diseases affecting the gastrointestinal tract. This includes the disorders of the esophagus, stomach, small intestine, liver, bile ducts, gallbladder, pancreas, colon, rectum, etc. Such disorders may include polyps and cancer, peptic ulcer disease, gastroesophageal reflux disease, pancreatitis, irritable bowel syndrome, etc. Some of the complex procedures in gastroenterology include endoscopic retrograde cholangiopancreatography, endoscopic mucosal resection, placement of internal drainage tubes, polypectomy, esophageal and intestinal dilation, etc. Hepatology is a specialization of gastroenterology. It is concerned with the management of the disorders of the liver, pancreas, gallbladder and biliary tree. Jaundice/hepatitis, liver disease, liver damage, storage disease of liver, hemochromatosis, etc. are some of the conditions that are under the scope of this field. Some of the procedures performed under this specialization include liver transplant, transjugular intrahepatic portosystemic shunt, transhepatic pancreato-cholangiography, etc. This book covers in detail some existing theories and innovative concepts revolving around gastroenterology and hepatology. Most of the topics introduced in this book cover new techniques and the applications of these fields. It is an essential guide for both academicians and those who wish to pursue these disciplines further.

Various studies have approached the subject by analyzing it with a single perspective, but the present book provides diverse methodologies and techniques to address this field. This book contains theories and applications needed for understanding the subject from different perspectives. The aim is to keep the readers informed about the progresses in the field; therefore, the contributions were carefully examined to compile novel researches by specialists from across the globe.

Indeed, the job of the editor is the most crucial and challenging in compiling all chapters into a single book. In the end, I would extend my sincere thanks to the chapter authors for their profound work. I am also thankful for the support provided by my family and colleagues during the compilation of this book.

Editor

1

The Frequency of Clinic Visits was not Associated with Medication Adherence or Outcome in Children with Inflammatory Bowel Diseases

Cheryl Kluthe,[1] Jenkin Tsui,[2] Donald Spady,[3] Matthew Carroll,[1] Eytan Wine,[1] and Hien Quoc Huynh[1]

[1]*Edmonton Pediatric IBD Clinic (EPIC), Edmonton, AB, Canada*
[2]*University of Edinburgh, Edinburgh, UK*
[3]*Division of Pediatric GI Nutrition, Stollery Children's Hospital, University of Alberta, Edmonton, AB, Canada*

Correspondence should be addressed to Hien Quoc Huynh; hien.huynh@ualberta.ca

Academic Editor: Fabio Grizzi

Background. Medication nonadherence is a challenge in pediatric patients with inflammatory bowel diseases (IBD). Poor adherence can result in disease flare-ups, disease complicationstherapy escalation, and the need for corticosteroids. The aim was to determine if clinic visit frequency was associated with treatment adherence. *Methods.* A retrospective chart review of patients attending the Edmonton Pediatric IBD Clinic (EPIC) at the Stollery Children's Hospital from January 2012 to December 2013 was completed. Correlations were made between frequency of clinic visit, percentage of prescriptions filled, percentage of requisitioned blood work completed, rural or urban residence, and steroid-free remission status of patients for the 6 months after the chart review. *Results.* 127 patients were reviewed with 82 patients diagnosed with Crohn's disease (CD) and 46 with ulcerative colitis (UC) which included one IBD-Unclassified. Mean age at diagnosis is 9.17 years and median duration of follow-up is 3.2 years. Almost all patients on infliximab infusions received them "within window." Immunomodulator median adherence rate was 88%. 5-ASA adherence was 82%. A median of 67% of patients had blood work completed as requested. Clinic visit frequency was not associated with adherence to blood work or to medications. Duration of disease was the only independent factor found to be associated with a reduction in blood work and immunomodulator adherence ("OR 0.86 and 95% CI: 0.74–0.99" and "OR 0.82 and 95% CI: 0.71–0.97") per year, respectively. Patients who remained corticosteroid-free in the 6 months after the 2 years' adherence review had an overall median medication adherence rate of 86% compared to only 53% for those who relapsed and required corticosteroids ($p = 0.01$). *Conclusion.* Clinic visit frequency was not associated with patient adherence to medications or blood work. However, disease duration was found to be associated with medication adherence. Adherent patients were more likely to remain in steroid-free remission.

1. Introduction

1.1. Background. Inflammatory bowel disease (IBD) is a chronic condition that leads to inflammation in the digestive tract. It is characterized by periods of disease activity and periods of disease remission [1]. Canada has one of the highest incidence rates of Crohn's disease (CD) and ulcerative colitis (UC) in the world: 13.4 and 11.8 cases over 100,000 persons for CD and UC [2]. Furthermore, the incidence of IBD in children under 10 years of age is increasing [3]. Currently, there is no cure for IBD, leading to the need for chronic treatment. Medication nonadherence is a challenging issue for patients with a chronic disease, including pediatric patients with IBD. Pediatric IBD is unique in that both the patients and the parents have a shared responsibility for administering medications [4]. Poor adherence can result in disease flare-ups, disease complications, therapy escalation, and need for corticosteroids. Previous studies indicate that nonadherent patients are 5.5 times more likely to experience a flare compared to individuals who are adherent [4]. Nonadherence rates range from 50 to 80% [4], with patients overestimating their oral medication intake rate by 23% [5].

Reasons often given for poor adherence include the following: forgetfulness, patient perceptions of side effects, and lack of education [6].

It has been shown that, by improving a patient's adherence rate, they can potentially decrease disease activity and improve long-term outcomes. Physicians commonly provide knowledge and education to their patients about disease management; however ultimately it is up to the patient to follow this advice. One factor in a patient's care that the physician can influence is the frequency of scheduled follow-up visits. The goal of this study was to investigate the association between frequency of clinic follow-up on adherence to medications and blood work and treatment outcomes.

2. Methods

2.1. Study Design. A retrospective chart review of patients attending the Edmonton Pediatric IBD Clinic (EPIC) at the Stollery Children's Hospital between January 2012 and December 2013 was conducted utilizing the EPIC research registry, "Global Outcomes in IBD." Written informed consent was obtained from all parents/legal guardians, and assent was obtained from children. Ethics approval was obtained from the University of Alberta Research Ethics Board.

Inclusions Criteria. Patients age must be between 2 and 17 years at time of diagnosis. IBD was diagnosed using standard criteria based on symptoms, endoscopy, and imaging findings and have at least a year of follow-up.

Exclusion Criteria. Patients who have less than 1 year of follow-up, patients listed for liver transplant (as they were also being followed by hepatologists), and patients living outside of the province of Alberta (their prescription and blood work data were not available on the provincial database) were excluded.

2.2. Variables. Information regarding disease diagnosis, age, gender, place of residence, baseline disease activity [Pediatric Crohn's Disease Activity Index (PCDAI) and Pediatric Ulcerative Colitis Activity Index (PUCAI)], and pharmaceutical managements were recorded for all eligible patients. Place of residence was broadly categorized as urban or rural using postal code (as specified by Census Canada), except for St Albert, Spruce Grove, Fort Saskatchewan, and Sherwood Park. Patients from these communities are adjacent to the immediate city limits of Edmonton and were therefore considered urban given their increased access to healthcare services. For the interim years (between time of diagnosis and 2012), any significant event such as flares, hospitalizations, or surgeries were recorded, as well as any change in maintenance therapy.

2.3. Data Source/Measurement. For the years 2012 and 2013, the frequency of clinic visits was extracted along with the corresponding clinical disease activity scores (PCDAI or PUCAI) for each visit. Disease flares were defined as any disease activity above a patient's normal status (i.e., PCDAI of >10 or PUCAI score > 10 compared to previous visit). In addition, any significant event such as emergency room visits, hospitalizations, or surgeries due to IBD were recorded. All IBD related medications (induction therapy and maintenance therapy) were noted along with any changes made to prescriptions during the study period. Using the Alberta provincial pharmacy database, all dispensed medications were recorded (initial dispensing plus refills). Episodes of laboratory investigations (individual blood work encounters) were determined using the Alberta Netcare electronic health record which collates all results from investigations performed in the province. The number of requisitioned laboratory encounters was determined by reviewing the electronic orders of individual patient encounters. This allowed "routine" laboratory encounters to be captured in addition to "unscheduled" encounters, such as those that may have been requested during a disease flare-up. For "routine" lab work, patients are given "standing order" blood work requisitions in clinic which specify frequency, thus obviating the need for new requisitions each time blood work is required.

2.4. Medication Adherence Rate. A medication adherence rate as a proportion was determined for each patient by comparing the number of prescriptions filled (days of medication dispensed) against the number of days of the year that a patient should have been taking the prescribed therapy over a 1-year period for both 2012 and 2013. This was a continuous variable determined for each patient.

2.4.1. Medication Adherence. As in previous studies, the medication adherence was defined as a patient having filled 80% or more of the prescribed medication [4]. This allowed adherence to be treated as a dichotomous variable in statistical analyses. Adherence to the antitumor necrosis factor α (anti-TNFα) therapy infliximab was defined as having received the medication "within window" (i.e., the prescribed frequency plus or minus 3 days). Nonadherence to infliximab was defined by a discrepancy of >72 hours between the scheduled date of infusion and the actual date of administration [7]. As stated by Ma et al., there is no widely accepted definition for adherence to an individual infliximab infusion. A 72-hour cut-off period was empirically decided on (between 3 days before and 3 days after their scheduled infusion date) as it was felt that this reflected a sufficient time to accommodate weekends, statutory holidays, infusion clinic availability, and minor personal reasons that may briefly delay or expedite the infusion schedule [7]. Any infusion given more than 3 days late was considered "out of window." If infliximab was administered early, held, or postponed under physician advice, it was not considered to be "out of window." No definition for Adalimumab "within window" was needed due to the extremely small number of patients receiving this subcutaneous form of anti-TNFα therapy.

2.5. Blood Work Adherence Rate. This was determined by comparing the number of completed laboratory encounters against the requisitioned number of encounters over a 1-year period for both 2012 and 2013. Patients are given "standing order" blood work requisitions in clinic with specify frequency, thus obviating the need for a new requisition each time blood work is required.

2.5.1. Steroid-Free Remission. Steroid-free remission was defined as the absence of enteral or parenteral corticosteroid use during the specified time period for patients who remained in clinical remission. After completion of primary data collection (December 2013), a further prospective 6-month follow-up period was performed to capture any patients who may have required courses of corticosteroids beyond the defined study period.

Data were analyzed looking at the population as a total group (all IBD) and then stratified by disease type (CD and UC). IBD-U was combined with UC. The following variables were assessed to determine association with adherence: clinic frequency, age, sex, address, disease type, severity of disease activity at diagnosis, duration, and exacerbations during the period of assessment (flares, hospitalization, or surgeries).

To analyze the effect of frequency of clinic visits on outcomes, we used both number of clinic appointments per year as a continuous variable and grouping patients into 3 categories based on the number of times they were seen in clinic per year: 0-1 time, 2-3 times, and 4 times or higher. These three categories were arbitrarily chosen but they correspond to standard practice of EPIC, where minimal follow-up would be considered 0-1 times, standard follow-up would be 2-3 times, and frequent follow-up would be 4 or more times per year.

3. Statistical Methods

3.1. Study Size. Study size was calculated using the University of British Columbia (UBC) power calculator inference for proportions (http://www.stat.ubc.ca/~rollin/stats/ssize/b2.html). An estimated adherence rate of 80% for frequently seen patients was utilized based on previous publications (Kitney et al.) whilst those seen infrequently were estimated to have an adherence rate of 55%. Using a 2-sided test, alpha cut-off of 0.05, we calculated a required sample size of 110 patients to achieve 80% power.

Categorical variables were expressed as proportions and compared using Chi square analysis. Continuous variables were calculated and reported as mean and standard deviation or median and interquartile range as indicated by their distribution. Correlations between primary variables were calculated using Pearson's correlation whilst nonparametric comparisons of continuous variables were calculated using the Mann–Whitney *U* test. To deal with the repeated outcome measures over the two-year study period and the problem of within-subject correlations, a generalized estimating equation (GEE) model was used. Repeated observations on the same data unit collected over successive time points were correlated over time. The GEE method accounts for this correlation using a semiparametric approach to such longitudinal analysis of categorical data. As the outcome variables were proportions type of data including 1 (or 100%), linear regression (1-inflated Beta regression when necessary) was performed. Analyses were conducted using Stata 13.1 software (StataCorp, LP, College Station, Texas). STATA/IC version 13.2 was used for the regression analysis. A p value less than 0.05 was considered statistically significant.

4. Results

4.1. Participants. One hundred and twenty-seven patients were reviewed; 81 patients were diagnosed with Crohn's disease (CD) and 46 with ulcerative colitis (UC) which included 1 IBD-Unclassified (Table 1). Patient demographics and disease characteristics and medication treatment were further described in Table 1. Sixty-five percent had an urban residence. Both diseases had very similar follow-up of over 3 years. Nearly 64% of patients were seen in clinic 4 or more times, 21.6% were seen 2 to 3 times, and 14.6% were seen only 0 to 1 time per year. Forty-three percent of UC patients were treated with 5-ASA alone versus 2% for CD. Immunomodulators were used in 67% of all patients. Methotrexate (MTX) was used in 55% of males and Azathioprine (AZA) was used in 83% of females (p = 0.002). Thirty-seven percent of patients were on immunomodulators only. Dual therapy with immunomodulators and anti-TNFα preparations (IFX or Adalimumab) were used in 25% of patients in 2012; this increased to 44% in 2013. Monotherapy, either with IFX or ADA, was used in 8 (6%) patients.

4.2. Medication and Blood Work Adherence Rates and Clinic Visits. Table 2 reviews the adherence rates to 3 key maintenance medications for IBD patients and their adherence to blood work. Only 3 patients were receiving Adalimumab. Almost all patients treated with anti-TNFα received infliximab and were infused within window (median of 100%). Patients taking immunomodulators had a median adherence rate of 88%; 5-ASA had the lowest median adherence rate of 82%. A median 67% of patients completed the blood work that was ordered.

Before categorizing the adherence rate and clinic visits, analysis in Figure 1 showed that there was no correlation between the adherence rates of immunomodulators, 5-ASA, and IFX infusion within window and number of clinic visits per year. There was a minimal correlation between blood work adherence and clinic visit frequency (r = 0.19 and p = 0.4).

Further analysis was carried out using conventional definition of adherence defined as filling 80% or more of the prescriptions or requisitioned blood work prescribed (Tables 3(a) and 3(b)). For anti-TNFα, adherence was defined as >80% given within window. Table 3(a) describes the categorical independent variables and Table 3(b) describes continuous independent variables in relation to adherence to immunomodulators, 5-ASA, and biologics as well as blood work adherence. Clinic visits were described in both tables as both continuous and categorical variables. The number of observations refers to the number of subjects that took the medication per year for 2 years (2012 and 2013). Table 4(a) describes the univariate analysis of the factors that could affect adherence. Overall age, gender, disease type, and disease exacerbation (flare, surgery, and hospitalization) during the influence period did not influence patient medication

TABLE 1: Patient demographics and medication treatment.

	Total group (%)	Crohn's (%)	Ulcerative colitis (%)
Total patients	127	82 (65)	46* (35)
Male patient	72 (57)	49 (60)	23 (50)
Age at diagnosis in years, mean (std. Dev.)	10.38 (4.00)	11.06 (3.47)	9.17 (4.54)
Disease activity at diagnosis PCDAI for CD, PUCAI for UC Mean (std. Dev.)	NA	21.7 (11.16)	31.9 (16.56)
Duration of disease since diagnosis in years: median (IQR)	3.2 (2 to 5.9)	3.1 (2.1 to 6.3)	3.2 (1.9 to 4.7)
5ASA therapy	39 (31)	10 (12)	30 (65)
AZA therapy	56 (44)	38 (46)	18 (39)
MTX therapy	29 (23)	25 (30)	4 (8.7)
Infliximab therapy	42 (33)	33 (40)	9 (20)
Adalimumab	3 (2.4)	2 (2.4)	1 (2.1)
5ASA monotherapy	22 (17)	2 (2.4)	20 (43)
AZA monotherapy w/o 5ASA	26 (20)	24 (29)	3 (6.5)
AZA monotherapy w 5ASA	12 (9.4)	4 (4.8)	9 (20)
AZA monotherapy w or w/o 5ASA	38 (30)	27 (33)	11 (24)
MTX monotherapy w/o 5ASA	8 (6.7)	8 (10)	2 (4.3)
MTX monotherapy w 5ASA	2 (1.6)	2 (2.4)	0 (0.0)
MTX monotherapy w or wo 5ASA	10 (79)	9 (11)	2 (4.3)
Infliximab monotherapy	7 (5.5)	7 (8.5)	0 (0.0)
Infliximab & AZA	18 (14)	11 (13)	7 (15)
Infliximab & AZA & 5ASA	4 (3.1)	2 (2.4)	3 (6.5)
Infliximab & MTX	17 (13)	15 (18)	2 (4.3)
Infliximab & MTX & 5ASA	2 (1.6)	1 (1.2)	1 (2.1)
Adalimumab monotherapy	1 (0.7)	0 (0.0)	1 (2.1)
Adalimumab & MTX	2 (1.6)	2 (2.4)	0 (0.0)

*1 subject has IBD-U. No patient on biologics and ASA alone. No patients on Adalimumab and AZA or Adalimumab and ASA alone.

TABLE 2: Adherence rates.

Therapy	*N* observations per year over 2 years	Median adherence rate	IQR (25–75)
Immunomodulators			
Total group	160	88%	58 to 100
Crohn's	120	88%	58 to 100
UC	40	87%	58 to 100
5-ASA			
Total group	72	82%	49 to 100
Crohn's	18	92%	46 to 100
UC	54	81%	49 to 100
Anti-TNFα			
Total group	80	100%	83 to 100
Crohn's	63	100%	82 to 100
UC	17	100%	86 to 100
Blood work			
Total group	250	67%	42 to 100
Crohn's	159	67%	42 to 92
UC	91	67%	33 to 100

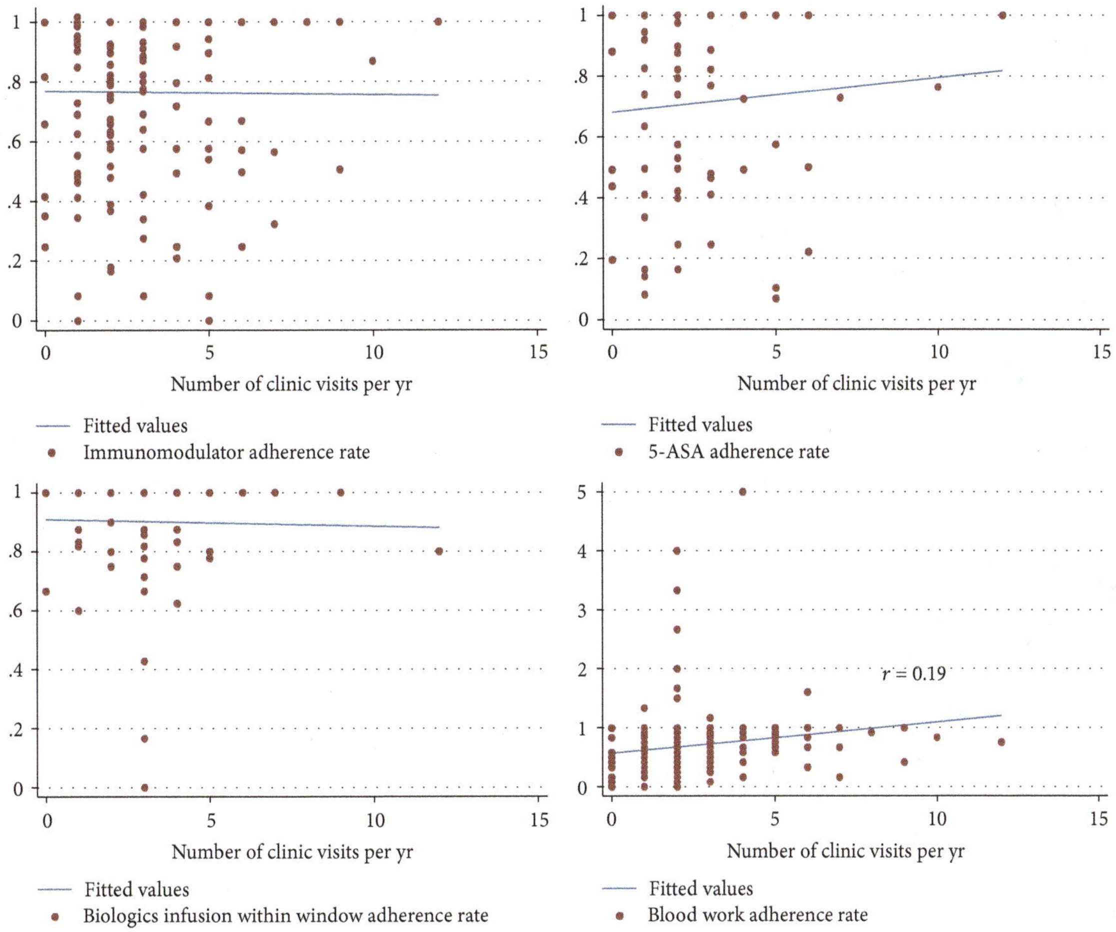

Figure 1: Lack of correlation between adherence rate and clinic visits.

adherence rates. Frequency of clinic visits did not appear to be associated with adherence to medications or blood work when clinic visits were analyzed as either a categorical or continuous variable.

Blood work adherence appeared to be associated with older age of diagnosis, shorter duration of disease, and exacerbation of disease during study period and more frequent clinic visits on univariate analysis. However, on multivariable analysis (Table 4(b)), only duration of disease was an independent factor that was associated with blood work adherence with a reduction of 14% per year (OR 0.86, 95% CI: 0.74–0.99), confirming the minimal correlation (r = 0.19) seen between blood work adherence rate and number of clinic visits per year in Figure 1. This correlation was confounded by duration from time of diagnosis.

Shorter duration from time of diagnosis also remained an independent factor associated with adherence to immunomodulators. With each year away from time of diagnosis, the odds ratio was reduced (OR 0.82, 95% CI: 0.71–0.97).

About three-quarters of patients taking 5-ASA had a diagnosis of UC. Disease severity and urban living were independent factors associated with 5-ASA adherence, for moderate disease when compared to mild disease (OR 3.2, 95% CI: 1.09–9.53) and urban patients when compared to rural patients (OR 3.6, 95% CI: 1.2–11) (see Table 4(b)).

4.3. Steroid-Free Remission and Adherence Rate. Table 5 shows that adherence rates affected patient outcomes. Patients adhering to all medications were more likely to remain in a steroid-free remission: those who remained corticosteroid-free had an overall median medication adherence rate of 86% compared to only 53% for those who relapsed and required corticosteroids (p = 0.01). Patients who adhered to their immunomodulators (median of 90%) remained without corticosteroids, versus only a median of 57% of those who used corticosteroids (p = 0.01). In fact, none of the UC patients that were adherent to 5-ASA and immunomodulators in the preceding 6 months required corticosteroids.

5. Discussion

The main purpose of this study was to explore the frequency of clinic appointments on adherence rates to medications and associated outcomes in IBD patients. Clinic visit frequency was not found to be associated with medication or blood work adherence. Univariate analysis appeared to show that

Table 3

(a) Univaried description of independent categorical variables and adherence

Categorical variables	Immunomodulators Number of observations per yr over 2 years	Immunomodulators Number with >80% adherence rate (%)	5-ASA Number of observations per yr over 2 years	5-ASA Number with >80% adherence rate (%)	Biologics Number of observations per yr over 2 years	Biologics Number with >80% adherence rate (%)	Blood work adherence Number of observations per yr over 2 years	Blood work adherence Number with >80% adherence rate (%)
Total	160	91 (57)	72	37 (51)	80	65 (81)	250	102 (41)
Sex								
Female	69	38 (55)	37	20 (54)	22	20 (91)	109	42 (39)
Male	91	53 (58)	35	17 (49)	58	45 (76)	141	60 (43)
Disease type								
Crohn's	120	68 (57)	18	10 (56)	63	51 (81)	159	64 (40)
Ulcerative colitis	40	23 (58)	54	27 (50)	17	14 (82)	91	38 (41)
Disease activity severity								
Mild	52	29 (56)	31	11 (35)	14	11 (79)	92	36 (39)
Moderate	81	46 (57)	31	20 (65)	44	35 (80)	112	49 (44)
Severe	27	16 (59)	10	6 (60)	21	18 (86)	44	15 (34)
Exacerbation								
No	126	74 (59)	52	28 (54)	64	52 (81)	202	76 (38)
Yes	34	17 (50)	20	9 (45)	16	13 (81)	48	26 (54)
Address								
Rural	57	31 (54)	30	10 (33)	24	21 (88)	88	29 (33)
Urban	103	60 (58)	42	27 (64)	56	44 (79)	162	73 (45)
Clinic visits per year								
0 (0-1 visit)	41	23 (56)	24	12 (50)	20	17 (85)	81	24 (30)
1 (2-3 visits)	41	21 (51)	18	9 (50)	17	16 (94)	66	27 (41)
2 (>3 visits)	78	47 (60)	30	16 (53)	43	32 (74)	103	51 (50)

(b) Univaried description of adherence and independent continuous variables. Adherence is defined as taking more than 80% of medication

Continuous variables	Age (yrs) of adherent patients	Age (yrs) of nonadherent patients	Number of clinic visits per year of adherent patients	Number of clinic visits per year of nonadherent patients	Duration of disease (yrs) of those adherence	Duration of disease (yrs) of those nonadherent
Immunomodulators						
n observations	91	69	91	69	91	69
Median	11.9	11.5	3	2	2.3	3.64
IQR	9.06 to 13.80	8.80 to 13.32	1.00 to 4.00	1.00 to 4.00	1.90 to 4.35	1.30 to 7.25
Mean	10.95	10.59	2.88	2.79	2.88	2.8
std. Dev.	3.79	4.07	2.11	1.91	2.11	1.91
5-ASA						
n observations	37	35	37	35	37	35
Median	13.18	10.99	2	2	2.4	2.92
IQR	7.47, 14.45	6.88, 13.18	1.00 to 3.00	1.00 to 4.00	2.00 to 3.25	1.88 to 4.43
Mean	11.12	10.46	2.7	2.69	3.26	3.63
std. Dev.	4.87	3.74	2.25	2.21	2.25	2.6
Biologics						
n observations	65	15	65	15	65	15
Median	11.20	11.19	2.00	3.00	3.76	5.52

(b) Continued.

Continuous variables	Age (yrs) of adherent patients	Age (yrs) of nonadherent patients	Number of clinic visits per year of adherent patients	Number of clinic visits per year of nonadherent patients	Duration of disease (yrs) of those adherence	Duration of disease (yrs) of those nonadherent
IQR	6.75 to 13.37	9.45 to 13.05	1.00 to 4.00	2.00 to 4.00	2.05 to 6.80	2.30 to 6.04
Mean	10.29	11.02	2.9	2.8	4.77	4.62
std. Dev.	4.14	2.48	2.06	1.47	3.26	1.98
Blood work						
n observations	102	148	102	148	102	148
Median	12.27	10.7	2.5	2	2.73	3.7
IQR	8.36 to 13.73	7.10 to 13.05	2.00 to 4.00	1.00 to 3.00	1.90 to 4.51	2.2 to 6.80
Mean	11.12	9.84	2.9	2.21	3.45	4.71
std. Dev.	3.9	4.01	1.89	1.82	2.33	3.03

increased clinic frequency was associated with blood work adherence but the association became insignificant when corrected for duration of disease and age of diagnosis. The increase in frequency of clinic visits is more related to early stage of the diagnosis, when patients are more likely to adhere to their blood work requirements.

The medication adherence rates of the patients in our population are similar to those found in previous studies [4]. Among the standard maintenance IBD medications, 5-ASA medications had a lower adherence rate with a median of 82%, which can often be associated with medications that have multiple daily dosing [8]. The fact that most patients on 5-ASA monotherapy had mild UC, and thus might be less concerned about flare-ups, may explain the low 5-ASA adherence. Adherence to 5-ASA was the only medication that was independently associated with disease severity when comparing moderate disease to mild one. Adherence was also much better among urban residents. The number of patients taking 5-ASA in our cohort is small, so these results need to be interpreted with caution. These two factors severity and rural/urban living were not observed be associated with adherence to immunomodulators, anti-TNFα, or blood work. Studies comparing medication adherence rates between urban and rural settings for other chronic diseases have not been consistent [9]. Patients with severe disease have been shown to be more motivated to perform proper health behaviour [10].

The median adherence rate to immunomodulators was 88%. More of our patients with Crohn's disease were treated with immunomodulators than are those with UC. Anti-TNFα adherence, with most receiving infliximab, was excellent with virtually all patients that received infusion within window. Blood work adherence rate was the lowest in our patients with a median of 67% in outpatients.

Duration of disease was found to be an independent predictor of adherence to immunomodulators and blood work. Increased adherence is often associated with increased belief in the need for a medication; this effect gradually diminishes over time as shown in the rheumatology literature [11]. However, we found no association between duration of disease and 5-ASA or anti-TNFα adherence. Our study, with fewer patients taking 5-ASA, may not have been sufficiently powered to show an association between 5-ASA adherence and duration of disease. We also did not observe any association between duration of disease and biologic use. The likely explanation for this is the very high adherence rate defined as given within window in the biologic group. It was no surprise that blood work adherence was independently associated with the recently diagnosed IBD children, that is, those with short duration from diagnosis and those who had exacerbation during the study period ($p = 0.09$). We generally request more blood work for these patients. Also, it is during this initial period when patients are often the most symptomatic and are relying on their medications to get them into remission. Once remission is achieved and patients have been "well," for a period, our data suggest that they are more likely to be nonadherent. The period of 1 to 2 years after diagnosis is an important time for medication education to occur to improve the patient's knowledge of the natural history of disease and to understand the importance of medication compliance in preventing relapses. Age, gender, and exacerbation (defined as having surgery or corticosteroid exposure due to IBD) during the study did not impact a patient's medication adherence rate.

Adherent patients are more likely to remain in a steroid-free remission in the following 6 months. This was observed in those taking immunomodulators as well as in the combining the medication adherence group. 5-ASA and anti-TNFα adherence was not significant in predicting steroid remission; this is again likely a reflection of low number needed for corticosteroids and the very high rate of adherence for anti-TNFα. Age group and gender did not have an impact. This is different from other studies, where these demographic variables were found to be associated with adherence rates [12]. Perhaps this can be attributed to the fact that we included only pediatric patients in whom it is the parents' responsibility to remind the child to take the medication.

Limitations to this study include a mixed population of eligible patients who attended the EPIC clinic including recently diagnosed patients (1 year after diagnosis), different

TABLE 4

(a) Univariate analysis of factors that were associated with medications and blood work adherence. (1 = reference)

Variables	Univaried											
	Immunomodulators			5-ASA			Biologics			Blood work		
	odd	95% CI	*p* value	odd	95% CI	*p* value	odd	95% CI	*p* value	odd	95% CI	*p* value
Age												
Year	1.01	0.91, 1.11	0.83	1.04	0.91, 1.18	0.56	0.95	0.85, 1.06	0.37	1.09	1.00, 1,17	0.04
Sex												
Female	1			1			1			1		
Male	1.03	0.42, 2.51	0.95	0.8	0.29, 2.29	0.69	0.4	0.08, 1.65	0.19	1.1	0.64, 2.04	0.66
Disease type												
Crohn's	1			1			1			1		
Ulcerative colitis	1.02	0.43, 2.41	0.96	0.8	0.23, 2.55	0.67	1.1	0.30, 4.07	0.89	1.1	0.58, 1.95	0.84
Duration of disease												
Each year diagnosed	0.83	0.71, 0.97	0.02	0.9	0.76, 1.14	0.52	1	0.88, 1.17	0.81	0.8	0.73, 0.96	0.01
Disease severity												
Mild	1			1			1			1		
Moderate	1.07	0.44, 2.62	0.88	3.2	1.04, 9.88	0.04	1.1	0.28, 4.03	0.93	1.2	0.64, 2.34	0.54
Severe	1.12	0.39, 3.26	0.83	2.6	0.49, 13.6	0.26	1.6	0.23, 11.5	0.62	0.8	0.32, 1.99	0.63
Exacerbation												
No	1			1			1			1		
Yes	0.94	0.46, 1.94	0.88	0.7	0.22, 2.21	0.53	1.1	0.24, 4.63	0.94	2	1.08, 3.59	0.03
Address												
Rural	1			1			1					
Urban	1.09	0.49, 2.42	0.84	3.5	1.18, 10.56	0.02	0.5	0.13, 1.91	0.32	1.6	0.87, 3.40	0.125
Clinic visits per year												
0 (0-1 visit)	1			1			1			1		
1 (2-3 visits)	0.84	0.41, 1.56	0.58	1.2	0.32, 4.26	0.82	2.9	0.27, 3.16	0.38	1.13	0.58, 2.24	0.71
2 (>3 visits)	0.95	0.55, 1.63	0.39	1.1	0.30, 4.33	0.85	0.5	0.12, 2.06	0.34	1.30	0.70, 2.45	0.05

(b) Multivariate analysis of factors that were significantly associated with medications and blood work adherence (1 = reference).

Variables	Multivariable analysis		
	Odd	95% CI	*p* value
		Immunomodulators	
Disease duration			
Year	**0.82**	**0.70, 0.97**	**0.02**
Sex			
Female	1		
Male	**1.02**	**0.42, 2.51**	**0.06**
		5-ASA	
Disease severity			
Mild	1		
Mod	**3.2**	**1.09, 9.53**	**0.03**
Severe	3.0	0.46, 23.8	0.24
Address			
Rural	1		
Urban	**3.6**	**1.20, 11.0**	**0.02**

(b) Continued.

Variables	Multivariable analysis Odd	95% CI	p value
		Blood work	
Disease Duration			
Year	**0.86**	**0.74, 0.99**	**0.04**
Exacerbation			
	1		
	1.7	**0.92, 3.29**	**0.09**

TABLE 5: Adherence to medication predicts 6-month steroid-free remission rates (using Wilcoxon rank-sum (Mann–Whitney) test with steroid-free remission as dependent variable and adherence rate as independent variables).

	Steroid-free remission group		Steroid use relapse group			
	Median adherence rate% (IQR)	n of observations	Median adherence rate% (IQR)	n of observations	Z	p value
Immunomodulators	90 (62 to 90)	150	57 (42 to 85)	10	−2.56	0.01
5ASA	82 (49 to 100)	64	48 (41 to 79)	8	−1.34	0.18
Biologics	100 (83 to 100)	79	71 (70 to 71)	1	−1.6	0.11
Combined all 3 drugs	86 (67 to 100)	198	53 (42 to 85)	15	−2.67	0.008
Blood work	67 (42 to 96)	232	67 (50 to 100)	18	0.72	0.47

age, and severity and chronicity of disease. Recently diagnosed patients are often more adherent to their treatment as the diagnosis is new and they are commonly experiencing symptoms. Their adherence at this time may be an unrealistic representation of what their adherence will be a few years into their disease. No socioeconomic and education status of the family was collected. The prescription refill information is available on the provincial pharmacy database; however, it is the pharmacy's responsibility to update the system with each prescription refill. In addition, there was no way to check the accuracy of the information or if information was missing.

Frequency of clinic appointments did not affect adherence rates for medications or blood work. Health care providers view clinic appointments as an excellent opportunity to reinforce education to patients and their families. Physicians may see their nonadherent patients more frequently in the hope of improving their adherence rates, but based on these data this strategy may not have the desired impact. Lack of disease education has been shown to be a barrier to medication adherence [6]; however our current way of running our IBD clinic and educating our patients through clinic appointments did not appear to improve treatment adherence. Patients on average will only remember 60% of the information that is told to them [13]. Therefore, families may only take away from the clinic appointment a few key points and forget the additional information that the doctor or nurse provided. The way we explain side effects and patient perception of side effects can also affect a patient's decision to take their medications [14]. Patients with a good relationship with the treatment team and the team's willingness to listen to the patient's concerns and involve them in the decision-making may make patients more willing to follow the treatment plan [5]. Patient preference is integral to decision-making regarding treatment decisions and can increase the success in treatment adherence and achieve a better health outcome [15].

IBD clinics should intend to develope strategies to enhance the above qualities that promote adherence. An example would be intentionally monitoring and reviewing blood work and other disease monitoring investigations with caregivers and patients at regular intervals, providing the reassurance that the medication is well tolerated and effective. The process where the patient's ability or desire to adhere to their medications when they return to their routine schedule is influenced by their environment such as family finance, beliefs about modern medicine, and how a patient fits their medications into their day-to-day life. A clear patient-specific understanding of these issues may be a better starting point to understand how healthcare providers can improve a patient's medication adherence rates.

In conclusion, medication adherence is an ongoing challenge in chronic illness, which was not associated with clinic visit frequency. It may be more likely influenced by the quality of those clinic visits. Qualitative research is required to explore the factors that really motivate patients to be adherent to their treatment plan.

Abbreviations

IBD: Inflammatory bowel disease
UC: Ulcerative colitis
IBD-U: Inflammatory bowel disease-unclassified
GEE: Generalized estimation equations
MTX: Methotrexate

AZA: Azathioprine
PCDAI: Pediatric Crohn's Disease Activity Index
PUCAI: Pediatric Ulcerative Colitis Activity Index
EPIC: Edmonton Pediatric IBD Clinic.

Authors' Contributions

All authors have participated in this research and agree with the content of the material.

Acknowledgments

Arun Pokhrel, a statistician from Women's and Children's Research Institute, is acknowledged for performing statistical analysis.

References

[1] W. N. Gray, L. A. Denson, R. N. Baldassano, and K. A. Hommel, "Treatment adherence in adolescents with inflammatory bowel disease: The collective impact of barriers to adherence and anxiety/depressive symptoms," *Journal of Pediatric Psychology*, vol. 37, no. 3, pp. 282–291, 2012.

[2] R. N. Fedorak, K. Wong, and R. Bridges, "Canadian digestive health foundation public impact series. Inflammatory bowel disease in Canada: incidence, prevalence, and direct and indirect economic impact," *Canadian Journal of Gastroenterology & Hepatology*, vol. 24, no. 11, pp. 651–655, 2010.

[3] Crohns and Colitis Foundation, "Annual Report. Crohns and Colitis Foundation of Canada," http://www.ccfa.ca.

[4] K. A. Hommel, L. A. Denson, and R. N. Baldassano, "Oral medication adherence and disease severity in pediatric inflammatory bowel disease," *Inflammatory Bowel Diseases*, vol. 19, no. 7, pp. 1534–1545, 2013.

[5] R. N. Greenley, J. H. Kunz, J. Walter, and K. A. Hommel, "Practical strategies for enhancing adherence to treatment regimen in inflammatory bowel disease," *Inflammatory Bowel Diseases*, vol. 19, no. 7, pp. 1534–1545, 2013.

[6] R. L. Hall, T. Willgoss, L. J. Humphrey, and J. H. Kongso, "The effect of medical device dose-memory functions on patients' adherence to treatment, confidence, and disease self-management," *Patient Preference and Adherence*, vol. 8, pp. 775–788, 2014.

[7] C. Ma, W. Evaschesen, and G. Gracias, "Inflammatory bowel disease patients are frequently non adherent to scheduled induction and maintenance therapy: A Canadian cohort study," *Canadian Journal of Gastroenterology and Hepatology*, vol. 29, no. 6, pp. 309–314, 2015.

[8] L. A. Feagins, R. Iqbal, and S. J. Spechler, "Case-control of factors that trigger inflammatory bowel disease flares," *World Journal of Gastroenterology*, vol. 20, no. 15, pp. 4329–4334, 2014.

[9] G. K. Murphy, F. A. McAlister, D. L. Weir, L. Tjosvold, and D. T. Eurich, "Cardiovascular medication utilization and adherence among adults living in rural and urban areas: a systematic review and meta-analysis," *BMC Public Health*, vol. 14, article 544, 2014.

[10] K. Kaspar, "A weighty matter: Heaviness influences the evaluation of disease severity, drug effectiveness, and side effects," *PLoS ONE*, vol. 8, no. 11, Article ID e78307, 2013.

[11] C. Morgan, J. McBeth, L. Cordingley et al., "The influence of behavioural and psychological factors on medication adherence over time in rheumatoid arthritis patients: A study in the biologics era," *Rheumatology*, vol. 54, no. 10, Article ID kev105, pp. 1780–1791, 2015.

[12] N. M. Sencan, A. Wertheimer, and C. B. Levine, "What determines the duration of patient medication compliance in patients with chronic disease: Are we looking in the wrong place?" *Southern Med Review*, vol. 4, no. 2, pp. 97–101, 2011.

[13] A. Cushing and R. Metcalfe, "Optimizing medicines management: From compliance to concordance," *Therapeutics and Clinical Risk Management*, vol. 3, no. 6, pp. 1047–1058, 2007.

[14] R. Horne and J. Weinman, "Patients' beliefs about prescribed medicines and their role in adherence to treatment in chronic physical illness," *Journal of Psychosomatic Research*, vol. 47, no. 6, pp. 555–567, 1999.

[15] G. Sylwestrzak, J. Liu, J. J. Stephenson, A. P. Ruggieri, and A. DeVries, "Considering patient preferences when selecting anti-tumor necrosis factor therapeutic options," *American Health and Drug Benefits*, vol. 7, no. 2, pp. 71–81, 2014.

2

Pleiotropic Effects of Heparins: From Clinical Applications to Molecular Mechanisms in Hepatocellular Carcinoma

Peyda Korhan,[1] Yeliz Yılmaz,[1,2] Ezgi Bağırsakçı,[1,3] Ayşim Güneş,[1] Hande Topel,[1,2] Brian I. Carr,[1] and Neşe Atabey[1]

[1] *Izmir Biomedicine and Genome Center, 35340, Turkey*
[2] *Medical Biology and Genetics, Heath Sciences Institute, Dokuz Eylul University, 35340, Turkey*
[3] *Izmir International Biomedicine and Genome Institute, Dokuz Eylul University, 35340, Turkey*

Correspondence should be addressed to Neşe Atabey; nese.atabey@ibg.edu.tr

Academic Editor: Pierluigi Toniutto

Hepatocellular carcinoma (HCC) is a major health problem worldwide and most cases are incurable because of late presentation. It is the most common primary neoplasm of the liver and often arises in the context of a chronic liver disease that impairs coagulation. Portal vein thrombosis (PVT) is a common complication of HCC that is associated with a poor prognosis. Heparin derivatives are widely used in the management of venous thromboembolism (VTE). Among them low molecular weight heparin (LMWH) favorably influences the survival in patients with advanced cancer, including HCC. Due to their pleiotropic function, heparins affect tumorigenesis in many ways and may promote or hamper tumorigenic transformation depending on the cancer type and cancer stage along with their structural properties and concentration. Thus, their application as an antithrombotic along with the conventional therapy regime should be carefully planned to develop the best management strategies. In this review, we first will briefly review clinical applications of heparin derivatives in the management of cancer with a particular focus on HCC. We then summarize the state of knowledge whereby heparin can crosstalk with molecules playing a role in hepatocarcinogenesis. Lastly, we highlight new experimental and clinical research conducted with the aim of moving towards personalized therapy in cancer patients at risk of thromboembolism.

1. Introduction

Worldwide, liver cancer is the sixth most common cancer and is the second leading global cause of cancer-related deaths [1, 2]. Among all primary liver cancers, HCC is the most prevalent malignancy, accounting for approximately 90% of cases [1–3]. The prognosis for HCC is very poor, with an incidence rate almost equaling the mortality rate (overall ratio of mortality to incidence of 0.95) [1]. The incidence of HCC increases progressively worldwide with advancing age in all populations, reaching a peak at 70 years [1]. The highest incidence and mortality rates of HCC are found in the less developed regions of the world, such as Southeast Asian countries [1], as compared to those in more developed regions in Europe and North America [1–3]. This global variation in incidence rates of HCC is closely related to the risk factors for HCC. HCC is common in patients with advanced hepatic fibrosis and cirrhosis, particularly with chronic damage caused by HBV or HCV infection, alcohol abuse, metabolic disease, and nonalcoholic fatty liver disease/obesity [4]. Tobacco smoke inhalation and dietary ingestion of fungal aflatoxins have been also recognized as major risk factors for HCC [4]. HCC originates as a result of an accumulation of genetic and epigenetic alterations, leading to an aberrant production of driver molecules. These altered expression profiles result in a multistep progression of precursor lesions to invasive/advanced HCC [4]. Importantly, Cancer Research, UK, has announced that 49% of liver cancer cases in the UK are preventable [5]. HBV vaccination, the establishment of treatments for HBV or HCV infections and widespread screening for hepatitis B or C viral infection, and interrupting the transmission of hepatitis virus infection via blood transfusion and blood products have all been shown to prevent liver cancer in high-incidence countries such as Japan [1, 5, 6].

Advances in science and technology have resulted in substantial opportunities for the management of HCC; however, prognosis of this disease is still poor due to the advanced stage at disease presentation, often due to absence of pathognomonic symptoms [7–10]. Larger tumor size, vascular invasion, poor liver functional status, and nodal metastasis are all associated with a poor prognosis [7–10]. Additionally, extraordinary inter- and intratumor heterogeneity of HCC contribute to drug resistance and recurrence, which pose a substantial bar to survival [11].

This complexity of HCC has led to the development of staging systems which combine both tumor and liver factors and a set of management guidelines, such as the Barcelona Clinic Liver Cancer (BCLC) guidelines recommended by the American Association for the Study of Liver Diseases (AASLD) and the European Association for the Study of the Liver (EASL) [8–10]. Surgical resection, transplantation, and ablation are potentially curative treatment options for HCC [8–10]. Unfortunately, less than 30% of patients globally who are diagnosed with early stage disease (Stage 0 or A) are eligible for these procedures [8–10]. For patients with intermediate stage disease (stage B), where patients are not eligible to be operated on, transarterial chemoembolisation (TACE) or transarterial radioembolisation (TARE) are recommended to establish local control and palliation [8–10]. TACE could potentially also be an adjuvant therapy for resectable HCC patients after hepatectomy, which could prevent recurrence and improve long-term survival [8–10]. Patients with advanced HCC which is considered as incurable have limited treatment options and chemotherapy provides minimal clinical benefit. Currently, Sorafenib, Lenvatinib, Regorafenib, or Opdivo, which are multitargeted kinase inhibitors or immune checkpoint inhibitors (Opdivo), are the only systemic agents demonstrated to extend overall survival (OS) compared with placebo in patients with advanced HCC by approximately three months [12–14].

Although TACE is relatively safe, it may cause liver damage complications, especially in presence of PVT [15]. In addition, like many cancers, HCC is also associated with hemostatic activation, with a reported incidence of PVT ranging from 20%-65% [16]. The presence of PVT in patients with HCC is associated with systemic VTE, worse hepatic function, intraarterial tumor invasion, portal hypertension, and poorer tolerance to undergoing treatment which are collectively lead to reduced survival [16, 17]. Not surprisingly, PVT is frequent in patients with liver cirrhosis which can be life-threatening [18]. Hemostatic alterations are well documented in liver disease: hemostasis is often impaired by thrombocytopenia and the reduced synthesis of coagulation factors that normally takes places in the liver [19]. These alterations can be worsened following surgery and chemotherapy even causing hemorrhagic complications [20, 21]. Thus, pharmacological prophylaxis of VTE is often needed in HCC patients. Despite the clinical relevance of the matter, there are no guidelines available on the administration of antithromboembolic prophylaxis in HCC patients. Currently, LMWH is strongly recommended for intervention in the prevention and management of thromboembolism complications [21–23]. Strikingly, several clinical and experimental studies have suggested that heparin derivatives affect cancer progression independent of their anticoagulant effects. Considering the fact that heparin derivatives are involved in a wide variety of biological activities, their application as an antithrombotic along with conventional therapy regime should be carefully planned to develop the best management strategies.

In this review, we firstly briefly review clinical applications of heparin derivatives in the management of cancer with a particular focus on HCC. Then we summarize the state of knowledge whereby heparin can cross-talk with molecules playing a role in hepatocarcinogenesis. Lastly, we highlight new experimental and clinical research conducted with the aim of moving towards personalized therapy in cancer patient at risk of thromboembolism.

2. Heparin Derivatives in the Management of Cancer

As mentioned above, patients with cancer are frequently treated with anti-coagulants, such as heparins, to treat or prevent thrombosis. Heparins are not absorbed orally, thus, they must be administrated parentally by intravenous infusion or subcutaneous injections [24]. UFH and other LMWHs, such as fondaparinux and danaparoid, do not possess intrinsic anticoagulant activity but potentiate antithrombin III that inhibits activated coagulation agents [25]. For many years unfractionated heparin (UFH) has been the standard treatment for initial anticoagulation [26]. However, recent randomized trials have demonstrated that LMWH is possibly superior to UFH in the initial treatment of VTE in people with cancer [26]. Moreover, LMWH provide other advantages versus UFH, including lower cost and simple dosing, and is associated with a lower risk for heparin-induced thrombocytopenia (HIT) [27]. Thus, LMWH is strongly recommended for intervention in the prevention and management of thromboembolism complications in cancer [21–23]. However, long-term use has been associated with bruising at injection sites, recurrent thromboembolism, thrombocytopenia, and bleeding which then causes interruption of essential cancer therapies [22, 26].

Importantly, randomized trials comparing LMWH to UFH for the treatment of thrombosis have also indicated that heparins may improve outcomes of patients with cancer, particularly in those with early stage disease cancer including HCC and in patients with small cell lung [28, 29]. The PROTECHT study (Prophylaxis of Thromboembolism during Chemotherapy; ClinicalTrials.gov Identifier: NCT00951574) has been designed to evaluate if prophylaxis with nadroparin (LMWH) conferred any additional benefit in terms survival, depending on whether chemotherapy disease control was achieved [30]. Notably, a statistically significant interaction between nadroparin treatment and response to chemotherapy was found, thus supporting the hypothesis difference in survival depends on the response to chemotherapy and nadroparin [30]. LMWHs lend themselves to such studies because of their pleiotropic effects and the relative ease of administration compared to UFH. A completed clinical trial, the results of which have not yet been released, investigated whether addition of LMWHs to TACE would improve HCC patient compared with TACE alone (ClinicalTrials.gov Identifier: NCT00827554). In addition, a current trial, which is not recruiting yet, aims to examine antithrombotic therapy with TACE in HCC to minimize mortality and to improve survival rate without provoking excessive bleeding (ClinicalTrials.gov Identifier: NCT02715492).

3. Heparin Derivatives

Heparin is a glycosaminoglycan that is synthesized by mast cells and basophils. Glycosaminoglycans are linear carbohydrate polymers that are composed of alternating uronate and hexosamine saccharides linked by glyosidic linkages [31]. Heparin undergoes extensive sulfation and rarely phosphorylation or carboxylation during synthesis and hence is a highly negatively charged biological molecule [32]. UHF is a naturally occurring mixture of glycosaminoglycan chains from porcine or bovine origin, each consisting of 200-300 saccharides units with molecular weights in the range of 12-14 kDa [33, 34]. LMWH consists of smaller fragments of UFH (nearly 18 saccharide units long, molecular weight approximately 5 kDa) produced by controlled enzymatic or chemical depolymerisation [33, 34]. Due to their structural differences, LMWH have relatively little antithrombotic activity compared to UFH [32].

4. Brief Review for Mechanisms of Heparin Affects Cancer Pathways

There are multiple experimental studies supporting the hypothesis that cancer progression can be influenced by heparins. Several *in vitro* and *in vivo* cancer models supported the idea that cancer cells exploit the coagulation system to facilitate cell growth, angiogenesis, immune evasion, and metastasis formation, by distinct mechanisms. In addition, numerous studies have demonstrated that heparins do not affect cancer only by their interaction with the coagulation cascade but also by various other ways, including by inhibition of cell-cell interaction by blocking cell-adhesion molecules (selectins), the inhibition of extracellular matrix proteinase heparanase, and the inhibition of angiogenesis.

Heparins are located primarily in the cell membrane and the extracellular matrix (ECM). They bind transiently with ECM-associated molecules, like the growth factors, cytokines, and enzymes, and alter their organization and functions [35]. One such example is heparin involvement in vascular epithelial growth factor- (VEGF-) fibronectin binding, where transient interaction of heparin with fibronectin promotes an open-conformation of fibronectin, which enhances binding to VEGF [36]. Consequently, VEGF binding to fibronectin is sufficient to mediate VEGF induced Erkl/2 activation, endothelial cell proliferation, and migration which are key steps in angiogenesis [37]. Moreover, blockage of the interaction between heparin and fibroblast growth factor (FGF), a well-known stimulator of angiogenesis, inhibits angiogenesis, tumor growth, and metastasis [38]. Duckworth et al. have shown that chemically modified heparin inhibits galectin-3-ligand binding and thereby prevents cancer-cell-endothelial adhesion and angiogenesis [39]. Also, heparin enhances ECM remodeling through the activation of metalloproteinase-2 and acts as a heparanase inhibitor that results in *in vitro* tubular morphogenesis of microvessels that is necessary for angiogenesis [33, 40]. Similarly, chemically modified nonanticoagulant species of heparin that specifically inhibit selectin-mediated heparanase enzymatic activity attenuate metastasis of melanoma cells [41]. It has been reported that heparin binds to platelets via P-selectin and prevents tumor invasion in lung cancer cells [42] Borsig et al. reported that heparin blocks P-selectin based platelet interactions through cell surface proteins such as mucins and thereby attenuates metastasis [42]. Furthermore, heparin binds L- and P-selectins to inhibit acute inflammation and thereby suppresses inflammatory processes in tumor microenvironment which is important for immune evasion. Moreover, heparin can also inhibit fibrin deposition around tumor cells for protecting cells from the immune system [43].

Another heparin interacting protein is factor 4 (CXCL4-PF4) which is released from activated platelets during platelet aggregation and promotes blood coagulation [44]. In addition, CXCL4-PF4 induces immune cells activation, differentiation, and migration but also inhibits endothelial cell migration, proliferation, and angiogenesis [44]. Relevant for this review are the effects of CXCL4-PF4 on the hemostatic system [44]. CXCL4-PF4 and heparin binding neutralise heparin on the endothelial surface of blood vessels, thereby inhibiting local antithrombin III activity and promoting coagulation [44]. In some patients exposed to heparin, CXCL4-PF4/heparin complex triggers an immunogenic response eventually leading to production of anti-CXCL4-PF4/heparin antibodies [44]. This may lead to a severe clinical condition characterized by platelet activation and aggregation, thrombocytopenia, and thrombocytopenia, which is commonly called heparin-induced thrombocytopenia (HIT). HIT typically develops 5-14 days after exposure to prophylactic or therapeutic doses of heparin [45]. In some cases, patients who previously had been exposed to heparin trigger HIT quicker [45].

In contrast to the anticarcinogenic effect above, heparin may also be involved in the activation of the metastatic cascade by forming a complex with midkine (MK). MK is highly expressed in HCC and in cancers of the stomach, colon, esophagus, pancreas lung, neuroblastoma, glioma, and urinary bladder [46–48]. MK is activated when it forms homodimers that are stabilised by heparin. Activated MK/heparin complex leads to metastasis and drug resistance [49]. Notably, Jia et al. demonstrated that LMWH significantly blocked coadhesion between connective tissue growth factor/CCN family 2 (CCN2) and low-density lipoprotein receptor-related protein 6 (LRP6) and enhanced chemotherapeutic effect of oxaliplatin on HCC [50]. CCN2 functions to orchestrate LRP6 which is coreceptor in Wnt signalling. Wnt signalling is key signaling related to stem-ness, and chemoresistance [50]. Combination treatment with oxaliplatin and LMWH showed improved response rates to chemotherapy [50] Likewise, Pfankuchen et al. reported that a therapeutic dosage of LMWH (tinzaparin) reversed cisplatin resistance in

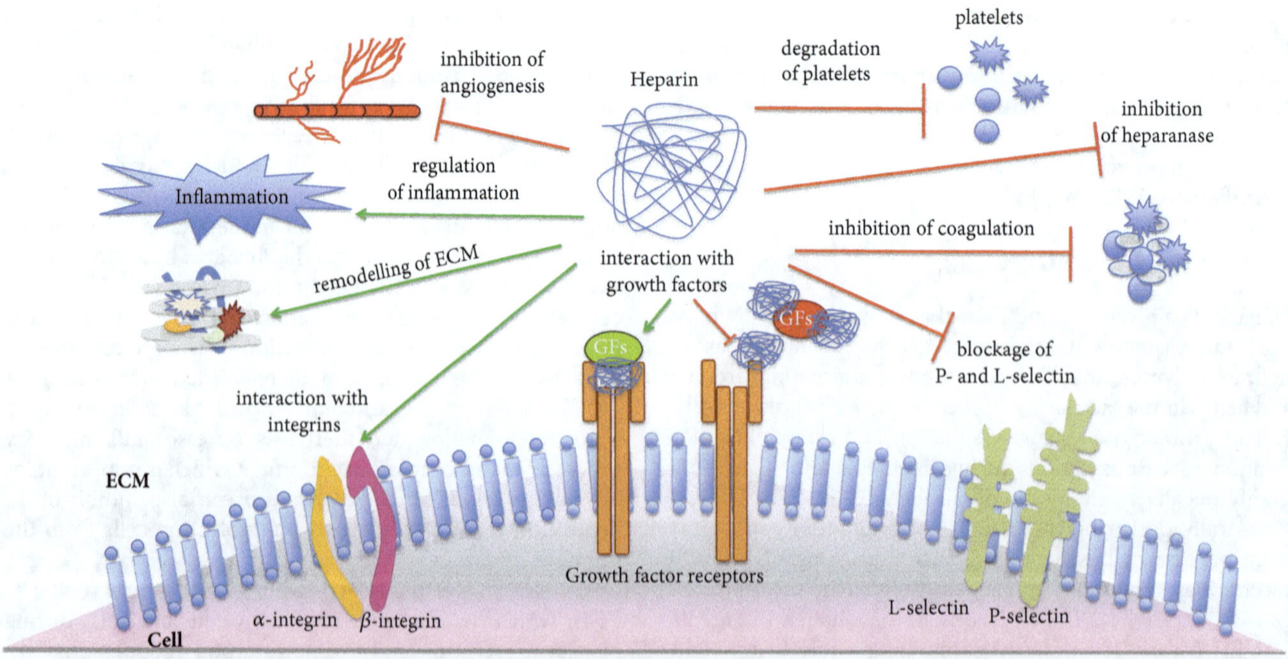

FIGURE 1: **Biological effects of heparin.** Heparin has inhibitory and activating roles in molecular and cellular mechanisms. It has a role in degradation of platelets, inhibition of coagulation, and angiogenesis. It also acts as a heparanase inhibitor and blocks P- and L-selectin to interact with platelets and prevents metastasis. Moreover, it interacts with ECM proteins and enhances remodeling of the ECM. It is involved in inflammatory processes and regulates inflammation. Heparin interacts with integrins and growth factors. However, in some growth factor signaling pathways it may have inhibitory as well as activating effects. For instance, it interacts with factors such as FGF, TGFB1, and MK and regulates the signaling positively. In contrast, it also interacts with FGF and HGF and regulates the signaling negatively (ECM: extracellular matrix; FGF: fibroblast growth factor; and HGF: hepatocyte growth factor.

a clone of ovarian cancer cell line to the level of sensitive cells [51, 52]. According to the follow up study, cisplatin resistant cells showed 3-fold higher Wnt signaling activity compared to wild type cells and Wnt pathway blockade increased cisplatin sensitivity. LMWH treatment reduced Wnt pathway activity and TCF-4 expression and enhanced cisplatin sensitivity in cisplatin resistant clones [51].

LMWH is also used as a nanocarrier to deliver drugs in cancer therapies. Modification of heparin molecules to generate nanocarriers become useful for applications like imaging, disease, and cancer treatments. Yan et al. prepared gambogic acid grafted low molecular weight heparin micelles to combine anti-tumor effect of gambogic acid with anti-angiogenic and anti-metastatic effect of heparin [53]. This *in vivo* study suggested that drugs grafted to LMWHs can be delivered to the liver and enhance their therapeutic effects by combining antitumor effects of heparin [53]. Furthermore, Du et al. modified LMWH to carry doxorubicin to overcome doxorubicin resistance in HCC [54].

5. Factors Influencing the Pleiotropic Role of Heparins

Due to their heterogeneity and natural location, heparins are able to interact with a wide variety molecules and mediate diverse biological processes (Figure 1). Therefore, it is not surprising that the role of heparins in tumor genesis is context dependent.

To clarify the various potential mechanisms of heparin anticancer activity, Niers et al. evaluated the data from preclinical studies (published between 1960 and 2005) in which heparins have been tested as anticancer therapy [32]. They suggested that heparin may affect the formation of metastasis rather than the growth of primary tumors. They also documented that chemically modified heparins with no or limited anticoagulant activity also showed antimetastatic properties [32]. They concluded with possible mechanisms to explain the effects on the process of metastasis include inhibition of blood coagulation, inhibition of cancer cell-platelet, and cancer cell-endothelial interactions by inhibition of cell invasion and angiogenesis [32]. They also documented interesting results highlighting the importance of types, duration, timing, and dose of heparin used, animal tumor model tested, and route of heparin administration in the course of disease [32]. Similarly, LMWH treatment was shown to inhibit FGF-induced mitogenesis of tumor derived endothelial cells in a time and concentration dependent manner [55]. Likewise, in Jha et al.'s study, to understand the effects of molecular weight and concentration of heparin on transforming growth factor (TGF)-β1 signaling, they used heparin-containing hyaluronic acid based hydrogels to analyze growth factor affinity and retention [56]. At equal concentrations, high molecular weight heparin has the highest amount of TGF-β1 retention from hydrogel compared to low molecular weight or unfractionated heparin. This response is critical for stem cell differentiation and lineage specification [56].

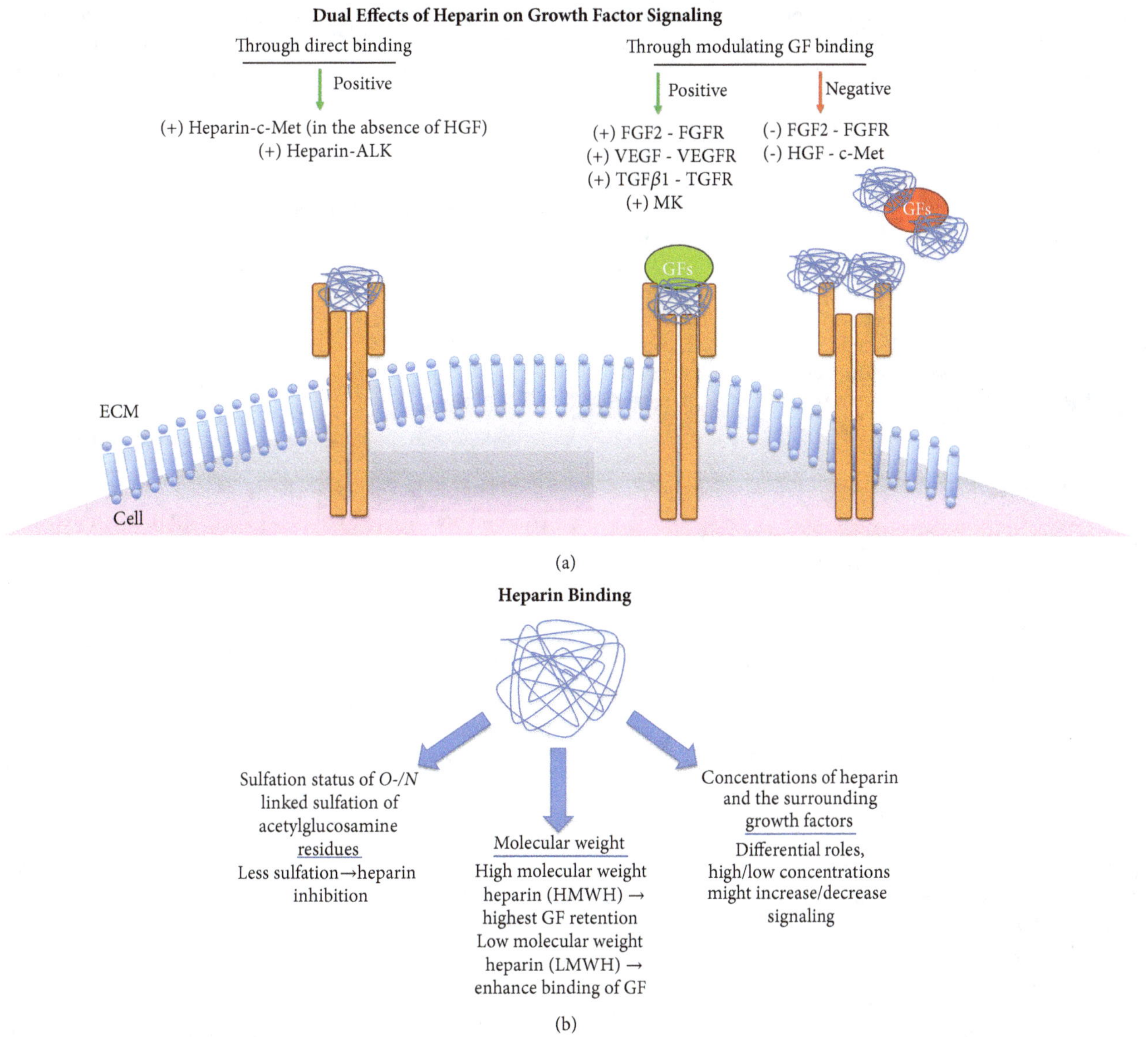

FIGURE 2: **Effects and effectors of heparin binding.** Heparin binding has context-dependent roles in Growth Factor (GF) signaling, it might directly bind to Growth Factor Receptors (GFRs) or it might modulate signaling positively or negatively through binding to both GFs and GFRs (a). Heparin binding to GFs and GFRs are affected by several factors including sulfation status, the molecular weight of heparin and the concentrations of both heparin and the GFs (b).

LaRochelle et al. determined that low concentrations of heparin enhance the binding of keratinocyte growth factor (KGF) to its receptor in CHO cells lacking HS proteoglycans but this effect is not observed in wild type CHO cells. In contrast higher heparin concentrations inhibit KGF signaling [57]. Furthermore, while heparins with short chain lengths are not able to activate anaplastic lymphoma kinase (ALK), heparins with longer chain lengths can induce dimerization and activation ALK in neuroblastoma cells [58]. Interestingly, in our previous studies, we showed that heparin can activate the c-Met signaling pathway by activating dimerization of c-Met receptor, which can then induce HCC cell invasion [59] However, when Hepatocyte Growth Factor (HGF), ligand of c-Met, is in the environment, heparin suppressed HGF/c-Met signaling mediated adhesion, motility, and invasion [59]. When we performed a microarray analysis to identify the molecular mechanisms behind heparin mediated biological responses, we observed that heparin modulates transcription of several genes involved in glucose metabolism, tumor angiogenesis, and EMT [60]. In our further analysis, we demonstrated that heparin controlled thioredoxin-interacting protein (TXNIP) gene expression through two mechanisms: (1) it can either directly bind to a unique carbohydrate response element located on the promoter of this gene or (2) it can trigger epigenetic modifications [60]. In either case, increased expression of TXNIP, which is a regulator glucose metabolism, accelerates migration and invasion abilities of HCC cells [60]. These data imply that, in addition to its regulatory role on receptor dimerization and ligand binding to its receptor, heparin also has a transcription regulatory role in HCC.

Overall, these studies emphasised that both intrinsic (such as tumor type) and extrinsic (such as heparin type) determinants play roles in the actions of heparin on tumors. For instance, while heparin administration increases tumor growth and metastasis in colon cancer, it reduces metastases in fibrosarcomas, lung, prostate, and mammary carcinomas [61–63]. These pleotropic effects of heparin might be related to expression or activation levels of growth factors and/or their receptors, as well as by heparin type and concentration. As summarized in Figure 2, heparin can directly bind to growth factor receptors or growth factors to stimulate signaling pathways, whereas it could block growth factor-receptor interaction as a context dependent manner.

6. Conclusions

The management of HCC along with other advanced-stage cancers remains a challenge. Venous thrombosis is a common complication in patients with cancer and indicates a poor prognosis. LMWH is widely used in the clinic as an anticoagulant as part of a treatment regimen in cancer patients to treat or control thrombosis. Many studies highlight the benefit of heparin derivatives in increasing patient survival, mostly through their antithrombotic effect. There is also a growing amount of evidence for the anticancer effects of heparin, which are mostly via its inhibition of metastasis rather than on primary tumor growth. However, there is also evidence revealing that heparin can act as a metastasis promoting agent. Clearly, due to its pleiotropic actions, heparin affects tumorigenesis in many ways and may promote or hamper cell transformation, depending on the cancer type and stage along with its structural properties and concentration. This phenomenon stresses the fact that heparin use in the clinic should be assessed carefully. In addition, the use of a same therapy approach for all patients might result in variable and unpredictable responses, because of heterogeneity among tumors and genotypic differences between patients. Hence, personalized medicine (PM) offers an attractive approach for cancer management and care. PM implements "-omic" sciences (genomics, epigenomics, transcriptomics, proteomics, etc.) to integrate various data sets with the aim of dissecting molecular signatures and functional pathways that help to classify tumor subtypes and determine their natural course, prognosis, and responsiveness to therapies [64]. Thus, stratification of the subset of patients who might respond to particular combinations of therapies is crucial in the management of cancer. For instance, mutations of the KDM6A, CUL9, FDG6, AKAp3, and RFN139 genes are associated with the development of PVT in advanced HBV-related HCC [65]. Since effective management of PVT may improve treatment results for HCC, these genes can be used for the identification or prediction of high-risk patients who will benefit most from antithrombotic therapy. Moreover, anti-CXCL4-PF4/heparin antibodies can be used as a predictive factor to identify patients who should avoid heparin treatment. Further studies are needed for better understanding of heparin and tumor biology and the determination of biomarkers for the planning of best evidence-based approaches that meet the needs of patients for disease treatment, reduction of symptoms, and improvement in quality of life.

Authors' Contributions

Peyda Korhan and Yeliz Yılmaz have equal contributions.

References

[1] "GLOBOCAN 2012, Cancer Incidence and Mortality Worldwide: IARC, vol. 11, International Agency for Research on Cancer, Lyon, France, 2018".

[2] "Globocan 2012 Liver Cancer Act Sheet, IARC: International Agency Research on Cancer, Lyon, 2012".

[3] G. Klöppel and World Health Organization Classification of Tumours, *Pathology and Genetics of Tumours of the Digestive System: Ductal Adenocarcinoma of the Pancreas*, International Agency for Research on Cancer Press, 2000.

[4] J. M. Llovet, J. Zucman-Rossi, E. Pikarsky et al., "Hepatocellular carcinoma," *Nature Reviews Disease Primers*, vol. 2, p. 16018, 2016.

[5] "Cancer Research UK Liver cancer risk factors," 2014, https://www.cancerresearchuk.org/health-professional/cancer-statistics/statistics-by-cancer-type/liver-cancer#heading-Three.

[6] M. Ikeda, S. Mitsunaga, S. Shimizu, I. Ohno, H. Takahashi et al., "Current status of hepatocellular carcinoma in Japan," *Chinese Clinical Oncology*, vol. 2, no. 4, p. 40, 2013.

[7] European Association for the Study of The Liver, "EASL-EORTC Clinical Practice Guidelines: management of hepatocellular carcinoma," *European Journal of Cancer*, vol. 48, no. 5, pp. 599–641, 2012.

[8] P. R. Galle, A. Forner, J. M. Llovet et al., "EASL Clinical Practice Guidelines: Management of hepatocellular carcinoma," *Journal of Hepatology*, vol. 69, no. 1, pp. 182–236, 2018.

[9] J. W. Park, M. Chen, M. Colombo et al., "Global patterns of hepatocellular carcinoma management from diagnosis to death: the BRIDGE Study," *Liver International*, vol. 35, no. 9, pp. 2155–2166, 2015.

[10] J. Bruix, M. Reig, and M. Sherman, "Evidence-based diagnosis, staging, and treatment of patients with hepatocellular carcinoma," *Gastroenterology*, vol. 150, no. 4, pp. 835–853, 2016.

[11] L. Li and H. Wang, "Heterogeneity of liver cancer and personalized therapy," *Cancer Letters*, vol. 379, no. 2, pp. 191–197, 2016.

[12] C. J. Wilhelm, R. A. Johnson, P. G. Lysko, A. J. Eshleman, and A. Janowsky, "Effects of methamphetamine and lobeline on vesicular monoamine and dopamine transporter-mediated dopamine release in a cotransfected model system," *The Journal of Pharmacology and Experimental Therapeutics*, vol. 310, no. 3, pp. 1142–1151, 2004.

[13] J. M. Llovet, S. Ricci, V. Mazzaferro et al., "Sorafenib in advanced hepatocellular carcinoma," *The New England Journal of Medicine*, vol. 359, no. 4, pp. 378–390, 2008.

[14] J. Bruix, S. Qin, P. Merle et al., "Regorafenib for patients with hepatocellular carcinoma who progressed on sorafenib

treatment (RESORCE): a randomised, double-blind, placebo-controlled, phase 3 trial," *The Lancet*, vol. 389, no. 10064, pp. 56–66, 2017.

[15] J. P. Silva, N. G. Berger, S. Tsai et al., "Transarterial chemoembolization in hepatocellular carcinoma with portal vein tumor thrombosis: a systematic review and meta-analysis," *HPB*, vol. 19, no. 8, pp. 659–666, 2017.

[16] G. C. Connolly, R. Chen, O. Hyrien et al., "Incidence, risk factors and consequences of portal vein and systemic thromboses in hepatocellular carcinoma," *Thrombosis Research*, vol. 122, no. 3, pp. 299–306, 2008.

[17] S. L. Chan, C. C. N. Chong, A. W. H. Chan, D. M. C. Poon, and K. S. H. Chok, "Management of hepatocellular carcinoma with portal vein tumor thrombosis: Review and update at 2016," *World Journal of Gastroenterology*, vol. 22, no. 32, pp. 7289–7300, 2016.

[18] L. von Köckritz, A. De Gottardi, J. Trebicka, and M. Praktiknjo, "Portal vein thrombosis in patients with cirrhosis," *Gastroenterology Report*, vol. 5, no. 2, pp. 148–156, 2017.

[19] T. Lisman and F. W. G. Leebeek, "Hemostatic alterations in liver disease: A review on pathophysiology, clinical consequences, and treatment," *Digestive Surgery*, vol. 24, no. 4, pp. 250–258, 2007.

[20] M. Vivarelli, M. Zanello, C. Zanfi et al., "Prophylaxis for venous thromboembolism after resection of hepatocellular carcinoma on cirrhosis: Is it necessary?" *World Journal of Gastroenterology*, vol. 16, no. 17, pp. 2146–2150, 2010.

[21] O. Negm, S. Abou Saif, M. El Gharib, M. Yousef, and S. Abd-Elsalam, "Role of low-molecular-weight heparins in prevention of thromboembolic complication after transarterial chemoembolization in hepatocellular carcinoma," *European Journal of Gastroenterology & Hepatology*, vol. 29, no. 3, pp. 317–321, 2017.

[22] S. Noble, A. Nelson, and S. Seaman, "Cancer-associated thrombosis, low-molecular-weight heparin, and the patient experience: a qualitative study," *Patient Preference and Adherence*, vol. 8, pp. 453–461, 2014.

[23] M. B. Hakoum, L. A. Kahale, I. G. Tsolakian et al., "Anticoagulation for the initial treatment of venous thromboembolism in people with cancer," *Cochrane Database of Systematic Reviews*, 2018.

[24] J. Hirsh, "Low molecular weight heparin," *Thrombosis and Haemostasis*, vol. 70, no. 1, pp. 204–207, 1993.

[25] J. Hirsh, K. A. Bauer, and M. B. Donati, "Parenteral anticoagulants: American College of Chest Physicians Evidence-Based Clinical Practice Guidelines (8th Edition)," *CHEST*, vol. 133, supplement 6, pp. 141S–159S, 2008.

[26] E. Donnellan and A. A. Khorana, "Cancer and venous thromboembolic disease: a review," *The Oncologist*, vol. 22, no. 2, pp. 199–207, 2017.

[27] N. Martel, J. Lee, and P. S. Wells, "Risk for heparin-induced thrombocytopenia with unfractionated and low-molecular-weight heparin thromboprophylaxis: a meta-analysis," *Blood*, vol. 106, no. 8, pp. 2710–2715, 2005.

[28] D. Sanford, A. Naidu, N. Alizadeh, and A. Lazo-Langner, "The effect of low molecular weight heparin on survival in cancer patients: An updated systematic review and meta-analysis of randomized trials," *Journal of Thrombosis and Haemostasis*, vol. 12, no. 7, pp. 1076–1085, 2014.

[29] N. Zhang, W. Lou, F. Ji, L. Qiu, B. K. Tsang, and W. Di, "Low molecular weight heparin and cancer survival: clinical trials and experimental mechanisms," *Journal of Cancer Research and Clinical Oncology*, vol. 142, no. 8, pp. 1807–1816, 2016.

[30] S. Barni, E. Bonizzoni, M. Verso et al., "To the editor: The effect of low-molecular-weight heparin in cancer patients: The mirror image of survival?" *Blood*, vol. 124, no. 1, pp. 155-156, 2014.

[31] S. Mohamed and D. Coombe, "Heparin Mimetics: Their Therapeutic Potential," *Pharmaceuticals*, vol. 10, no. 4, p. 78, 2017.

[32] T. M. H. Niers, C. P. W. Klerk, M. DiNisio et al., "Mechanisms of heparin induced anti-cancer activity in experimental cancer models," *Critical Review in Oncology/Hematology*, vol. 61, no. 3, pp. 195–207, 2007.

[33] S. M. Smorenburg and C. J. F. Van Noorden, "The complex effects of heparins on cancer progression and metastasis in experimental studies," *Pharmacological Reviews*, vol. 53, no. 1, pp. 93–105, 2001.

[34] S. A. Mousa, R. Linhardt, J. L. Francis, and A. Amirkhosravi, "Anti-metastatic effect of a non-anticoagulant low-molecular-weight heparin versus the standard low-molecular-weight heparin, enoxaparin," *Thrombosis and Haemostasis*, vol. 96, no. 6, pp. 816–821, 2006.

[35] F. Peysselon and S. Ricard-Blum, "Heparin-protein interactions: From affinity and kinetics to biological roles. Application to an interaction network regulating angiogenesis," *Matrix Biology*, vol. 35, pp. 73–81, 2014.

[36] M. Mitsi, K. Forsten-Williams, M. Gopalakrishnan, and M. A. Nugent, "A catalytic role of heparin within the extracellular matrix," *The Journal of Biological Chemistry*, vol. 283, no. 50, pp. 34796–34807, 2008.

[37] E. S. Wijelath, S. Rahman, M. Namekata et al., "Heparin-II domain of fibronectin is a vascular endothelial growth factor-binding domain: Enhancement of VEGF biological activity by a singular growth factor/matrix protein synergism," *Circulation Research*, vol. 99, no. 8, pp. 853–860, 2006.

[38] S. M. Plum, J. W. Holaday, A. Ruiz, J. W. Madsen, W. E. Fogler, and A. H. Fortier, "Administration of a liposomal FGF-2 peptide vaccine leads to abrogation of FGF-2-mediated angiogenesis and tumor development," *Vaccine*, vol. 19, no. 9-10, pp. 1294–1303, 2000.

[39] C. A. Duckworth, S. E. Guimond, P. Sindrewicz et al., "Chemically modified, non-anticoagulant heparin derivatives are potent galectin-3 binding inhibitors and inhibit circulating galectin-3-promoted metastasis," *Oncotarget* , vol. 6, no. 27, pp. 23671–23687, 2015.

[40] L. Ling, S. K. Tan, T. H. Goh et al., "Targeting the heparin-binding domain of fibroblast growth factor receptor 1 as a potential cancer therapy," *Molecular Cancer*, vol. 14, no. 1, article no. 136, 2015.

[41] N. Hostettler, A. Naggi, G. Torri et al., "P-selectin- and heparanase-dependent antimetastatic activity of non-anticoagulant heparins," *The FASEB Journal*, vol. 21, no. 13, pp. 3562–3572, 2007.

[42] L. Borsig, R. Wong, J. Feramisco, D. R. Nadeau, N. M. Varki, and A. Varki, "Heparin and cancer revisited: mechanistic connections involving platelets, P-selectin, carcinoma mucins, and tumor metastasis," *Proceedings of the National Acadamy of Sciences of the United States of America*, vol. 98, no. 6, pp. 3352–3357, 2001.

[43] H. Engelberg, "Actions of heparin that may affect the malignant process," *Cancer*, vol. 85, no. 2, pp. 257–272, 1999.

[44] P. M. Sandset, "CXCL4-platelet factor 4, heparin-induced thrombocytopenia and cancer," *Thrombosis Research*, vol. 129, pp. S97–S100, 2012.

[45] N. Lubenow, R. Kempf, A. Eichner, P. Eichler, L. E. Carlsson, and A. Greinacher, "Heparin-induced thrombocytopenia: Temporal

pattern of thrombocytopenia in relation to initial use or reexposure to heparin," *CHEST*, vol. 122, no. 1, pp. 37–42, 2002.

[46] J. Yao, W.-Y. Li, and S.-G. Gao, "The advances of Midkine with peripheral invasion in pancreatic cancer," *American Journal of Cancer Research*, vol. 5, no. 9, pp. 2912–2917, 2015.

[47] Y. Xu, X. Qu, X. Zhang et al., "Midkine positively regulates the proliferation of human gastric cancer cells," *Cancer Letters*, vol. 279, no. 2, pp. 137–144, 2009.

[48] B. Sun, C. Hu, Z. Yang et al., "Midkine promotes hepatocellular carcinoma metastasis by elevating anoikis resistance of circulating tumor cells," *Oncotarget* , vol. 8, no. 20, pp. 32523–32535, 2017.

[49] K. Kadomatsu, S. Kishida, and S. Tsubota, "The heparin-binding growth factor midkine: the biological activities and candidate receptors," *The Journal of Biochemistry*, vol. 153, no. 6, pp. 511–521, 2013.

[50] Q. Jia, Y. Bu, Z. Wang et al., "Maintenance of stemness is associated with the interation of LRP6 and heparin-binding protein CCN2 autocrined by hepatocellular carcinoma," *Journal of Experimental & Clinical Cancer Research*, vol. 36, no. 1, article 117, 2017.

[51] D. B. Pfankuchen, F. Baltes, T. Batool, J. Li, M. Schlesinger, and G. Bendas, "Heparin antagonizes cisplatin resistance of A2780 ovarian cancer cells by affecting the Wnt signaling pathway," *Oncotarget*, vol. 8, no. 40, pp. 67553–67566, 2017.

[52] D. B. Pfankuchen, D. P. Stölting, M. Schlesinger, H.-D. Royer, and G. Bendas, "Low molecular weight heparin tinzaparin antagonizes cisplatin resistance of ovarian cancer cells," *Biochemical Pharmacology*, vol. 97, no. 2, pp. 147–157, 2015.

[53] X. Yan, Y. Yang, L. He, D. Peng, and D. Yin, "Gambogic acid grafted low molecular weight heparin micelles for targeted treatment in a hepatocellular carcinoma model with an enhanced anti-angiogenesis effect," *International Journal of Pharmaceutics*, vol. 522, no. 1-2, pp. 110–118, 2017.

[54] H. Du, M. Liu, A. Yu, J. Ji, and G. Zhai, "Insight into the role of dual-ligand modification in low molecular weight heparin based nanocarrier for targeted delivery of doxorubicin," *International Journal of Pharmaceutics*, vol. 523, no. 1, pp. 427–438, 2017.

[55] S. L. Smiley, D. O. Henry, and M. K. Wong, "The mechanism of low molecular weight heparin (LMWH) inhibition of tumor growth," *Journal of Clinical Oncology*, vol. 24, supplement 18, pp. 13093-13093, 2006.

[56] A. K. Jha, A. Mathur, F. L. Svedlund, J. Ye, Y. Yeghiazarians, and K. E. Healy, "Molecular weight and concentration of heparin in hyaluronic acid-based matrices modulates growth factor retention kinetics and stem cell fate," *Journal of Controlled Release*, vol. 209, pp. 308–316, 2015.

[57] W. J. LaRochelle, K. Sakaguchi, N. Atabey et al., "Heparan sulfate proteoglycan modulates keratinocyte growth factor signaling through interaction with both ligand and receptor," *Biochemistry*, vol. 38, no. 6, pp. 1765–1771, 1999.

[58] P. B. Murray, I. Lax, A. Reshetnyak et al., "Heparin is an activating ligand of the orphan receptor tyrosine kinase ALK," *Science Signaling*, vol. 8, no. 360, pp. ra6–ra6, 2015.

[59] E. Ozen, A. Gozukizil, E. Erdal, A. Uren, D. P. Bottaro, and N. Atabey, "Heparin inhibits Hepatocyte growth factor induced motility and invasion of hepatocellular carcinoma cells through early growth response protein 1," *PLoS ONE*, vol. 7, no. 8, article e42717, 2012.

[60] A. Gunes, E. Iscan, H. Topel et al., "Heparin treatment increases thioredoxin interacting protein expression in hepatocellular carcinoma cells," *The International Journal of Biochemistry & Cell Biology*, vol. 65, pp. 169–181, 2015.

[61] C. Lim, H. Multhaupt, and J. R. Couchman, "Cell surface heparan sulfate proteoglycans control adhesion and invasion of breast carcinoma cells," *Molecular Cancer*, vol. 14, no. 1, article no. 15, 2015.

[62] G.-X. Zhong, Y. Gong, C.-J. Yu et al., "Significantly inhibitory effects of low molecular weight heparin (Fraxiparine) on the motility of lung cancer cells and its related mechanism," *Tumor Biology*, vol. 36, no. 6, pp. 4689–4697, 2015.

[63] A. Takeuchi, Y. Yamamoto, S. Munesue et al., "Low molecular weight heparin suppresses receptor for advanced glycation end products-mediated expression of malignant phenotype in human fibrosarcoma cells," *Cancer Science*, vol. 104, no. 6, pp. 740–749, 2013.

[64] P. Korhan, R. Verkerk, and W. R Critchley, "Scientific rationale for integrative and personalised strategies for pancreatic ductal adenocarcinoma management," *Integrative Molecular Medicine*, vol. 4, no. 5, pp. 1–32, 2017.

[65] J. Huang, Q. Deng, Q. Wang et al., "Exome sequencing of hepatitis B virus-associated hepatocellular carcinoma," *Nature Genetics*, vol. 44, no. 10, pp. 1117–1121, 2012.

3

The Correlation between miR-122 and Lipoprotein Lipase Expression in Chronic Hepatitis C Patients

Malgorzata Sidorkiewicz, Martyna Grek-Kowalinska, and Anna Piekarska

Medical University of Lodz, Poland

Correspondence should be addressed to Malgorzata Sidorkiewicz; malgorzata.sidorkiewicz@umed.lodz.pl

Academic Editor: Tetsuro Shimakami

Chronic HCV infection is strictly associated with host lipid/lipoprotein metabolism disorders. The study aimed to analyze the relationship between viral load, lipid profile, IFNγ, and the expression of miR-122 and LPL in the liver and PBMCs. Sera, PBMCs, and matching liver biopsies from 17 chronic hepatitis C patients were enrolled in this study. Collected data shows that liver (not PBMCs) miR-122 expression is positively correlated with HCV RNA load and IFNγ and reversely with LPL expression in CHC patients. Presented, for the first time, in this study, the reverse correlation of miR-122 and LPL expression in liver; miR-122 and LPL seem to be important factors of CHC infection.

1. Introduction

Hepatitis C virus (HCV), with an estimated over 185 million people infected worldwide [1], is the major etiological cause of chronic hepatitis. Chronic hepatitis C (CHC) is directly associated with development of liver cirrhosis and hepatoma. HCV RNA triggers production of interferon gamma (IFNγ) but is often abrogated in CHC patients [2]. Reduced IFNγ level implicates an immunological impairment that in turn consolidates the state of chronicity.

HCV infection affects host lipids/lipoproteins homeostasis. Alteration of metabolism seems to be essential for the HCV entire "life cycle": entry, replication, and the secretory pathway [3]. Circulating HCV virions are associated with VLDL and LDL, designated as lipo-viro-particles. Lipoprotein lipase (LPL) that catalyzes triglyceride (TG) hydrolysis of chylomicrons and VLDL has been identified as a promising host factor against HCV infection [4]. Lipo-viro HCV particles constitute effective substrate for LPL; thus reduction of HCV infectivity can be achieved by modifying the virion-associated lipid composition [5]. Additionally, LPL increases the binding capacity of HCV particles and reduces infectivity of the virus, possibly by blocking virions on the surface of cells [6]. Also, LPL-induced peroxisomal proliferators-activated receptor-α (PPAR-α) signaling pathway activation was suggested as a factor that suppresses HCV infection [7].

Previous reports underscore the importance of miR-122 in liver biology and in the control of HCV infection (for review [8]). miR-122 exerts in vitro a positive effect on HCV replication through a direct interaction with 5'UTR region of viral genome. Inhibition of miR-122 reduces serum cholesterol level [9]. HCV RNA sequences were detected in vivo, not only in hepatocytes but also in fresh peripheral blood mononuclear cell (PBMC) preparations from HCV-infected patients as well as cultured PBMCs [10]. In previous studies we showed not only changes in serum lipid profile in CHC patients but also in cholesterol expression in PBMCs [11]. Neither this lipid's alteration nor HCV RNA presence in cells was related to miR-122 expression in PBMCs.

This study compares miR-122 and lipoprotein lipase expression in the liver and PBMCs and investigates how these parameters are associated with lipid profile, with HCV load and IFN-gamma, revealing the reverse correlation between lipoprotein lipase and miR-122 expression in the liver of CHC patients. To the best of our knowledge this study represents the first attempt to evaluate the relationship between miR-122 and LPL expression.

2. Materials and Methods

2.1. Participant Enrollment. This study recruited 17 patients with CHC (genotype 1) and 26 healthy donors (HD). Blood samples obtained from both groups, CHC patients and healthy donors, were used for PBMCs and sera isolation. Serum HCV RNA was detected by the Amplicor HCV test, version 2.0 (Roche Diagnostics). In case of CHC patients, matching human liver specimens from fine needle biopsies were collected. The study was approved by the Bioethical Committee of the Medical University of Lodz (RNN/93/07/kB); signed informed consent from all participants was obtained.

2.2. Determination of Biochemical Parameters in Sera and PBMCs. We followed the methods of Sidorkiewicz et al. 2017 [12]. Serum total cholesterol (TC), high-density lipoprotein-cholesterol (HDL-C), low-density lipoprotein-cholesterol (LDL-C), and triglycerides (TG) were measured enzymatically in Olympus AU 640 and the kits of Olympus. The IFNγ concentration in sera was measured using Human IFNγ ELISA kit (BioVendor).

Intracellular cholesterol level in PBMC (IC) was evaluated using the cholesterol assay kit, Cholesterol CHOD-PAP (BIOLABO S.A., France) as per manufacturer's recommendation, and the results were normalized to the protein concentration in cell lysates and presented as relative expression of (r.e. IC).

2.3. miR-122 Analysis. For miR-122 analysis, RNA fraction <200 nt was extracted from PBMCs, using mirVana miRNA Isolation Kit (Ambion), and total RNA from biopsy samples using TRIzol Reagent (Invitrogen) according to the manufacturer's instructions. The reverse transcription (RT) was done, on 10 ng of RNA using the TaqMan MicroRNA Assay specific for miRNA-122 (Applied Biosystems). RT product (3.3 μL) was used in Real-Time PCR with miRNA-122-specific primers/probe mix and TaqMan Universal PCR Master Mix (Applied Biosystems). The reaction was performed on the ABI Prism 7900 Fast Real-Time PCR System (Applied Biosystems). Relative expression (r.e.) of miR-122 presents the mean Ct value for miRNA-122 Ct, calculated from triplicate reactions and normalized to average Ct values, obtained for snRNA U6.

2.4. Determination of LPL Expression. LPL expression was determined by Western Blotting. A total of 50 μg of protein from PBMCs lysates was subjected to SDS-PAGE, transferred into nitrocellulose, and incubated with rabbit anti-LPL primary antibodies (sc-32885, Santa Cruz Biotechnology, dilution 1:300) and secondary goat anti-rabbit antibodies (sc-2004, Santa Cruz Biotechnology, dilution 1:4000). As a control, goat antibodies against β-actin (sc-1615, Santa Cruz Biotechnology, dilution 1:300) were used with secondary rabbit anti-goat (1:10000) from Sigma. The positive bands were detected using enhanced chemiluminescence system (ECL) and were quantitatively analyzed using the Bio-Rad Quantity One System. Relative expression (r.e.) of LPL was calculated by normalization to the actin expression for each sample.

2.5. Statistical Analysis. Statistical analysis was performed with STATISTICA 8,0 PL software (StatSoft). Groups were compared using the Mann-Whitney *U* test. Spearman's correlation analysis was applied to measure the strength of relationship between parameters. Differences were considered statistically significant at p<0,05.

All origin data supporting the results reported in this paper are collected and available in the Department of Medical Biochemistry.

Table 1: Comparison of analyzed parameters in the group of CHC patients and healthy donors.

Analyzed parameters (mean values)	CHC patients	Healthy donors	p value
Number (M/F)	17 (13/4)	26 (15/11)	n.a.
Age (ys)	22,7	23,2	n.a.
ALT (IU/ml)	69,18	20,6	0,003
IFN gamma (pg/ml)	4,41	5,52	0,015
TC (mmol/L)	2,55	3,61	<0,0001
LDL-C (mmol/L)	1,4	2,03	0,003
HDL-C (mmol/L)	0,8	1,09	0,002
TG (mmol/L)	0,77	1,1	0,16 (ns)
r.e. IC (PBMCs)	1,12	1,76	<0,0001
HCV RNA load (IU/ml)	$3{,}79 \times 10^5$	n.a.	n.a.
r.e. LPL (PBMCs)	2,37	1,32	0,008
r.e. LPL (Liver)	3,12	n.a.	n.a.
r.e. miR-122 (PBMCs)	0,88	0,76	0,001
r.e. miR-122 (Liver)	1,15	n.a.	n.a.

ALT: alanine aminotransferase; F: female; M: male; n.a.: not analyzed; ns: not statistically confirmed result; r.e.: relative expression; ys: years.

3. Results

This study recruited 17 patients with CHC (genotype 1) and 26 healthy donors (HD). General characteristics of studied subjects are included in Table 1. As presented, the level of total cholesterol, LDL, and HDL fractions in sera as well as intracellular cholesterol level in PBMCs were significantly lower in CHC patients compared to healthy donors. Similarly, serum IFNγ was significantly lower in CHC patients than in HD. Observed decreased level of triglycerides in CHC patients was not statistically significant. Comparison of LPL and miR-122 expression in PBMCs showed, for both parameters, a higher expression in cells from CHC patients than from HD.

Spearman rank correlation analysis performed on data collected from CHC patients (Table 2) indicated strong reverse correlation for miR-122 expression between liver and PBMCs as well as for LPL expression between these two origins. miR-122 expression in liver was positively correlated with serum HCV RNA load and IFNγ and reversely correlated with hepatic LPL expression. We found also the tendency for hepatic LPL expression to be reversely correlated with viral load. Neither for miR-122 nor for LPL expression in PBMCs of CHC patients, significant correlation with HCV

TABLE 2: The list of correlations (Spearman rank correlation test) found for data obtained by the analysis of sera (S), liver biopsies (L), and PBMCs (P) samples collected from CHC patients.

Compared parameters	Correlation coefficient value	P value
miR-122 (L) vs HCV RNA (S)	+0,63	0,006
miR-122 (L) vs IFN γ (S)	+0,54	0,024
miR-122 (P) vs HCV RNA (S)	-0,81	0,026
miR-122 (P) vs miR-122 (B)	-0,93	0,001
LPL (L) vs LPL (P)	-0,56	0,028
LPL (L) vs miR-122 (B)	-0,47	0,014
LPL (L) vs HCV RNA (S)	-0,31	0,06*
LPL (P) vs HCV RNA (S)	+0,42	0,036

* - indicates a tendency.

RNA load was revealed. Additionally, in the group of healthy donors, strong reverse correlation was found between serum IFNγ and both TC ($r= -0{,}52$, $p=0{,}008$) and LDL ($r= -0{,}42$, $p=0{,}039$), not detected in the group of CHC patients.

4. Discussion

The strategic role of hepatitis C virus in manipulating of host lipids/lipoproteins metabolism was described [3] as essential for the entry, secretion, and replication of virus. Our results showed that TC, LDL, and HDL fractions, as well as intracellular cholesterol level in PBMCs, were significantly decreased in CHC patients compared to healthy donors. These data remain in line with previous observations that associates CHC infections not only with liver steatosis but also with decreased cholesterol expression [13, 14]. HCV may modulate lipid metabolism in host cells in order to create a more hospitable environment for its own "life cycle".

Concerning IFN, we observed that serum IFNγ level was significantly reduced in CHC patients compared to healthy donors, which remains in agreement with earlier reports [15, 16]. Additionally, we found that serum IFNγ was reversely correlated with total cholesterol and LDL level, but only in the group of healthy donors. Lack of such a relationship in the group of CHC patients may suggest perturbation between cholesterol metabolism and IFNγ signaling. It was shown by others [17] that the alteration of cholesterol pathway may abrogate the IFN-gamma-dependent immune response.

Lipoprotein lipase, which plays a main role in lipoprotein/lipid homeostasis, emerged recently as a host-protecting factor against HCV infection. Indeed, a strong tendency to opposite correlation between HCV RNA load and hepatic expression of lipoprotein lipase seems to confirm these observations in our study. Lack of such a relationship for LPL in PBMCs can be explained by opposite correlation between LPL expression in liver and PBMCs. Interestingly, while LPL may regulate TG metabolism, no correlation was found between LPL expression and TG level.

According to the suggested role of miR-122 in HCV replication [8], our results demonstrated the positive correlation between the HCV RNA load and miR-122 expression in liver (not in PBMCs). Like in case of LPL, miR-122 showed also opposite expression in the liver and in PBMCs. Hepatic miR-122 was reversely correlated with the expression of lipoprotein lipase. It is especially interesting observation as liver-specific miR-122 is known to promote hepatitis C virus replication and lipoprotein lipase to protect the host from HCV infection.

As was mentioned earlier, LPL may suppress HCV infectivity by the breakdown of viral lipid coat and bridging between HCV and hepatocytes that blocks the viral entry to the cell [4, 6]. The third mechanism of anti-HCV action of LPL is based on activation of peroxisomal proliferators-activated receptor-α (PPAR-α) signaling pathway [7]. After LPL hydrolysis free fatty acids create ligands for this pathway in target cells. That in turn may cause an antiviral action in infected patients via reduction of viral assembly and secretion. Independently of LPL activity, the same pathway may be triggered directly by alteration of miR-122 expression. The study of Gatfield [18] demonstrated that the knockdown of miR-122 expression resulted in the activation of PPAR-α signaling pathway.

Additionally, we found that miR-122 expression in liver (not in PBMCs) is positively correlated with IFNγ concentration. Interestingly, it was found earlier that IFNγ is involved in lipoprotein lipase inhibition, at the level of LPL gene transcription [19]. Thus, we cannot exclude that, in CHC patients, IFN-gamma may participate in reducing of LPL expression along with miR-122.

In conclusion, this study provides evidence for opposite expression of both miR-122 and lipoprotein lipase in liver and PBMCs. Hepatic miR-122 expression in CHC patients seems to be of high importance for HCV infection which was evidenced by strong positive relationship between miR-122 and HCV RNA load. The reverse relationship between miR-122 and lipoprotein lipase in liver suggests that the modulation of lipoprotein lipase may be another manifestation of the proinfective action of miR-122. Therefore, a future study attempting to explain the mechanism of cross-reactivity between miR-122 and LPL is worth considering.

Acknowledgments

This study was conducted with the financial support of the Ministry of Science and Higher Education of Poland

(N N401098536) and the statutory funds of Department of Medical Biochemistry (503/6-086-01/503-61-001) of Medical University of Lodz.

References

[1] A. P. Thrift, H. B. El-Serag, and F. Kanwal, "Global epidemiology and burden of HCV infection and HCV-related disease," *Nature Reviews Gastroenterology & Hepatology*, vol. 14, no. 2, pp. 122–132, 2017.

[2] L. M. Pfeffer, M. A. Madey, C. A. Riely, and J. F. Fleckenstein, "The induction of type i interferon production in hepatitis C-infected patients," *Journal of Interferon & Cytokine Research*, vol. 29, no. 5, pp. 299–306, 2009.

[3] C.-I. Popescu, L. Riva, O. Vlaicu, R. Farhat, Y. Rouillé, and J. Dubuisson, "Hepatitis C virus life cycle and lipid metabolism," *Biology*, vol. 3, no. 4, pp. 892–921, 2014.

[4] Y. Shimizu, T. Hishiki, K. Sugiyama et al., "Lipoprotein lipase and hepatic triglyceride lipase reduce the infectivity of hepatitis C virus (HCV) through their catalytic activities on HCV-associated lipoproteins," *Virology*, vol. 407, no. 1, pp. 152–159, 2010.

[5] Y. Shimizu, T. Hishiki, S. Ujino, K. Sugiyama, K. Funami, and K. Shimotohno, "Lipoprotein component associated with hepatitis C virus is essential for virus infectivity," *Current Opinion in Virology*, vol. 1, no. 1, pp. 19–26, 2011.

[6] P. Maillard, M. Walic, P. Meuleman et al., "Lipoprotein lipase inhibits hepatitis C virus (HCV) infection by blocking virus cell entry," *PLoS ONE*, vol. 6, no. 10, Article ID e26637, 2011.

[7] H.-Y. Sun, C.-C. Lin, P.-J. Tsai et al., "Lipoprotein lipase liberates free fatty acids to inhibit HCV infection and prevent hepatic lipid accumulation," *Cellular Microbiology*, vol. 19, no. 4, Article ID e12673, 2017.

[8] S. Bandiera, S. Pfeffer, T. Baumert, and M. Zeisel, "miR-122 a key factor and therapeutic target in liver disease," *Journal of Hepatology*, vol. 62, pp. 448–457, 2015.

[9] C. Esau, S. Davis, S. F. Murray et al., "miR-122 regulation of lipid metabolism revealed by in vivo antisense targeting," *Cell Metabolism*, vol. 3, no. 2, pp. 87–98, 2006.

[10] I. Castillo, E. Rodríguez-Iñigo, J. Bartolomé et al., "Hepatitis C virus replicates in peripheral blood mononuclear cells of patients with occult hepatitis C virus infection," *Gut*, vol. 54, no. 5, pp. 682–685, 2005.

[11] M. Sidorkiewicz, M. Grek, B. Jozwiak, and A. Piekarska, "Decreased level of intracellular cholesterol in peripheral blood mononuclear cells is associated with chronic hepatitis C virus infection," *Virus Research*, vol. 178, no. 2, pp. 539–542, 2013.

[12] M. Sidorkiewicz, M. Grek, B. Jozwiak, A. Krol, and A. Piekarska, "The impact of chronic hepatitis C infection on cholesterol metabolism in PBMCs is associated with microRNA-146a expression," *European Journal of Clinical Microbiology & Infectious Diseases*, vol. 36, no. 4, pp. 697–702, 2017.

[13] D. Siagris, M. Christofidou, G. J. Theocharis et al., "Serum lipid pattern in chronic hepatitis C: Histological and virological correlations," *Journal of Viral Hepatitis*, vol. 13, no. 1, pp. 56–61, 2006.

[14] D. J. Felmlee, M. L. Hafirassou, M. Lefevre, T. F. Baumert, and C. Schuster, "Hepatitis C virus, cholesterol and lipoproteins—impact for the viral life cycle and pathogenesis of liver disease," *Viruses*, vol. 5, no. 5, pp. 1292–1324, 2013.

[15] Y. Kondo, V. M. Sung, K. Machida, M. Liu, and M. M. Lai, "Hepatitis C virus infects T cells and affects interferon-γ signaling in T cell lines," *Virology*, vol. 361, no. 1, pp. 161–173, 2007.

[16] M. Malaguarnera, I. Di Fazio, A. Laurino, G. Pistone, S. Restuccia, and B. A. Trovato, "Decrease of interferon gamma serum levels in patients with chronic hepatitis C," *Biomedicine & Pharmacotherapy*, vol. 51, no. 9, pp. 391–396, 1997.

[17] J. M. Jameson, J. Cruz, A. Costanzo, M. Terajima, and F. A. Ennis, "A role for the mevalonate pathway in the induction of subtype cross-reactive immunity to influenza A virus by human $\gamma\delta$ T lymphocytes," *Cellular Immunology*, vol. 264, no. 1, pp. 71–77, 2010.

[18] D. Gatfield, G. Le Martelot, C. E. Vejnar et al., "Integration of microRNA miR-122 in hepatic circadian gene expression," *Genes & Development*, vol. 23, no. 11, pp. 1313–1326, 2009.

[19] S. M. Harris, E. J. Harvey, T. R. Hughes, and D. P. Ramji, "The interferon-γ-mediated inhibition of lipoprotein lipase gene transcription in macrophages involves casein kinase 2- and phosphoinositide-3-kinase-mediated regulation of transcription factors Sp1 and Sp3," *Cellular Signalling*, vol. 20, no. 12, pp. 2296–2301, 2008.

4

Prognostic Impact of Cirrhosis in Patients with Intrahepatic Cholangiocarcinoma following Hepatic Resection

Seogsong Jeong,[1] Lei Gao,[2] Ying Tong,[1] Lei Xia,[1] Ning Xu,[1] Meng Sha,[1] Jianjun Zhang,[1] Xiaoni Kong,[1] Jinyang Gu,[1] and Qiang Xia[1]

[1]*Department of Liver Surgery, Renji Hospital, School of Medicine, Shanghai Jiao Tong University, Shanghai 200127, China*
[2]*Institute of Liver Diseases, 81st Hospital of People's Liberation Army, Nanjing 210002, China*

Correspondence should be addressed to Jinyang Gu; gjynyd@126.com and Qiang Xia; 2870166877@qq.com

Academic Editor: Pierluigi Toniutto

Background. Prognostic impact of cirrhosis in patients with intrahepatic cholangiocarcinoma (ICC) upon hepatic resection remains unclear due to lack of studies in the literature. *Methods.* A total of 106 resected patients with ICC were reviewed, including 25 patients (23.6%) with cirrhosis and 81 noncirrhotic patients (76.4%). Subgroups of cirrhotic patients with and without hepatitis B virus (HBV) infection were studied. *Results.* The impact of cirrhosis on the overall survival (OS) (hazard ratio [HR], 0.901; 95% confidence interval [CI], 0.510 to 1.592; $P = 0.720$) and the relapse-free survival (RFS) (HR, 0.889; 95% CI, 0.509 to 1.552; $P = 0.678$) revealed no statistical significance. Furthermore, HBV-associated cirrhotic patients and the other cirrhotic patients demonstrated no statistical difference on survival outcomes (1 yr OS, 60.0% versus 70.0%; 5 yr OS, 10.0% versus 0%; $P = 0.744$; 1 yr RFS, 53.3% versus 30.0%; 5 yr RFS, 10.0% versus 0%; $P = 0.279$). In patients with cirrhosis, tumor size larger than 5 cm was found to be the foremost factor that was independently associated with poor prognosis. *Conclusion.* The presence of liver cirrhosis did not significantly affect prognosis of patients with ICC after resection. Downstaging modality may be in need for patients with ICC underlying cirrhosis, which remains to be validated in future studies.

1. Introduction

Intrahepatic cholangiocarcinoma (ICC) is the second most common primary liver cancer after hepatocellular carcinoma (HCC) that originates from epithelial cells of intrahepatic bile ducts [1]. To date, surgical resection remains the only curative treatment that has been generally recognized for ICC [2]. However, clinical manifestation of ICC is usually late and unspecific, leading most ICC to be advanced at the time of diagnosis [3]. Consequently, approximately one-third of patients with ICC are not recommended to be candidates for hepatic resection due to high postoperative recurrence rates, even after extended hepatectomy [4]. Another major concern that limits patients with ICC to receive hepatic resection is underlying liver disease, including primary biliary cirrhosis in western countries and hepatitis B virus- (HBV-) associated cirrhosis in eastern countries [5]. A few previous publications indicated that the presence of cirrhosis was independently associated with reduced long-term survival outcomes in patients with HCC [6, 7]. In addition, Li et al. [8] demonstrated that cirrhosis is an independent predictor for poor prognosis in patients with ICC after resection. In another study of 514 patients with ICC who underwent hepatic resection, cirrhosis was also found to be an unfavorable prognostic factor so that they subjected the presence of cirrhosis into the nomogram predicting prognosis [9]. On the contrary, Zhang et al. [10] reported that the presence of cirrhosis showed no impact in the prognosis of patients with ICC ($P = 0.730$). Therefore, the exact relationship of liver cirrhosis with the prognosis of ICC remains to be further elucidated.

Herein, we conducted the present study to evaluate prognostic impact of liver cirrhosis on ICC. All the enrolled patients were divided according to the presence of liver cirrhosis as well as HBV infection, which would especially focus on HBV-associated liver cirrhosis frequently in China. Furthermore, a statistical analysis was carried out to identify foremost factors significantly affecting long-term survival outcomes of cirrhotic patients.

2. Methods

2.1. Patients. From January 2007 to July 2015, 106 consecutive patients with ICC underwent hepatic resection at the Department of Liver Surgery, Renji Hospital (Shanghai, China). The patients were included according to the following criteria: (1) pathological confirmation of ICC; (2) single type of tumor; (3) Child-Pugh score of A or B; (4) hepatic resection, and (5) not having distant metastasis at the time of surgery.

2.2. Definition of Subgroups. The enrolled patients were stratified into 4 subgroups according to the presence of HBV infection and liver cirrhosis. The first group (Group 1; $n = 15$) was comprised of cirrhotic patients with HBV infection, and noncirrhotic patients with HBV-associated ICC were defined as Group 2 ($n = 27$). Group 3 ($n = 10$) was consisted of the cirrhotic patients without seropositivity of HBV infection, and the others were subjected into Group 4 ($n = 54$).

2.3. Data Collection. Prospectively collected ICC database was used for the description of baseline characteristics and survival analyses. HBV infection was defined as positivity of either hepatitis B surface antigen (HBsAg) or hepatitis B core antibody (HBcAb) and confirmed by serological examinations. Liver cirrhosis was collected from results of imaging studies and further confirmed by Sirius Red staining from liver specimens after hepatic resection. Preoperative levels of alpha fetoprotein (AFP) and carbohydrate antigen (CA) 19-9 were collected within one week before operation. Tumor size was defined as a maximal diameter of the principal tumor nodule. Histologic grade was classified by the Edmondson-Steiner criteria ((I) well; (II) moderate; (III) poor) [11]. The follow-up investigation was carried out ranging from 17 to 118 months. The endpoints of the study were the survival outcomes of the patients.

2.4. Surgical Procedures. All the patients underwent hepatic resection with regional lymph node dissection. The types of resection included minor hepatectomy (partial or less than a half of liver) and major hepatectomy (hemihepatectomy or extended hemihepatectomy). The indication for major hepatectomy was an indocyanine green clearance rate at 15 min rate of less than 10%. All the surgical operations were performed with informed consents.

2.5. Statistical Analysis. SPSS for Windows version 19.0 (SPSS Inc., Chicago, Illinois, US) was applied in statistical analyses. Categorical data were analyzed with the use of Pearson's chi-square test. Survival curves were presented with the use of Kaplan-Meier method. Between-group differences were evaluated by Log-rank method. The univariate and multivariate analyses were applied in assessing prognostic value of variables and identifying independent prognostic factors, which were presented with hazard ratio (HR) and 95% confidence interval (CI). Statistical significance was defined as a P value of less than 0.05.

3. Results

3.1. Patient Characteristics. The mean age was 60.0 ± 10.34 with a 58.5% of male distribution (Table 1). The age was significantly younger in HBV-associated cirrhotic patients compared with the cirrhotic patients without HBV infection (54.9 ± 7.4 yrs versus 71.2 ± 8.4 yrs, $P < 0.001$) with a predominance of male patients ($P = 0.013$; Table 2). The mean age of cirrhotic patients without HBV infection revealed to be older than the noncirrhotic patients without HBV infection (71.2 ± 8.4 yrs versus 62.0 ± 9.8 yrs, $P = 0.011$). Elevation of AFP was found in 29 patients (26.4%), whereas more than two-thirds (68.9%) of the patients had an elevated level of CA19-9. Minor and major hepatectomy were performed in 49 (45.3%) and 58 (54.7%) patients, respectively. More than a half of ICC patients (57.5%) had a larger than 5 cm of maximal diameter of tumor. Eighty-nine patients (84.0%) showed a single tumor nodule and the other 17 patients (16.0%) presented with multiple nodules. Almost all the patients ($n = 100$, 94.3%) displayed Child-Pugh score of A. Fifty-two (49.1%) patients belonged to well or moderate differentiation, whereas the other 54 (50.9%) were poorly differentiated. Vascular invasion and lymph node metastasis were found in 28 (26.4%) and 48 (45.3%) patients, respectively. Further specific between-group differences are shown in Table 2.

3.2. Prognostic Factors of All Resected Patients with ICC. As for the cumulative OS of all the resected patients, HBsAg, preoperative level of CA19-9, tumor size, Child-Pugh score, vascular invasion, and lymph node metastasis revealed significance in the univariate analysis and were employed into the multivariate analysis. Tumor size larger than 5 cm (HR, 1.923; 95% CI, 1.147 to 3.226; $P = 0.013$), Child-Pugh score of B (HR, 3.349; 95% CI, 1.387 to 8.090; $P = 0.007$), vascular invasion (HR, 1.867; 95% CI, 1.103 to 3.159; $P = 0.020$), and lymph node metastasis (HR, 2.790; 95% CI: 1.628 to 4.781; $P < 0.001$) were found to be independently associated with decreased OS (Table 3).

Seropositivity of HBsAg, tumor size, Child-Pugh score, lymph node metastasis, and tumor number were found to affect RFS. Among them, the seropositivity of HBsAg was associated with prolonged RFS (HR, 0.505; 95% CI, 0.279 to 0.914; $P = 0.024$), whereas tumor size larger than 5 cm (HR, 1.947; 95% CI, 1.177 to 3.219; $P = 0.009$), Child-Pugh score of B (HR, 3.067; 95% CI, 1.293 to 7.275; $P = 0.011$), and lymph node metastasis (HR, 2.188; 95% CI, 1.310 to 3.654; $P = 0.003$) negatively influenced the RFS.

3.3. Survival Outcomes. Survival outcomes of the cirrhotic patients and noncirrhotic patients are presented in Figure 1. As shown in Figures 1(a) and 1(b), the presence of cirrhosis revealed no significant impact on the OS (HR, 0.882; 95% CI, 0.501 to 1.552; $P = 0.664$) and RFS (HR, 0.869; 95% CI, 0.499 to 1.513; $P = 0.619$). When the patients were stratified into 4 groups, the OS indicated no significant between-group differences, whereas the RFS showed a statistically significant difference between Groups 2 and 4 (1-yr, 55.6% versus 29.6%; 5-yr, 16.7% versus 10.4; $P = 0.011$; Table 4; Figure 2).

TABLE 1: Clinicopathological characteristics of the patients according to the presence of HBV infection and cirrhosis.

Variables	Overall patients (n = 106)	Group 1 (n = 15)	Group 2 (n = 27)	Group 3 (n = 10)	Group 4 (n = 54)
Age	60.0 ± 10.34	54.9 ± 7.4	54.7 ± 9.1	71.2 ± 8.4	62.0 ± 9.8
Gender					
Male	62 (58.5)	14 (93.3)	14 (51.9)	5 (50.0)	29 (53.7)
Female	44 (41.5)	1 (6.7)	13 (48.1)	5 (50.0)	25 (46.3)
Preoperative AFP					
>9 ng/ml	28 (26.4)	8 (53.3)	9 (33.3)	2 (20.0)	9 (16.7)
≤9 ng/ml	78 (73.6)	7 (46.7)	18 (66.7)	8 (80.0)	45 (83.3)
Preoperative CA19-9					
>35 U/ml	73 (68.9)	9 (60.0)	19 (70.4)	7 (70.0)	38 (70.4)
≤35 U/ml	33 (31.1)	6 (40.0)	8 (29.6)	3 (30.0)	16 (29.6)
Resection type					
Minor hepatectomy	48 (45.3)	10 (66.6)	10 (37.0)	6 (60.0)	22 (40.7)
Major hepatectomy	58 (54.7)	5 (33.4)	17 (63.0)	4 (40.0)	32 (59.3)
Tumor size					
>5 cm	61 (57.5)	7 (46.7)	21 (77.8)	4 (40.0)	29 (53.7)
≤5 cm	45 (42.5)	8 (53.3)	6 (22.2)	6 (60.0)	25 (46.3)
Tumor number					
Single	89 (84.0)	13 (86.7)	23 (85.2)	9 (90.0)	44 (81.5)
Multiple	17 (16.0)	2 (13.3)	4 (14.8)	1 (10.0)	10 (18.5)
Child-Pugh score					
A	100 (94.3)	13 (86.7)	26 (96.3)	9 (90.0)	52 (96.3)
B	6 (5.7)	2 (13.3)	1 (3.7)	1 (10.0)	2 (3.7)
Histologic grade					
Well or moderate	52 (49.1)	5 (33.4)	12 (44.4)	4 (40.0)	31 (57.4)
Poor	54 (50.9)	10 (66.6)	15 (55.6)	6 (60.0)	23 (42.6)
Vascular invasion					
Present	28 (26.4)	8 (53.3)	8 (29.6)	3 (30.0)	9 (16.7)
Absent	78 (73.6)	7 (46.7)	19 (70.4)	7 (70.0)	45 (83.3)
Lymph node metastasis					
Present	48 (45.3)	6 (40.0)	9 (33.3)	6 (60.0)	27 (50.0)
Absent	58 (54.7)	9 (60.0)	18 (66.7)	4 (40.0)	27 (50.0)

Group 1, patients with HBV infection and cirrhosis; Group 2, patients with HBV infection but without cirrhosis; Group 3, patients with cirrhosis but without HBV infection; Group 4, patients without both HBV infection and cirrhosis; AFP, alpha-fetoprotein; CA19-9, carbohydrate antigen 19-9.

3.4. Prognostic Factors of Cirrhotic Patients with ICC. Minor hepatectomy (versus major hepatectomy), tumor size > 5 cm (versus ≤5 cm), and lymph node metastasis showed a significant association with the survival outcomes in the univariate analysis. In addition, major hepatectomy showed a HR of 4.194, 95% CI of 1.447 to 12.093, and a P value of 0.008 for the OS, and a HR of 3.159, 95% CI of 1.164 to 8.576, and a P value of 0.024 for the RFS. However, the type of hepatectomy and lymph node metastasis revealed no significantly independent association with both the OS and RFS. Only the tumor size larger than 5 cm was found to be independently reduced in the OS (HR, 16.435; 95% CI, 2.211 to 122.179; P = 0.006) and RFS (HR, 10.264; 95% CI, 1.881 to 55.987; P = 0.007) of the cirrhotic patients (Table 5). Furthermore, among the 11 cirrhotic patients with tumor size larger than 5 cm, 8 patients had relapse of the tumor within 6 months after surgical operation and the other 3 patients developed recurrence at the 9th, 10th, and 12th month.

TABLE 2: Between-group comparison of the clinicopathological characteristics.

Variables	*P* values					
	I versus II	I versus III	I versus IV	II versus III	II versus IV	III versus IV
Age	NS	<0.001	0.014	<0.001	0.003	0.011
Gender	0.006	0.013	0.005	NS	NS	NS
Preoperative AFP	NS	NS	0.004	NS	NS	NS
Preoperative CA19-9	NS	NS	NS	NS	NS	NS
Resection type	NS	NS	NS	NS	NS	NS
Tumor size	0.04	NS	NS	0.029	0.036	NS
Tumor number	NS	NS	NS	NS	NS	NS
Child-Pugh score	NS	NS	NS	NS	NS	NS
Histologic differentiation	NS	NS	NS	NS	NS	NS
Vascular invasion	NS	NS	0.004	NS	NS	NS
Lymph node metastasis	NS	NS	NS	NS	NS	NS

NS, not significant; AFP, alpha-fetoprotein; CA19-9, carbohydrate antigen 19-9.

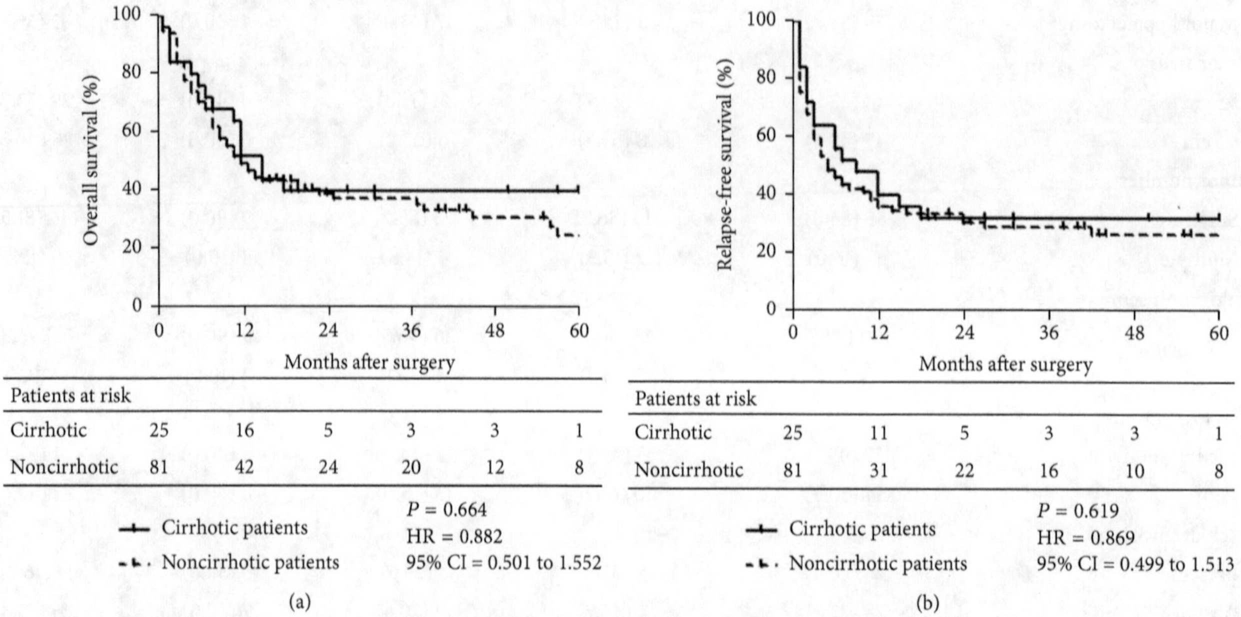

FIGURE 1: Survival outcomes of the patients with and without cirrhosis. Shown are the impact of cirrhosis on the OS (Panel (a)) and RFS (Panel (b)) of the entire cohort. The data revealed that the presence of cirrhosis showed no association with the OS (HR, 0.882; 95% CI, 0.501 to 1.552; $P = 0.664$) and RFS (HR, 0.869; 95% CI, 0.499 to 1.513; $P = 0.619$) of the patients.

4. Discussion

Although hepatic resection provides patients with ICC an opportunity of long-term survival, the prognosis of this group of patients remains dismal [12, 13]. In eastern countries, numerous patients present with underlying liver disease, such as liver cirrhosis, due to a high prevalence of viral hepatitis that limits surgical approaches [14]. As known widely, liver cirrhosis may contribute to severe complications, including deterioration of liver function and gastrointestinal bleeding [15]. However, our data showed no significant correlation between the prognosis and the presence of liver cirrhosis in ICC patients. As stratified according to the presence of HBV infection and cirrhosis, the HBV-associated patients achieved relatively prolonged RFS and the presence of cirrhosis revealed no statistically significant prognostic impact. Moreover, a subgroup analysis of cirrhotic patients indicated a tumor size larger than 5 cm to be the foremost factor that significantly reduced the prognosis of cirrhotic patients with ICC.

In the present study, the 1- and 5-year OS rates of 106 patients after hepatic resection were merely at 54.7% and 11.4%, respectively. These survival outcomes might be affected by the patient characteristics, including advanced tumor size and a high proportion of patients with vascular invasion and lymph node metastasis, which were found to be the

TABLE 3: Univariate and multivariate analysis of variables that significantly affected the survival outcomes.

Variables	Overall survival					Relapse-free survival				
	Univariate analysis			Multivariate analysis		Univariate analysis			Multivariate analysis	
	1 yr	5 yr	P value	HR (95% CI)	P value	1 yr	5 yr	P value	HR (95% CI)	P value
HBsAg										
Positive	70.0	25.0	0.025	0.665 (0.363–1.220)	0.188	63.3	25.0	0.002	0.505 (0.279–0.914)	0.024
Negative	48.7	6.8				30.3	6.3			
Tumor size										
>5 cm	44.3	5.9	0.002	1.923 (1.147–3.226)	0.013	26.2	5.7	0.003	1.947 (1.177–3.219)	0.009
≤5 cm	68.9	21.4				57.8	19.4			
Child-Pugh score										
A	56.0	12.3	0.005	3.349 (1.387–8.090)	0.007	41.0	11.5	0.017	3.067 (1.293–7.275)	0.011
B	33.3	0				16.7	0			
Vascular invasion										
Present	39.3	4.3	0.049	1.867 (1.103–3.159)	0.020			NS		
Absent	60.3	14.3								
Lymph node metastasis										
Present	37.5	0	<0.001	2.790 (1.628–4.781)	<0.001	18.8	0	<0.001	2.188 (1.310–3.654)	0.003
Absent	69.0	25.0				56.9	22.5			
Tumor number										
Single			NS			43.8	13.2	0.046	1.150 (0.638–2.071)	0.643
Multiple						17.6	0			

HR, hazard ratio; CI, confidence interval; HBsAg, hepatitis B surface antigen; NS, not significant.

TABLE 4: Comparison of the survival curves.

	OS (%)			P values				RFS (%)			P values			
	1 yr	5 yr	MS	Versus I	Versus II	Versus III	Versus IV	1 yr	5 yr	MS	Versus I	Versus II	Versus III	Versus IV
Group 1	60.0	10.0	12	/	0.540	0.744	0.447	53.3	10.0	12	/	0.718	0.279	0.106
Group 2	66.7	16.7	37	/	/	0.575	0.079	55.6	16.7	24	/	/	0.082	0.011
Group 3	70.0	0	16.5	/	/	/	0.503	30.0	0	6	/	/	/	0.885
Group 4	44.4	11.1	10.5	/	/	/	/	29.6	10.4	3	/	/	/	/

OS: overall survival; MS: median survival month; RFS: relapse-free survival.

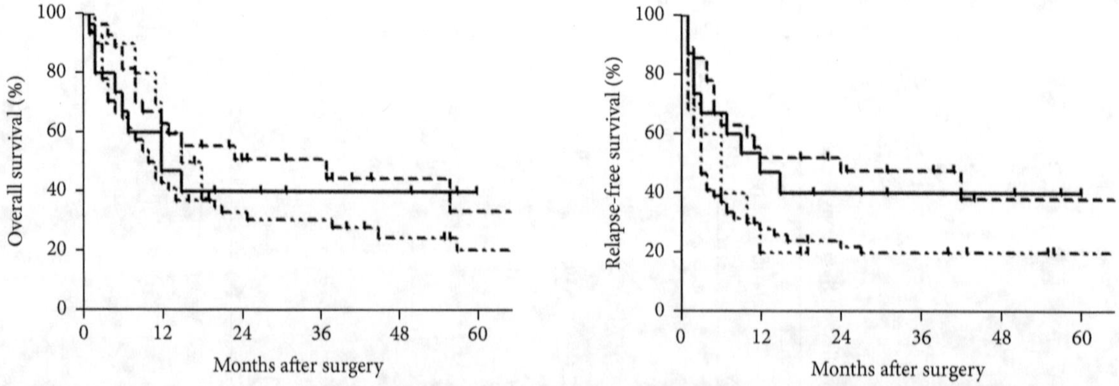

(a) Patients at risk

Patients at risk						
Group 1	15	9	5	3	3	1
Group 2	27	18	11	8	4	3
Group 3	10	7	0	0	0	0
Group 4	54	24	13	12	8	5

(b) Patients at risk

Patients at risk						
Group 1	15	8	5	3	3	1
Group 2	27	15	11	7	3	3
Group 3	10	3	0	0	0	0
Group 4	54	16	11	9	7	5

Group 1 Group 3 Group 2 Group 4

FIGURE 2: Survival curves of the patients according to the presence of HBV infection and cirrhosis. Shown are the survival curves of the HBV-associated cirrhotic patients (Group 1), HBV-associated noncirrhotic patients (Group 2), HBV-negative cirrhotic patients (Group 3), and HBV-negative noncirrhotic patients (Group 4) on the OS (Panel (a)) and RFS (Panel (b)). The curves demonstrated no significant between-group differences except for Group 2 and Group 4 in the RFS ($P = 0.011$). The most favorable prognosis was found in Group 2 (1-yr OS, 66.7%; 5-yr OS, 16.7%; median survival for OS, 37 months; 1-yr RFS, 55.6%; 5-yr RFS, 16.7%; median survival for RFS, 24 months) and Group 4 showed the worst prognosis (1-yr OS, 44.4%; 5-yr OS, 11.1%; median survival for OS, 10.5 months; 1-yr RFS, 29.6%; 5-yr RFS, 10.4%; median survival for RFS, 3 months).

independent factors that showed significant association with decreased OS. On the other hand, several previous publications demonstrated that HBV infection is associated with survival outcomes of patients with ICC after resection [16–18]. However, due to conflicting results, prognostic impact of HBV infection in ICC remained controversial [19, 20]. In the present study, the recurrence of the tumor was significantly decreased in the HBV carriers (seropositive for HBsAg). In addition, a recent meta-analysis regarding prognostic value of viral hepatitis indicated that HBV infection was associated with relatively low incidence of lymph node metastasis (odd ratio, 0.39; 95% CI, 0.25 to 0.58), which was also found to be an unfavorable prognostic factor for the RFS in this study [21]. Therefore, our data regarding prognostic value of HBV-associated cirrhosis might be affected by inhibiting lymph node metastasis in HBV-associated patients.

To date, information regarding survival outcomes and prognostic factors of cirrhotic ICC remains insufficient due to limited number of studies. A previous relevant publication indicated that hypoalbuminemia, vascular invasion, positive surgical margins, and perioperative blood transfusion are the independent predictors for poor prognosis of cirrhotic ICC [22]. Another study from France indicated that, among 10 patients with unrecognized ICC complicating liver cirrhosis, 5 patients (50%) developed recurrence of the tumor after liver transplantation, suggesting that cirrhosis is associated with more frequent recurrence and poor prognosis in patients with ICC [23]. However, our data revealed that only the tumor size was independently associated with poor prognosis, which was also found to be an independent predictor for the high recurrence rate of the tumor in the entire cohort, rendering us to elucidate that the survival outcomes of the cirrhotic

TABLE 5: Subgroup analysis of cirrhotic patients (n = 25).

Variables	Overall survival					Relapse-free survival				
	Univariate analysis			Multivariate analysis		Univariate analysis			Multivariate analysis	
	1 yr	5 yr	*P* value	HR (95% CI)	*P* value	1 yr	5 yr	*P* value	HR (95% CI)	*P* value
Resection type										
Minor hepatectomy	75.0	14.3	0.004	0.297 (0.051–1.746)	0.179	50.0	11.1	0.019	0.402 (0.093–1.734)	0.222
Major hepatectomy	44.4	0				22.2	0			
Tumor size										
>5 cm	27.3	0	<0.001	16.435 (2.211–122.179)	0.006	9.1	0	<0.001	10.264 (1.881–55.987)	0.007
≤5 cm	92.9	20.0				64.3	14.3			
Lymph node metastasis										
Present	41.7	0	0.002	2.505 (0.595–10.536)	0.210	16.7	0	0.007	2.345 (0.696–7.900)	0.169
Absent	84.6	20.0				61.5	14.3			

HR: hazard ratio, CI: confidence interval.

patients with ICC were mainly affected by the recurrence of the tumor. In recent years, preoperative downstaging treatments have been suggested to be performed for patients with HCC in order to meet the Milan criteria or to prevent dropout from the liver transplantation waiting list, as validated by the United Network for Organ Sharing (UNOS) [24]. A previous publication including 35 patients with locally advanced ICC from the University of California, Los Angeles (UCLA), demonstrated that the patients who received both neoadjuvant therapy and adjuvant therapy resulted in relatively better prognosis compared with the patient who received adjuvant therapy only or no therapy (47% versus 33% versus 20%, $P = 0.03$) [25]. More recently, Rayar et al. [26] reported a patient with a huge and locally advanced ICC through preoperative yttrium-90 radioembolization successfully reduced tumor size and then received liver transplantation. Three-year follow-up investigation confirmed that liver function of the patient remained normal and no sign of recurrence was found. Therefore, implementing downstaging treatment for patients with ICC upon hepatic resection might also significantly improve long-term survival of patients with ICC, including patients underlying cirrhosis, which awaits confirmation by future prospective trials.

On the other hand, our results showed no significant difference on prognostic impact between minor hepatectomy and major hepatectomy; the survival outcomes of the patients who received minor hepatectomy revealed to be relatively more favorable without statistical significance. As we performed further subgroup analysis on cirrhotic patients, the impact of major hepatectomy revealed to be a risk factor that significantly reduced both the OS and RFS. However, major hepatectomy was not found to be an independent prognostic factor, which might be on account of the limited number of patients. Hence, we call for future large-scaled trials to verify whether major hepatectomy could be effectively and safely performed in cirrhotic patients with ICC.

Another important factor that significantly affected the survival outcomes was lymph node metastasis, which is a representative hallmark of ICC [27]. Prophylactic lymph node dissection has been considered as a benign factor that might improve the prognosis of patients with ICC [28, 29]. A case report from Japan demonstrated that wide lymph node dissection with hemihepatectomy, including regional and para-aortic lymph nodes, was found to be curative in the first 5-year survival of periductal-infiltrating advanced ICC with para-aortic lymph nodes metastases [30]. In addition, we previously found that there was no significant difference in 5-year survival rates between patients with para-aortic lymph node metastasis and patients with regional nodal metastasis and contended that micrometastases of para-aortic nodes may also play a significant role in the prognosis of patients with biliary cancer [31]. In the present study, the presence of lymph node metastasis showed strong relationship with poor survival outcomes in the entire cohort ($P < 0.001$). In addition, lymph node metastasis also revealed significant difference in the univariate analysis of cirrhotic patients. The survival outcomes of the cirrhotic patients without lymph node metastasis were remarkably higher than the others (1 yr and 5 yr OS: 84.6% and 20.0% versus 41.7% and 0%). Hence, future prospective trials need to focus on the effective and precise detection of lymph node metastasis.

This study had a few underlying limitations. First, this is a retrospective single-center investigation. Limited number of patients might be a weakness. Second, the most common etiological factor for the development of cirrhosis was HBV infection, which is endemic in Asian countries. Therefore, our results need to be validated in large-scaled studies on the basis of other type of cirrhosis, such as primary biliary cirrhosis in western populations.

In conclusion, the presence of cirrhosis in patients with ICC showed no association with the survival outcomes. Tumor size of larger than 5 cm was found to be the foremost factor that significantly influenced long-term survival outcomes. Our results suggest that hepatic resection itself cannot derive favorable prognosis of cirrhotic patients with ICC of larger than 5 cm. Neoadjuvant therapy might improve prognosis of patients with ICC size of larger than 5 cm underlying liver cirrhosis.

Authors' Contributions

Seogsong Jeong and Lei Gao equally contributed to this work.

Acknowledgments

This work was supported by the National Natural Science Foundation of China (81772507, 81472243, and 81670598).

References

[1] N. Razumilava and G. J. Gores, "Cholangiocarcinoma," *The Lancet*, vol. 383, no. 9935, pp. 2168–2179, 2014.

[2] A. Ruzzenente, S. Conci, A. Valdegamberi, C. Pedrazzani, and A. Guglielmi, "Role of surgery in the treatment of intrahepatic cholangiocarcinoma," *European Review for Medical and Pharmacological Sciences*, vol. 19, no. 15, pp. 2892–2900, 2015.

[3] J. Bridgewater, P. R. Galle, S. A. Khan et al., "Guidelines for the diagnosis and management of intrahepatic cholangiocarcinoma," *Journal of Hepatology*, vol. 60, no. 6, pp. 1268–1289, 2014.

[4] A. Doussot, M. Gonen, J. K. Wiggers et al., "Recurrence Patterns and Disease-Free Survival after Resection of Intrahepatic Cholangiocarcinoma: Preoperative and Postoperative Prognostic Models," *Journal of the American College of Surgeons*, vol. 223, no. 3, pp. 493–505.e2, 2016.

[5] H. Zhang, T. Yang, M. Wu, and F. Shen, "Intrahepatic cholangiocarcinoma: Epidemiology, risk factors, diagnosis and surgical management," *Cancer Letters*, vol. 379, no. 2, pp. 198–205, 2016.

[6] E. C. Lee, S. H. Kim, H. Park, S. D. Lee, S. Lee, and S. Park, "Survival analysis after liver resection for hepatocellular carcinoma: A consecutive cohort of 1002 patients," *Journal of Gastroenterology and Hepatology*, vol. 32, no. 5, pp. 1055–1063, 2017.

[7] F. Conti, F. Buonfiglioli, A. Scuteri et al., "Early occurrence and recurrence of hepatocellular carcinoma in HCV-related cirrhosis treated with direct-acting antivirals," *Journal of Hepatology*, vol. 65, no. 4, pp. 727–733, 2016.

[8] Y.-Y. Li, H. Li, P. Lv et al., "Prognostic Value of Cirrhosis for Intrahepatic Cholangiocarcinoma After Surgical Treatment," *Journal of Gastrointestinal Surgery*, vol. 15, no. 4, pp. 608–613, 2011.

[9] O. Hyder, H. Marques, C. Pulitano et al., "A nomogram to predict long-term survival after resection for intrahepatic cholangiocarcinoma: an Eastern and Western experience," *JAMA Surgery*, vol. 149, no. 5, pp. 432–438, 2014.

[10] L. Zhang, J.-Q. Cai, J.-J. Zhao et al., "Impact of hepatitis B virus infection on outcome following resection for intrahepatic cholangiocarcinoma," *Journal of Surgical Oncology*, vol. 101, no. 3, pp. 233–238, 2010.

[11] H. A. Edmondson and P. E. Steiner, "Primary carcinoma of the liver: a study of 100 cases among 48,900," *Cancer*, vol. 7, no. 3, pp. 462–503, 1954.

[12] H. M. Park, S. P. Yun, E. C. Lee et al., "Outcomes for Patients with Recurrent Intrahepatic Cholangiocarcinoma After Surgery," *Annals of Surgical Oncology*, vol. 23, no. 13, pp. 4392–4400, 2016.

[13] T. Yoh, E. Hatano, K. Yamanaka et al., "Is Surgical Resection Justified for Advanced Intrahepatic Cholangiocarcinoma?" *Liver Cancer*, vol. 5, no. 4, pp. 280–289, 2016.

[14] C. de Martel, D. Maucort-Boulch, M. Plummer, and S. Franceschi, "World-wide relative contribution of hepatitis B and C viruses in hepatocellular carcinoma," *Hepatology*, vol. 62, no. 4, pp. 1190–1200, 2015.

[15] P. S. Ge and B. A. Runyon, "Treatment of patients with cirrhosis," *The New England Journal of Medicine*, vol. 375, no. 8, pp. 767–777, 2016.

[16] H.-B. Zhou, H. Wang, Y.-Q. Li et al., "Hepatitis B virus infection: a favorable prognostic factor for intrahepatic cholangiocarcinoma after resection," *World Journal of Gastroenterology*, vol. 17, no. 10, pp. 1292–1303, 2011.

[17] Z.-F. Wu, X.-Y. Wu, N. Zhu et al., "Prognosis after resection for hepatitis B virus-associated intrahepatic cholangiocarcinoma," *World Journal of Gastroenterology*, vol. 21, no. 3, pp. 935–943, 2015.

[18] S. Jeong, Y. Tong, M. Sha, J. Gu, and Q. Xia, "Hepatitis B virus-associated intrahepatic cholangiocarcinoma: A malignancy of distinctive characteristics between hepatocellular carcinoma and intrahepatic cholangiocarcinoma," *Oncotarget* , vol. 8, no. 10, pp. 17292–17300, 2017.

[19] L.-Y. Tao, X.-D. He, and D.-R. Xiu, "Hepatitis B virus is associated with the clinical features and survival rate of patients with intrahepatic cholangiocarcinoma," *Clinics and Research in Hepatology and Gastroenterology*, vol. 40, no. 6, pp. 682–687, 2016.

[20] C. Ahn, S. Hwang, Y. Lee et al., "Prognostic impact of hepatitis B virus infection in patients with intrahepatic cholangiocarcinoma," *ANZ Journal of Surgery*, 2016.

[21] Z. Wang, Y.-Y. Sheng, Q.-Z. Dong, and L.-X. Qin, "Hepatitis B virus and hepatitis C virus play different prognostic roles in intrahepatic cholangiocarcinoma: A meta-analysis," *World Journal of Gastroenterology*, vol. 22, no. 10, pp. 3038–3051, 2016.

[22] H. Li, J.-S. Wu, X.-T. Wang et al., "Factors predicting surgical resection in patients with intrahepatic cholangiocarcinoma and cirrhosis," *Journal of Investigative Surgery*, vol. 27, no. 4, pp. 219–225, 2014.

[23] M. Vallin, N. Sturm, G. Lamblin et al., "Unrecognized intrahepatic cholangiocarcinoma: an analysis of 993 adult cirrhotic liver explants," *Clinical Transplantation*, vol. 27, no. 3, pp. 403–409, 2013.

[24] M. N. G. J. A. Braat, M. Samim, M. A. A. J. van den Bosch, and M. G. E. H. Lam, "The role of 90Y-radioembolization in downstaging primary and secondary hepatic malignancies: a systematic review," *Clinical and Translational Imaging*, vol. 4, no. 4, pp. 283–295, 2016.

[25] J. C. Hong, C. M. Jones, J. P. Duffy et al., "Comparative analysis of resection and liver transplantation for intrahepatic and hilar cholangiocarcinoma: a 24-year experience in a single center," *JAMA Surgery*, vol. 146, no. 6, pp. 683–689, 2011.

[26] M. Rayar, G. B. Levi Sandri, P. Houssel-Debry, C. Camus, L. Sulpice, and K. Boudjema, "Multimodal therapy including yttrium-90 radioembolization as a bridging therapy to liver transplantation for a huge and locally advanced intrahepatic cholangiocarcinoma," *Journal of Gastrointestinal and Liver Diseases*, vol. 25, no. 3, pp. 401–404, 2016.

[27] Z. Jutric, W. C. Johnston, H. M. Hoen et al., "Impact of lymph node status in patients with intrahepatic cholangiocarcinoma treated by major hepatectomy: a review of the National Cancer Database," *HPB*, vol. 18, no. 1, pp. 79–87, 2016.

[28] S.-B. Choi, K.-S. Kim, J.-Y. Choi et al., "The prognosis and survival outcome of intrahepatic cholangiocarcinoma following surgical resection: association of lymph node metastasis and lymph node dissection with survival," *Annals of Surgical Oncology*, vol. 16, no. 11, pp. 3028–3056, 2009.

[29] T. Adachi and S. Eguchi, "Lymph node dissection for intrahepatic cholangiocarcinoma: A critical review of the literature to date," *Journal of Hepato-Biliary-Pancreatic Sciences*, vol. 21, no. 3, pp. 162–168, 2014.

[30] Y. Murakami, T. Yokoyama, Y. Takesue et al., "Long-term survival of peripheral intrahepatic cholangiocarcinoma with metastasis to the para-aortic lymph nodes," *Surgery*, vol. 127, no. 1, pp. 105-106, 2000.

[31] J. Gu, L. Xia, B. Xu et al., "Clinical prognostic significance of regional and extended lymphadenectomy for biliary cancer with para-aortic lymph node metastasis: A systematic review and meta-analysis," *Digestive and Liver Disease*, vol. 48, no. 7, pp. 717–725, 2016.

5

Efficacy and Safety of Lumen Apposing Self-Expandable Metal Stents for EUS Guided Cholecystostomy

Nikhil R. Kalva,[1] Vishwas Vanar,[1] David Forcione,[2] Matthew L. Bechtold,[3] and Srinivas Reddy Puli[1]

[1]*Internal Medicine, University of Illinois College of Medicine at Peoria, Peoria, IL, USA*
[2]*Interventional Endoscopy Services, Gastrointestinal Unit, Massachusetts General Hospital, Harvard Medical School, Boston, MA, USA*
[3]*Division of Gastroenterology and Hepatology, University of Missouri-Columbia, Columbia, MO, USA*

Correspondence should be addressed to Srinivas Reddy Puli; srinivas.puli@osfhealthcare.org

Academic Editor: Yousuke Nakai

Background. Patients with acute cholecystitis are treated with early cholecystectomy. A subset of patients are unfit for surgery due to comorbidities and late presentation. Prompt gall bladder drainage (GBD) with percutaneous or endoscopic approach remains a viable therapeutic option for nonoperative candidates. Endoscopic ultrasound (EUS) guided transluminal gall bladder drainage (EUS-GBD) continues to evolve as an alternative approach to percutaneous drainage. With continued refinement in stent technology, lumen apposing self-expandable metal stent (LAMS) offers several advantages. We performed a pooled analysis on the efficacy and safety of EUS-GBD with LAMS in nonoperative candidates with acute cholecystitis. *Methods.* Extensive English language literature search was performed in Medline, Embase, Cochrane Central, and Google Scholar using keywords "endoscopic ultrasound", "stent", "gallbladder", "acute cholecystitis", and "cholecystostomy" from Jan 2000 to Dec 2016. Fixed and random effects models were used to calculate the pooled proportions. *Results.* Data was extracted from 13 studies that met the inclusion criteria ($n = 233$). Pooled proportion of technical success was 93.86% (95% CI = 90.56 to 96.49) and clinical success was 92.48% (95% CI = 88.9 to 95.42). Overall complication rate was 18.31% (95% CI = 13.49 to 23.68) and stent related complication rate was 8.16% (95% CI = 4.03 to 14.96) in the pooled percentage of patients. Pooled proportion for perforation was 6.71% (95% CI 3.65 to 10.6) and recurrent cholangitis/cholecystitis was noted in 4.05% (95% CI = 1.64 to 7.48). Publication bias calculated using Harbord-Egger bias indicator gave a value of −0.61 (95% CI = −1.39 to 0.16, $p = 0.11$). The Begg-Mazumdar indicator for bias gave Kendall's tau b value of −0.42 ($p \geq 0.05$). *Conclusions.* EUS-GBD with LAMS is a safe and alternative treatment modality for patients needing gallbladder drainage, with acceptable intraprocedural and postprocedural complications. However, due to the limited data and lack of direct comparison with other methods, further controlled trials are necessary to estimate the overall efficacy and safety and the role of EUS-GBD with LAMS in management of nonoperative patients with acute cholecystitis.

1. Introduction

Cholecystectomy remains first-line treatment for acute cholecystitis due to stone disease or malignant cystic duct obstruction in patients who are considered good surgical candidates. Early laparoscopic cholecystectomy performed within two days of clinical presentation has favorable clinical outcome and remains highly cost effective [1]. In acutely ill patients unfit for surgery, percutaneous gallbladder drainage (PTGBD) with prompt decompression has shown evidence of reducing the risk of severe sepsis, gall bladder perforation, or even death [2]. Since its introduction in 1980s, the technique of PTGBD has undergone refinements with acceptable perioperative complication rates. Despite its highly successful insertion and improvement in short-term mortality, drain related issues continue to negatively impact outcomes due to accidental dislodgement, pain and discomfort, and quality of life [3]. PTGBD remains widely used because of its ease of placement either as destination therapy or as two-staged approach for patients who are future candidates for cholecystectomy.

Endoscopic ultrasound (EUS) now has a well-established role in transmural drainage of extraluminal fluid collections from complicated pancreatitis with excellent success in the management of pseudocysts and walled-off necrosis (WON). Despite several shortcomings of the earlier stents, the availability of the lumen apposing metal stents or LAMS (Axios; Xlumena, Inc., Mountain View, California, USA) has furthered our capacity to perform successful transmural drainage under EUS and image guidance [4]. The practical advantages of larger flanges at the end are the following: when fully expanded they permit excellent tissue apposition and resist stent migration. The larger inner diameter facilitates adequate drainage and a silicone covering assists in maintaining adequate seal between the gall bladder and the bowel. Additional advantages of the silicone covering include resistance to tissue ingrowth aiding in subsequent stent removal following maturation of the cholecystoenteric fistula. With continued expansion of therapeutic EUS, alternative transmural drainage of the gall bladder is entertained to overcome the recognized challenges in PTGBD [5]. Kwan et al. first described the novel transgastric/transduodenal (transmural) drainage of the gall bladder under EUS guidance with subsequent series reporting clinical success by various authors using plastic biliary stents across the tract [6, 7]. Stent migration, bile peritonitis, and pneumoperitoneum became an apparent following tract dilation at the time of stent deployment, limiting its wider adaptation and clinical use. Self-expandable metal stents (SEMS) with flanges at the end could overcome the flaws from tract dilation and prevent spontaneous stent migration [8]. Finally, with significant advancements in the stent technology and remarkable success of LAMS in the management of pancreatic fluid collections, various authors now have assessed feasibility of transmural drainage of the gall bladder in both retrospective and prospective cohorts.

The aim of our analysis is to assess the efficacy and safety of EUS-GBD using the newer LAMS in the management of inoperable patients with acute cholecystitis.

2. Material and Methods

2.1. Study Selection. The study was conducted based on the Preferred Reporting Items for Systematic Reviews and Meta-analysis guidelines (PRISMA guideline) [9]. A study protocol was developed by the study team prior to the initiation of the study. Studies evaluating the use of EUS for gall bladder drainage and stenting with lumen apposing stents that reported clinical success and complications were selected. Articles were searched using Medline, Embase, Cochrane Central, and Google Scholar and limited to English language. The last date of the search was December 2016. The search terms used include endoscopic ultrasound, stents, acute cholecystitis, gall bladder, and cholecystostomy. The citations were imported into EndNote and duplicates were removed. Articles were reviewed by title, abstracts, and full texts by two independent reviewers (N.R.K, S.R.P). Differences were resolved by mutual consensus. The agreement among reviewers for the collected data was quantified using Cohen's alpha [10]. Data from the studies were extracted into Excel spreadsheet for further analysis and performing statistical analysis.

2.2. Statistical Methods. This study was performed by calculating the pooled proportions (i.e., pooled proportion of patients with primary outcomes). First, the individual study proportion of outcome was transformed into a quantity using Freeman–Tukey variant of the arcsine square root transformed proportion. The pooled proportion is calculated as the back transform of the weighted mean of the transformed proportions using the inverse arcsine variance weights for the fixed effect model and the DerSimonian–Laird weights for the random-effect model [11]. Forrest plots were drawn to show the point estimates in each study in relation to the summary pooled estimate. The width of the point estimates in the Forrest plots indicated the assigned weight to the independent study. The heterogeneity among studies was tested using Cochran's Q test based on inverse variance weights [12]. If $p > 0.10$, it rejects the null hypothesis that the studies are heterogeneous. The effects of publication and selection bias on the summary estimates were tested using both the Harbord-Egger bias indicator and Begg-Mazumdar bias indication [13, 14]. Funnel plots were also constructed to evaluate publication bias using the standard error [14].

2.3. Assessment of Study Quality. There are no internationally agreed quality reporting scales for use in systematic reviews and meta-analysis using observational studies. We used the Strengthening the Reporting of Observational Studies in Epidemiology (STROBE) guidelines as a template for assessment of quality of each study [15]. We identified key elements that could potentially introduce bias and include selection bias and confounding bias.

3. Results

The initial search identified 659 reference articles, of which 58 relevant articles were selected and reviewed. A total of 13 studies were selected for data extraction that met our inclusion criteria, with 233 patients included in the analysis [8, 16–27]. Figure 1 shows the flow diagram for the meta-analysis. The study characteristics are included in Table 1. The interrater reliability of the included studies using Cohen's Kappa gave a value of 0.81 suggesting excellent agreement among the study authors.

The diagnosis of acute cholecystitis used in the studies was based on clinical and radiographic criteria. All the patients included in the reference studies were unfit for surgery. Patients with calculous and acalculous cholecystitis and malignant cystic duct obstruction were included in the analysis. Primary analysis of the study is predefined and include technical and clinical success and overall complication rates. The technical success is defined as successful stent deployment between the stomach or duodenum and the gallbladder. The pooled proportion of technical success using fixed effect model for endoscopic ultrasound guided

TABLE 1: Study characteristics.

Author	Year	Number of patients	Study type	Type of stent
Walter et al.	2015	30	Prospective	Axios
Law et al.	2016	7	Retrospective	Axios
Takagi et al.	2016	16	Retrospective	BONA
Chan et al.	2016	25	Retrospective	Axios
Choi et al.	2016	14	Case control	Regular stent
Ge et al.	2016	7	Retrospective	Micro Tech
Song et al.	2010	8	Prospective	Regular stent
Song et al.	2012	15	Prospective	BONA
Itoi et al.	2012	5	Retrospective	Axios
Serna-Higuera et al.	2013	13	Prospective	Axios
Jang et al.	2012	15	Prospective	BONA
Irani et al.	2015	15	Retrospective	Axios
Choi et al.	2014	63	Retrospective	BONA

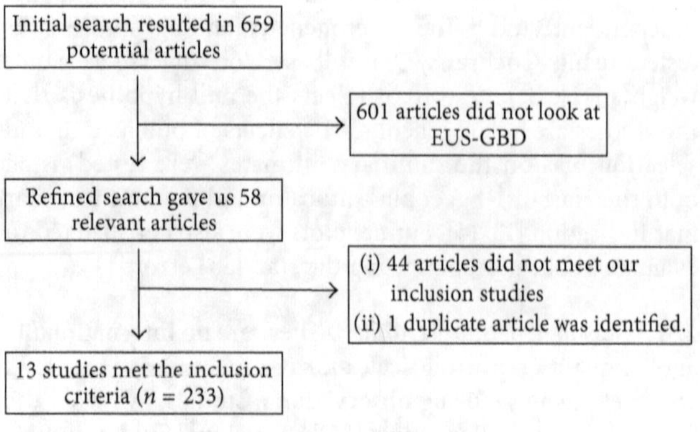

FIGURE 1: Flowchart of study selection.

gall bladder drainage (EUS-GBD) was 93.86% (95% CI; 90.56–96.49). Individual study proportions of technical success using fixed effect model are depicted in the Forrest plot and shown in Figure 2. The clinical success is defined as resolution of symptoms of acute cholecystitis following achieving successful gallbladder stenting. The pooled proportion of clinical success was 92.48% (95% CI; 88.90–95.42). Individual study proportions of clinical success using fixed effect model are depicted in the Forrest plot and shown in Figure 3.

The overall complication rate was 18.31% (95% CI; 13.49–23.68) and stent related complication rate was 8.16% (95% CI; 4.03 to 14.96) in the pooled percentage of patients. The individual study proportions of overall complications are depicted in the Forrest plot and shown in Figure 4. Pooled proportion for perforation was 6.71% (95% CI; 3.65–10.6) and recurrent cholangitis/cholecystitis was noted in 4.05% (95% CI; 1.64–7.48).

Publication bias calculated using Harbord-Egger bias indicator gave a value of −0.61 (95% CI; 1.39–0.16, $p = 0.11$). The Begg-Mazumdar indicator gave Kendall's tau b value of −0.42 ($p \geq 0.05$). Both these indicators showed that there was no publication bias. Additionally, Figure 5 represents funnel plot to assess and screen for publication bias for various outcomes that were analyzed for this study.

4. Discussion

EUS-GBD is a technically challenging procedure even with experienced endoscopists. Unlike walled-off pancreatic cysts including necrosis which are fixed to the gastric wall, the gallbladder is a mobile structure making the transmural puncture challenging. The technique consists of a multistep process which includes imaging of the gallbladder from the prepyloric antrum or the duodenal bulb [6, 7]. The body or the neck of the gallbladder is selected as an ideal site of entry over the fundus. The shortest distance from the enteral lumen to the gallbladder is selected and color flow Doppler is used to exclude interposing vessels. A 19-gauge needle is used to puncture after selection and, following needle entry, a guidewire (0.035 inch) is coiled into the gallbladder. Subsequently a cautery or mechanical track dilation is performed. An appropriate sized LAMS is selected and deployed from distal to proximal bowel wall under endoscopic and fluoroscopic control to achieve lumen apposition.

Our analysis is thus far the largest reported pooled data on the technical and clinical success rate in EUS-GBD with placement of LAMS with results approaching close to 95%. Most studies used Axios or BONA LAMS in the management. There are several advantages with use of LAMS in this setting when compared to use of either plastic or SEMS without the lumen apposing features. The large diameter of the LAMS stent facilitates adequate gallbladder drainage decreasing the risk of stent obstruction due to thick bilious or purulent secretions. Additionally, the prompt lumen apposition of the gallbladder with the lumen reduces the risk of bile leak peritonitis in addition to minimizing distal stent migration. With further refinement of the technique and stent technology, additional cholecystoscopy using smaller caliber or standard endoscopes with cholecystolithotomy could be considered [19]. The efficacy seems to be mostly in the immediate setting as long-term outcomes are not reported except in one study that was included in our analysis [18]. The study by Choi et al. assessed long-term efficacy outcomes of recurrent acute cholecystitis and need for reintervention

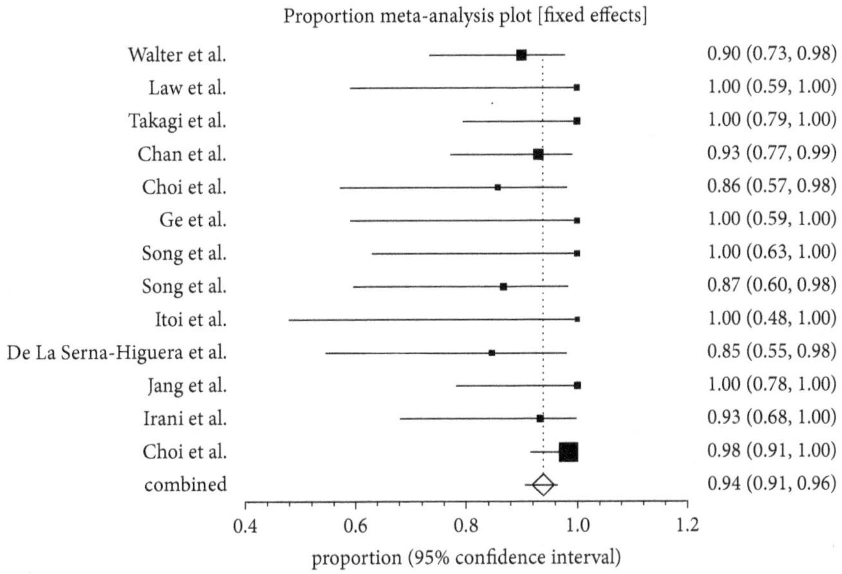

FIGURE 2: Forrest plot showing the individual study proportion of technical success in EUS-GBD.

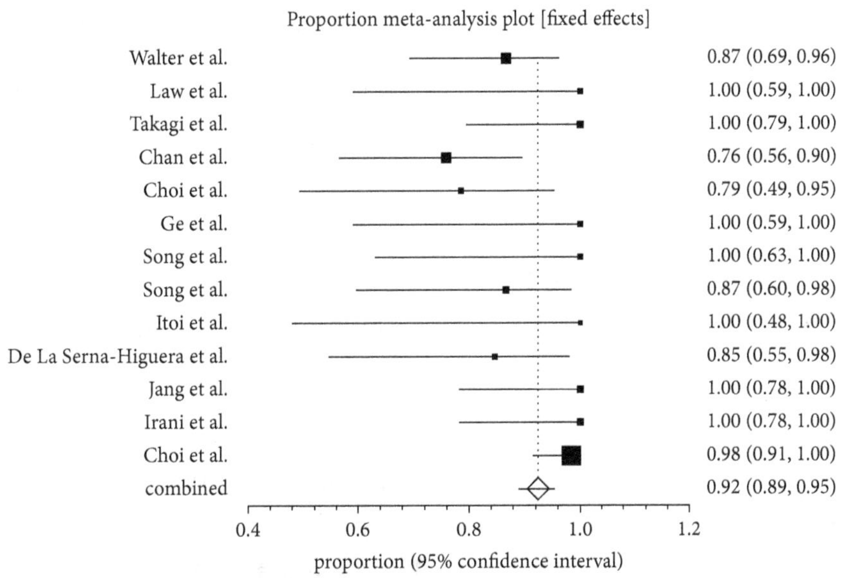

FIGURE 3: Forrest plot showing the individual study proportion of clinical success in EUS-GBD using fixed effect model.

after a median follow-up of approximately 275 days [18]. The rates of late stent related outcomes including distal migration and occlusion requiring reintervention were reported to be around 7.1% in the same study with relatively long-term stent patency rates close to 90% even at the end of 3 years in patients who survived the episode of acute cholecystitis. Subsequent management following formation of the mature cholecystoenteric fistula remains unclear for the published studies to draw a meaningful conclusion. The gallbladder can be accessed both from the prepyloric antrum and the duodenal bulb as described for successful stent deployment. Any drawn conclusions on the safety and efficacy remain unclear. In patients who have undergone PTGBD and remain unfit for future cholecystectomy, Law et al. have reported excellent rates of conversion to EUS-GBD with internalization with similar outcomes [23].

Transluminal drainage and stenting with LAMS have clear advantages in the management of these patients. Despite these important findings on efficacy, our analysis has also shown overall complications rates to be around 18% with direct stent and procedure related complication to be close to 8%. Though the overall complication rates are important they account for both the procedure related and independent outcomes. The more important outcome we believe is stent and procedure related outcome which appears to be acceptable. Recurrence rate of acute cholecystitis appears to be due to obstruction of the stent due to food material and is reported to be about 4% which could be managed with

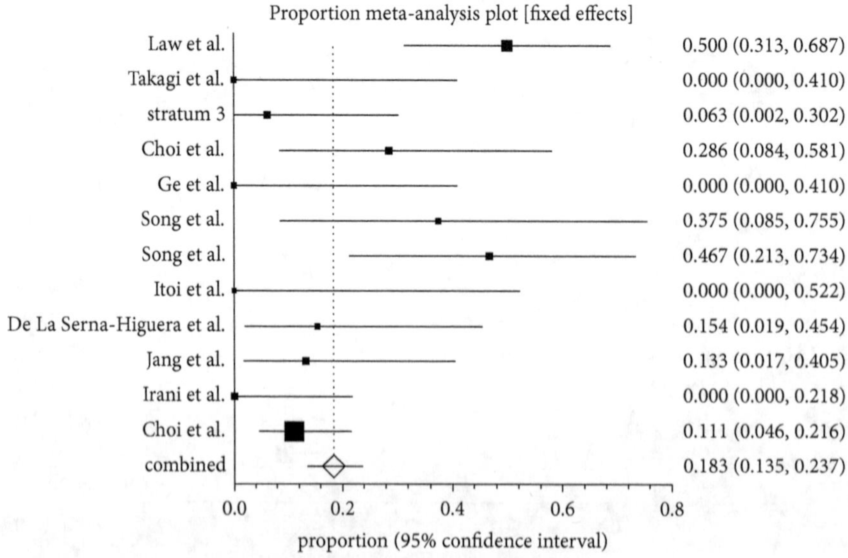

FIGURE 4: Forrest plot showing the individual study proportion of overall complications in EUS-GBD using fixed effect model.

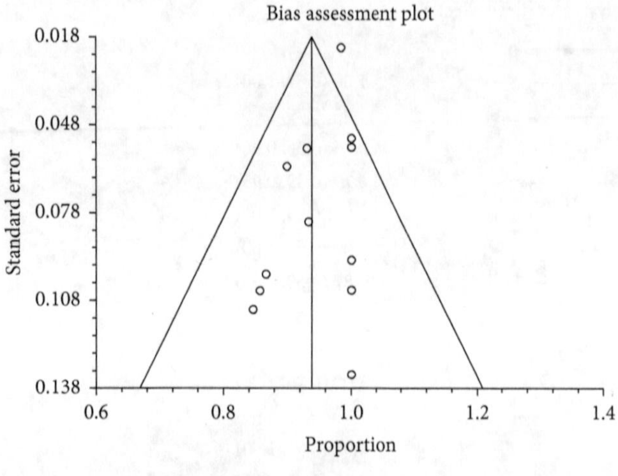

FIGURE 5: Funnel plot evaluating the effect of publication bias on studies investigating technical success in patients undergoing EUS-GBD.

repeat endoscopy with manipulation to clear the stent of the debris. Other unusual stent related adverse events that are reported include self-limiting pneumoperitoneum, distal stent migration into the gall bladder, and tissue ingrowth at variable frequencies.

5. Limitations

Despite encouraging results in short-term clinical success with EUS-GBD and stenting in acute cholecystitis patients, the long-term efficacy of this approach in definitive management remains unclear as a subset of these patients remain indefinitely unfit for surgical cholecystectomy. The theoretical risk of entry of ingested food entry into the gall bladder with subsequent obstruction of the cystic duct and the common bile duct leading to acute cholecystitis and biliary sepsis remain with unknown frequency. This problem could be overcome by targeting the distal end of the LAMS to the neck of the gallbladder there by obstructing the cystic duct. This has an advantage by minimizing the entry of ingested food material into the common bile duct via the way of the cystic duct.

One of the major limitations of the analysis is the inclusion of only small retrospective case series from tertiary centers. The inclusion of small case series could greatly enhance the effect size compared to larger prospective studies. Additionally, the patients are carefully selected resulting in introduction of selection bias in the studies that were included. We systematically attempted to exclude the biases by performing Egger bias indicator and construction of the funnel plot. In our present analysis, we used both the Egger and Begg-Mazumdar bias indicators which showed no statistically significant bias [13, 14]

6. Conclusions

EUS-GBD using LAMS offers an alternative to PTGBD with good short-term technical and clinical success rate. Despite the reported complications, albeit managed conservatively, EUS-GBD using LAMS appears to be higher than most routine gastrointestinal endoscopic procedures. Further long-term prospective studies comparing its efficacy to transpapillary gallbladder stenting and mini-invasive strategies are needed before wide spread adaptation of this technique. In spite of the complexity of the procedure, it should be offered in highly specialized centers with the expertise in advanced therapeutic endoscopy with capacity to manage complications if they arise.

Disclosure

The manuscript was presented as a poster presentation at the Annual Scientific Meeting of the American Society of

Gastrointestinal Endoscopy in conjunction with the Digestive Disease Week in Chicago, May 2017.

References

[1] S. N. Zafar, A. Obirieze, B. Adesibikan, E. E. Cornwell, T. M. Fullum, and D. D. Tran, "Optimal time for early laparoscopic cholecystectomy for acute cholecystitis," *JAMA Surgery*, vol. 150, no. 2, pp. 129–136, 2015.

[2] C.-K. Chou, K.-C. Lee, C.-C. Chan et al., "Early percutaneous cholecystostomy in severe acute cholecystitis reduces the complication rate and duration of hospital stay," *Medicine (United States)*, vol. 94, no. 27, p. e1096, 2015.

[3] A. McKay, M. Abulfaraj, and J. Lipschitz, "Short- and long-term outcomes following percutaneous cholecystostomy for acute cholecystitis in high-risk patients," *Surgical Endoscopy*, vol. 26, no. 5, pp. 1343–1351, 2012.

[4] R. J. Shah, J. N. Shah, I. Waxman et al., "Safety and Efficacy of Endoscopic Ultrasound-Guided Drainage of Pancreatic Fluid Collections With Lumen-Apposing Covered Self-Expanding Metal Stents," *Clinical Gastroenterology and Hepatology*, vol. 13, no. 4, pp. 747–752, 2015.

[5] A. Y. B. Teoh, C. Serna, I. Penas et al., "Endoscopic ultrasound-guided gallbladder drainage reduces adverse events compared with percutaneous cholecystostomy in patients who are unfit for cholecystectomy," *Endoscopy*, vol. 49, no. 2, pp. 130–138, 2017.

[6] V. Kwan, P. Eisendrath, F. Antaki, O. Le Moine, and J. Devière, "EUS-guided cholecystenterostomy: a new technique (with videos)A figure is presented," *Gastrointestinal Endoscopy*, vol. 66, no. 3, pp. 582–586, 2007.

[7] S. S. Lee, D. H. Park, C. Y. Hwang et al., "EUS-guided transmural cholecystostomy as rescue management for acute cholecystitis in elderly or high-risk patients: a prospective feasibility study," *Gastrointestinal Endoscopy*, vol. 66, no. 5, pp. 1008–1012, 2007.

[8] J. W. Jang, S. S. Lee, D. H. Park, D.-W. Seo, S.-K. Lee, and M.-H. Kim, "Feasibility and safety of EUS-guided transgastric/transduodenal gallbladder drainage with single-step placement of a modified covered self-expandable metal stent in patients unsuitable for cholecystectomy," *Gastrointestinal Endoscopy*, vol. 74, no. 1, pp. 176–181, 2011.

[9] D. Moher, D. G. Altman, A. Liberati, and J. Tetzlaff, "PRISMA statement," *Epidemiology*, vol. 22, no. 1, p. 128, 2011.

[10] P. Brennan and A. Silman, "Statistical methods for assessing observer variability in clinical measures," *British Medical Journal*, vol. 304, no. 6840, pp. 1491–1494, 1992.

[11] R. DerSimonian and N. Laird, "Meta-analysis in clinical trials," *Controlled Clinical Trials*, vol. 7, no. 3, pp. 177–188, 1986.

[12] J. J. Deeks, "Systematic reviews of evaluations of diagnostic and screening tests," *BMJ*, vol. 323, no. 7305, p. 157, 2001.

[13] R. M. Harbord, M. Egger, and J. A. Sterne, "A modified test for small-study effects in meta-analyses of controlled trials with binary endpoints," *Statistics in Medicine*, vol. 25, no. 20, pp. 3443–3457, 2006.

[14] C. B. Begg and M. Mazumdar, "Operating characteristics of a rank correlation test for publication bias," *Biometrics*, vol. 50, no. 4, pp. 1088–1101, 1994.

[15] J. P. Vandenbroucke, "Strengthening the Reporting of Observational Studies in Epidemiology (STROBE): Explanation and Elaboration," *Annals of Internal Medicine*, vol. 147, no. 8, p. W, 2007.

[16] S. M. Chan, A. Y. B. Teoh, H. C. Yip, V. W. Y. Wong, P. W. Y. Chiu, and E. K. W. Ng, "Feasibility of per-oral cholecystoscopy and advanced gallbladder interventions after EUS-guided gallbladder stenting (with video)," *Gastrointestinal Endoscopy*, 2016.

[17] J. H. Choi, H. W. Kim, J.-C. Lee et al., "Percutaneous transhepatic versus EUS-guided gallbladder drainage for malignant cystic duct obstruction," *Gastrointestinal Endoscopy*, vol. 85, no. 2, pp. 357–364, 2017.

[18] J.-H. Choi, S. S. Lee, J. H. Choi et al., "Long-term outcomes after endoscopic ultrasonography-guided gallbladder drainage for acute cholecystitis," *Endoscopy*, vol. 46, no. 8, pp. 656–661, 2014.

[19] C. De La Serna-Higuera, M. Pérez-Miranda, P. Gil-Simón et al., "EUS-guided transenteric gallbladder drainage with a new fistula-forming, lumen-apposing metal stent," *Gastrointestinal Endoscopy*, vol. 77, no. 2, pp. 303–308, 2013.

[20] N. Ge, S. Sun, S. Sun, S. Wang, X. Liu, and G. Wang, "Endoscopic ultrasound-assisted transmural cholecystoduodenostomy or cholecystogastrostomy as a bridge for per-oral cholecystoscopy therapy using double-flanged fully covered metal stent," *BMC Gastroenterology*, vol. 16, no. 1, article no. 9, 2016.

[21] S. Irani, T. H. Baron, I. S. Grimm, and M. A. Khashab, "EUS-guided gallbladder drainage with a lumen-apposing metal stent (with video)," *Gastrointestinal Endoscopy*, vol. 82, no. 6, pp. 1110–1115, 2015.

[22] T. Itoi, K. F. Binmoeller, J. Shah et al., "Clinical evaluation of a novel lumen-apposing metal stent for endosonography-guided pancreatic pseudocyst and gallbladder drainage (with videos)," *Gastrointestinal Endoscopy*, vol. 75, no. 4, pp. 870–876, 2012.

[23] R. Law, I. S. Grimm, J. M. Stavas, and T. H. Baron, "Conversion of Percutaneous Cholecystostomy to Internal Transmural Gallbladder Drainage Using an Endoscopic Ultrasound-Guided, Lumen-Apposing Metal Stent," *Clinical Gastroenterology and Hepatology*, vol. 14, no. 3, pp. 476–480, 2016.

[24] T. J. Song, Y. S. Hyun, S. S. Lee et al., "Endoscopic ultrasound-guided choledochoduodenostomies with fully covered self-expandable metallic stents," *World Journal of Gastroenterology*, vol. 18, no. 32, pp. 4435–4440, 2012.

[25] T. J. Song, D. H. Park, J. B. Eum et al., "EUS-guided cholecystoenterostomy with single-step placement of a 7F double-pigtail plastic stent in patients who are unsuitable for cholecystectomy: a pilot study (with video)," *Gastrointestinal Endoscopy*, vol. 71, no. 3, pp. 634–640, 2010.

[26] W. Takagi, T. Ogura, T. Sano et al., "EUS-guided cholecystoduodenostomy for acute cholecystitis with an anti-stent migration and anti-food impaction system; a pilot study," *Therapeutic Advances in Gastroenterology*, vol. 9, no. 1, pp. 19–25, 2016.

[27] D. Walter, A. Y. Teoh, T. Itoi et al., "EUS-guided gall bladder drainage with a lumen-apposing metal stent: A prospective long-term evaluation," *Gut*, vol. 65, no. 1, pp. 6–8, 2016.

6

Serum Albumin is Independently Associated with Persistent Organ Failure in Acute Pancreatitis

Wandong Hong,[1] Suhan Lin,[1] Maddalena Zippi,[2] Wujun Geng,[3] Simon Stock,[4] Zarrin Basharat,[5] Bicheng Cheng,[6] Jingye Pan,[7] and Mengtao Zhou[8]

[1] *Department of Gastroenterology and Hepatology, The First Affiliated Hospital of Wenzhou Medical University, Wenzhou, Zhejiang, China*
[2] *Unit of Gastroenterology and Digestive Endoscopy, Sandro Pertini Hospital, Rome, Italy*
[3] *Department of Anesthesiology, The First Affiliated Hospital of Wenzhou Medical University, Wenzhou, Zhejiang, China*
[4] *Department of Surgery, World Mate Emergency Hospital, Battambang, Cambodia*
[5] *Microbiology & Biotechnology Research Lab, Department of Environmental Sciences, Fatima Jinnah Women University, Rawalpindi 46000, Pakistan*
[6] *Zhejiang Provincial Top Key Discipline in Surgery, Wenzhou Key Laboratory of Surgery, Department of Surgery, The First Affiliated Hospital, Wenzhou Medical University, Wenzhou, Zhejiang, China*
[7] *Intensive Care Unit, The First Affiliated Hospital of Wenzhou Medical University, Wenzhou, Zhejiang, China*
[8] *Department of Surgery, The First Affiliated Hospital of Wenzhou Medical University, Wenzhou, Zhejiang, China*

Correspondence should be addressed to Mengtao Zhou; studyzhoumengtao@sina.com

Academic Editor: Yousuke Nakai

Background and Aims. To investigate the association between serum albumin levels within 24 hrs of patient admission and the development of persistent organ failure in acute pancreatitis. *Methods.* A total of 700 patients with acute pancreatitis were enrolled. Multivariate logistic regression and subgroup analysis determined whether decreased albumin was independently associated with persistent organ failure and mortality. The diagnostic performance of serum albumin was evaluated by the area under Receiver Operating Characteristic (ROC) curves. *Results.* As levels of serum albumin decrease, the risk of persistent organ failure significantly increases ($P_{trend} < 0.001$). The incidence of organ failure was 3.5%, 10.6%, and 41.6% in patients with normal albumin and mild and severe hypoalbuminaemia, respectively. Decreased albumin levels were also proportionally associated with prolonged hospital stay ($P_{trend} < 0.001$) and the risk of death ($P_{trend} < 0.001$). Multivariate analysis suggested that biliary etiology, chronic concomitant diseases, hematocrit, blood urea nitrogen, and the serum albumin level were independently associated with persistent organ failure. Blood urea nitrogen and the serum albumin level were also independently associated with mortality. The area under ROC curves of albumin for predicting organ failure and mortality were 0.78 and 0.87, respectively. *Conclusion.* A low serum albumin is independently associated with an increased risk of developing of persistent organ failure and death in acute pancreatitis. It may also be useful for the prediction of the severity of acute pancreatitis.

1. Introduction

Though most patients with acute pancreatitis (AP) have a benign clinical course, approximately 10%–20% of patients develop persistent organ failure (defined as organ failure lasting for ≥48 hours) associated with significant mortality of at least 30% [1, 2]. Recent international consensus identified that persistent organ failure is the key determinant of severity regardless of the presence or absence of local pancreatic complications [3]. Early identification of patients likely to develop persistent organ failure would help physicians to select those patients who would benefit the most from close surveillance or aggressive intervention [4]. Existing scoring system such as the Bedside index of severity in acute pancreatitis (BISAP) [5] and the Harmless acute pancreatitis score (HAPS) [6] have moderate diagnostic accuracy in the prediction of persistent organ failure [2]. More recently, attention has also focused on assessing the association between persistent organ failure in acute pancreatitis and individual laboratory parameters such as admission hematocrit ≥ 44%, rise in blood urea nitrogen (BUN) at 24 hours [7], serum triglycerides [8], and high-density lipoprotein [9].

Albumin is exclusively synthesized in the liver. Low serum albumin (<35 g/L) is often observed in hospitalized elderly patients [10] or patients with decompensated liver cirrhosis, malnutrition, nephrotic syndrome, diabetes, heart failure, cancer, and sepsis [11, 12]. Hypoalbuminemia has been proposed as a useful predictor of morbidity and mortality in many different clinical settings such as community-acquired pneumonia [12] and hemodialysis and coronary heart disease [13]. As a negative acute phase protein, initial serum albumin was also independently associated with disease progression to severe sepsis [14] and 30-day mortality in emergency medical patients, irrespective of the cause [15, 16].

A few studies have evaluated hypoalbuminemia as predictor of severe acute pancreatitis [17–19]. However, these studies are limited due to small sample size with low statistical power and inconsistent definitions of severity ranging from severe pancreatitis based on the Atlanta criteria to mortality. Although a recent study by Li et al. [20] had used persistent organ failure of acute pancreatitis as the primary outcome, the results of that study [20], as well as the above-mentioned studies [17–19], are biased due to lack of adjustment for confounding factors such as etiology and chronic concomitant diseases. Furthermore, to the best of our knowledge, no study has performed a complete overview of the association between serum albumin levels at admission and outcomes in acute pancreatitis up until now. Therefore, the aim of this study was to investigate whether serum albumin levels within 24 hrs of patient admission correlate with clinical outcomes in acute pancreatitis.

2. Materials and Methods

Patients with AP who were admitted (index admissions) to our hospital within 72 hours of the onset of symptoms between January 2012 and January 2015 were enrolled for the study. Acute pancreatitis was defined as described previously [4]. Organ failure [1] was defined as having a Marshall score ≥ 2 for at least one of the three organs (respiratory, cardiovascular, and renal failure) involved. Duration of organ failure was defined as persistent if it lasted for >48 hours [1, 3]. Exclusion criteria included [21] patients that had developed organ failure before data collection, recurrent or not first-time pancreatitis, previous pancreatic surgery, ERCP or trauma-induced pancreatitis, chronic pancreatitis, pancreatic cancer, pleural effusions preceding the development of AP, and pleural effusions resulting from concomitant diseases (e.g., pneumonia, chronic heart failure), patients with albumin infusion before data collection in our hospital, hypoalbuminemia due to malnutrition, chronic renal disease, albuminuria, hepatitis, bleeding/coagulation disorders, chronic alcoholism, and liver cirrhosis, and patients for whom completed data was unavailable. Chronic concomitant diseases [12] were classified as neurologic (stroke), cardiovascular (coronary heart disease and arrhythmia), pulmonary (emphysema and chronic bronchitis), diabetes mellitus, hypertension, hepatitis virus carrier, and fatty liver. This study protocol was approved by the Ethics Committee of the First Affiliated Hospital of Wenzhou Medical College.

Age, gender, body mass index (BMI), time from pain onset to admission, and biochemical parameters were recorded within 12 hours of admission before the development of persistent organ failure [4, 21]. Serum albumin levels were measured within 24 hours of admission [12]. If patients had multiple albumin measurements within 24 hrs, only the first-time measurement was picked. Hypoalbuminemia was defined by a serum albumin < 35 g/l [11]. Similar to previous studies [8, 22], patients with hypoalbuminemia were further divided into mild (<35 g/l but ≥30 g/l) and severe (<30 g/l) groups according to the serum albumin level.

2.1. Statistical Analysis. Sample size calculation was based on identifying independent dichotomous predictors in a multivariable logistic regression analysis for persistent organ failure [23]. With an α risk of 0.05 (α is the probability of rejecting a true null hypothesis) and β risk of 0.2 (β is the probability of accepting a false null hypothesis), and a bilateral test, the sample size was calculated for the following hypotheses: assuming a prevalence of persistent organ failure at 10% and a low correlation between the predictor and other covariates ($R^2 = 0.10$) (R-squared, namely, the coefficient of determination, which is equal to the squared correlation coefficient and provides an estimate of the percent of variation in one variable that is explained by the other variables [24]). A sample of 668 patients would provide 80% power of detecting an adjusted odds ratio of 2.0 for a predictor with an overall prevalence of 35%.

A Shapiro-Wilk test was used to evaluate whether the continuous data was a normal distribution. According to the results of Shapiro-Wilk test, continuous values were expressed by mean ± standard deviation (SD) or median and interquartile range (IQR) and compared using one-way analysis of variance or the Kruskal-Wallis nonparametric test. Categorical values were described by count and proportions and compared by the χ^2 test or Fisher's exact test.

Linear trend of categorical and continuous variables was tested by a Royston extension of the Cochran-Armitage test [25] and a nonparametric Wilcoxon rank sum test [26], respectively.

Univariate logistic regression analysis was used to identify potential independent predictors of persistent organ failure and death. Except for serum albumin level and the time from pain onset to admission [8], all other variables, namely, age (≥60 years) [8], male sex [27], BMI (≥30) [28], biliary etiology (yes versus no), chronic concomitant diseases (yes versus no) [12], hematocrit (≥44%) [7], total bilirubin (≥2 mg/dL), alanine aminotransferase (ALT > 50 units/L) [29], glucose (≥150 mg/dL) [28], and blood urea nitrogen (BUN) (>25 mg/dL) [5], were used as dichotomous/categorical variable when performing logistic regression analysis. Variables reaching statistical difference among patients with different albumin levels or between patients with and without organ failure in univariate logistic regression analysis were included

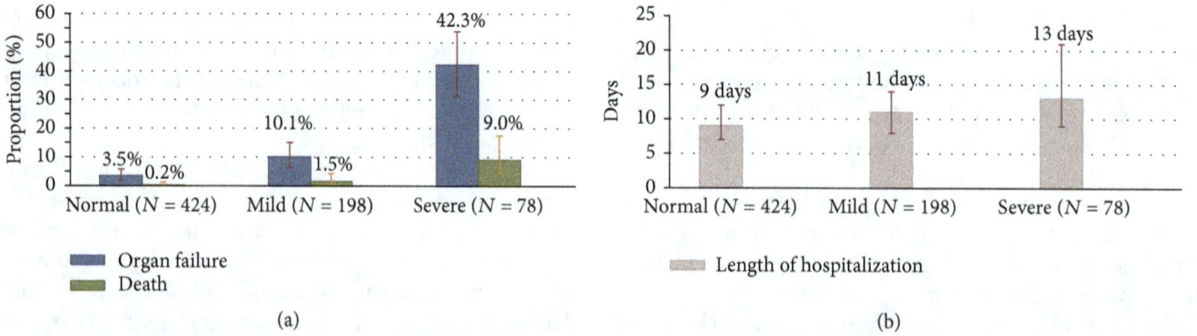

FIGURE 1: Trends of median hospital days, incidence of persistent organ failure, and mortality in acute pancreatitis patients with normal, mild, and severe low serum albumin.

in the multivariate logistic regression analysis. Multivariate logistic regression was used to evaluate the relationship between patients with different albumin levels and persistent organ failure and death adjusted for potential risk factors and confounding factors. Odds ratios (OR) were calculated, with 95% CI [30]. Multicollinearity was considered to be significant if the largest variance inflation factor exceeded 10 [4].

The area under the Receiver Operating Characteristic Curve (AUC) was used to evaluate the performance of predictions. The serum albumin level was used as a continuous rather than categorical variable when performing Receiver Operating Characteristic (ROC) curve analysis. A variable with an AUC above 0.7 was considered useful, while an AUC between 0.8 and 0.9 indicated excellent diagnostic accuracy [31]. As described by Maksimow et al. [32], the best cut-off point was selected based on that where the number of false positives is as low as possible (specificity > 90%) by selecting a threshold value at a point where the longest increase in the sensitivity of the slope declines since ICU beds are limited. The sensitivity, specificity, negative predictive value, positive predictive value, positive likelihood ratio, negative likelihood ratio, and diagnostic accuracy were calculated for corresponding cut-off values.

Differences were considered to be statistically significant if the two-tailed P value was less than 0.05.

3. Results

3.1. Characteristics of Study Subjects. A total of 700 patients were included in the study. 435 (62.1%) were male, with a median age of 48 (IQR 37–63) years. The mean time interval between onset and admission was 1.8 ± 0.8 days. The median value of albumin within 24 hrs of admission was 36.2 g/L (IQR: 32.9–39.7). The overall prevalence of hypoalbuminemia (<35 g/L) was 39.4% (276/700). Of these, 198 had mild hypoalbuminemia, while 78 had severe hypoalbuminemia.

In all the patients, the most common etiology of AP was biliary (42.7%). 24 patients had combined biliary and alcohol etiology and 9 patients had combined biliary and hypertriglyceridemia etiology. Nearly 57.4% (402/700) of patients had ≥1 comorbidities, mainly fatty liver (257/700, 36.7%), hypertension (160/700, 22.9%), and diabetes mellitus (105/700, 15.0%). 68 (9.7%) patients developed persistent OF, which was multiple (≥1) OF, in 31 (45.6%) patients. Respiratory failure (82.4%) was the most frequent OF. Eleven (1.6%) patients with OF died from AP, seven during the first week in hospital.

3.2. Clinical Features and Results of Patients with Different Serum Albumin Levels. The demographic, clinical, and laboratory findings at hospital admission of patients with different serum albumin levels are shown in Table 1. A greater increase in age (P_{trend} = 0.012) and longer time from pain onset to admission ($P_{trend} < 0.001$) were associated with decreased serum albumin level. No significant difference was observed among patients with different albumin levels with respect to gender, BMI, and alcohol etiology.

There was also a trend for increasing rates of overall incidence of chronic concomitant diseases with a lower serum albumin level though it did not reach statistical significance (P = 0.134). However, there was a significant statistical difference among patients with different albumin levels with respect to biliary etiology and concomitant neurologic disease though it occurred in a few patients. Regarding laboratory findings, decline in serum albumin level was associated with a decrease in hematocrit (P = 0.001), alanine aminotransferase (P = 0.001), glucose (P = 0.003), and BUN ($P < 0.001$).

As shown in Table 1 and Figure 1, persistent organ failure developed in 3.5% (15/424) patients with normal albumin, 10.1% (20/198) patients with mild hypoalbuminemia, and 42.3% (33/78) with severe hypoalbuminemia when patients were divided into three groups according to different albumin levels. This indicated that a greater decrease in serum albumin level was associated with increased organ failure rate ($P_{trend} <$ 0.001). There was also a statistically significant trend for increasing rates of mortality ($P_{trend} < 0.001$) and prolonged hospital stay ($P_{trend} < 0.001$) with a lower serum albumin level.

TABLE 1: Baseline clinical characteristics and outcomes among patients with different albumin levels.

Characteristic	Normal (N = 424)	Hypoalbuminemia Mild (N = 198)	Hypoalbuminemia Severe (N = 78)	P value
Median age, years (IQR)	46.5 (37–60)	50 (39–67)	47.5 (36–70)	0.012
Male sex, N (%)	273 (64.4)	116 (58.6)	46 (59.0)	0.316
Time from pain onset to admission (days)	1.75 ± 0.77	1.88 ± 0.79	2.10 ± 0.82	<0.001
BMI ≥ 30, N (%)	23 (5.4)	12 (6.1)	4 (5.1)	0.934
Etiology*				
Biliary, N (%)	198 (46.7)	87 (43.7)	23 (30.0)	0.024
Alcohol, N (%)	56 (13.2)	29 (14.6)	11 (14.3)	0.888
Hypertriglyceridemia, N (%)	21 (5.0)	8 (4.0)	8 (10.1)	0.094
Idiopathic, N (%)	145 (34.2)	68 (34.2)	33 (42.9)	0.323
Other, N (%)	9 (2.1)	9 (4.5)	4 (5.2)	0.153
Chronic concomitant diseases◆	240 (56.6)	116 (58.3)	53 (68.8)	0.134
Neurologic, N (%)	4 (0.9)	1 (0.5)	5 (0.5)	0.004
Cardiovascular, N (%)	13 (3.1)	13 (6.5)	4 (5.2)	0.126
Pulmonary, N (%)	5 (1.2)	4 (2.0)	2 (2.6)	0.385
Diabetes mellitus, N (%)	66 (15.6)	27 (13.6)	12 (15.6)	0.800
Hypertension, N (%)	92 (21.7)	48 (24.1)	20 (26.0)	0.365
Hepatitis virus carrier, N (%)	16 (3.8)	7 (3.5)	2 (2.6)	0.721
Fatty liver, N (%)	162 (38.2)	63 (31.7)	27 (35.1)	0.279
Laboratory findings				
Hematocrit	0.43 (0.38–0.46)	0.41 (0.37–0.45)	0.40 (0.37–0.45)	0.001
Bilirubin, mg/dL (IQR)	1.17 (0.82–1.70)	1.23 (0.82–1.81)	1.053 (0.64–1.81)	0.805
ALT, U/L (IQR)	43 (21–160)	34 (16–92)	36 (19–57)	0.001
Glucose, mg/dL (IQR)	139 (114–182)	150 (119–200)	171 (117–216)	0.003
BUN, mg/dL (IQR)	12.7 (10.1–16.2)	15.1 (11.2–19.6)	16.0 (10.6–29.4)	<0.001
Outcomes				
Median hospital days (IQR)	9 (7–12)	11 (8–14)	13 (9–21)	<0.001
Organ failure N (%)	15 (3.5)	20 (10.1)	33 (42.3)	<0.001
Death, N (%)	1 (0.2)	3 (1.5)	7 (9.0)	<0.001

*Subjects may have more than one etiology. ◆Subjects may have more than one chronic concomitant disease.

3.3. Independent Predictors of Organ Failure and Mortality. As shown in Figure 2, univariate analysis revealed that biliary etiology, chronic concomitant diseases, hematocrit, glucose, BUN, and the serum albumin level were significantly associated with the development of persistent organ failure. Multivariable logistic regression identified biliary etiology (OR: 0.44; 95% CI: 0.22–0.87; P = 0.018), chronic concomitant diseases (OR: 5.26; 95% CI: 2.07–11.31; P < 0.001), hematocrit ≥ 44% (OR: 2.92; 95% CI: 1.55–5.51; P = 0.001), BUN > 25 mg/dL (OR: 8.30; 95% CI: 4.05–17.01; P < 0.001), and the serum albumin level (OR: 0.81; 95% CI: 0.76–0.87; P < 0.001) were independently associated with persistent organ failure.

As shown in Figure 3, factors considered potentially relevant to mortality were analyzed by univariate and multivariate logistic regression. Multivariate logistic regression identified that BUN > 25 mg/dL (OR: 5.06; 95% CI: 1.37–18.67; P = 0.015) and the serum albumin level (OR: 0.79; 95% CI: 0.69–0.91; P = 0.001) were independently associated with mortality. Multicollinearity between covariates did not exist, and the variance inflation factor was less than 10 for all variables.

3.4. Subgroup Analysis. Subgroup analysis confirmed the strong association between the serum albumin level and persistent organ failure across subgroups of age, gender, the time from pain onset to admission, different etiology, chronic concomitant diseases, total bilirubin, ALT, hematocrit, glucose, and BUN (Figure 4). As to association between the serum albumin level and mortality, subgroup analysis confirmed that these associations were stronger in subgroups of patients with one day from pain onset to admission,

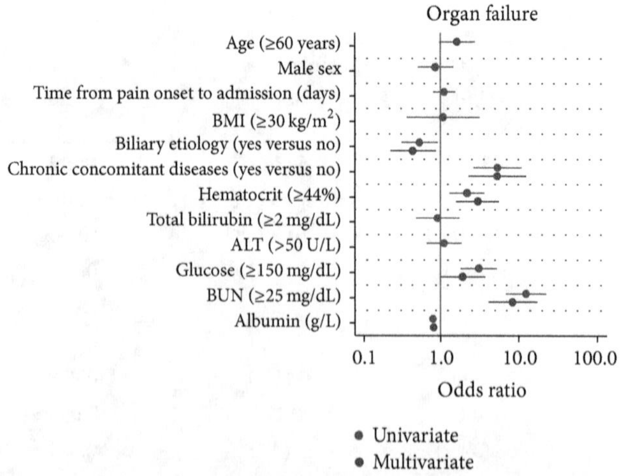

FIGURE 2: Univariate and multivariate logistic regression plot of odds ratios and 95% confidence intervals for evaluation of the relationship between serum albumin level and persistent organ failure in acute pancreatitis.

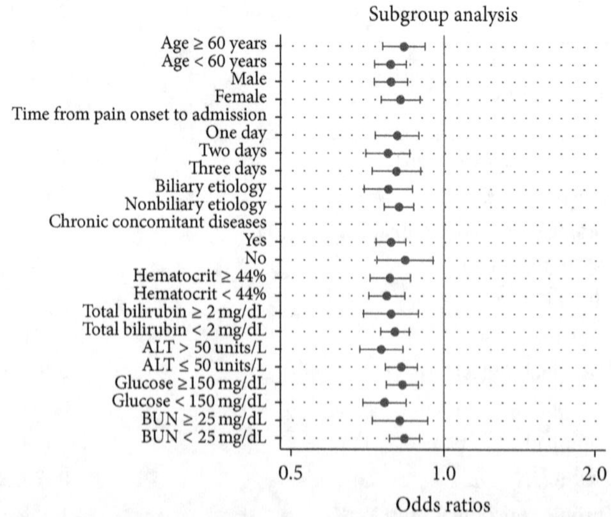

FIGURE 4: Logistic regression plot of odds ratios and 95% confidence intervals; subgroup analysis of relationship between serum albumin level and risk of persistent organ failure in acute pancreatitis.

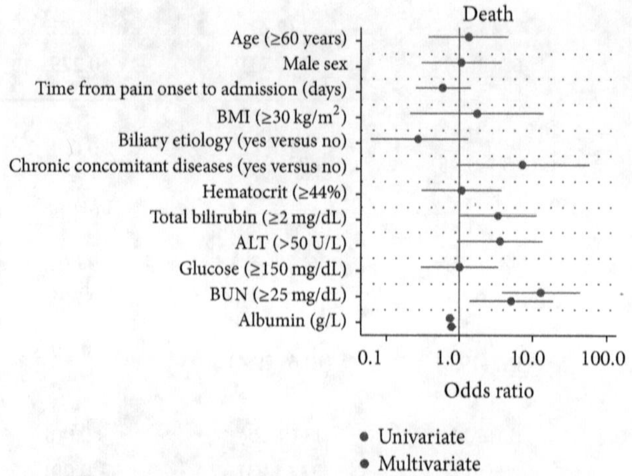

FIGURE 3: Univariate and multivariate logistic regression plot of odds ratios and 95% confidence intervals for evaluation of the relationship between serum albumin level and death in acute pancreatitis.

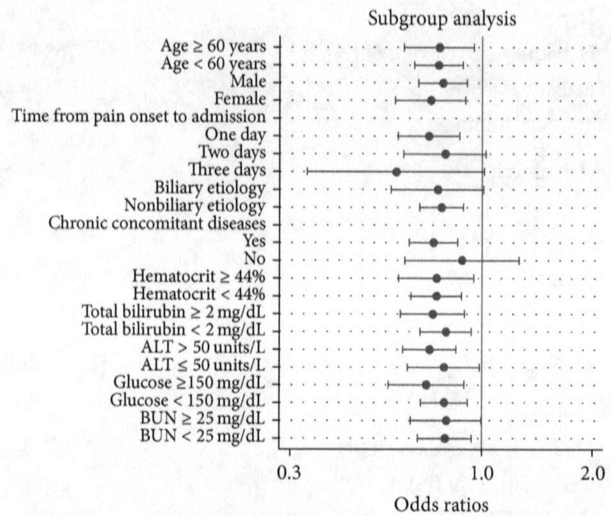

FIGURE 5: Logistic regression plot of odds ratios and 95% confidence intervals; subgroup analysis of relationship between serum albumin level and mortality in acute pancreatitis.

nonbiliary etiology, and chronic concomitant diseases than those in subgroups with two or three days from pain onset to admission and biliary etiology and without chronic concomitant diseases (Figure 5).

3.5. Albumin as Early Predictor of Persistent Organ Failure and Mortality. The ROC curve for albumin for the prediction of persistent organ failure and mortality is shown in Figure 6. The AUC of albumin for predicting organ failure and mortality were 0.78 (95% CI: 0.72–0.85) and 0.87 (95% CI: 0.78–0.95), respectively. As shown in Table 2, the best cut-off points to predict organ failure and mortality were albumin level ≤ 30.8 g/L and ≤29 g/L, respectively.

4. Discussion

The results of the present study demonstrated the following: (i) persistent organ failure and early hypoalbuminemia occurred in 9.7% and 39.3% of patients with acute pancreatitis, respectively; (ii) as a risk factor, low serum albumin levels within 24 hours of admission are independently associated with the development of persistent organ failure and mortality in acute pancreatitis. Furthermore, this association is proportional; meaning the lower the serum albumin level, the greater the likelihood for persistent organ failure and mortality. The associations between the serum albumin level and mortality were stronger in subgroups of patients with one day from pain onset to admission, nonbiliary etiology,

TABLE 2: The best cut-off values of albumin levels to predict organ failure and death in patients with acute pancreatitis.

	Organ failure	Death
AUC (95% CI)	0.78 (95% CI: 0.72–0.85)	0.87 (95% CI: 0.78–0.95)
Albumin level (cutoff point)	≤30.8 g/L	≤29 g/L
Sensitivity	0.53	0.55
Specificity	0.90	0.92
Positive likelihood ratio	5.40	6.83
Negative likelihood ratio	0.52	0.49
Positive predictive value	0.37	0.10
Negative predictive value	0.95	0.99
Diagnostic accuracy	0.87	0.91

AUC = area under the curve of the Receiver Operating Characteristic Curve.

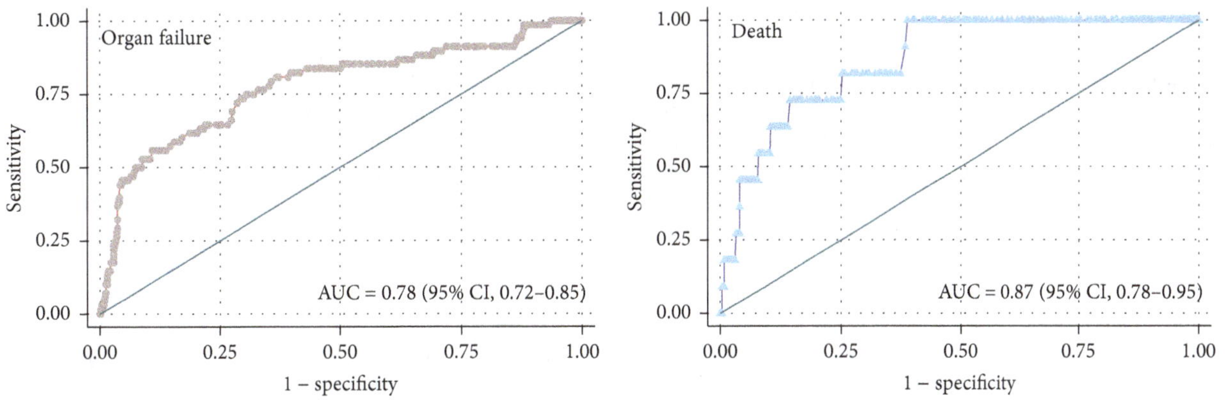

(a) (b)

FIGURE 6: Receiver operating characteristic curves for serum albumin to predict the development of persistent organ failure and occurring of death in acute pancreatitis.

and chronic concomitant diseases than those in subgroups with two or three days from pain onset to admission and biliary etiology and without chronic concomitant diseases; (iii) as a predictor, the serum albumin had moderate and excellent performance for prediction of persistent organ failure (AUC: 0.78) and mortality (AUC: 0.87) in acute pancreatitis, respectively.

The mechanisms of hypoalbuminemia in acute pancreatitis are diverse [11, 33, 34]: (i) a decrease in energy or amino acid supply due to fasting and increased tissue catabolism in acute pancreatitis, (ii) excessive release of inflammatory cytokines such as interleukin-1, interleukin-6, and tumor necrosis factor α in the early stage of acute pancreatitis resulting in a decreased albumin synthesis in the liver, and (iii) active inflammatory cytokines also injuring microvascular endothelial cells which result in increased capillary permeability leading to a redistribution of albumin from the intravascular to the interstitial space.

Albumin has many physiologic roles including maintaining osmotic pressure, protecting the microvasculature and mitigating increased vascular permeability, binding of endogenous and exogenous substances, antioxidant and scavenging free radicals, anticoagulant effect, maintenance of acid base status, anti-inflammatory effects, and antiapoptosis [12, 33]. Therefore, hypoalbuminemia may be causally linked to the development of persistent organ failure rather than serving simply as a marker of severity of acute pancreatitis. The persistent organ failure in acute pancreatitis mainly includes respiratory, cardiovascular, and renal failure [3]. Albumin may improve oxygenation in patients with acute respiratory distress syndrome by reduced alveolar-capillary permeability, decreased inflammatory cell infiltration, enhanced total plasma antioxidant capacity, and faster hemodynamic stabilization [35, 36]. A study in chronic obstructive pulmonary disease suggested that hypoalbuminemia is independently associated with the development of acute respiratory failure [37]. On the other hand, hypoalbuminemia is associated with decreased colloid osmotic pressure, which can lead to the development of pulmonary edema and exacerbation of acute heart failure [38]. The causal relationship between hypoalbuminemia and acute kidney injury is now confirmed [39]. Albumin may improve renal perfusion and glomerular filtration through prolonged renal vasodilation [40, 41], stimulation of the proliferation of proximal renal tubular epithelial cells by activation of mitogenic pathways [42], and inhibition of apoptosis of renal tubular cells by scavenging of reactive oxygen species [43]. Therefore, the fact that hypoalbuminemia is associated with prolonged hospital stay and increased morbidity and mortality has been noted in many clinical scenarios regardless of the implicated disease [10, 11, 13, 15, 16, 27]. On the other hand, positive protective effects of human albumin solutions have been noted in several clinical scenarios such as septic shock [44] and liver cirrhosis with hepatorenal syndrome [45] or with spontaneous bacterial peritonitis, a disease that shares important pathophysiological features with severe sepsis [46]. It is unknown whether administration of albumin would improve the clinical outcomes of acute pancreatitis with hypoalbuminemia though severe acute pancreatitis has many similarities to sepsis syndrome and septic shock [47]. Therefore, it would be interesting to conduct a randomized clinical trial to assess the effect of the correction of hypoalbuminemia on acute pancreatitis in the future.

A few reports have also attempted to study the effect of serum albumin levels on the clinical outcomes of acute pancreatitis. Xue et al. [18] suggested that hypoalbuminemia in the early stage can accelerate the deterioration in pathophysiology of severe acute pancreatitis and it was associated with a high incidence of infection and mortality. Gonzalvez-Gasch et al. [19] use albumin < 25 g/L as a point in the prediction score for complicated acute pancreatitis. A recent study by Li et al. [20], which used persistent organ failure as primary outcome, proposed that serum albumin was a good indicator of persistent organ failure in acute pancreatitis. However, all the above-mentioned have small sample sizes with low statistical power and the results were not adjusted for confounding factors such as age, gender, the time from pain onset to admission, etiology, and chronic concomitant disorders. In addition, no subgroup analysis was performed in these studies. Therefore, these studies were not comparable to our current study. The current study showed that the risk of persistent organ failure significantly increases as levels of serum albumin decrease ($P_{trend} < 0.001$) (Figure 1). Decreased albumin levels were also proportionally associated with prolonged hospital stay ($P_{trend} < 0.001$) and an increased risk of mortality ($P_{trend} < 0.001$). Multivariate logistic regression analysis suggested that an increase of 1 g/L in serum albumin level was associated with a statistically significant 19% (OR: 0.81; 95% CI: 0.76–0.87) reduction in the odds of persistent organ failure after adjusting for potential confounders (Figure 2). Similarly, multivariate logistic regression analysis suggested that an increase of 1 g/L in serum albumin level was associated with a statistically significant 21% (OR: 0.79; 95% CI: 0.69–0.91; $P = 0.001$) reduction in the odds of mortality after adjusting for potential confounders (Figure 3). Subgroup analysis confirmed the strong association between the serum albumin level and persistent organ failure across subgroups of age, gender, the time from pain onset to admission, different etiology, chronic concomitant diseases, total bilirubin, ALT, hematocrit, glucose, and BUN (Figure 4). As to association between the serum albumin level and mortality, subgroup analysis confirmed that these associations were stronger in subgroups of patients with one day from pain onset to admission, nonbiliary etiology, and chronic concomitant diseases than in those subgroups with two or three days from pain onset to admission and biliary etiology and without chronic concomitant diseases (Figure 5).

The area under ROC curves of albumin for predicting organ failure and mortality were 0.78 (95% CI: 0.72–0.85) and 0.87 (95% CI: 0.78–0.95), respectively (Figure 6). These results suggest that albumin may be used as an early predictor of persistent organ failure and mortality. As shown in Table 2, with a cut-off value of ≤30.8 g/L, albumin had a sensitivity of 53% and a specificity of 90% with an overall accuracy of 87% for prediction of organ failure. With a cut-off value of ≤29 g/L, albumin had a sensitivity of 55% and a specificity of 91% with an overall accuracy of 93% for prediction of death. Both cut-off values had low sensitivity, which means that some of these patients who were at high risk of developing persistent organ failure and death may not have a low serum albumin level. However, both cut-off values had high negative predictive value, which is important in emergency for identification of patients not at risk for the development of persistent organ failure and death.

The existing scoring systems have shown moderate accuracy in predicting persistent organ failure but are cumbersome to use in the clinical setting [2]. Xu et al. [48] suggested that fatty liver assessed by computed tomography was associated with severity of acute pancreatitis. Mikolasevic et al. [49] showed that presence of nonalcoholic fatty liver was related to more severe forms of acute pancreatitis. Therefore, it is no surprise that chronic concomitant disease (OR: 5.26; 95% CI: 2.07–11.31) was independently associated with persistent organ failure since fatty liver was the most common chronic concomitant disease in our study (Table 1). Cho et al. [50] reported that patients with alcoholic acute pancreatitis have a longer hospital stay and higher incidence of persistent organ failure compared to those with biliary acute pancreatitis. As expected, our results indicated that patients with biliary etiology had a statistically significant 56% (OR: 0.44; 95% CI: 0.22–0.87) reduction in the odds of persistent organ failure compared to patients without biliary etiology. Simple, routine biomarkers such as hematocrit [7] and blood urea nitrogen (BUN) [7, 51–53] have been proposed as markers of disease severity. Koutroumpakis et al. [7] suggested that admission hematocrit ≥ 44% and rise in BUN at 24 hrs may be the optimal predictive tools in clinical practice among existing laboratory parameters and scoring systems. Mounzer et al. [2] showed that BUN had similar accuracy in comparison with more complex scoring systems in predicting organ failure. As expected, our results suggested that hematocrit ≥ 44% (OR: 2.92; 95% CI: 1.55–5.51) and BUN > 25 mg/dL (OR: 8.30; 95% CI: 4.05–17.01) were independently associated with persistent organ failure. BUN > 25 mg/dL was also associated with a higher mortality risk in acute pancreatitis compared to patients with BUN ≤ 25 mg/dL (OR: 5.06; 95% CI: 1.37–18.67; $P = 0.015$), which is consistent with a previous report [5]. Additionally, contrary to the report by Kumaravel et al. [54], our study showed that BMI was not associated with organ failure and mortality in acute pancreatitis. These differences may be due to the variations among studies regarding the proportion of different etiology and number of obese patients, as evidenced by the fact that only a small proportion of patients with alcohol etiology and obesity were enrolled in our study (Table 1). The drawbacks in currently available data are that risk factors such as blood urea nitrogen are not necessarily pathophysiologically linked to the development of the organ failure and, therefore, elevation of these markers simply reflects ongoing organ failure [9]. Theoretically, pathophysiologically relevant biomarkers may perform better in this clinical setting. In this regard, serum albumin may provide important prognostic information and help risk stratification. The advantage of using of serum albumin levels for predicting outcomes is that it is an objective variable which is easily performed, being inexpensive and available in most hospital laboratories [12].

The strengths of our study include the following: (i) this is the first study to investigate albumin not only as a risk factor but also as a predictor of persistent organ failure and mortality of acute pancreatitis by multivariable logistic regression analysis and subgroup analysis; (ii) exhaustive efforts were made to collect all clinical and laboratory data (including serum albumin and its related confounding factors) in the early stage of acute pancreatitis and a large sample with adequate power enabled us to evaluate the relationship between serum albumin and organ failure of acute pancreatitis; (iii) we have taken serum albumin levels within 24 hours of admission and excluded patients with albumin infusion before data collection so that artifactual influence on serum albumin levels due to intravenous fluid treatment would be minimized [55]. In addition, we also excluded patients with hypoalbuminemia due to malnutrition, chronic renal disease, albuminuria, bleeding/coagulation disorders, chronic alcoholism, hepatitis, and liver cirrhosis. Limitations of our study are as follows. (i) This is a retrospective study, which may have selection bias. Because of the retrospective design, we did not investigate other risk factors of severe acute pancreatitis such as lipase [56], prealbumin/fibrinogen [57], and red cell distribution width [58]. (ii) Data were collected in a single tertiary care hospital, which may not be generalized to a local clinic or a community hospital. Therefore, a prospective external validation of our results is mandatory before its application in the future. (iii) Serum albumin level may have been affected by fluid administration since it was measured within 24 hours of admission [12]. Therefore, another important limitation of current study is that we had no data on the volume of resuscitation or IV fluid therapy due to the retrospective study design. As a remediation, we have evaluated hematocrit and blood urea nitrogen, which often were used as the markers of hemoconcentration [59], as confounding factors of hypoalbuminemia in our multivariate logistic regression analysis.

In summary, as a risk factor, hypoalbuminemia within 24 hrs of hospital admission is independently associated with increased risk of development of persistent organ failure and death in acute pancreatitis. An increase in serum albumin level was associated with a statistically significant reduction in the odds of persistent organ failure and mortality of acute pancreatitis after adjusting for potential confounders. The association between the serum albumin level and mortality was stronger in subgroups of patients with one day from pain onset to admission, nonbiliary etiology, and chronic concomitant diseases than in those subgroups with two or three days from pain onset to admission and biliary etiology and without chronic concomitant diseases. As a predictor, low albumin had a high negative predictive value and allowed identification of patients not at risk of developing persistent organ failure, thereby eliminating the need for intensive care.

Ethical Approval

This study protocol was approved by the Ethic Committee of the First Affiliated Hospital of Wenzhou Medical University. This study was performed according to the principles expressed in the Declaration of Helsinki.

Authors' Contributions

Wandong Hong joined in the design of the study and carried out the studies; Wandong Hong, Suhan Lin, Wujun Geng, and Jingye Pan participated in data collection. Wandong Hong conducted data analysis and drafted the manuscript. Maddalena Zippi, Simon Stock, Zarrin Basharat, Bicheng Cheng, and Mengtao Zhou helped to finalize the manuscript. All of the authors read and approved the manuscript. Wandong Hong, Wujun Geng, Bicheng Cheng, and Jingye Pan contributed equally to this work.

References

[1] P. G. Lankisch, M. Apte, and P. A. Banks, "Acute pancreatitis," *The Lancet*, vol. 386, no. 9988, pp. 85–96, 2015.

[2] R. Mounzer, C. J. Langmead, B. U. Wu et al., "Comparison of existing clinical scoring systems to predict persistent organ failure in patients with acute pancreatitis," *Gastroenterology*, vol. 142, no. 7, pp. 1476–1482, 2012.

[3] P. A. Banks, T. L. Bollen, C. Dervenis et al., "Classification of acute pancreatitis–2012: revision of the Atlanta classification and definitions by international consensus," *Gut*, vol. 62, no. 1, pp. 102–111, 2013.

[4] W. Hong, L. Dong, Q. Huang, W. Wu, J. Wu, and Y. Wang, "Prediction of severe acute pancreatitis using classification and regression tree analysis," *Digestive Diseases and Sciences*, vol. 56, no. 12, pp. 3664–3671, 2011.

[5] B. U. Wu, R. S. Johannes, X. Sun, Y. Tabak, D. L. Conwell, and P. A. Banks, "The early prediction of mortality in acute pancreatitis: a large population-based study," *Gut*, vol. 57, no. 12, pp. 1698–1703, 2008.

[6] P. G. Lankisch, B. Weber-Dany, K. Hebel, P. Maisonneuve, and A. B. Lowenfels, "The Harmless Acute Pancreatitis Score: A Clinical Algorithm for Rapid Initial Stratification of Nonsevere Disease," *Clinical Gastroenterology and Hepatology*, vol. 7, no. 6, pp. 702–705, 2009.

[7] E. Koutroumpakis, B. U. Wu, O. J. Bakker et al., "Admission hematocrit and rise in blood urea nitrogen at 24 h outperform

other laboratory markers in predicting persistent organ failure and pancreatic necrosis in acute pancreatitis: a post hoc analysis of three large prospective databases," *American Journal of Gastroenterology*, vol. 110, no. 12, pp. 1707–1716, 2015.

[8] H. Nawaz, E. Koutroumpakis, J. Easler et al., "Elevated serum triglycerides are independently associated with persistent organ failure in acute pancreatitis," *American Journal of Gastroenterology*, vol. 110, no. 10, pp. 1497–1503, 2015.

[9] Y.-S. Peng, Y.-C. Chen, Y.-C. Tian et al., "Serum levels of apolipoprotein A-I and high-density lipoprotein can predict organ failure in acute pancreatitis," *Critical Care*, vol. 19, p. 88, 2015.

[10] M. A. Marinella and R. J. Markert, "Admission serum albumin level and length of hospitalization in elderly patients," *Southern Medical Journal*, vol. 91, no. 9, pp. 851–854, 1998.

[11] A. Gatta, A. Verardo, and M. Bolognesi, "Hypoalbuminemia," *Internal and Emergency Medicine*, vol. 7, no. 3, pp. 193–199, 2012.

[12] D. Viasus, C. Garcia-Vidal, A. Simonetti et al., "Prognostic value of serum albumin levels in hospitalized adults with community-acquired pneumonia," *Journal of Infection*, vol. 66, no. 5, pp. 415–423, 2013.

[13] P. Goldwasser and J. Feldman, "Association of serum albumin and mortality risk," *Journal of Clinical Epidemiology*, vol. 50, no. 6, pp. 693–703, 1997.

[14] A. L. Holder, N. Gupta, E. Lulaj et al., "Predictors of early progression to severe sepsis or shock among emergency department patients with nonsevere sepsis," *International Journal of Emergency Medicine*, vol. 9, no. 1, article no. 10, pp. 1–11, 2016.

[15] M. E. Jellinge, D. P. Henriksen, P. Hallas, and M. Brabrand, "Hypoalbuminemia is a strong predictor of 30-day all-cause mortality in acutely admitted medical patients: a prospective, observational, cohort study," *PLoS ONE*, vol. 9, no. 8, Article ID e105983, 2014.

[16] O. Lyons, B. Whelan, K. Bennett, D. O'Riordan, and B. Silke, "Serum albumin as an outcome predictor in hospital emergency medical admissions," *European Journal of Internal Medicine*, vol. 21, no. 1, pp. 17–20, 2010.

[17] M. P. Holliday, D. Shaw, W. M. Thomas, and T. Leese, "Threshold for albumin as a prognostic marker in acute pancreatitis," *British Journal of Surgery*, vol. 76, no. 5, pp. 472-473, 1989.

[18] P. Xue, Z. W. Huang, Y. H. Li et al., "Clinical study on severe acute pancreatitis associated with hypoalbuminemia in early stage," *Zhong Xi Yi Jie He Xue Bao*, vol. 3, no. 6, pp. 443–445, 2005.

[19] A. Gonzalvez-Gasch, G. García de Casasola, R. Barba Martín, B. Herreros, and C. Guijarro, "A simple prognostic score for risk assessment in patients with acute pancreatitis," *European Journal of Internal Medicine*, vol. 20, no. 3, pp. e43–e48, 2009.

[20] S. Li, Y. Zhang, M. Li, C. Xie, and H. Wu, "Serum albumin, a good indicator of persistent organ failure in acute pancreatitis," *BMC Gastroenterology*, vol. 17, no. 1, 2017.

[21] W.-D. Hong, X.-R. Chen, S.-Q. Jin, Q.-K. Huang, Q.-H. Zhu, and J.-Y. Pan, "Use of an artificial neural network to predict persistent organ failure in patients with acute pancreatitis," *Clinics*, vol. 68, no. 1, pp. 27–31, 2013.

[22] A. Michaud, G. B. Marchand, M. Nadeau et al., "Biliopancreatic Diversion with Duodenal Switch in the Elderly: Long-Term Results of a Matched-Control Study," *Obesity Surgery*, vol. 26, no. 2, pp. 350–360, 2016.

[23] P. C. Schroy, J. B. Wong, M. J. O'Brien, C. A. Chen, and J. L. Griffith, "A risk prediction index for advanced colorectal neoplasia at screening colonoscopy," *American Journal of Gastroenterology*, vol. 110, no. 7, pp. 1062–1071, 2015.

[24] J. Peat, B. Barton, and E. Elliott, *Statistics Workbook for Evidence-Based Healthcare*, Blackwell, Malden, MA, USA, 2008.

[25] P. Royston, "PTREND: stata module for trend analysis for proportions," 2014, https://ideas.repec.org/c/boc/bocode/s426101.html.

[26] J. Cuzick, "A wilcoxon-type test for trend," *Statistics in Medicine*, vol. 4, no. 1, pp. 87–90, 1985.

[27] G. Grimm, H. Haslacher, T. Kampitsch et al., "Sex differences in the association between albumin and all-cause and vascular mortality," *European Journal of Clinical Investigation*, vol. 39, no. 10, pp. 860–865, 2009.

[28] E. De-Madaria, P. A. Banks, N. Moya-Hoyo et al., "Early Factors Associated With Fluid Sequestration and Outcomes of Patients With Acute Pancreatitis," *Clinical Gastroenterology and Hepatology*, vol. 12, no. 6, pp. 997–1002, 2014.

[29] P. Mentula, M.-L. Kylänpää, E. Kemppainen et al., "Early prediction of organ failure by combined markers in patients with acute pancreatitis," *British Journal of Surgery*, vol. 92, no. 1, pp. 68–75, 2005.

[30] R. L. Grant, "Converting an odds ratio to a range of plausible relative risks for better communication of research findings," *British Medical Journal*, vol. 348, no. jan24 1, pp. f7450–f7450, 2014.

[31] W.-D. Hong, Q.-H. Zhu, Z.-M. Huang et al., "Predictors of esophageal varices in patients with HBV-related cirrhosis: a retrospective study," *BMC Gastroenterology*, vol. 9, article 11, 2009.

[32] M. Maksimow, L. Kyhälä, A. Nieminen et al., "Early prediction of persistent organ failure by soluble CD73 in patients with acute pancreatitis*," *Critical Care Medicine*, vol. 42, no. 12, pp. 2556–2564, 2014.

[33] J.-L. Vincent, J. A. Russell, M. Jacob et al., "Albumin administration in the acutely ill: What is new and where next," *Critical Care*, vol. 18, no. 6, article no. 630, p. 231, 2014.

[34] Y.-J. Zheng, B. Zhou, G. Ding et al., "Effect of serum from patients with severe acute pancreatitis on vascular endothelial permeability," *Pancreas*, vol. 42, no. 4, pp. 633–639, 2013.

[35] C. Uhlig, P. L. Silva, S. Deckert, J. Schmitt, and M. G. de Abreu, "Albumin versus crystalloid solutions in patients with the acute respiratory distress syndrome: a systematic review and meta-analysis," *Critical Care*, vol. 18, no. 1, article R10, 2014.

[36] G. J. Quinlan, S. Mumby, G. S. Martin, G. R. Bernard, J. M. C. Gutteridge, and T. W. Evans, "Albumin influences total plasma antioxidant capacity favorably in patients with acute lung injury," *Critical Care Medicine*, vol. 32, no. 3, pp. 755–759, 2004.

[37] C.-W. Chen, Y.-Y. Chen, C.-L. Lu et al., "Severe hypoalbuminemia is a strong independent risk factor for acute respiratory failure in COPD: A nationwide cohort study," *International Journal of COPD*, vol. 10, pp. 1147–1154, 2015.

[38] T. B. Horwich, K. Kalantar-Zadeh, R. W. MacLellan, and G. C. Fonarow, "Albumin levels predict survival in patients with systolic heart failure," *American Heart Journal*, vol. 155, no. 5, pp. 883–889, 2008.

[39] C. J. Wiedermann, W. Wiedermann, and M. Joannidis, "Causal relationship between hypoalbuminemia and acute kidney injury," *World Journal of Nephrology*, vol. 6, no. 4, p. 176, 2017.

[40] M. A. Kaufmann, I. Castelli, H. Pargger, and L. J. Drop, "Nitric oxide dose-response study in the isolated perfused rat

kidney after inhibition of endothelium-derived relaxing factor synthesis: the role of serum albumin," *Journal of Pharmacology and Experimental Therapeutics*, vol. 273, no. 2, pp. 855–862, 1995.

[41] E. H. Lee, S. H. Baek, and J. H. Chin, "Preoperative hypoalbuminemia is a major risk factor for acute kidney injury following off-pump coronary artery bypass surgery," *Intensive Care Medicine*, vol. 38, no. 9, pp. 1478–1486, 2012.

[42] R. Dixon and N. J. Brunskill, "Activation of mitogenic pathways by albumin in kidney proximal tubule epithelial cells: implications for the pathophysiology of proteinuric states," *Journal of the American Society of Nephrology*, vol. 10, no. 7, pp. 1487–1497, 1999.

[43] J. Iglesias, V. E. Abernethy, Z. Wang, W. Lieberthal, J. S. Koh, and J. S. Levine, "Albumin is a major serum survival factor for renal tubular cells and macrophages through scavenging of ROS," *The American Journal of Physiology—Renal Physiology*, vol. 277, no. 5, pp. F711–F722, 1999.

[44] P. Caironi, G. Tognoni, and L. Gattinoni, "Albumin replacement in severe sepsis or septic shock.," *The New England journal of medicine*, vol. 371, no. 1, p. 84, 2014.

[45] F. Salerno, R. J. Navickis, and M. M. Wilkes, "Albumin treatment regimen for type 1 hepatorenal syndrome: A dose-response meta-analysis," *BMC Gastroenterology*, vol. 15, no. 1, article no. 167, 2015.

[46] F. Salerno, R. J. Navickis, and M. M. Wilkes, "Albumin infusion improves outcomes of patients with spontaneous bacterial peritonitis: a meta-analysis of randomized trials," *Clinical Gastroenterology and Hepatology*, vol. 11, no. 2, pp. 123–130, 2013.

[47] P. G. Wilson, M. Manji, and J. P. Neoptolemos, "Acute pancreatitis as a model of sepsis," *Journal of Antimicrobial Chemotherapy*, vol. 41, pp. 51–63, 1998.

[48] C. Xu, Z. Qiao, Y. Lu et al., "Influence of fatty liver on the severity and clinical outcome in acute pancreatitis," *PLoS ONE*, vol. 10, no. 11, Article ID e0142278, 2015.

[49] I. Mikolasevic, L. Orlic, G. Poropat et al., "Nonalcoholic fatty liver and the severity of acute pancreatitis," *European Journal of Internal Medicine*, vol. 38, pp. 73–78, 2017.

[50] J. H. Cho, T. N. Kim, and S. B. Kim, "Comparison of clinical course and outcome of acute pancreatitis according to the two main etiologies: alcohol and gallstone," *BMC Gastroenterology*, vol. 15, no. 1, article no. 87, 2015.

[51] B. U. Wu, O. J. Bakker, G. I. Papachristou et al., "Blood urea nitrogen in the early assessment of acute pancreatitis: an international validation study," *Archives of Internal Medicine*, vol. 171, no. 7, pp. 669–676, 2011.

[52] W. Hong, S. Lin, M. Zippi et al., "High-density lipoprotein cholesterol, blood urea nitrogen, and serum creatinine can predict severe acute pancreatitis," *BioMed Research International*, vol. 2017, pp. 1–7, 2017.

[53] S. Lin, W. Hong, Z. Basharat, Q. Wang, J. Pan, and M. Zhou, "Blood urea nitrogen as a predictor of severe acute pancreatitis based on the revised atlanta criteria: timing of measurement and cutoff points," *Canadian Journal of Gastroenterology and Hepatology*, vol. 2017, Article ID 9592831, 7 pages, 2017.

[54] A. Kumaravel, T. Stevens, G. I. Papachristou et al., "A Model to Predict the Severity of Acute Pancreatitis Based on Serum Level of Amylase and Body Mass Index," *Clinical Gastroenterology and Hepatology*, vol. 13, no. 8, pp. 1496–1501, 2015.

[55] D. B. Gundpatil, B. L. Somani, T. K. Saha, and M. Banerjee, "Serum Urea: Albumin ratio as a prognostic marker in critical patients with non-chronic kidney disease," *Indian Journal of Clinical Biochemistry*, vol. 29, no. 1, pp. 97–100, 2014.

[56] V. V. Gumaste, P. B. Dave, D. Weissman, and J. Messer, "Lipase/amylase ratio. A new index that distinguishes acute episodes of alcoholic from nonalcoholic acute pancreatitis," *Gastroenterology*, vol. 101, no. 5, pp. 1361–1366, 1991.

[57] W. Yue, Y. Liu, W. Ding et al., "The predictive value of the prealbumin-to-fibrinogen ratio in patients with acute pancreatitis," *International Journal of Clinical Practice*, vol. 69, no. 10, pp. 1121–1128, 2015.

[58] D. Wang, J. Yang, J. Zhang et al., "Red cell distribution width predicts deaths in patients with acute pancreatitis," *Journal of Research in Medical Sciences*, vol. 20, no. 5, pp. 424–428, 2015.

[59] G. A. Cote, S. V. Sagi, S. E. Schmidt et al., "Early measures of hemoconcentration and inflammation are predictive of prolonged hospitalization from post - Endoscopic retrograde cholangiopancreatography pancreatitis," *Pancreas*, vol. 42, no. 5, pp. 850–854, 2013.

7

Predictive Value of a Noninvasive Serological Hepatic Fibrosis Scoring System in Cirrhosis Combined with Oesophageal Varices

Feiyue Zhang,[1] **Tong Liu**,[1] **Pan Gao**,[1] **and Sujuan Fei**[2]

[1]*Department of Gastroenterology, Xuzhou Medical University, Xuzhou, Jiangsu 221000, China*

[2]*Department of Gastroenterology, The Affiliated Hospital of Xuzhou Medical University, Xuzhou, Jiangsu 221000, China*

Correspondence should be addressed to Sujuan Fei; xyfyfeisj99@163.com

Academic Editor: Mingyu Sun

Objective. In recent years, the noninvasive serological scoring system has become a research hotspot in predicting hepatic fibrosis and has achieved good results. However, it has rarely been applied to the prediction of oesophageal varices. The aim of the study was to evaluate the predictive value of the four following scoring systems in cirrhosis combined with oesophageal varices: aspartate and platelet ratio index (APRI), aspartate aminotransferase-alanine aminotransferase ratio (AAR), FIB-4, and S index. *Methods.* A total of 153 patients with cirrhosis were categorized into groups with or without oesophageal varices. In addition, cirrhosis patients with oesophageal varices were further divided into mild, moderate, and severe grades. The rank sum test was used to compare the significant differences of APRI, AAR, FIB-4, and S index between the two groups of cirrhosis patients with or without oesophageal varices. A ROC curve was generated to compare the area under the curve of the three groups and to obtain the corresponding optimal prediction value. Moreover, multivariate logistic regression analysis was employed to assess the predictive factors for cirrhosis combined with oesophageal varices. *Results.* 44 patients had no oesophageal varices and 108 patients had oesophageal varices. Of the 108 patients with oesophageal varices, 43 were mild, 32 were moderate, and 33 were severe. The rank sum test indicated that the APRI, FIB-4, and S index were statistically significant between two groups ($P < 0.05$), while no significant difference was detected in terms of AAR between the two groups ($P > 0.05$). In addition, all four scoring systems were statistically significant between nonoesophageal varices group and severe oesophageal varices group ($P < 0.05$). In the ROC curve of oesophageal varices, the AUC values of APRI, FIB-4, and S index for predicting oesophageal varices were 0.681, 0642, and 0.673, respectively. However, in the ROC curve of severe oesophageal varices, the AUC values of APRI, AAR, FIB-4, and S index were 0.729, 0.648, 0.673, and 0.695, respectively. Multivariate logistic regression analysis indicated that APRI and FIB-4 were predictors of disease progression ($P < 0.05$). *Conclusion.* AAR harboured a poor predictive value for oesophageal varices, APRI can be used as a reference index for the prediction of severe oesophageal varices, and the S index harboured potential value in predicting the degree of progression of cirrhosis.

1. Introduction

Liver cirrhosis, a common chronic liver disease, is caused by long-term or repeated damage to liver tissue due to one or more causes, leading to diffuse degeneration and necrosis of hepatocytes, regenerative nodules, and fibrous tissue hyperplasia. Portal hypertension is observed in the advanced stage of cirrhosis. When the portal vein pressure increases to a certain degree, oesophageal varices can occur, while, in severe cases, oesophageal variceal bleeding will emerge, which is the most common and severe complication of cirrhosis and cirrhotic portal hypertension, as well as the most common cause of death for cirrhosis [1]. In the 1990s, the mortality rate after the onset of oesophageal variceal bleeding was as high as 50% [2]. With the development and advancements of medical technology and equipment, along with a further understanding of the disease, the mortality rate has decreased; however, new statistics indicate that the 6-week mortality rate is still as high as 20% [3]. Digestive endoscopy is considered the gold standard for the screening and diagnosis of oesophageal varices [4]. However, as an invasive examination, there are potential risks, such

Table 1: Grading method of oesophageal varices [8].

Grade)	EV morphology (F)	EV red-color sign (RC)
mild (G1)	EV Straight or slightly tortuous (F1)	no
moderate (G2)	EV Straight or slightly tortuous (F1)	yes
	EV Swelling and distortion like snake (F2)	no
severe (G3)	EV Swelling and distortion like snake (F2)	yes
	EV Bead-like, nodular or tumor-like (F3)	yes/no

as bleeding and anaesthesia accidents during operation, and repeated monitoring can introduce more pain, leading to poor compliance, which makes it difficult to conduct clinical observations on patients with oesophageal varices. In recent years, the exploration of noninvasive methods for predicting oesophageal varices has become a research focus, aiming to selectively assess patients with a relatively high risk of oesophageal varices to further effectively monitor the degree of varices, to administer selective interventions, and to reduce the pain and burden of patients to some extent. Recently, the application noninvasive serological examinations in the prediction and diagnosis of the degree of hepatic fibrosis has become a hotspot. Among them, the classic ones, including APRI and FIB-4 scores, have been recommended by the World Health Organization (WHO) guidelines for assessing hepatic fibrosis [5]. In addition, it has also been shown that AAR is 0.8 in healthy individuals, and AAR > 1 indicates the presence of cirrhosis. Chinese scholars have established an S index in the analysis of risk factors for hepatic fibrosis in chronic hepatitis B virus (HBV), which harbours a higher accuracy in the assessment of hepatic fibrosis in HBV [6]. The above four scoring methods are simple and easy to obtain in clinical practice. However, few studies have applied it in the prediction of cirrhosis and oesophageal varices. Hence, in this study, we aimed to explore and compare the predictive value of the APRI, AAR, FIB-4, and S index scoring systems in oesophageal varices.

2. Subjects and Methods

2.1. Subject. We retrospectively analysed patients with cirrhosis who were admitted to the Affiliated Hospital of Xuzhou Medical University from January 2010 to September 2017. The inclusion criteria were as follows: ① all patients met the diagnostic criteria for cirrhosis in the Guidelines for Chronic Hepatitis B Prevention and Treatment (2015 Update) by the Chinese Medical Association, 2015 Edition) [7] (gastroscopy and serum biochemical examination were performed after admission). The exclusion criteria were as follows: ① a history of hepatic carcinoma; ② prior hepatic operation and splenectomy; ③ prior transjugular intrahepatic portosystemic shunt; ④ prior sclerotherapy or ligation for oesophageal varices; ⑤ the existence of other factors that might affect the platelet count and spleen size; ⑥ patients with severe heart, lung, and kidney disease; ⑦ patients who have used drugs that inhibit or promote bone marrow haematopoiesis or that decrease portal vein pressure and albumin in the last six months; ⑧ the emergence of upper gastrointestinal bleeding during previous and current admission.

2.2. Methods. We recorded the age of the patients and the levels of AST, ALT, albumin, and PLT in peripheral blood. In addition, patients were divided into slight, moderate, and severe groups according to the morphology of oesophageal varices (EV) and the severity of haemorrhage under gastroscopy (shown in Table 1).

2.3. Calculation. APRI = (AST/upper limit of normal)×100/PLT (10^9/L); AAR = AST/ALT; FIB-4 = (year of age × AST)/(PLT × the square root of ALT); S index: 1000∗GGT/(PLT∗ albumin^2).

2.4. Statistical Analysis. SPSS22.0 statistical software was used for all data processing and analysis. The chi-square test was used for enumeration data, the median (quartile) was used for nonnormally distributed measurement data, and the rank sum test was employed for comparisons between groups. $P < 0.05$ represented statistical significance. The combination with or without oesophageal varices in cirrhosis was taken as the demarcation point, and the diagnostic criteria of gastroesophageal varices under gastroscopy were considered the gold standard to investigate whether the four scoring systems of APRI, AAR, FIB-4, and S index were statistically significant between cirrhosis without oesophageal varices and cirrhosis with oesophageal varices. Whether cirrhosis was combined with oesophageal varices or with severe oesophageal varices or not was taken as two demarcation points. The ROC curve was generated, followed by the use of the AUC value to evaluate the predictive accuracy of three scores in cirrhosis combined with oesophageal varices or severe oesophageal varices. The optimal demarcation point was detected, which corresponded to the maximum value by adding sensitivity and specificity on the ROC curve. AUC values > 0.7 indicated clinical value, AUC values of 0.8-0.9 suggested relatively good clinical value, and AUC values > 0.9 indicated very good clinical value. Nonconditional multivariate logistic regression analysis was performed on multiple sets of data. A $P < 0.05$ was considered to represent statistical significance.

3. Results

3.1. General State. A total of 153 patients with cirrhosis who met the requirements were collected (shown in Table 2). Of them, there were 109 patients with HBV cirrhosis, 11 patients with hepatitis C virus (HCV) cirrhosis, 10 patients with alcoholic cirrhosis, 10 patients with autoimmune cirrhosis, and 13 patients with other causes (drug-induced cirrhosis, mixed cirrhosis, and cryptogenic cirrhosis). There were

TABLE 2: General state of the 153 patients with cirrhosis.

General information	no	mild	moderate	severe
Number of cases	44	43	32	33
Mean age	51.0±12.6	48.8±12.7	52.9±11.3	47.5±9.3
Male (cases)	25	31	19	24
Female (cases)	19	12	13	9
APRI	1.0 (0.6,3.5)	1.7 (1.1,2.9)	2.2 (1.4,4.9)	2.7 (1.9,4.2)
AAR	1.1 (0.8,1.2)	1.0 (0.8,1.4)	1.1 (0.9,1.4)	1.2 (0.9,1.4)
FIB-4	102. (55.5,562.7)	196.3 (104.9,392.2)	324.3 (165.9,708.1)	244.0 (153.3,518.1)
S index	0.3 (0.1,1.0)	0.7 (0.2,1.3)	0.9 (0.4,1.9)	0.8 (0.4,1.9)

44 cirrhosis patients without oesophageal varices (nonoesophageal varices group), 43 with mild oesophageal varices (mild group), 31 with moderate oesophageal varices (moderate group), and 32 patients with severe oesophageal varices (severe group). There was no significant difference in age or gender between patients in each group (all $P > 0.05$).

3.2. APRI, AAR, FIB-4, and S Index. Due to the nonnormal distribution of the data, median (M) and quartile range (Q) were used. The group and data of each group are shown in Table 2.

3.3. Comparison of the Nonoesophageal Varices Group and Oesophageal Varices Group. APRI: 1.0 (0.6-3.5) versus 2.2 (1.5-3.8); AAR: 1.1 (0.8-1.2) versus 1.1 (0.9-1.4); FIB-4: 102.6 (55.5-562.7) versus 247.8 (130.2-529.4); S index: 0.3 (0.1-1.0) versus 0.8 (0.4-1.8). The rank sum test was used to compare the nonoesophageal varices group and oesophageal varices group, which revealed that APRI scoring system statistically significant ($P < 0.001$), and the P values of AAR, FIB-4, and S index were 0.078, 0.006, and 0.001; in other words, all three scoring systems were statistically significant (all $P < 0.05$).

3.4. Comparison of the Nonoesophageal Varices Group and Severe Oesophageal Varices Group. APRI: 1.0 (0.6-3.5) versus 2.7 (1.9- 4.2); AAR: 1.1 (0.8-1.2) versus 1.2 (0.9-1.4); FIB-4: 102.6 (55.5-562.7) versus 244.0 (153.3-518.1); S index: 0.3 (0.1-1.0) versus 0.8 (0.4,1.9). The rank sum test was used to compare the nonoesophageal varices group and severe oesophageal varices group, which revealed P values of 0.001, 0.026, 0.009, and 0.003, respectively; in other words, all four scoring systems were statistically significant (all $P < 0.05$).

3.5. Predictive Value of APRI, FIB-4, and S Index in Oesophageal Varices (Shown in Figure 1). ROC curve analysis showed that the AUC values of APRI, FIB-4, and S index in predicting oesophageal varices were 0.681, 0.642, and 0.673, respectively (shown in Table 3). The optimal demarcation point of blood APRI in predicting cirrhosis combined with oesophageal varices was 1.29, and the corresponding sensitivity and specificity were 0.815 and 0.600, respectively. The optimal demarcation point of FIB-4 in predicting cirrhosis combined with oesophageal varices was 103.7, with a corresponding sensitivity and specificity of 0.843 and 0.511, respectively. The optimal demarcation point of the S index in predicting cirrhosis combined with oesophageal varices was

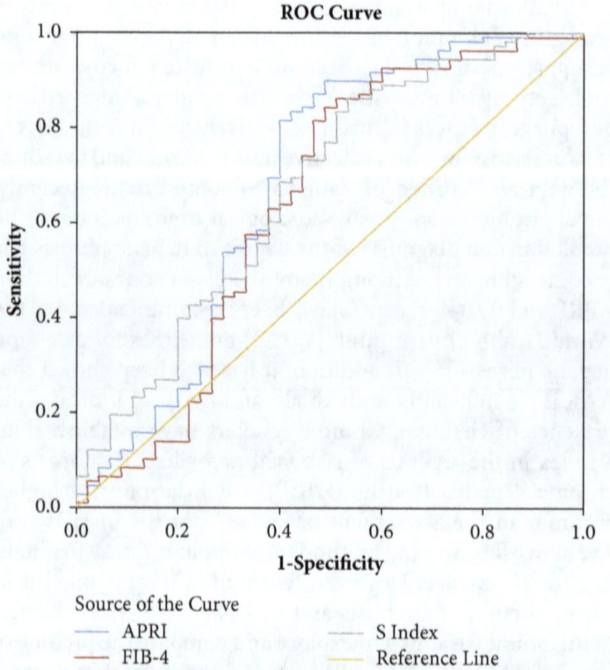

FIGURE 1: Receiver operating characteristic curve of APRI, FIB-4, and S index in diagnosis of cirrhosis combined with oesophageal varices. APRI: aspartate aminotransferase and platelet ratio; FIB-4: fibrosis index based on factor-4.

0.23, with a corresponding sensitivity and specificity of 0.861 and 0.467, respectively.

3.6. Predictive Value of APRI, AAR, FIB-4, and S Index in Severe Oesophageal Varices (Shown in Figure 2). ROC curve analysis showed that the AUC values of APRI, AAR, FIB-4, and S index in predicting severe oesophageal varices were 0.729, 0.648, 0.673, and 0.695, respectively (shown in Table 4). The optimal demarcation point of blood APRI in predicting cirrhosis combined with oesophageal varices was 1.4, with the corresponding sensitivity and specificity being 0.939 and 0.600, respectively. The optimal demarcation point of AAR in predicting cirrhosis combined with oesophageal varices was 1.3, with a corresponding sensitivity and specificity of 0.394 and 0.933, respectively. The optimal demarcation point of FIB-4 in predicting cirrhosis combined with oesophageal varices was 113.4, with a corresponding

TABLE 3: The predictive value of noninvasive serological hepatic fibrosis scoring system in cirrhosis combined with oesophageal varices.

indicator	AUC	Cut-off	sensitivity	specificity	PPV	NPV
APRI	0.681	1.29	0.815	0.600	0.832	0.578
FIB-4	0.642	103.7	0.843	0.511	0.805	0.564
S index	0.673	0.23	0.861	0.467	0.793	0.613

APRI: aspartate aminotransferase and platelet ratio; FIB-4: fibrosis index based on factor-4; AUC: area under the curve; PPV: positive predictive value; NPV: negative predictive value.

TABLE 4: The predictive value of noninvasive serological hepatic fibrosis scoring system in cirrhosis combined with severe oesophageal varices.

indicator	AUC	Cut-off	sensitivity	specificity	PPV	NPV
APRI	0.729	1.4	0.939	0.600	0.640	0.963
AAR	0.648	1.3	0.394	0.933	0.667	0.661
FIB-4	0.673	113.4	0.939	0.533	0.588	0.885
S index	0.695	0.27	0.861	0.467	0.545	0.864

APRI: aspartate aminotransferase and platelet ratio; FIB-4: fibrosis index based on factor-4; AUC: area under the curve; PPV: positive predictive value; NPV: negative predictive value.

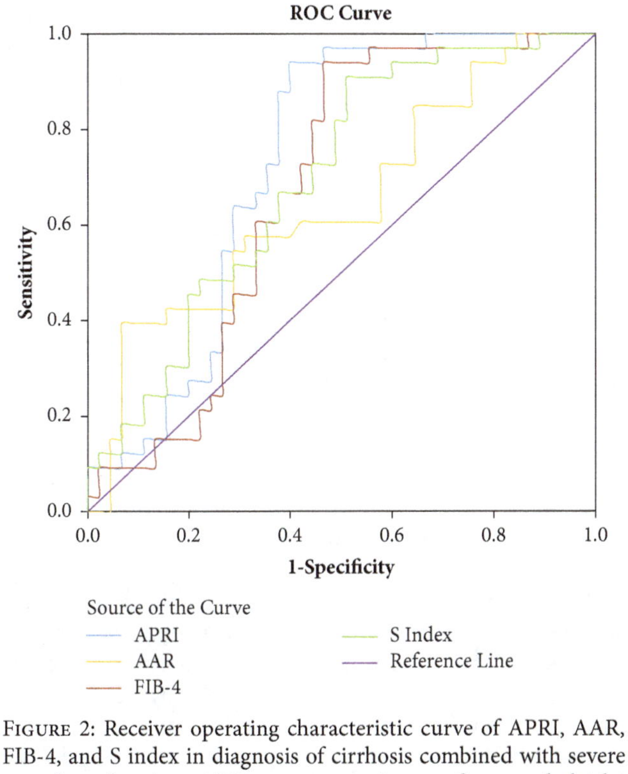

FIGURE 2: Receiver operating characteristic curve of APRI, AAR, FIB-4, and S index in diagnosis of cirrhosis combined with severe oesophageal varices. APRI: aspartate aminotransferase and platelet ratio; FIB-4: fibrosis index based on factor-4; AAR: aspartate aminotransferase-alanine aminotransferase ratio.

sensitivity and specificity of 0.939 and 0.533, respectively. The optimal demarcation point of the S index in predicting cirrhosis combined with oesophageal varices was 0.27, with a corresponding sensitivity and specificity of 0.861 and 0.467, respectively.

3.7. Nonconditional Multivariate Logistic Regression Analysis of APRI, FIB-4, and S Index for Oesophageal Varices. According to whether cirrhosis was combined with oesophageal varices, which was a two-class response variable, nonconditional logistic regression analysis was used to construct a predictive model for the three values. The introduction criterion was $P < 0.05$, and the elimination criterion was $P > 0.10$. As a result, APRI and FIB-4 could be used as an independent predictive model for cirrhosis combined with oesophageal varices (shown in Table 5).

3.8. Nonconditional Multivariate Logistic Regression Analysis of APRI, AAR, FIB-4, and S Index for Severe Oesophageal Varices. According to whether cirrhosis was combined with severe oesophageal varices, which was a two-class response variable, nonconditional logistic regression analysis was used to construct a predictive model for the four values. The introduction criterion was $P < 0.05$, and the elimination criterion was $P > 0.10$. Consistently, APRI and FIB-4 could be used as independent predictive models for cirrhosis combined with severe oesophageal varices (shown in Table 6).

4. Discussion

Oesophageal variceal bleeding is the most lethal complication of cirrhotic portal hypertension. However, in most cirrhosis patients, no obvious clinical manifestations are present, even at decompensation period. This is especially true of oesophagogastric varices, which is difficult to detect if gastroscopy is not performed. Gastroscopy and portal vein pressure testing harbour a relatively good predictive value for the degree of oesophagogastric varices, but they are invasive procedures that are not easily tolerated by patients due to the pain. In addition, their safety is relatively low; hence, their clinical application is limited [3, 9]. In recent years, the noninvasive prediction of oesophagogastric varices has become a hotspot of research. In consideration of the emergence of portal hypertension due to the progression of hepatic fibrosis, noninvasive biochemical markers of hepatic fibrosis have been used to predict the incidence rate of oesophageal varices in patients with cirrhosis [10]. The noninvasive serological hepatic fibrosis score has the advantages of accurate data,

TABLE 5: Logistic regression analysis of APRI, FIB-4, and S index in prediction of cirrhosis combined with oesophageal varices.

	B	S.E.	Wald	df	Sig.	Exp(B)
APRI	.731	.264	7.647	1	.006	2.077
FIB-4	-.002	.001	8.961	1	.003	.998
S Index	.280	.205	1.855	1	.173	1.323
constant	-.187	.350	.286	1	.593	.829

TABLE 6: Logistic regression analysis of APRI, AAR, FIB-4, and S index in prediction of cirrhosis combined with oesophageal varices.

	B	S.E.	Wald	df	Sig.	Exp(B)
APRI	2.833	.762	13.814	1	.000	16.990
AAR	.016	.937	.000	1	.986	1.017
FIB-4	-.012	.003	12.302	1	.000	.988
S Index	.173	.148	1.375	1	.241	1.189
constant	-2.967	1.117	7.057	1	.008	.051

good repeatability, and little effect on patients, which can avoid sampling errors and interpretation errors of imaging examinations; however, its evaluation effect is not clear yet.

Cheung et al. [11] demonstrated that glutamic-oxaloacetic transaminase/glutamic-pyruvic transaminase and AAR index > 1 generally indicate the occurrence of cirrhosis. Iwata et al. [12] reported that AAR is associated with the severity of oesophageal varices. In this study, there was no significant difference in the AAR index between cirrhosis without oesophageal varices and cirrhosis combined with oesophageal varices. In the prediction of severe oesophageal varices, the AUC value of AAR was the lowest of the four scores. Hence, we demonstrate that the AAR index harboured limited predictive value for oesophageal varices.

The APRI index and FIB-4 are two classic scores and harbour good diagnostic efficiency for cirrhosis [13–15]. In this study, the AUC value of APRI for oesophageal varices and severe oesophageal varices was higher than those of the other three indexes. Notably, the AUC in the prediction of severe oesophageal varices was > 0.7 (AUC = 0.729) and the negative predictive value (NPV) was 0.963. In severe oesophageal varices, an APRI value < 1.4 was only detected in two patients, accounting for 6% of the severe oesophageal varices. Therefore, APRI > 1.4 can be used as a reference indicator for the early intervention of severe oesophageal varices. Although the FIB-4 index was found to be an independent predictor of oesophageal varices in an unconditional logistic regression analysis, the AUC value was less than 0.7; hence, FIB-4 failed to harbour a clinical diagnostic value.

The S index was proposed by Chinese scholars. In this study, the AUC value of the S index was higher than that of the FIB-4 index. However, the S index was not detected as an independent predictor of oesophageal varices by the unconditional logistic regression analysis (all $P > 0.01$). The calculation formula was 1 000×GGT/(PLT×albumin^2). Of the albumin, GGT, and PLT established by this model, PLT and albumin have been confirmed to be associated with the severity of cirrhosis [6, 16]. GGT mainly originated from liver and is generated by the mitochondria of hepatocytes, confined to the cytoplasm and intrahepatic bile duct epithelium. However, GGT levels can be significantly elevated in the cases of fatty liver, alcoholic liver disease, and biliary system diseases [17, 18]. In this study, patients with alcoholic liver disease and autoimmune liver disease were included, which may have a certain impact on the experimental results. Additionally, ALT and AST are associated with the degree of liver damage. Intriguingly, GGT was replaced with ALT and AST in the formula of 1000×ALT/(PLT×albumin^2) and 1000×AST/(PLT×albumin^2), which revealed that the AUC value of predicting oesophageal varices was 0.681 and 0.663, respectively, and that the AUC value of predicting severe oesophageal varices was 0.718 and 0.701, respectively. All the AUC values were greater than 0.7. However, it was not considered as an independent risk factor for oesophageal varices by further unconditional logistic regression analysis. Therefore, whether the formula can be applied to the diagnosis and evaluation of the degree of fibrosis and hepatic lesions remains unknown.

Thus, in the four scoring systems, the AAR score harboured a poor diagnostic efficiency for oesophageal varices, while APRI scores have clinical value for the prediction of severe oesophageal varices. APRI>1.4 may be used as a reference index for early intervention in severe oesophageal varices. The S index cannot effectively predict the degree of oesophageal varices, which is possibly affected by the aetiology of cirrhosis. However, we demonstrated that the modified formula after replacing AST and ALT with GGT can be used as a potential predictive formula to assess the degree of cirrhosis progression.

References

[1] S. Augustin, A. González, and J. Genescà, "Acute esophageal variceal bleeding: Current strategies and new perspectives," *World Journal of Hepatology*, vol. 2, no. 7, pp. 261–274, 2010.

[2] B. Bernard, D. Lebrec, P. Mathurin, P. Opolon, and T. Poynard, "Beta-adrenergic antagonists in the prevention of gastroin-

testinal rebleeding in patients with cirrhosis: A meta-analysis," *Hepatology*, vol. 25, no. 1, pp. 63–70, 1997.

[3] I. Haq and D. Tripathi, "Recent advances in the management of variceal bleeding," *Gastroenterology Report*, vol. 5, no. 2, pp. 113–126, 2017.

[4] D. M. Jensen, "Endoscopic screening for varices in cirrhosis: Findings, implications, and outcomes," *Gastroenterology*, vol. 122, no. 6, pp. 1620–1630, 2002.

[5] C. Stasi and S. Milani, "Non-invasive assessment of liver fibrosis: Between prediction/prevention of outcomes and cost-effectiveness," *World Journal of Gastroenterology*, vol. 22, no. 4, pp. 1711–1720, 2016.

[6] K. Zhou, C. Gao Y, and H. Liu L, "Simpler score of routine laboratory tests predicts liver fibrosis in patients with chronic hepatitis B," *Journal of Gastroenterology and Hepatology*, vol. 25, no. 9, pp. 1569–1577, 2010.

[7] Hepatology Branch of Chinese Medical Association, "Guidelines for Chronic Hepatitis B Prevention and Treatment," *Chinese Journal of Virus*, vol. 31, no. 6, pp. 1941–1960, 2015.

[8] Portal hypertension group and Surgery Branch of Chinese Medical Association, "Consensus on Diagnosis and Treatment of bleeding in esophagogastric varices due to cirrhotic portal hypertension," *Chinese Journal of Surgery*, vol. 53, no. 12, pp. 917–921, 2015.

[9] G. D'Amico, G. Garcia-Tsao, and L. Pagliaro, "Natural history and prognostic indicators of survival in cirrhosis: a systematic review of 118 studies," *Journal of Hepatology*, vol. 44, no. 1, pp. 217–231, 2006.

[10] G. Sebastiani, D. Tempesta, G. Fattovich et al., "Prediction of oesophageal varices in hepatic cirrhosis by simple serum non-invasive markers: Results of a multicenter, large-scale study," *Journal of Hepatology*, vol. 53, no. 4, pp. 630–638, 2010.

[11] R. C. Cheung, S. Currie, H. Shen et al., "Can we predict the degree of fibrosis in chronic hepatitis C patients using routine blood tests in our daily practice?" *Journal of Clinical Gastroenterology*, vol. 42, no. 7, pp. 827–834, 2008.

[12] Y. Iwata, H. Enomoto, Y. Sakai et al., "Elevation of the AST to ALT ratio in association with the severity of esophageal varices in patients with HCV-related compensated liver cirrhosis," *Hepato-Gastroenterology*, vol. 60, no. 122, pp. 149–152, 2013.

[13] S. Mansoor, L. Yerian, R. Kohli et al., "The Evaluation of Hepatic Fibrosis Scores in Children with Nonalcoholic Fatty Liver Disease," *Digestive Diseases and Sciences*, vol. 60, no. 5, pp. 1–8, 2015.

[14] W. G. Shin, S. H. Park, M. K. Jang et al., "Aspartate aminotransferase to platelet ratio index (APRI) can predict liver fibrosis in chronic hepatitis B," *Digestive and Liver Disease*, vol. 40, no. 4, pp. 267–274, 2008.

[15] A. Valletpichard, V. Mallet, and S. Pol, "FIB-4: a simple, inexpensive and accurate marker of fibrosis in HCV-infected patients," *Hepatology*, vol. 44, no. 3, pp. 769-770, 2006.

[16] S. M. Sumon, S. R. Sutradhar, M. Chowdhury et al., "Relation of different grades of esophageal varices with Child-Pugh classes in cirrhosis of liver," *Mymensingh medical journal*, vol. 22, no. 1, pp. 37–41, 2013.

[17] I. J. Perry, S. G. Wannamethee, and A. G. Shaper, "Prospective study of serum γ-glutamyltransferase and risk of NIDDM," *Diabetes Care*, vol. 21, no. 5, pp. 732–737, 1998.

[18] Y. Matsuda, M. Tsuchishima, Y. Ueshima, S. Takase, and A. Takada, "The relationship between the development of alcoholic liver and pancreatic diseases and the induction of gamma glutamyl transferase," *Alcohol and Alcoholism*, vol. 28, no. 1B, pp. 27–33, 1993.

8

The Ethanol Supernatant Extracts of Liushenwan Could Alleviate Nanodiethylnitrosamine-Induced Liver Cancer in Mice

Xi-Zhen Chen,[1] Wei Kevin Zhang,[1] He-Bin Tang,[1] Xiao-Jun Li,[1] Gui-Hua Tian,[2] Hong-Cai Shang,[2] and Yu-Sang Li[1]

[1]*Department of Pharmacology, School of Pharmaceutical Sciences, South-Central University for Nationalities, Wuhan, China*
[2]*Key Laboratory of Chinese Internal Medicine of MOE, Beijing Dongzhimen Hospital, Beijing University of Chinese Medicine, Beijing, China*

Correspondence should be addressed to Gui-Hua Tian; rosetgh@163.com and Yu-Sang Li; liys2006@mail.scuec.edu.cn

Academic Editor: Pascal Lapierre

Liver cancer is one of the leading causes of cancerous deaths worldwide. At present, the treatment of hepatocellular carcinoma (HCC) remains to be a problem globally. Liushenwan (LSW), an ancient Chinese medicine previously used to treat localized infections, was recently reported to possess anticancer activity. Here in this study, we aim to examine the effect of LSW-ET (LSW-ET is the supernatant fraction of LSW from ultrasound assisted ethanol extraction) in prevention and treatment on nanodiethylnitrosamine- (nanoDEN-) induced HCC in mice. In nanoDEN-induced HCC mice treated with LSW-ET by oral (po) or intragastric gavage (ig), we observed an alleviation of serum ALT and AST levels, amelioration in histopathological stainings, and an inhibition in liver tumor growth. In addition, compared with the nanoDEN group, downregulation of multiple pivotal factors (COX-2, β-catenin, PCNA, and HMGB-1) was observed in LSW-ET-po and LSW-ET-ig groups. Taken together, the delivery of LSW-ET by oral could be a potential prevention and treatment of liver cancer.

1. Introduction

Liver cancer, also called hepatocellular carcinoma (HCC), has been and would remain to be one of the leading causes of cancerous deaths worldwide nowadays and in the near future [1]. In China particular, liver diseases affect approximately 300 million people, which contributes much to the global burden of liver diseases [2]. A large fraction of these patients would probably progress into liver cancer at advanced stages due to late diagnoses [3]. In addition, large variability of treatment choices and disease-relate survival also confirmed such heterogeneity. However, a so-called "best" choice for patients with HCC could be quite hard [4]. Thus, alternative agents with better efficacy and less detriment for the management (prevention and treatment included) of HCC are urgently needed [5].

Traditional Chinese Medicine has been widely used for anticancer treatment in China with a long history and many substances possess application prospect, such as bufadienolide [6, 7]. Liushenwan (LSW), a well-known heat clearing and detoxifying herbal preparation, is composed of Niu-huang (Calculus bovis), She-xiang (Moschus), Chan-shu (Bufonis venenum), Xiong-huang (Realgar), Zhen-zhu (Margarita), and Bing-pian (Camphora). This ancient prescription is quite effective in treating localized infections and inflammation associated pain [8]. During the past 200 years, many other applications of LSW have been uncovered, including the treatment of diphtheria, scarlet fever, pharyngotonsillitis, acute tonsillitis, purulent parotitis, encephalitis B, and leukemia [9, 10]. Recently, it was also reported that LSW had a potential anticancer activity [9]. In the meantime, LSW has also been suggested to be associated with some toxicity due to the constituents of Realgar and Bufonis venenum, both of which were found to be hazardous once administered alone [11]. In our previous study, we demonstrated that the ethanol fraction of LSW (LSW-ET), which maintained its analgesic and anticancer activities, possessed a minimum side effect to a normal human hepatic cell line L02, while inhibiting cell proliferation and inducing apoptosis of the human cancerous cell line HepG2 in a dose-dependent manner via the downregulation of NK-1 receptor [12]. However, experiments on cancerous animal models were required to investigate the efficacy of LSW-ET in vivo.

It would be quite complicated for the occurrence and development of liver cancer, which could be separated into multiple stages and involved key regulatory factors and signaling pathways [13–16]. Abnormal expressions of canonical Wnt/β-catenin signaling pathway was closely related to malignancies, and its role in liver biology had come to the forefront over the last several years [17]. Under hepatic pathological conditions, an aberrant activation of β-catenin was evident in chronic inflammation, steatosis, fibrosis, and subsequently tumors of the liver [18, 19]. Another "active player", COX-2, a key protein involved in the inflammation process [20], had also been suggested to play important roles in the relationship between inflammation and cancer. Studies had shown that the expression of COX-2 in para-carcinoma tissues was higher than that of tumor tissues and was also positively correlated with the degree of differentiation for liver tumor, suggesting a promoting role in the carcinogenesis of early stage [21]. Meanwhile, PCNA (a protein recently related with tumor formation [22]) and HMGB-1 (acts extracellularly as a cytokine to promote cell migration [23]) had been shown to be associated with liver cancer as well.

Therefore, in this study, to further evaluate the efficacy and detriment of LSW-ET in vivo, we employed a nanoDEN-induced liver cancer model of mice previously introduced by us [24] and examined the tumor growth rate, hepatotoxicity, and histopathological changes after the treatment of LSW-ET. Furthermore, we investigated expression changes of several pivotal factors during the progression of HCC via histochemical stainings, including β-catenin, COX-2, PCNA, and HMGB-1.

2. Materials and Methods

2.1. Materials. LSW was purchased from shanghai ley's pharmaceutical Co., Ltd. (Shanghai, China). Diethylnitrosamine (DEN) was purchased from Tokyo Chemical Industry Co., Ltd. (Tokyo, Japan). Tween-80 was kindly provided by Amresco®. (Amresco, USA). Lecithin from egg yolk was purchased from Sinopharm Chemical Reagent Co., Ltd. (Shanghai, China). Sesame oil was kindly provided by Blessing Mill (Wuhan, China). Glycerol ReagentPlus (Gas chromatography [GC] grade) were obtained from Sigma-Aldrich Co. (St Louis, MO, USA). Ultrapure deionized water (Heal Force Bio-Meditech Holdings Ltd., Shanghai, China) was used for all the experiments. All other reagents were of analytical grade. Primary antibodies used in this study included antibodies against β-catenin, PCNA, HMGB-1, and COX-2 (Abcam Inc., Cambridge, MA, USA).

2.2. HPLC Analysis of LSW-ET. The chemical components of LSW-ET were detected by HPLC DionexTM Ultimate 3000 system (Thermo Fischer Scientific, Inc., USA) equipped with an Ultimate 3000 pump, an Ultimate 3000 autosampler, and an Ultimate 3000 column compartment. Separation was performed using a C18 column (4.6 × 250 mm, 5 μm, Kromasil) and an optimized mobile phase composed of acetonitrile (solvent A) and 0.2% formic acid water solution (solvent B, v/v). For the combinative elution, elution was achieved using the following conditions: 0-3 min, 9% solvent A; 3-13 min, 9-12% solvent A; 13-15 min, 12-20% solvent A; 15-25 min, 20-30% solvent A; 25-30 min, 30-51% solvent A; 30-50 min, 51% solvent A (total run time 50 min). The detection wavelength was set at 296 nm and the flow rate was 0.8 mL/min. The column temperature was set at 30°C and the injection volume was 10 μL.

2.3. Animal Care. Male Kunming mice (18–22 g) were acclimatized for seven days under SPF conditions before the initiation of experiments. The animals were kept in a temperature controlled laboratory (22–25°C) with a 12-hour light–dark cycle. The care and use of animals and experimental protocols for this study were performed according to the Committee of Research Facilities for Laboratory Animal Sciences. All studies on mice were approved by the Committee on the Ethics of Animal Experiments of the South-Central University for Nationalities, Wuhan, China (permit number: 2012-SCUEC-AEC-005).

2.4. Evaluation of the Tumor Growth Inhibition. A liver cancer model induced by nanoDEN with modifications was employed according to a previous study [24]. In brief, 128 male Kunming mice were randomly divided into four groups: the control, model, LSW-ET-ig, and LSW-ET-po groups. All groups were orally given nanoDEN (16.5 mg / kg) once a week for twenty consecutive weeks, except for the control group which was applied with vehicle treatment. Meanwhile, LSW-ET-ig or LSW-ET-po (9.639 mg/kg in sesame oil) group was treated with LSW-ET intragastrically or orally respectively, twice a week for thirty weeks. Body weights were measured daily until the mice were sacrificed at week 10, 15, 20, and 30 (the day of the first administration of LSW-ET and nanoDEN was week 0). Liver samples from all mice were collected. While a part of each liver was used for histopathological analysis, the rest of the liver was stored at −80°C fridge.

2.5. Liver Blood Tests of Mice. Blood (1 ml) for each mouse was collected at sacrifice and centrifuged at 1000 rpm for 5 min. Serum was stored at −20°C for serum chemistry profile analysis. The levels of alanine aminotransferase (ALT), aspartate aminotransferase (AST), total bilirubin (TBIL), alkaline phosphatase (ALP), triglycerides (TRIG), and low-density lipoprotein-cholesterol (LDL-C) were determined using DRI-CHEM 7000i automated clinical chemistry analyzer (Fujifilm Corporation, Tokyo, Japan).

2.6. Histopathological Analysis of Liver Tissues. Fresh liver tissue pieces were fixed in 10% formalin, dehydrated, paraffin embedded successively, sliced at 2 μm, and subsequently followed by sectioning and hematoxylin and eosin (H&E) by standard techniques. Histopathologic examinations of the liver sections were conducted using a Nikon 50i light

TABLE 1

No	Ret Time min	Area MAU∗min	Mass (m/z) Measure	Mass (m/z) Calculated	Compound
1	5.170	13.064	219.1490	219.1502	5-HTQ
2	6.033	21.191	177.1026	177.1033	5-HT ∗
3	26.913	5.752	417.2270	417.2282	Ψ-Bufarenogin
4	27.977	5.755	403.2476	403.2489	Gamabufotali
5	29.733	6.611	217.2270	417.2282	Bufarenogin
6	31.343	9.517	417.2268	417.2282	Arenobufagin
7	31.540	8.257	417.2268	417.2282	Desacetylcinobufotalin∗
8	33.757	9.192	403.2476	403.2489	Telocinobufagin ∗
9	34.130	4.021	401.2322	401.2322	Desacetylcinobufagin
10	34.400	12.225	445.2581	445.2584	Bufotaline ∗
11	35.190	12.599	459.2370	459.2377	Cinobufotalin ∗
12	37.187	17.828	387.2524	387.2529	Bufalin ∗
13	40.767	28.922	443.2421	443.2428	Cinobufagin ∗
14	41.437	28.623	385.2368	385.2372	Resibufogenin∗

∗Identities of these peaks were additionally verified with correspondent reference substances.

microscope (Nikon Inc., Tokyo, Japan) by a pathologist and peer-reviewed.

2.7. Immunohistochemical of Liver Tissues. Samples were deparaffinized, hydrated, and blocked with 3% hydrogen peroxide for 15 min. Then specimens were subjected to antigen retrieval by immersing in 0.01 M boiling citrate buffer and heating in a microwave oven for 10 min. After blocking by 5% BSA (Boster, Wuhan, China) for 1 hour, the sections were incubated overnight at 4°C with primary antibodies against β-catenin (1:200), COX-2 (1:200), PCNA (1:6000), and HMGB-1 (1:1000), respectively. After incubation with horseradish peroxidase- (HRP-) conjugated secondary antibodies (Boster, Wuhan, China) at 37°C for 1 hour, the expression was visualized by 3,3′-diaminobenzidine tetrahydrochloride (Boster, Wuhan, China) staining. Hematoxylin was used as a nuclear counterstain in tissue sections. Stained slides were dehydrated by sequential steps through a graded series of alcohol washes and mounted using coverslips. Multispectral images was obtained using the Nuance Multispectral Imaging System (Cambridge Research and Instrumentation Inc., Woburn, MA) as described in our previous study [25]. Briefly, spectral optical density data were automatically acquired from 420 to 720 nm in 10 nm increments. Spectral unmixing was accomplished by the Nuance software (v3.0.2) and pure spectral libraries of individual chromogens. Nonspecific background staining was subtracted from each image individually. For the quantification in each experiment, three equal-sized fields of each photograph per group were randomly chosen.

2.8. Statistical Analysis. All results were presented as mean ± SEM. Statistical analysis was carried out by a one-way analysis of variance (ANOVA, followed by Bonferroni post hoc tests if necessary) in Origin8.0 (Origin lab Corp., MA, USA). $P < 0.05$ was considered to be statistically significant, and the levels of differences were indicated in the legend of each figure as follows: compared with the normal group, $*P < 0.05$, $**P < 0.01$, $***P < 0.001$, and $\dagger P > 0.05$; compared with the nanoDEN group, $\#P < 0.05$, $\#\#P < 0.01$, $\#\#\#P < 0.001$, and $\ddagger P > 0.05$.

3. Results

3.1. Component Analysis of LSW-ET. As shown in Figure 1 and Table 1, with the help of LC-MS and reference substances, telocinobufagin, bufotaline, cinobufotalin, bufalin, cinobufagin, and resibufogenin had been identified as main components of LSW-ET, most of which have been reported to possess anti-inflammatory, antitumor, and cardiotonic effects [26–28].

3.2. Oral Uptake of LSW-ET Phenotypically Relieved Liver Damage in Mice. To explore the effect of LSW-ET on liver cancer in vivo, a model induced by nanoDEN was employed. In our experiments, we observed a severe damage in livers of mice after the application of nanoDEN as shown in Figure 2. Phenotypically, mice in each group were almost identical with others in the first 15 weeks. By careful measurement of their weight, mice with all treatments were identical to each other, suggesting a relative equal intake of food and water among mice in different groups. However, at the 20th week, the hair of mice in the nanoDEN group appeared to be dull and yellowish, while they were also thinner and lighter compared with other treatment groups (Figure 2(a)). The differences of body weight could be due to the occurrence of liver tumor, which affected the appetite of these mice.

Moreover, significant toxicity was observed in the nanoDEN group by weight loss while LSW-ET-ig and LSW-ET-po treatments relieved a bit (Figures 2(b) and 2(c)). As shown in Table 2, the levels of alanine transaminase (ALT), aspartate transaminase (AST), and alkaline phosphatase (ALP) were

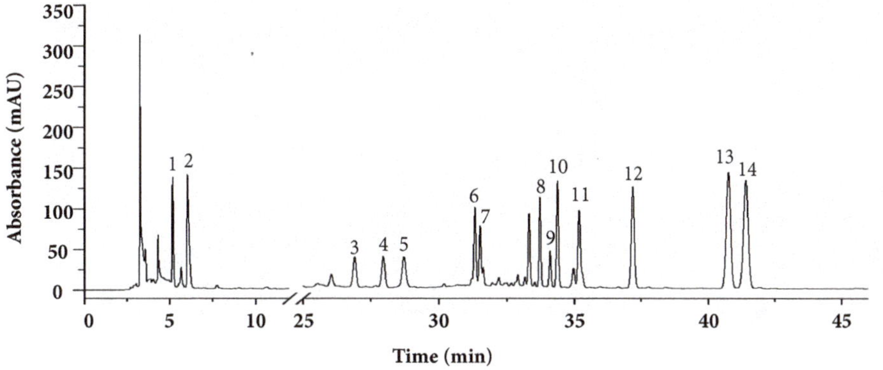

FIGURE 1: Separation of the alcohol-soluble extractants of LSW by using HPLC.

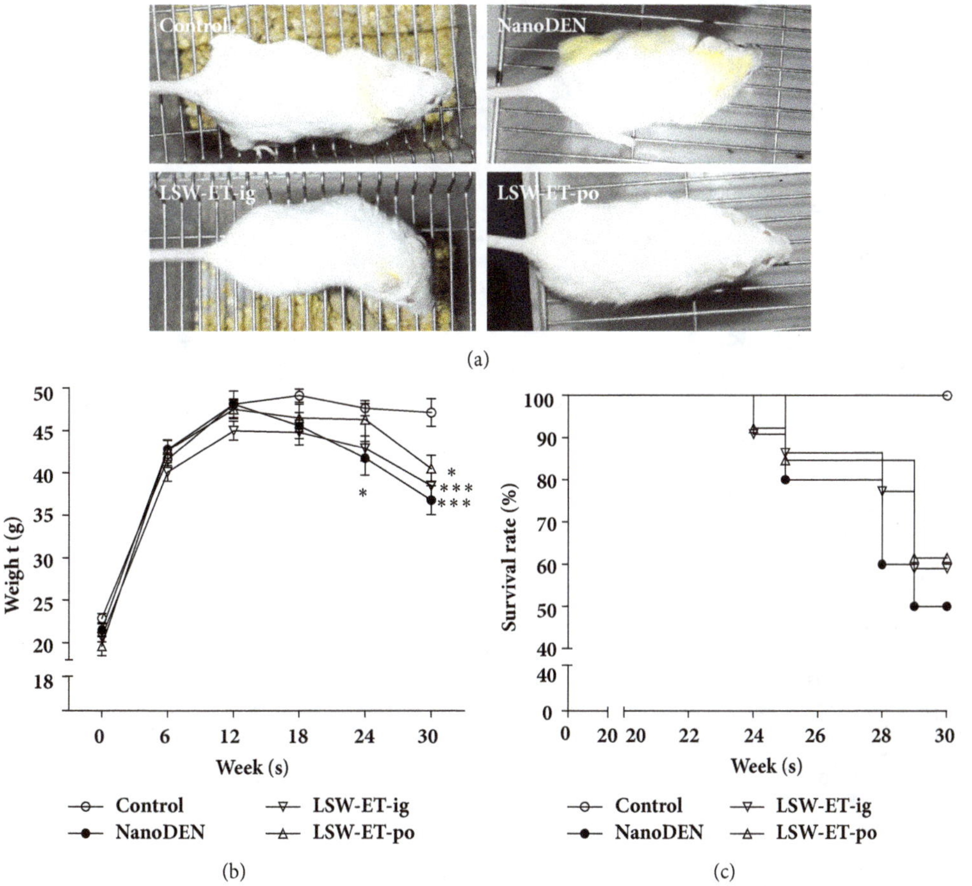

FIGURE 2: **The overviews of mice with different treatments.** (a) General view of the mice. (b) Gain of body weight in different groups during the experiment. (c) Survival rates of mice in various groups during the liver carcinogenesis. ∗ and ∗ ∗ ∗, $P < 0.05$ and 0.001, respectively; †, $P > 0.01$ compared with the control group; ‡, $P > 0.01$ compared with the nanoDEN group.

significantly elevated in the nanoDEN group suggesting that nanoDEN, as demonstrated previously, could cause the hematologic disorders. In comparison, treatments of LSW-ET-po and LSW-ET-ig could alleviate this nanoDEN-induced liver cytotoxicity. It would also be interesting to note that LDL-C level was significantly decreased in nanoDEN-treated group but recovered after both treatments of LSW-ET-ig and LSW-ET-po.

Liver specimens of mice in different treatment groups were harvested at weeks 10, 15, 20, and 30. In Figure 3(a), we could observe from the representative histopathological stainings in the week 30 mice that there were severe inflammatory infiltration and weakly extensive collagen deposition and pseudo-lobular formation in nanoDEN group, whereas liver cancer (80%; 4/5) occurred frequently with an increased nuclear-to-cytoplasmic index, enlarged and hyperchromatic

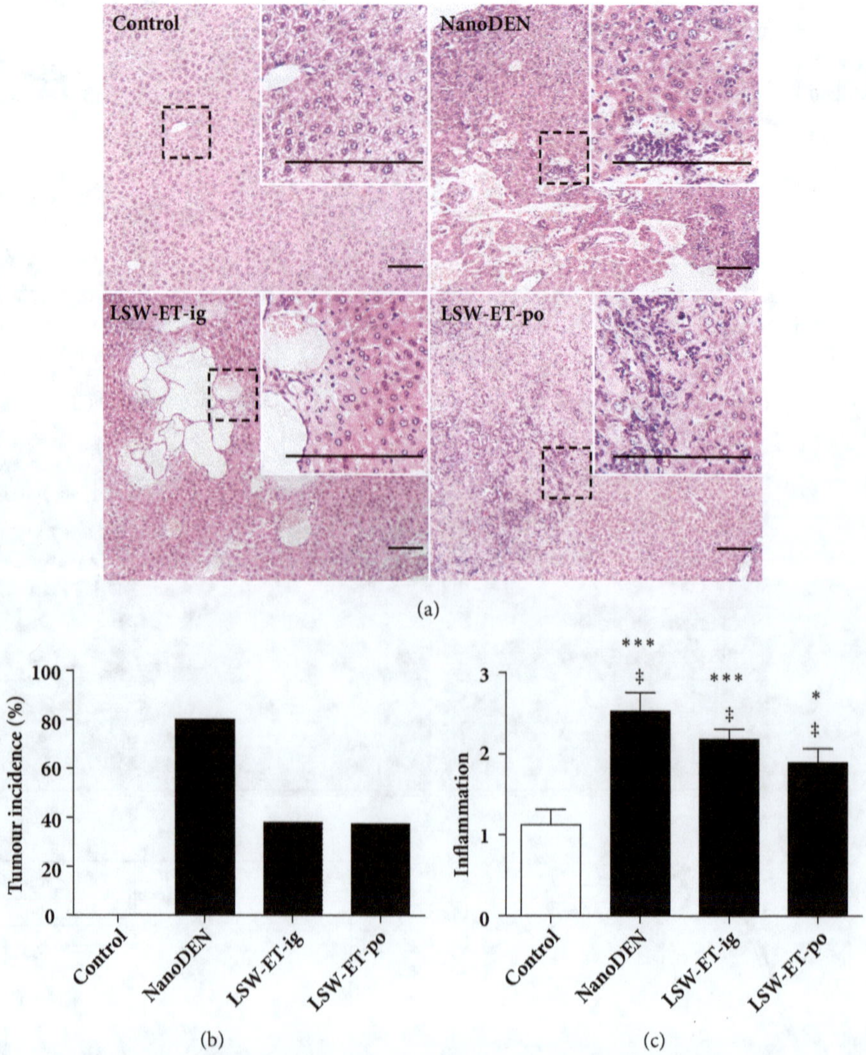

FIGURE 3: **The anticancer efficacy of different administration of LSW-ET in nanoDEN-induced HCC in mice.** (a) Histological analysis of livers from the control group, nanoDEN group, LSW-ET-ig, and LSW-ET-po group at the 30th week. Histological analysis of the livers was performed by hematoxylin and eosin staining. Part of the arbor (stippled outline, 100×) is shown enlarged in the inset (400×) in the top right corner. Scale bar, 50 μm. (b) The probability of occurrence of tumor in each group. (c) Scores of inflammation of liver samples. $*$ and $***$, $P < 0.05$ and 0.001, respectively, compared with the control group; ‡, $P > 0.01$ compared with the nanoDEN group.

nuclei, and expansive growth. In the contrary, intragastric injection of LSW-ET decreased the development of tumor nodules, but their inflammatory infiltration and hepatocyte necrosis were noted in the adjacent tissues. However, oral treatment of LSW-ET decreased the development of tumor nodules. In the meantime, normal architecture of the adjacent tissues remains intact.

These results indicated an in vivo antitumor effect of ethanol extracts of LSW, especially after oral treatment. To further quantify the difference among different treatments, scores of inflammation were introduced as reported previously [29]. The results showed that the inflammatory infiltration (inflammatory score: 2.52 ± 0.23) in the nanoDEN group was significantly increased at the thirtieth week compared with the control group, and the degree of inflammation in the liver tissues of mice treated with LSW-ET group (LSW-ET-ig group: 2.18 ± 0.13; LSW-ET-po group: 1.89 ± 0.18) was decreased, suggesting an anti-inflammatory effect of LSW-ET on liver. The overall scores of inflammation and incidence of tumor further strengthen the idea that ethanol extracts of LSW could alleviate nanoDEN-induced cancer (Figures 3(b) and 3(c)).

3.3. Expressions of Inflammatory and Tumor-Related Proteins Were Decreased after LSW-ET Treatment In Vivo. To further demonstrate the efficacy and efficiency of LSW-ET, we monitored changes of several pivotal factors, which had already been demonstrated to be greatly increased in liver samples of nanoDEN-treated mice [18, 24]. As shown in the following figures, expressions of all these four factors were elevated as

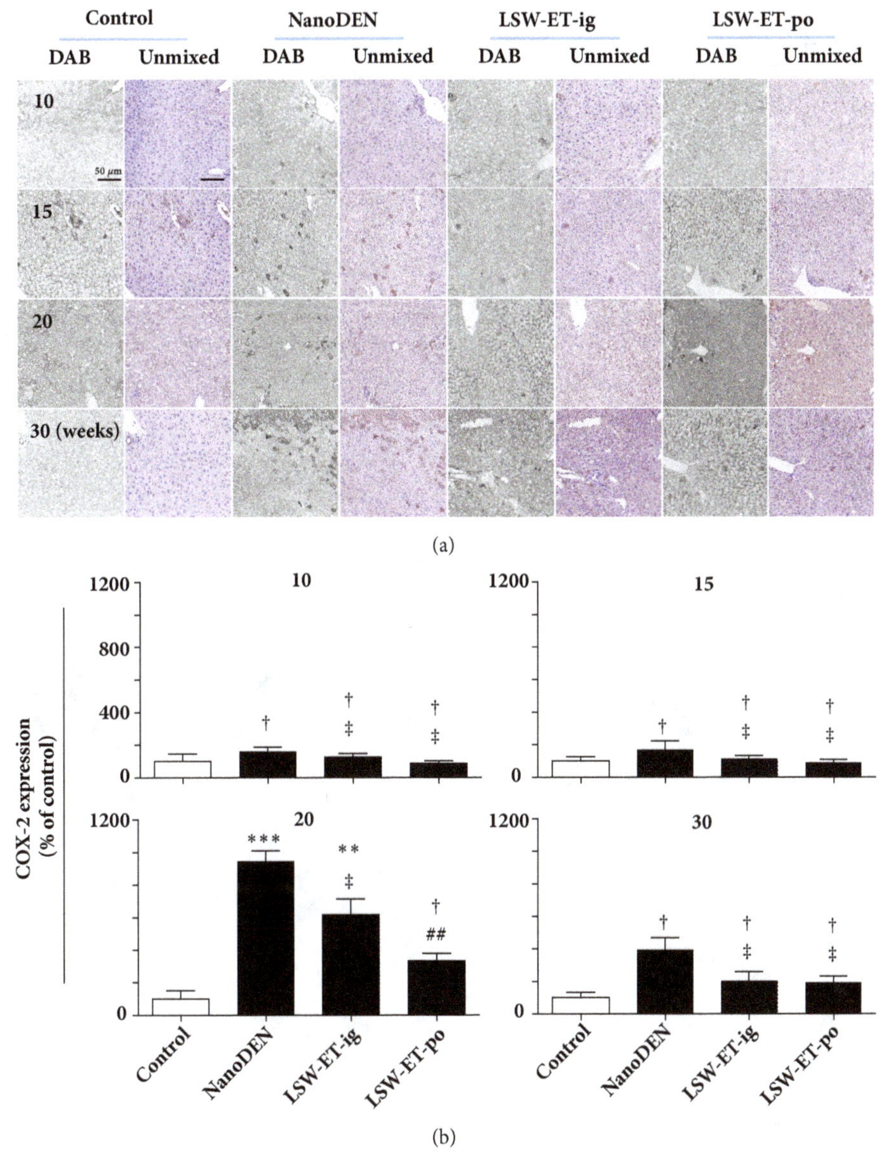

FIGURE 4: **Oral application of LSW-ET decreased the nanoDEN-induced COX-2 expression in mice.** (a) Expression of COX-2 by immunohistochemistry. Scale bar, 50 μm. (b) Quantitative expression of COX-2 determined by immunohistochemistry. (Results were expressed as the mean ± SEM. ∗, $P < 0.05$; ∗∗, $P < 0.01$; ∗ ∗ ∗, $P < 0.001$; †, $P > 0.01$, compared with the control group. #, $P < 0.05$; ##, $P < 0.01$; ###, $P < 0.001$; ‡, $P > 0.01$, respectively, compared with the nanoDEN group.)

well in the nanoDEN-treated group during the progress of the experiment at the 10th, 15th, 20th, and 30th week. In a good comparison, LSW-ET treatment, particularly the oral treatment, could dramatically decrease expressions of these factors in mice.

In accordance with our previous result that the inflammatory infiltration of mice in nanoDEN group was more severe and LSW-ET treatment could attenuate that, the expression pattern of COX-2 protein levels in liver tissues of nanoDEN group (942 ± 68% and 391 ± 77% of control at the 20th and 30th weeks, respectively) was much stronger than that in LSW-ET-ig group (618 ± 97% and 200 ± 59% of control at the 20th and 30th weeks, respectively). More importantly, the COX-2 expression in the LSW-ET-po group (333 ± 46% and 190 ± 41% of control at the 20th and 30th weeks, respectively) reduced significantly, as shown in Figure 4.

Aberrant accumulation of β-catenin had been suggested to be quite important during the progression of liver tumor. Therefore, we quantified our liver samples with a multi-spectrum imaging system to see the difference of nuclear localization of β-catenin. As we can see in Figure 5, compared to nanoDEN group (477 ± 32%, 805 ± 72%, 1963 ± 167%, and 2579 ± 232% of control at the 10th, 15th, 20th, and 30th weeks, respectively), the protein level of nuclear β-catenin obviously decreased in liver tissue after LSW-ET oral treatment (192 ± 20%, 466 ± 20%, 1075 ± 240%, and 1506 ± 54% at the 10th, 15th, 20th, and 30th weeks, respectively). Similar result was

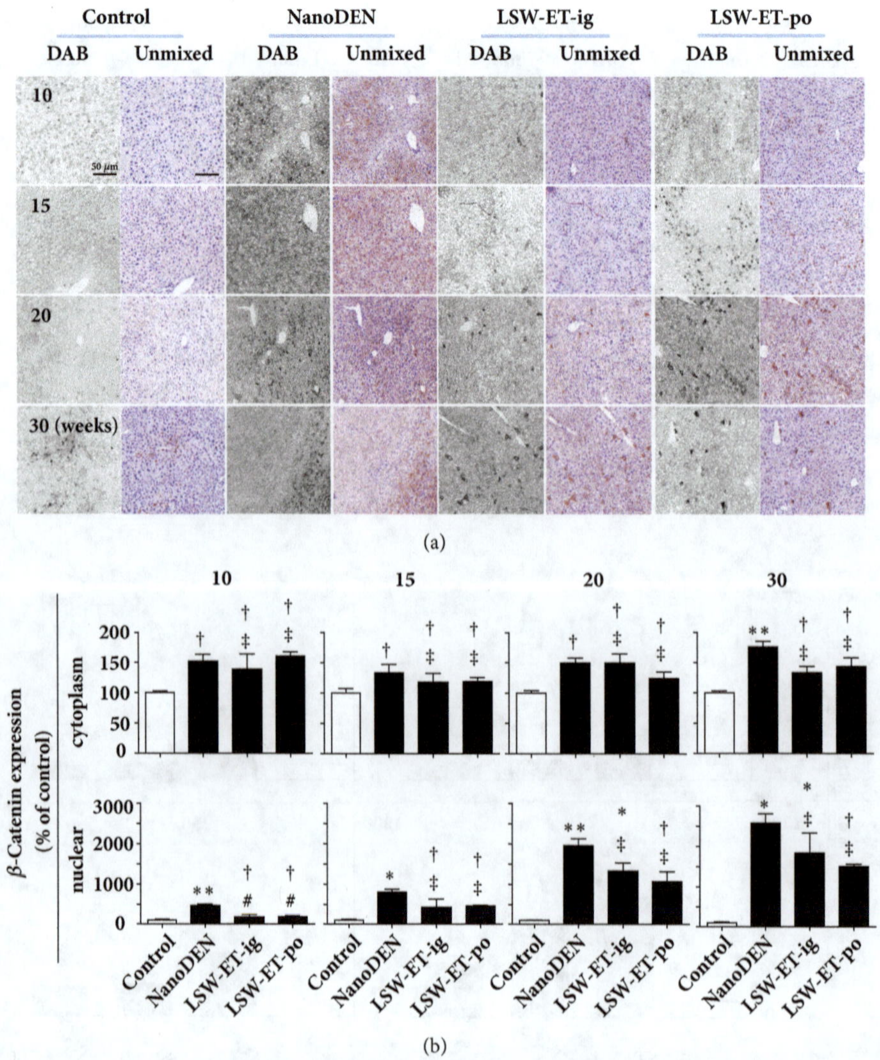

FIGURE 5: **Oral application of LSW-ET decreased the nanoDEN-induced β-catenin expression in mice.** (a) The expression of β-catenin by immunohistochemistry. Scale bar, 50 μm. (b) Quantitative expression of the cytoplasmic and nuclear expression of β-catenin determined by immunohistochemistry.

observed in the expression pattern of COX-2 in LSW-ET-ig group (1334 ± 198% and 1838 ± 495% of control at the 20th and 30th weeks, respectively).

Consistently, oral LSW-ET treatment induced decreases in protein levels of PCNA (560 ± 113% and 1937 ± 194% of control at the 20th and 30th weeks, respectively) and HMGB-1 (nuclear: 449 ± 178% of control; cytoplasm: 132 ± 28% of control, at 30th week, respectively) in mice in comparison to that in the nanoDEN group (Figures 6 and 7).

It is also interesting to notice that the decrease of COX-2, β-catenin, PCNA, and HMGB-1 expression in the LSW-ET-po group was lower than in the LSW-ET-ig group at week 30, further demonstrating a better antitumor effect of LSW-ET oral application.

4. Discussion

According to a recent investigation, hepatocellular carcinoma (HCC), which accounted for approximately 90% of primary liver cancers, became the second most common cause of cancer-related death with an average annual occurrence of about 850 K new cases worldwide [30]. Sorafenib was approved as a first-line systemic therapy for advanced HCC with associated extrahepatic spread and/or vascular invasion in 2007. However, there were several limitations associated with sorafenib therapy. And it extended the survival of advanced HCC patients by only approximately three months compared with placebo [31, 32]. These data underscored the urgent need to develop more effective therapies against liver cancer. Recently, many potential new compounds have been demonstrated to possess anticancer cell abilities, including ailanthone [33], botulin [34], and matrine [35]. However, in vivo experiments were still needed for better illustration of their efficacies.

Here, for the first time, we demonstrated that the LSW-ET, the alcoholic extract of Liushenwan, an herbal preparation in the Traditional Chinese Medicine, could reduce the occurrence and relieve the phenotype of nanoDEN-induced

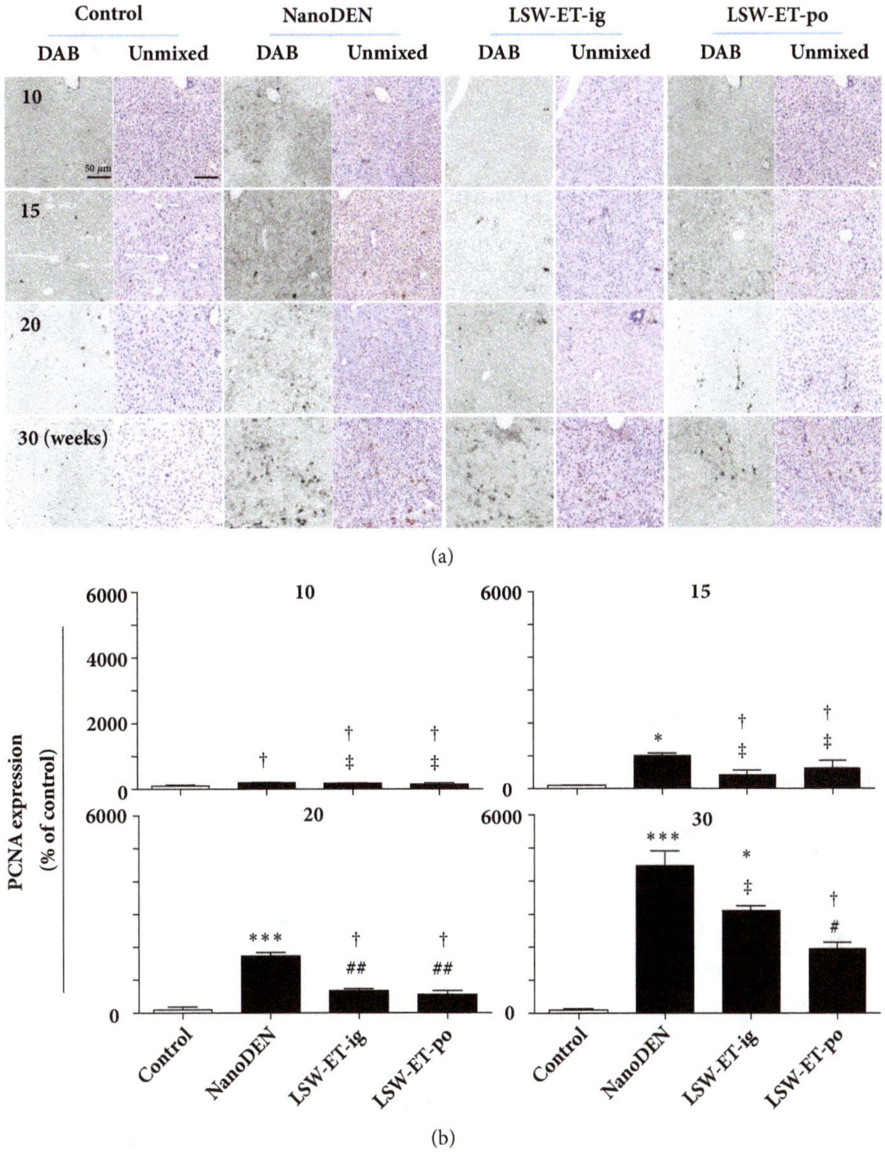

FIGURE 6: **Oral application of LSW-ET decreased the nanoDEN-induced PCNA expression in mice.** (a) Expression of PCNA by immunohistochemistry. Scale bar, 50 μm. (b) Quantitative expression of PCNA determined by immunohistochemistry.

liver cancer in mice. Two different administration methods were used in this study for the delivery of LSW-ET. Results showed that oral administration might be better to reduce the inflammation of livers since it was more efficient in alleviating upregulation of pivotal factors. It is not surprising because most components of LSW-ET (other than 5-HTQ and 5-HT), as can be seen in LC-MS, were of low polarities and hence would be easier to be intake in mouth. This fits well with the traditional usage of Liushenwan, since it was recommended to be taken sublingually.

We previously demonstrated that COX-2, β-catenin, and PCNA were upregulated in the liver of tumorous mice induced by nanoDEN. Here, we showed that after the uptake of LSW-ET, these three factors were all recovered (at least partly) compared with the nanoDEN-treated model group. Moreover, elevation of nuclear β-catenin in the model group was largely inhibited especially after the oral uptake of LSW-ET. We also examined the expression level of HMGB-1, the expression of which had been demonstrated to control liver cancer initiation via YAP-HIF1α pathway. Results showed that, particularly in week 30, when tumors were observed, the nuclear and cytoplasmic expressions of HMGB-1 in LSW-ET-treated groups were greatly reduced compared with the model group, which further strengthened the notion that LSW-ET was effective in preventing the initiation of liver cancer. It is also interesting to note that the inflammation scores of livers were reduced in LSW-ET-po group, which is in accordance with the COX-2 expression levels in liver specimens, suggesting that LSW-ET was not only effective in preventing tumor but also capable of alleviating inflammations in liver. This is not surprised though, since the components of LSW-ET, as demonstrated via LC-MS,

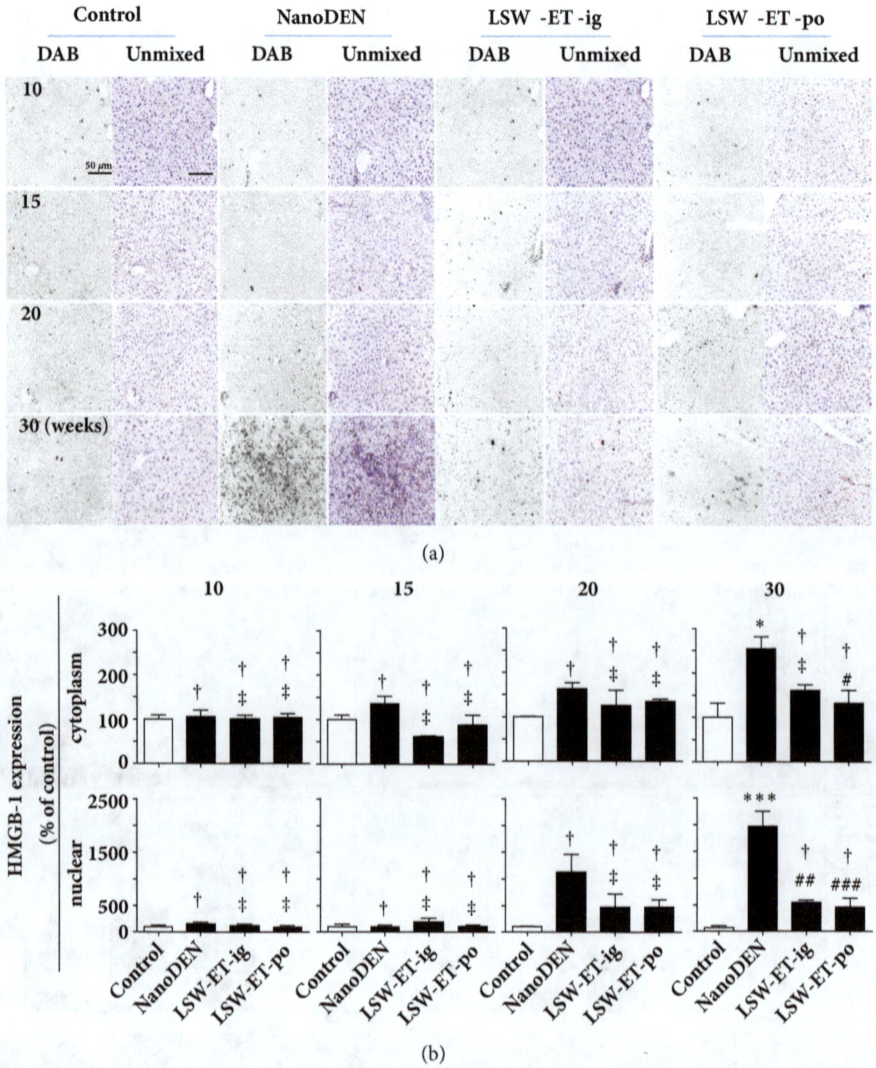

FIGURE 7: **Oral application of LSW-ET decreased the nanoDEN-induced HMGB-1 expression in mice.** (a) Expression of HMGB-1 by immunohistochemistry. Scale bar, 50 μm. (b) Quantitative expression of the cytoplasmic and nuclear expression of HMGB-1 determined by immunohistochemistry.

possessed anti-inflammatory effect. Nevertheless, this could potentially be insightful since the occurrence of hepatitis, whether virus or alcohol-induced, was not rare, and LSW-ET may contribute to the cure of them.

Another interesting aspect of this study is that, as shown in Table 2, plasmatic LDL-C concentration of the model group is significantly reduced compared with the control group, which is in accordance with the observation that the hair of mice in the nanoDEN group appeared to be dull and yellowish, suggesting an imbalance of lipid metabolism in cancerous mice induced by nanoDEN. In addition, LSW-ET treatment totally reversed the reduction of plasmatic LDL-C concentration indicating that LSW-ET is potentially capable of maintaining the balance of lipid metabolism. More investigations could be conducted to analyze the phenomena and illustrated the possible detailed mechanism.

5. Conclusion

In this study, we observed antitumor activity of LSW-ET in nanoDEN-induced HCC in mice. Pathology analysis indicated that modulation on inflammatory-, proliferation-, apoptosis-, and migration-related proteins may contribute together to the enhanced activity of LSW-ET. Our studies suggest that orally uptake of LSW-ET might be a promising prevention and treatment for liver cancer.

Authors' Contributions

Yu-Sang Li, Wei Kevin Zhang, and He-Bin Tang conceived and designed the experiments. Xi-Zhen Chen, Wei Kevin Zhang, and Yu-Sang Li performed the experiments. Xi-Zhen Chen, Wei Kevin Zhang, Yu-Sang Li, He-Bin Tang, Xiao-Jun Li, and Gui-Hua Tian analyzed the data. Wei Kevin Zhang and Yu-Sang Li contributed reagents/materials/analysis tools. Xi-Zhen Chen, Wei Kevin Zhang, Yu-Sang Li, He-Bin Tang, Xiao-Jun Li, and Gui-Hua Tian wrote the paper. Xi-Zhen Chen and Wei Kevin Zhang contributed equally to this work.

TABLE 2: Results of the serum chemistry profile analysis in the week 30 mice. The changes in serum ALT, AST, TBIL, and ALP levels directly or indirectly reflect the damage, and the changes in serum TRIG and LDL-C levels reflect the lipid accumulation and metabolism of livers in groups under different treatments. Data were presented as mean ± SEM. Comparing with the control group, * and ** represent $P < 0.05$ and 0.01, respectively, while comparing with the nanoDEN group, # represents $P < 0.05$.

	ALT (U/L)	AST (U/L)	TBIL (μmol/L)	ALP (U/L)	TRIG (mmol/L)	LDL-C (mmol/L)
Control	23 ± 3	75 ± 6	8.2 ± 1.1	30.9 ± 2.5	1.52 ± 0.12	1.86 ± 0.14
nanoDEN	36.7 ± 2.1*	117 ± 25	11.0 ± 1.1	84 ± 11**	1.33 ± 0.07	1.12 ± 0.07*
LSW-ET-ig	33 ± 3	111 ± 20	8.9 ± 1.2	48 ± 7#	1.34 ± 0.08	1.99 ± 0.24#
LSW-ET-po	26.6 ± 2.0	91 ± 7	11.6 ± 2.7	62 ± 14	1.77 ± 0.23	2.03 ± 0.10#

Acknowledgments

This work was supported by the National Natural Science Foundation of China (81573887, 81673711, and 81674050).

References

[1] R. Siegel, J. Ma, Z. Zou, and A. Jemal, "Cancer statistics, 2014," *CA: A Cancer Journal for Clinicians*, vol. 64, no. 1, pp. 9–29, 2014.

[2] F.-S. Wang, J.-G. Fan, Z. Zhang, B. Gao, and H.-Y. Wang, "The global burden of liver disease: the major impact of China," *Hepatology*, vol. 60, no. 6, pp. 2099–2108, 2015.

[3] A. Villanueva and J. M. Llovet, "Targeted therapies for hepatocellular carcinoma," *Gastroenterology*, vol. 140, no. 5, pp. 1410–1426, 2011.

[4] G. G. di Costanzo and R. Tortora, "Intermediate hepatocellular carcinoma: How to choose the best treatment modality?" *World Journal of Hepatology*, vol. 7, no. 9, pp. 1184–1191, 2015.

[5] L. Berliner, H. U. Lemke, E. vanSonnenberg et al., "Model-guided therapy for hepatocellular carcinoma: a role for information technology in predictive, preventive and personalized medicine," *EPMA Journal*, vol. 5, no. 1, 2014.

[6] S. Zhang, D. Tang, W. Zang et al., "Synergistic inhibitory effect of traditional Chinese medicine astragaloside IV and curcumin on tumor growth and angiogenesis in an orthotopic nude-mouse model of human hepatocellular carcinoma," *Anticancer Reseach*, vol. 37, no. 2, pp. 465–474, 2017.

[7] L.-J. Deng, Q.-L. Peng, L.-H. Wang et al., "Arenobufagin intercalates with DNA leading to G2 cell cycle arrest via ATM/ATR pathway," *Oncotarget*, vol. 6, no. 33, pp. 34258–34275, 2015.

[8] M. Kimura, E. Osada, T. Matsui, and C. Kobayashi, "Fundamental research for the pharmacological activity of Oriental drugs. IX. On the combined action of several crude drugs consisting in "Rokusingan" for the anti-inflammatory effect," *Journal of the Pharmaceutical Society of Japan*, vol. 88, no. 2, pp. 135–139, 1968.

[9] H.-Y. Ma, J.-P. Kou, J.-R. Wang, and B.-Y. Yu, "Evaluation of the anti-inflammatory and analgesic activities of Liu-Shen-Wan and its individual fractions," *Journal of Ethnopharmacology*, vol. 112, no. 1, pp. 108–114, 2007.

[10] S. Q. Zhang, "Tongue temperature of healthy persons and patients with yin deficiency by using thermal video," *Zhong Xi Yi Jie He Za Zhi*, vol. 10, no. 12, pp. 732-709, 1990.

[11] J. Liu, S.-X. Liang, Y.-F. Lu, J.-W. Miao, Q. Wu, and J.-S. Shi, "Realgar and realgar-containing Liu-Shen-Wan are less acutely toxic than arsenite and arsenate," *Journal of Ethnopharmacology*, vol. 134, no. 1, pp. 26–31, 2011.

[12] X.-J. Li, M.-M. Jia, Y.-S. Li, Y.-L. Yang, X.-Q. Mao, and H.-B. Tang, "Involvement of substance P/neurokinin-1 receptor in the analgesic and anticancer activities of minimally toxic fraction from the traditional Chinese medicine Liu-Shen-Wan *in vitro Biological & Pharmaceutical Bulletin*, vol. 37, no. 3, pp. 431–438, 2014.

[13] Y. Liang, Y. Feng, M. Zong et al., "β-catenin deficiency in hepatocytes aggravates hepatocarcinogenesis driven by oncogenic β-catenin and MET," *Hepatology*, vol. 67, no. 5, pp. 1807–1822, 2018.

[14] L.-B. Jeng, B. K. Velmurugan, H.-H. Hsu et al., "Fenofibrate induced PPAR alpha expression was attenuated by oestrogen receptor alpha overexpression in Hep3B cells," *Environmental Toxicology*, vol. 33, no. 2, pp. 234–247, 2018.

[15] A. de Conti, J. F. Ortega, V. Tryndyak et al., "MicroRNA deregulation in nonalcoholic steatohepatitisassociated liver carcinogenesis," *Oncotarget*, vol. 8, no. 51, pp. 88517–88528, 2017.

[16] S. Tian, X. Hui, Z. Fan et al., "Suppression of hepatocellular carcinoma proliferation and hepatitis B surface antigen secretion with interferon-λ1 or PEG-interferon-λ1," *The FASEB Journal*, vol. 28, no. 8, pp. 3528–3539, 2014.

[17] J. Behari, "The Wnt/beta-catenin signaling pathway in liver biology and disease," *Expert Rev Gastroenterol Hepatol*, vol. 4, no. 6, pp. 745–756, 2010.

[18] Y. Li, C. Leng, M. Chen et al., "Mouse hepatic neoplasm formation induced by trace level and low frequency exposure to diethylnitrosamine through β-catenin signaling pathway," *Toxicology Research*, vol. 5, no. 1, pp. 210–223, 2016.

[19] Y. Kim, C. Park, H. Kim et al., "Genetic alterations of Wnt signaling pathway-associated genes in hepatocellular carcinoma," *Journal of Gastroenterology and Hepatology*, vol. 23, no. 1, pp. 110–118, 2008.

[20] E. A. Bayomi, A. B. Barakat, M. A. El-Bassuoni et al., "Cyclooxygenase-2 expression is associated with elevated aspartate aminotransferase level in hepatocellular carcinoma," *Journal of Cancer Research and Therapeutics*, vol. 11, no. 4, pp. 786–792, 2015.

[21] H. Chen, W. Cai, E. S. H. Chu et al., "Hepatic cyclooxygenase-2 overexpression induced spontaneous hepatocellular carcinoma formation in mice," *Oncogene*, vol. 36, no. 31, pp. 4415–4426, 2017.

[22] S. Srigopalram, I. A. Jayraaj, B. Kaleeswaran et al., "Ellagic acid normalizes mitochondrial outer membrane permeabilization and attenuates inflammation-mediated cell proliferation in experimental liver cancer," *Applied Biochemistry and Biotechnology*, vol. 173, no. 8, pp. 2254–2266, 2014.

[23] V. Chandrashekaran, R. K. Seth, D. Dattaroy et al., "HMGB1-RAGE pathway drives peroxynitrite signaling-induced IBD-like

inflammation in murine nonalcoholic fatty liver disease," *Redox Biology*, vol. 13, pp. 8–19, 2017.

[24] W. K. Zhang, H. Gu, X. Li et al., "The dark side of "the force" – lipid nanoparticles enhance the oncogenesis of diethylnitrosamine and result in liver cancer in mice," *Nanomedicine: Nanotechnology, Biology and Medicine*, vol. 13, no. 2, pp. 701–711, 2017.

[25] Y. S. Li, J. X. Wang, M. M. Jia, M. Liu, X.-J. Li, and H.-B. Tang, "Dragon's blood inhibits chronic inflammatory and neuropathic pain responses by blocking the synthesis and release of substance P in rats," *Journal of Pharmacological Sciences*, vol. 118, no. 1, pp. 43–54, 2012.

[26] F. Qi, A. Li, L. Zhao et al., "Cinobufacini, an aqueous extract from Bufo bufo gargarizans Cantor, induces apoptosis through a mitochondria-mediated pathway in human hepatocellular carcinoma cells," *Journal of Ethnopharmacology*, vol. 128, no. 3, pp. 654–661, 2010.

[27] D.-M. Zhang, J.-S. Liu, M.-K. Tang et al., "Bufotalin from Venenum Bufonis inhibits growth of multidrug resistant HepG2 cells through G2/M cell cycle arrest and apoptosis," *European Journal of Pharmacology*, vol. 692, no. 1-3, pp. 19–28, 2012.

[28] D.-M. Zhang, J.-S. Liu, and L.-J. Deng, "Arenobufagin, a natural bufadienolide from toad venom, induces apoptosis and autophagy in human hepatocellular carcinoma cells through inhibition of PI3K/Akt/mTOR pathway," *Carcinogenesis*, vol. 34, no. 6, pp. 1331–1342, 2013.

[29] D. E. Kleiner, E. M. Brunt, M. van Natta et al., "Design and validation of a histological scoring system for nonalcoholic fatty liver disease," *Hepatology*, vol. 41, no. 6, pp. 1313–1321, 2005.

[30] M. Pavel and J. Fuster, "Expansion of the hepatocellular carcinoma Milan criteria in liver transplantation: Future directions," *World Journal of Gastroenterology*, vol. 24, no. 32, pp. 3626–3636, 2018.

[31] J. M. Llovet, S. Ricci, V. Mazzaferro et al., "Sorafenib in advanced hepatocellular carcinoma," *The New England Journal of Medicine*, vol. 359, no. 4, pp. 378–390, 2008.

[32] M. Reig and J. Bruix, "Sorafenib for hepatocellular carcinoma: global validation," *Gastroenterology*, vol. 137, no. 3, pp. 1171–1173, 2009.

[33] Z. Zhuo, J. Hu, X. Yang et al., "Ailanthone inhibits huh7 cancer cell growth via cell cycle arrest and apoptosis in vitro and in vivo," *Scientific Reports*, vol. 5, no. 1, 2015.

[34] Z. Zhuo, M. Xiao, H. Lin, J. Luo, and T. Wang, "Novel betulin derivative induces anti-proliferative activity by G2/M phase cell cycle arrest and apoptosis in Huh7 cells," *Oncology Letters*, vol. 15, no. 2, pp. 2097–2104, 2017.

[35] J. Cao, R. Wei, and S. Yao, "Matrine has pro-apoptotic effects on liver cancer by triggering mitochondrial fission and activating Mst1-JNK signalling pathways," *The Journal of Physiological Sciences*, pp. 1–14, 2018.

9

Percutaneous Radiofrequency Ablation of Small (1–2 cm) Hepatocellular Carcinomas Inconspicuous on B-Mode Ultrasonographic Imaging: Usefulness of Combined Fusion Imaging with MRI and Contrast-Enhanced Ultrasonography

Min Woo Lee,[1,2] Hyo Keun Lim,[1,2] Hyunchul Rhim,[1,2] Dong Ik Cha,[1] Tae Wook Kang,[1] Kyoung Doo Song,[1] Ji Hye Min,[1] Geum-Youn Gwak,[3] Seonwoo Kim,[4] and David S. K. Lu[5]

[1]*Department of Radiology and Center for Imaging Science, Samsung Medical Center, Sungkyunkwan University School of Medicine, Seoul 06351, Republic of Korea*
[2]*Department of Health Sciences and Technology, SAIHST, Sungkyunkwan University, Seoul 06351, Republic of Korea*
[3]*Department of Medicine, Samsung Medical Center, Sungkyunkwan University School of Medicine, Seoul 06351, Republic of Korea*
[4]*Statistics and Data Center, Samsung Medical Center, Seoul 06351, Republic of Korea*
[5]*Department of Radiological Sciences, David Geffen School of Medicine at UCLA, 757 Westwood Plaza, Los Angeles, CA 90095, USA*

Correspondence should be addressed to Hyo Keun Lim; rfalim@skku.edu

Academic Editor: Michele Molinari

Purpose. To assess usefulness of adding contrast-enhanced ultrasonography (CEUS) to fusion imaging (FI) for percutaneous radiofrequency ablation (RFA) of hepatocellular carcinomas (HCCs) inconspicuous on FI alone. Therapeutic outcomes of RFA under CEUS-added FI guidance for HCCs inconspicuous on FI alone were also evaluated. *Methods.* This prospective study was approved by the institutional review board and informed consent was obtained from all patients. Planning US was performed with FI for 126 patients with a single HCC (1–2 cm) to evaluate the feasibility of RFA by grading lesion conspicuity score using a four-point scale. RFA was performed under CEUS-added FI guidance for HCCs inconspicuous on FI alone. We evaluated how many HCCs initially inconspicuous on FI became conspicuous after adding CEUS. After CEUS-added FI-guided RFA, therapeutic outcomes including rates of technical success, primary technique efficacy, major complications, and local tumor progression were assessed. *Results.* After adding CEUS, 90.5% (19/21) of all tumors initially inconspicuous on FI became conspicuous, thus enabling direct targeting for RFA. Technical success and primary technique efficacy rates were 94.7% (18/19) and 100% (19/19), respectively. No major complications were observed after RFA. Cumulative local tumor progression rates after RFA were estimated to be 5.3%, 10.8%, and 10.8% at 1, 2, and 3 years, respectively. *Conclusion.* Adding CEUS to FI is useful for improving the conspicuity of HCCs inconspicuous on FI alone, thus enabling successful percutaneous RFA with excellent therapeutic outcomes.

1. Introduction

It can be challenging to ablate small hepatocellular carcinomas (HCCs) under B-mode ultrasonography (US) guidance as small HCCs sometimes have poor sonographic conspicuity [1]. Fusion imaging (FI) of B-mode US and pre-acquired computed tomography (CT)/magnetic resonance imaging (MRI) has emerged as a useful guidance modality for percutaneous radiofrequency ablation (RFA) of small HCCs [2–5]. FI increases the confidence of a subtle lesion by colocalizing it to pre-acquired CT/MRI. However, when a tumor is completely isoechoic compared to surrounding normal liver, FI can only estimate the location of what is in essence a "virtual target," and incomplete ablation can occur even after FI-guided RFA [6]. This shortcoming is due to the inherent registration error that occurs when applying rigid registration to a deformable organ during motion.

Contrast-enhanced US (CEUS) using Sonazoid (gaseous perflubutane, GE Healthcare, New York City, NY) has emerged as a promising technique for localizing small HCCs and guiding percutaneous RFA [7, 8]. HCCs can be localized with high confidence using the post-vascular phase unique to Sonazoid [9].

CEUS is now often combined with FI for percutaneous RFA of challenging small HCCs [10, 11]. This combination has been shown to enhance the feasibility of percutaneous RFA for HCCs inconspicuous on FI alone [11, 12] and also better assess the ablation zone [13]. However, most of these studies had retrospective designs. They included heterogeneous mixtures of liver tumors and only evaluated the value of CEUS-added FI for localizing liver tumors without sufficient follow-up data [11, 12, 14, 15]. To our knowledge, there are no solid data regarding how many tumors initially inconspicuous on FI become conspicuous after adding CEUS, thus enabling direct targeting for RFA.

Therefore, the primary endpoint of this trial was to assess the value of adding CEUS to FI for improving lesion conspicuity and the technical feasibility of percutaneous RFA of HCCs (1–2 cm) inconspicuous on FI alone. The secondary endpoint was to assess the therapeutic outcomes of RFA under CEUS-added FI guidance for HCCs inconspicuous on FI alone.

2. Materials and Methods

2.1. Sample Size Estimation. The detection rate of very-early-stage HCC [Barcelona Clinic Liver Cancer (BCLC) stage 0, single nodule ≤ 2 cm] on FI has been reported to be approximately 85% [16]. Assuming that 15% are discordant pairs analyzed using the exact binomial test, a sample size of 101 is required with a 5% significance level and 80% power. Considering a drop-out rate of 20%, the minimum sample size was determined to be 126.

2.2. Patients. This prospective study was approved by the Institutional Review Board of Samsung Medical Center, a tertiary referral center. Informed consent was obtained from all patients prior to enrollment. Between August 2013 and January 2015, a total of 126 patients satisfying the following inclusion criteria underwent planning US to assess the feasibility of percutaneous RFA in our department. Inclusion criteria were as follows: (a) a treatment-naïve, single HCC 1–2 cm in diameter on contrast-enhanced MRI with gadoxetic acid (Gd-EOB-DTPA), (b) classification as Child-Pugh class A or B, (c) normal coagulation status, and (d) absence of vascular invasion and extrahepatic metastasis on MRI at the time of diagnosis. Exclusion criteria were as follows: (a) patients who did not undergo CEUS despite inconspicuous tumors on FI, (b) artificial ascites used instead of CEUS to improve sonographic window, (c) RFA infeasible due to reasons other than lesion conspicuity, (d) other treatments performed instead of RFA, and (e) patients who did not agree to participate in this study or who were lost to follow-up.

Treatment modality was determined based on recommendations from a multidisciplinary tumor board. Among these 126 patients, 34 patients were determined to have HCCs inconspicuous on FI alone; 19 of these patients who finally underwent percutaneous RFA under CEUS-added FI guidance were included in the evaluation of therapeutic outcomes after RFA.

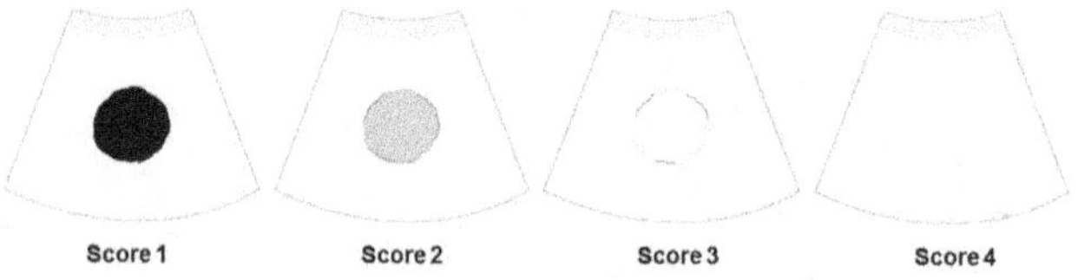

Figure 1: A schema showing the conspicuity score.

Diagnosis of HCC was based on typical imaging features according to the American Association for the Study of Liver Disease guidelines [20] obtained on MRI. Scans were acquired using a 3.0-T system (Intera Achieva 3.0-T, Philips Healthcare, Best, The Netherlands) equipped with a 32-channel phased-array coil.

2.3. Planning US with Fusion Imaging. Planning US was performed to evaluate whether percutaneous RFA was feasible by one of three experienced radiologists (H.K.L., H.R., and M.W.L. with 15, 15, and 10 years of clinical experience with percutaneous RFA, respectively). For planning US, FI (Volume Navigation; GE Healthcare, Waukesha, WI) of the LOGIQ E9 system (GE Healthcare) was routinely used with a 1–5-MHz convex probe regardless of the initial US conspicuity of the tumor. The process of image fusion between B-mode US and MRI was similar to the methods of previous studies [2, 16]. After image fusion, the HCC conspicuity score on B-mode US was graded by the radiologist performing planning US using a four-point scale at the time of US examination (Figure 1 and Table 1). Lesions with a score of 1 or 2 were regarded as conspicuous HCCs, while those with a score of 3 or 4 were regarded as inconspicuous HCCs. The technical feasibility of RFA was also evaluated based on the expected electrode path, adjacent organ vulnerable to thermal injury, and heat-sink effect [17].

2.4. Percutaneous RFA. Percutaneous RFA was performed using a 200-W RF generator (VIVA RF system; STARmed, Goyang, Korea) and a length-adjustable RF electrode (Proteus; STARmed) by the radiologists who performed planning US. Additional CEUS was applied for HCCs inconspicuous on FI to increase lesion conspicuity, and RFA was performed if feasible under CEUS-added FI guidance. When CEUS was added to FI, image fusion between B-mode US and MRI was first performed to estimate the location of the index tumor before applying CEUS. Then, the US image was switched from B-mode to CEUS mode and displayed side by side with the fused MRI. Contrast harmonic imaging technique with a default setting of a mechanical index level of 0.24 was used. The focal zone was placed in the posterior margin of the liver. Sonazoid was injected intravenously at a dose of 0.015 mL/kg, followed by a flush with 10 mL of normal saline. Images were obtained during each phase: arterial (10–40 seconds after contrast injection), portal (60–90 seconds), and delayed phase (3 minutes) and post-vascular phase (more than 10 minutes) [11]. If the index tumor was not clearly identified on the arterial phase but was visible on the post-vascular

TABLE 1: Scoring criteria for evaluation of tumor conspicuity.

Score	Criteria
1	The echogenicity of the index tumor is definitely different from that of the surrounding liver and more than 90% of the tumor has a well-defined margin
2	The echogenicity of the index tumor is slightly different from that of the surrounding liver and more than 50% of the tumor has a well-defined margin
3	The index tumor is nearly isoechoic to the surrounding liver and less than 50% of the tumor has a well-defined margin
4	Definitely unidentifiable

This scoring system was described in our previous study [11] and was established after reviewing previous relevant studies regarding planning US for RFA and making necessary updates [17–19].

phase, Sonazoid was reinjected in the post-vascular phase to visualize arterial enhancement of the target lesion [9]. The conspicuity score of the index tumor after adding CEUS was reassessed by the aforementioned scoring system based on the post-vascular phase as the temporal window of the post-vascular phase is long and the RF electrode is inserted during the phase. When the index tumor was definitely unidentifiable even after adding CEUS, percutaneous RFA was not attempted. Instead, an alternative treatment or imaging follow-up was considered.

The technical goals of RFA were to eradicate the tumor and to achieve a minimum 0.5-cm ablative margin where feasible. The energy deposition algorithm was based on the manufacturer's recommended protocol. Overlapping ablation was performed when needed. Although the standard ablation time recommended by the manufacturer was 12 minutes, RFA was finished earlier when the echogenic zone created was large enough to achieve a sufficient ablative margin or collateral thermal injury was suspected. The electrode path was cauterized during electrode removal at the end of the ablation session to avoid tract bleeding or tumor seeding.

2.5. Assessment of the Effects of Adding CEUS to FI and the Therapeutic Efficacy of RFA. For tumors inconspicuous on FI alone, we evaluated how initially inconspicuous HCCs became conspicuous after adding CEUS to FI, thus enabling direct targeting of percutaneous RFA. The rate of conspicuous HCCs on FI was compared with that on CEUS-added FI. Lesions conspicuous on FI alone were also regarded as conspicuous on CEUS-added FI, even though additional CEUS was not performed.

For patients who underwent RFA, therapeutic efficacy and complications were assessed using multiphase liver CT obtained within 12 hours after RFA. In addition, chest radiography, multiphase liver CT or MRI, and laboratory tests including serum α-fetoprotein were performed one month after initial discharge and every 3–4 months thereafter. Assessments were performed according to standardized terminology and reporting criteria for image-guided tumor ablation [21]. Technical success was defined as when the index tumor was treated according to our treatment protocol and was covered by ablation zone completely on the immediate post-RFA CT images [21]. The treatment course included all RFA sessions performed within one month to eradicate any residual tumor. Primary technique efficacy was assessed based on follow-up CT images taken one month after ablation. Local tumor progression (LTP) was defined as when foci of untreated disease appeared in tumors that were initially considered to be completely ablated on follow-up CT or MRI. A major complication was defined as any event that resulted in substantial morbidity and disability, an increased level of care, or substantial lengthening of hospital stay [21]. All other complications were regarded as minor.

2.6. Statistical Analysis. The conspicuity scores of inconspicuous HCCs on FI alone before versus after adding CEUS were compared using the Wilcoxon signed rank test. The rate of conspicuous HCCs on FI alone was compared with the rate of conspicuous HCCs on CEUS-added FI. Improvement of conspicuity score with the addition of CEUS was tested with the exact binomial test. Cumulative LTP rates of CEUS-added FI-guided RFA were estimated using the Kaplan-Meier method. All statistical analyses were performed using the SPSS Statistics software package (version 18.0; SPSS, Chicago, IL). A p value less than 0.05 was considered statistically significant.

3. Results

3.1. Patient and Lesion Characteristics. Of 126 patients, 92 (73.0%) patients had a lesion conspicuity score of 1 or 2, whereas 34 (27.0%) patients had a conspicuity score of 3 or 4 on FI (Figure 2). Of the 34 patients with a score of 3 or 4, 13 did not undergo CEUS due to the following reasons: percutaneous RFA was infeasible due to reasons other than lesion conspicuity ($n = 7$); artificial ascites fluid was used to enhance lesion conspicuity ($n = 4$); or other treatments were performed instead of percutaneous RFA ($n = 2$). The remaining 21 patients with conspicuity score of 3 or 4 also underwent CEUS (Figure 2). The conspicuity score of the 21 HCCs (mean ± standard deviation [SD], 1.2 ± 0.2 cm; median, 1.1 cm; range, 1.0–1.8 cm) was significantly higher after adding CEUS (before CEUS; median, 3; range, 3–4 versus after CEUS; median, 1; range, 1–4; $p < 0.001$) (Figure 3). Of the 21 lesions inconspicuous on FI alone, 19 (90.5%) became conspicuous after adding CEUS (16 on both arterial and post-vascular phase, two in post-vascular phase, and one in arterial phase) (Table 2). The rate of conspicuous HCCs on CEUS-added FI was significantly higher than that on FI alone [(92+19)/(92+21), 98.2% versus 92/(92+21), 81.4%; $p < 0.001$].

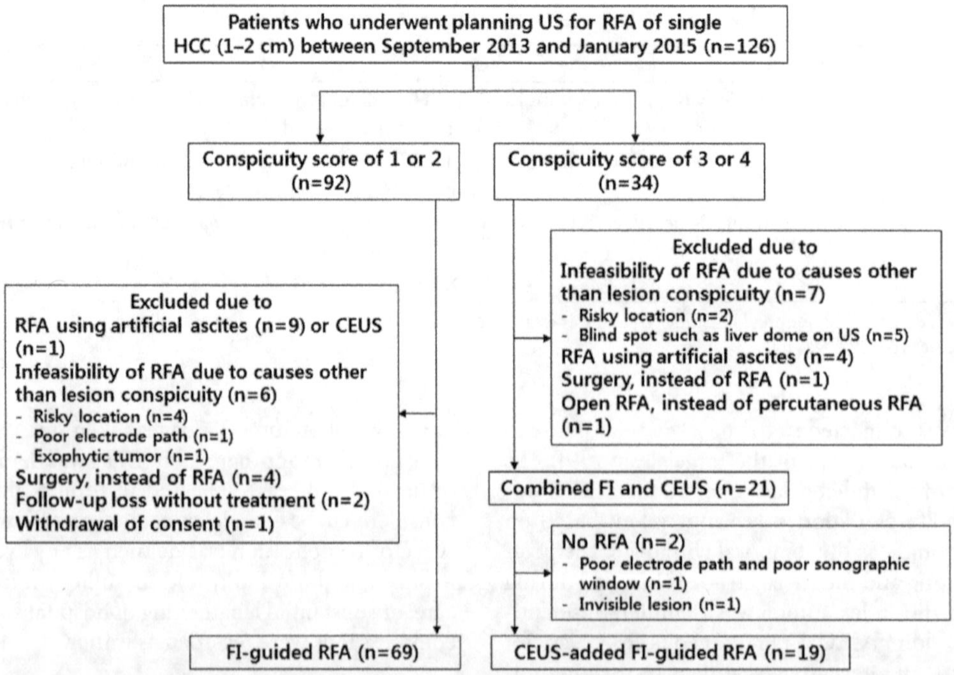

FIGURE 2: Flow diagram of the patient enrollment process. US = ultrasonography; HCC = hepatocellular carcinoma; RFA = radiofrequency ablation; FI = fusion imaging; CEUS = contrast-enhanced ultrasonography.

TABLE 2: Conspicuity score before and after CEUS in the 21 patients with fusion imaging-inconspicuous HCCs.

Before CEUS	After CEUS
3 ($n = 13$)	1 ($n = 8$)
	2 ($n = 4$)
	3 ($n = 1$)
4 ($n = 8$)	1 ($n = 4$) [a]
	2 ($n = 3$) [b]
	4 ($n = 1$) [c]

CEUS = contrast-enhanced ultrasonography; HCC = hepatocellular carcinoma.
[a] Residual tumor was noted after the first RFA session in one patient in whom the tumor was located in the subcapsular area in segment 5, just below the right rib. Technique efficacy was achieved after the second RFA session.
[b] In one patient, although the lesion was identified after CEUS was added, both the expected electrode path and sonographic window were poor. Therefore, chemoembolization was performed instead of percutaneous RFA.
[c] In this patient, the target lesion was not identified on the arterial or postvascular phase. Therefore, instead of treatment, this patient was followed up with CT/MRI. Eventually, the lesion disappeared on 8-month follow-up MRI, indicating that it was a pseudolesion.

Among the 21 patients who underwent CEUS-added FI, one underwent chemoembolization instead of RFA due to poor electrode path and poor sonographic window due to perihepatic fat thickness, even though the index tumor was identified after adding CEUS (conspicuity score: 2). Another patient did not undergo RFA due to invisibility of the target lesion, even after adding CEUS. The latter patient was followed up with CT/MRI and the lesion had disappeared on 8-month follow-up MRI, indicating that it had been a pseudolesion. Eventually, direct targeting for percutaneous RFA was possible in 90.5% (19/21) of tumors initially inconspicuous on FI alone after adding CEUS (Figure 2).

3.2. Percutaneous RFA and Its Therapeutic Outcomes. The baseline characteristics of the 19 patients who underwent RFA under CEUS-added FI guidance are summarized in Table 3. Tumor size was 1.2 ± 0.2 cm. After RFA, a residual tumor was detected in one patient at CT, requiring a second ablation session to complete the treatment course. In this patient, the tumor (1.2 cm in diameter) was located in the subcapsular area of segment 5, just below the right rib. Although the conspicuity score of the tumor increased from 4 to 1 after adding CEUS, the sonographic window was poor due to the overlying rib shadow.

Meanwhile, incomplete ablation was avoided by adding CEUS in one case where a subtle lesion on FI was initially thought to be a true lesion that corresponded to the tumor nodule on MRI (Figure 4).

The therapeutic outcomes are summarized in Table 4. The technical success rate was 94.7% (18/19). No major complications were identified after CEUS-added FI-guided RFA. No residual tumors were identified in any patient on CT obtained one month after RFA (primary technique efficacy rate: 100%, 19/19). The cumulative LTP rates after CEUS-added FI-guided RFA were estimated to be 5.3%, 10.8%, and 10.8% at 1, 2, and 3 years, respectively.

4. Discussion

In general, FI can enhance the detectability of small HCCs inconspicuous on B-mode US and reduce false-positive

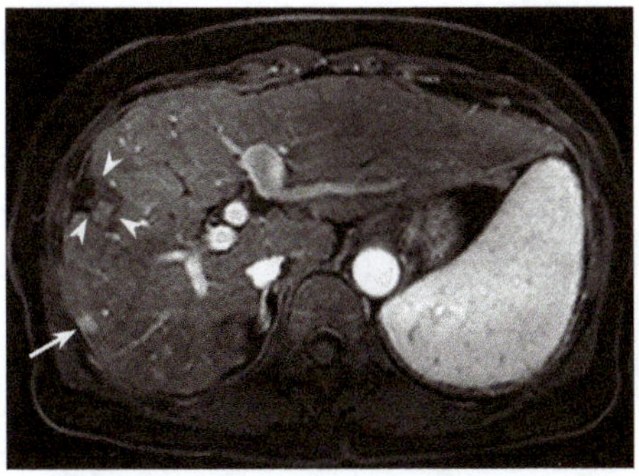

(a) Arterial-phase MRI showing a small hypervascular HCC (arrow) in segment 5 of the liver. Arrowheads indicate a previous RFA zone

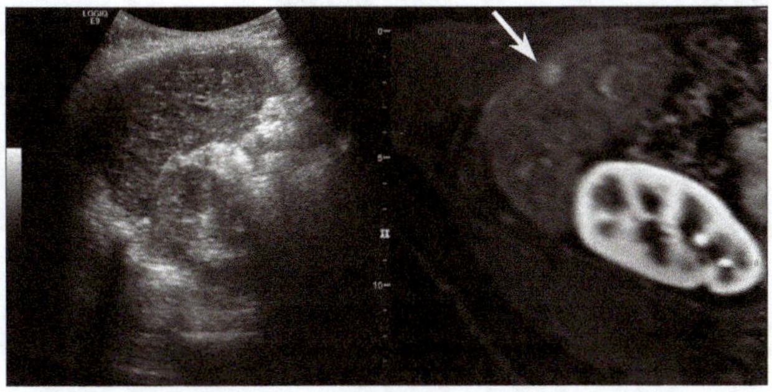

(b) After fusion imaging, the HCC nodule could not be identified on B-mode US imaging at the corresponding site on fused MRI (arrow). Therefore, the index tumor was given a conspicuity score of 4 on fusion imaging as it was definitely unidentifiable

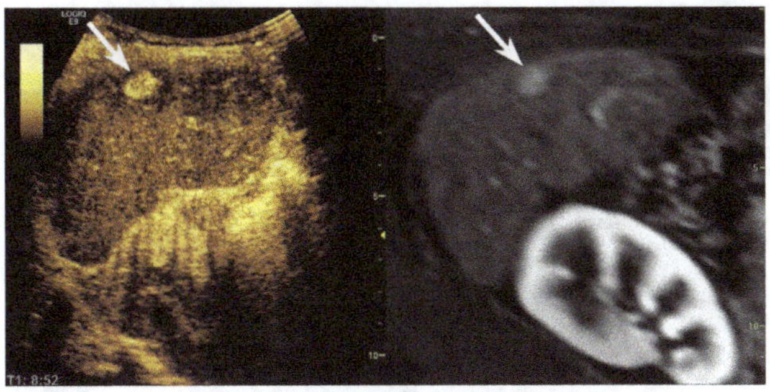

(c) On arterial-phase imaging obtained after the second injection of Sonazoid, a small enhanced lesion (arrow) was clearly identifiable at the corresponding location on fused MRI. After the first injection of the contrast agent, the optimal arterial phase was not obtained due to irregular respiration of the patient

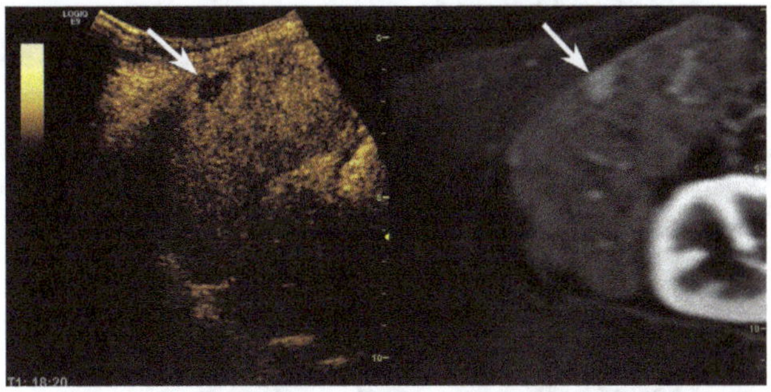

(d) On post-vascular-phase imaging, the index tumor (arrow) was clearly identified as a perfusion defect at the corresponding site (arrow) on fused MRI. Therefore, the index tumor was given a conspicuity score of 1 on CEUS-added fusion imaging

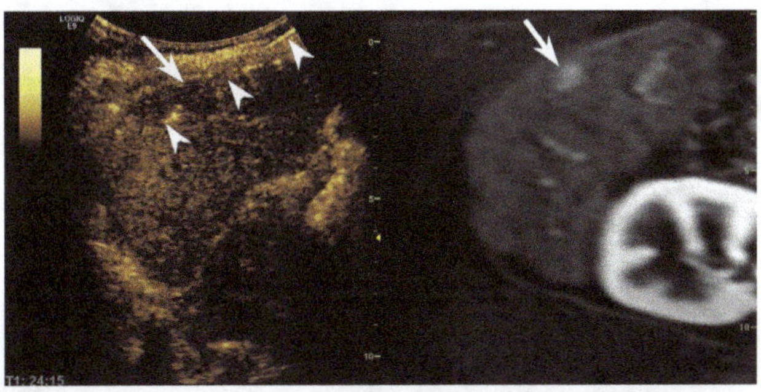

(e) An RF electrode (arrowheads) was inserted into the index tumor (arrow) under CEUS-added fusion imaging guidance, after which RF energy was applied

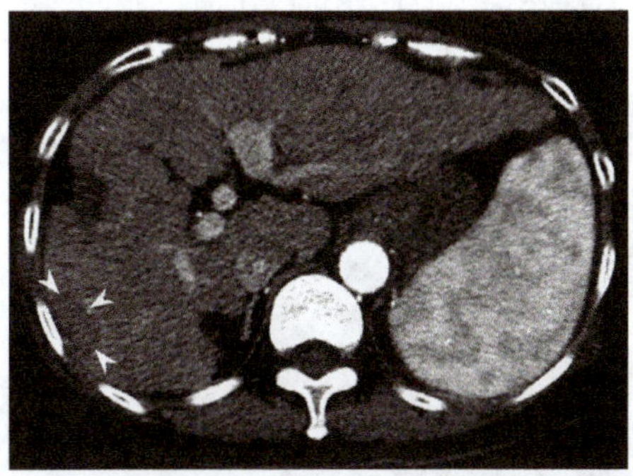

(f) Arterial-phase CT image obtained immediately after RFA revealed technical success with sufficient ablative margins (arrowheads). LTP was not identified on follow-up MRI obtained 32 months after RFA (not shown here)

FIGURE 3: Images from a 59-year-old woman with a 1.1-cm HCC and hepatitis B virus-related liver cirrhosis who had previously undergone percutaneous RFA of HCC.

detection of HCCs on B-mode US [16, 22]. In a previous study [16], false-positive detection on B-mode US was as high as 9.1% (9 of 99) for HCCs (1–2 cm) based on FI findings. In this context, we have adopted FI as the routine guiding modality for percutaneous RFA of HCCs. However, FI is not always sufficient for localizing small HCCs. Actually, 31.3% (76/243) of HCCs (mean size, 1.5 cm; range, 0.3–5.0 cm) were invisible on FI in a recent study [5].

Our study demonstrated that adding CEUS to FI improved the conspicuity of HCCs inconspicuous on FI of real-time US and MRI (Table 2). Consequently, it enabled percutaneous RFA of HCCs inconspicuous on FI alone in most cases (90.5%, 19/21). Moreover, unnecessary RFA was avoided in one case, which was later identified as a pseudolesion based on added CEUS and follow-up imaging findings. Furthermore, therapeutic outcomes including rates

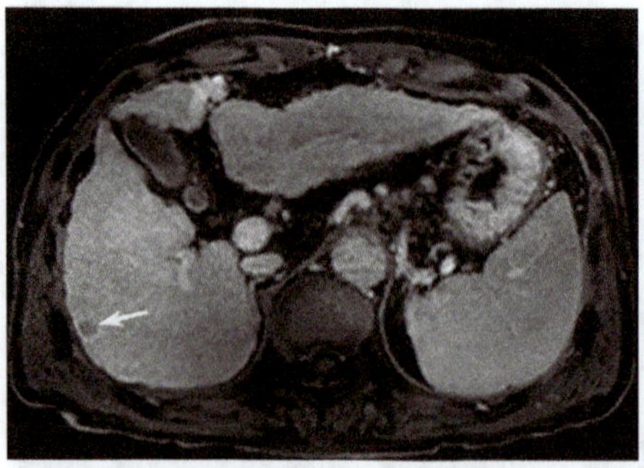

(a) Delayed-phase MRI obtained three minutes after contrast injection showing a 1.1-cm hypointense nodule (arrow) with peripheral rim enhancement in segment 6. Note that the tumor abuts the liver capsule and is located close to the right rib

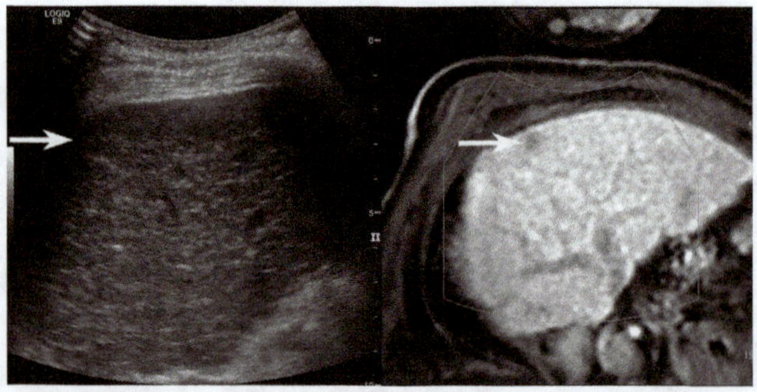

(b) On planning US with fusion imaging, a subtle hypoechoic lesion (arrow) was identified at a similar location (arrow) on fused MRI; the lesion was given a conspicuity score of 3 as it was nearly isoechoic to the surrounding liver and less than 50% of the tumor had a well-defined margin

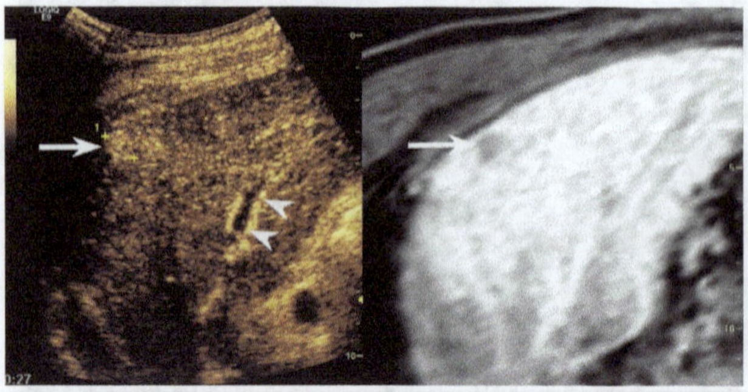

(c) On arterial-phase CEUS, the lesion identified on the previous fusion images did not show arterial enhancement. When the patient breathed in slightly, the liver moved somewhat downwards and the true enhanced lesion (arrow), which was initially located below the right rib, appeared. Note that a portal vein branch (arrowheads) is not seen on US in (**b**), indicating that the image plane is different from that of (**b**) even though the US image was obtained at the same intercostal space

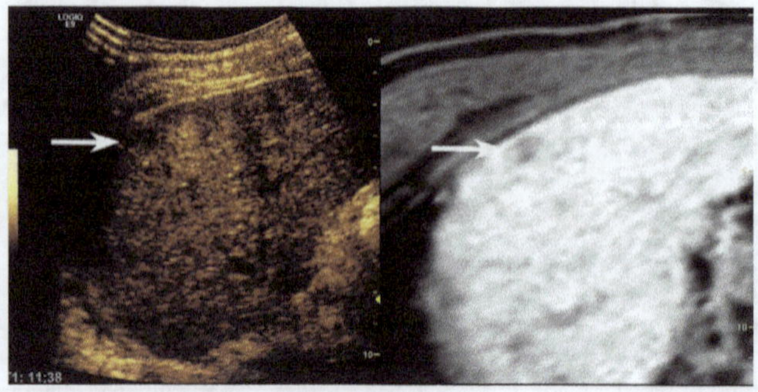

(d) The lesion was seen as a defect (arrow) on the post-vascular phase and the tumor was given a conspicuity score of 1 on CEUS-added fusion imaging

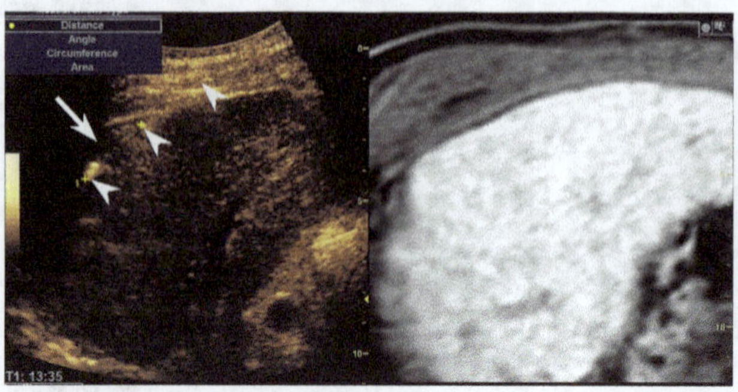

(e) An RF electrode (arrowheads) was positioned in the index tumor (arrow) with confidence under CEUS-added fusion imaging guidance, after which RF energy was applied

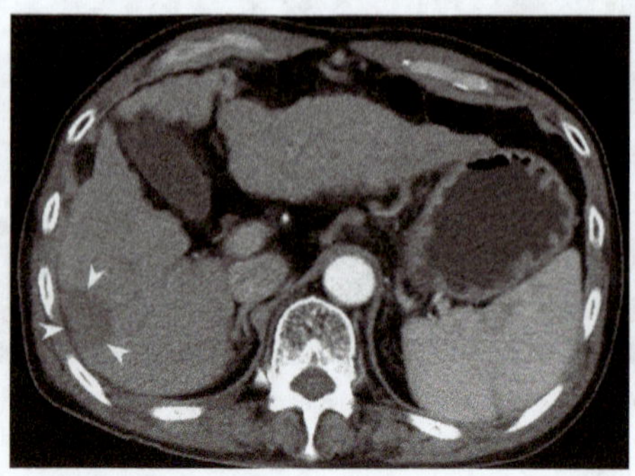

(f) Arterial-phase image of post-RFA CT revealed complete ablation of the tumor with sufficient ablative margins (arrowheads)

FIGURE 4: Images from a 65-year-old man with a recurrent HCC and hepatitis B virus-related liver cirrhosis who had previously undergone chemoembolization for HCC.

of technical success, primary technique efficacy, major complications, and LTP were excellent. Therefore, we propose that adding CEUS is a valuable strategy for accurate guidance of RFA for small (1–2 cm) HCCs inconspicuous on FI alone.

FI has been used in combination with CEUS for guidance of percutaneous RFA of HCCs in previous studies [10–12, 15, 23]. However, these studies were limited by selection bias due to their retrospective nature. Moreover, although they demonstrated the technical feasibility of combined FI and CEUS guidance, few studies have evaluated long-term therapeutic outcomes such as LTP rate [10]. When applying both FI and CEUS, no standardized method has been suggested by any society of interventional radiology or international working group on image-guided tumor ablation. In one

TABLE 3: Baseline characteristics of 19 patients who underwent percutaneous CEUS-added FI-guided RFA.

Characteristics	$n = 19$
Age (mean ± SD, y) (range)	63.9 ± 9.3 (50–81)
Sex (female) [number (%)]	5 (26.3)
Etiology (HBV/HCV/other) [number (%)]	10 (52.6)/2 (10.5)/7 (36.8)
Liver cirrhosis [number (%)]	10 (52.6)
HCC history [number (%)]	
None	3(15.8)
Resection	3(15.8)
RFA	2(10.5)
TACE	6(31.6)
Other	5(26.3)
Child-Pugh class (A/B) [number (%)]	19 (100)/0 (0)
Albumin (mean ± SD, g/dl)	4.1 ± 0.4
Total bilirubin (mean ± SD, mg/dl)	1.0 ± 0.5
PT (mean ± SD, INR)	1.14 ± 0.11
Serum AFP (mean ± SD, ng/ml)	8.5 ± 7.3
Tumor size (mean ± SD, cm) (range)	1.2 ± 0.2 (1.0–1.8)
Segment [number (%)]	
I	0 (0)
II	1 (5.3)
III	2 (10.5)
IV	1 (5.3)
V	6 (31.6)
VI	3 (15.8)
VII	4 (21.1)
VIII	2 (10.5)
Subcapsular location[a] (yes) [numbers (%)]	5 (26.3)
Subphrenic location[b] (yes) [numbers (%)]	5 (26.3)
Time interval between MR imaging and planning US (mean ± SD, days) (range)	12.4 ± 6.8 (2–31)
Time interval between planning US and RFA (mean ± SD, days) (range)	12.9 ± 8.0 (0–32)
Conspicuity score (median, range)	3, 3–4 (before CEUS) 1, 1–4 (after CEUS)
Follow-up after RFA (median, range) (months)	30.2, 14.0–36.9

Data are presented as the number of patients or tumors with percentages in parentheses, unless otherwise specified.
AFP = α-fetoprotein; FI = fusion imaging; HBV = hepatitis B virus; HCV = hepatitis C virus; INR = international normalized ratio; PT = prothrombin time; RFA = radiofrequency ablation; TACE = transcatheter arterial chemoembolization; SD = standard deviation.
[a] Subcapsular location was defined as when the index tumor abutted the liver capsule.
[b] Subphrenic location was defined as when the index tumor was located within 1 cm from the diaphragm [6].

TABLE 4: Therapeutic outcomes after CEUS-added FI-guided RFA.

Outcome	$n = 19$
Number of ablation sessions (mean ± SD)	1.1 ± 0.2
Technical success rate (%)	94.7% (18/19)
Primary technique efficacy rate (%)	100% (19/19)
Major complication rate (%)	0% (0/19)
Local tumor progression rate (%)	10.5% (2/19)

study, CEUS was applied first, followed by FI [14], whereas in other studies, FI was applied first, followed by CEUS [11, 15, 23]. Both methods have also been used in a single study [10]. Although no data have been obtained to evaluate which method is better, we propose that FI be applied first because it requires no additional cost related to contrast agents in most cases. As demonstrated in our study, many small HCCs can still be identified using only FI. In addition, the overall procedure time of CEUS-guided RFA can be substantially decreased if FI is applied first.

This is because the location of the target lesion can be estimated based on fused CT/MRI, which obviates the need for a second injection of Sonazoid to obtain the optimal arterial phase of the target lesion [11]. Moreover, when FI is applied first, image fusion can be performed within 3–4 minutes using manual registration methods [2, 5]. Nowadays, automatic registration methods facilitate easier and faster image fusion [24, 25]. Therefore, this procedure is much faster than typical CEUS performed using Sonazoid, in which a waiting period of about 10 minutes is needed after the initiation of contrast agent injection to obtain optimal post-vascular phase imaging.

Tumor size is one of the most important factors affecting lesion conspicuity on both B-mode US and FI of B-mode US and CT/MRI [1, 16, 26]. As expected, the mean size of tumors inconspicuous on FI was only 1.2 cm in our cohort. However, the rate of primary technique efficacy after percutaneous CEUS-added FI-guided RFA was 100% (19/19) and the LTP rate at 3 years was 10.8%. This implies that small HCCs (BCLC stage 0) can be ablated effectively once they are accurately localized.

According to a previous study [6], subphrenic or subcapsular tumor location is an important factor affecting mistargeting after FI-guided RFA of HCCs. Peripheral tumor location implies that large anatomic landmarks such as the portal vein branch cannot be used to locate the tumor. In addition, some tumors can be obscured by the rib shadow. Moreover, liver deformation and movement due to a patient's breathing or heart beat may be more apparent in peripheral liver than in central liver [6, 27]. This technical difficulty of percutaneous RFA of tumors in peripheral locations was also observed in our study. Residual tumor was noted in one patient with a tumor located in the subcapsular area, just below the right rib. Nevertheless, mistargeting or incomplete ablation can be avoided after CEUS, as seen in one of our cases (Figure 4).

Our study did have several limitations. First, this was a single-center study conducted at a tertiary academic hospital with a large volume of RFAs. In general, outcomes after RFA depend on operator experience. Also, 75% (66/88) of the study population had hepatitis B-related liver disease; thus, the results of this study may not be generalizable to other institutions or countries where hepatitis B virus is not the primary cause of liver cirrhosis or HCC. Second, lesion conspicuity was graded by one of three experienced radiologists and interobserver agreement was not assessed because the conspicuity score was graded in a prospective manner at the time of US examination. Third, more patients were excluded than expected before initiating the study. For example, four patients in whom artificial ascites was used during RFA were excluded from our final patient population because artificial ascites can enhance lesion conspicuity by improving the sonographic window [28]. Since we sought to determine the direct effect of CEUS on lesion conspicuity during percutaneous FI-guided RFA, this exclusion criterion may not have significantly affected our study outcome. Fourth, CEUS was selectively applied to a small number of patients with HCCs inconspicuous on FI alone because FI was sufficient for guidance of RFA of HCCs in many cases [5, 16]. Therefore, comparing the rate of conspicuous HCCs between FI alone and CEUS-added FI may yield limited insight. Applying CEUS to the entire study sample could have provided a more comprehensive understanding of the advantages and disadvantages of combined FI and CEUS.

In conclusion, adding CEUS to FI significantly improved the conspicuity of HCCs inconspicuous on FI alone, which enabled direct targeting for percutaneous RFA. This led to successful percutaneous RFA with excellent therapeutic outcomes.

Acknowledgments

This study was supported in part by a grant from GE Healthcare.

References

[1] M. W. Lee, Y. J. Kim, H. S. Park et al., "Targeted sonography for small hepatocellular carcinoma discovered by CT or MRI: Factors affecting sonographic detection," *American Journal of Roentgenology*, vol. 194, no. 5, pp. W396–W400, 2010.

[2] J. H. Min, M. W. Lee, H. Rhim et al., "Radiofrequency ablation for viable hepatocellular carcinoma around retained iodized oil after transcatheter arterial chemoembolization: Usefulness of biplane fluoroscopy plus ultrasound guidance," *Korean Journal of Radiology*, vol. 13, no. 6, pp. 784–794, 2012.

[3] G. Mauri, L. Cova, S. De Beni et al., "Real-Time US-CT/MRI Image Fusion for Guidance of Thermal Ablation of Liver Tumors Undetectable with US: Results in 295 Cases," *CardioVascular and Interventional Radiology*, vol. 38, no. 1, pp. 143–151, 2015.

[4] Y. Minami, H. Chung, M. Kudo et al., "Radiofrequency ablation of hepatocellular carcinoma: Value of virtual CT sonography with magnetic navigation," *American Journal of Roentgenology*, vol. 190, no. 6, pp. W335–W341, 2008.

[5] S. J. Ahn, J. M. Lee, D. H. Lee et al., "Real-time US-CT/MR fusion imaging for percutaneous radiofrequency ablation of hepatocellular carcinoma," *Journal of Hepatology*, vol. 66, no. 2, pp. 347–354, 2017.

[6] S. Lim, M. W. Lee, H. Rhim et al., "Mistargeting after fusion imaging-guided percutaneous radiofrequency ablation of hepatocellular carcinomas," *Journal of Vascular and Interventional Radiology*, vol. 25, no. 2, pp. 307–314, 2014.

[7] R. Masuzaki, S. Shiina, R. Tateishi et al., "Utility of contrast-enhanced ultrasonography with Sonazoid in radiofrequency ablation for hepatocellular carcinoma," *Journal of Gastroenterology and Hepatology*, vol. 26, no. 4, pp. 759–764, 2011.

[8] Y. Minami, M. Kudo, K. Hatanaka et al., "Radiofrequency ablation guided by contrast harmonic sonography using perfluorocarbon microbubbles (Sonazoid) for hepatic malignancies: An initial experience," *Liver International*, vol. 30, no. 5, pp. 759–764, 2010.

[9] M. Kudo, K. Hatanaka, and K. Maekawa, "Newly developed novel ultrasound technique, defect reperfusion ultrasound imaging, using Sonazoid in the management of hepatocellular carcinoma," *Oncology*, vol. 78, no. 1, pp. 40–45, 2010.

[10] T. Minami, Y. Minami, H. Chishina et al., "Combination guidance of contrast-enhanced us and fusion imaging in radiofrequency ablation for hepatocellular carcinoma with poor con-

spicuity on contrast-enhanced US/fusion imaging," *Oncology (Switzerland)*, vol. 87, pp. 55–62, 2014.

[11] J. H. Y. Min, H. K. E. Lim, S. Lim et al., "Radiofrequency ablation of very-early-stage hepatocellular carcinoma inconspicuous on fusion imaging with B-mode US: value of fusion imaging with contrast-enhanced US," *Clinical and Molecular Hepatology*, vol. 20, no. 1, pp. 61–70, 2014.

[12] X.-W. Bo, H.-X. Xu, D. Wang et al., "Fusion imaging of contrast-enhanced ultrasound and contrast-enhanced CT or MRI before radiofrequency ablation for liver cancers," *British Journal of Radiology*, vol. 89, no. 1067, Article ID 20160379, 2016.

[13] G. Mauri, E. Porazzi, L. Cova et al., "Intraprocedural contrast-enhanced ultrasound (CEUS) in liver percutaneous radiofrequency ablation: Clinical impact and health technology assessment," *Insights into Imaging*, vol. 5, no. 2, pp. 209–216, 2014.

[14] Y. Dong, W.-P. Wang, F. Mao, Z.-B. Ji, and B.-J. Huang, "Application of imaging fusion combining contrast-enhanced ultrasound and magnetic resonance imaging in detection of hepatic cellular carcinomas undetectable by conventional ultrasound," *Journal of Gastroenterology and Hepatology*, vol. 31, no. 4, pp. 822–828, 2016.

[15] E. M. Jung, C. Friedrich, P. Hoffstetter et al., "Volume navigation with contrast enhanced ultrasound and image fusion for percutaneous interventions: First results," *PLoS ONE*, vol. 7, no. 3, Article ID e33956, 2012.

[16] M. W. Lee, H. Rhim, D. Ik Cha, Y. Jun Kim, and H. K. Lim, "Planning US for percutaneous radiofrequency ablation of small hepatocellular carcinomas (1-3 cm): Value of fusion imaging with conventional US and CT/MR Images," *Journal of Vascular and Interventional Radiology*, vol. 24, no. 7, pp. 958–965, 2013.

[17] H. Rhim, D. Choi, Y.-S. Kim, H. K. Lim, and B.-K. Choe, "Ultrasonography-guided percutaneous radiofrequency ablation of hepatocellular carcinomas: A feasibility scoring system for planning sonography," *European Journal of Radiology*, vol. 75, no. 2, pp. 253–258, 2010.

[18] H. Rhim, H. L. Mi, Y.-S. Kim, D. Choi, J. L. Won, and H. K. Lim, "Planning sonography to assess the feasibility of percutaneous radiofrequency ablation of hepatocellular carcinomas," *American Journal of Roentgenology*, vol. 190, no. 5, pp. 1324–1330, 2008.

[19] J.-E. Kim, Y.-S. Kim, H. Rhim et al., "Outcomes of patients with hepatocellular carcinoma referred for percutaneous radiofrequency ablation at a tertiary center: Analysis focused on the feasibility with the use of ultrasonography guidance," *European Journal of Radiology*, vol. 79, no. 2, pp. e80–e84, 2011.

[20] J. Bruix and M. Sherman, "Management of hepatocellular carcinoma: an update," *Hepatology*, vol. 53, no. 3, pp. 1020–1022, 2011.

[21] M. Ahmed, L. Solbiati, C. L. Brace et al., "Image-guided tumor ablation: standardization of terminology and reporting criteria–a 10-year update," *J Vasc Interv Radiol*, vol. 25, no. 11, pp. 1691–1705, 2014.

[22] M. W. Lee, H. Rhim, D. I. Cha et al., "Percutaneous radiofrequency ablation of hepatocellular carcinoma: Fusion imaging guidance for management of lesions with poor conspicuity at conventional sonography," *American Journal of Roentgenology*, vol. 198, no. 6, pp. 1438–1444, 2012.

[23] M. W. Lee, "Fusion imaging of real-time ultrasonography with CT or MRI for hepatic intervention," *Ultrasonography*, vol. 33, no. 4, pp. 227–239, 2014.

[24] G. Mauri, S. De Beni, L. Forzoni et al., "Virtual navigator automatic registration technology in abdominal application," *Conference proceedings : ... Annual International Conference of the IEEE Engineering in Medicine and Biology Society. IEEE Engineering in Medicine and Biology Society. Annual Conference*, vol. 2014, pp. 5570–5574, 2014.

[25] D. I. Cha, M. W. Lee, A. Y. Kim et al., "Automatic image fusion of real-time ultrasound with computed tomography images: A prospective comparison between two auto-registration methods," *Acta Radiologica*, vol. 58, no. 11, pp. 1349–1357, 2017.

[26] Y. Kunishi, K. Numata, M. Morimoto et al., "Efficacy of fusion imaging combining sonography and hepatobiliary phase MRI with Gd-EOB-DTPA to detect small hepatocellular carcinoma," *American Journal of Roentgenology*, vol. 198, no. 1, pp. 106–114, 2012.

[27] M. W. Lee, H. J. Park, T. W. Kang et al., "Image Fusion of Real-Time Ultrasonography with Computed Tomography: Factors Affecting the Registration Error and Motion of Focal Hepatic Lesions," *Ultrasound in Medicine & Biology*, vol. 43, no. 9, pp. 2024–2032, 2017.

[28] H. Rhim, H. K. Lim, Y.-S. Kim, and D. Choi, "Percutaneous radiofrequency ablation with artificial ascites for hepatocellular carcinoma in the hepatic dome: Initial experience," *American Journal of Roentgenology*, vol. 190, no. 1, pp. 91–98, 2008.

Gastric Peroral Endoscopic Myotomy (G-POEM) as a Treatment for Refractory Gastroparesis: Long-Term Outcomes

Jiaxin Xu,[1] Tianyin Chen,[1] Shaimaa Elkholy,[2] Meidong Xu,[1] Yunshi Zhong,[1] Yiqun Zhang,[1] Weifeng Chen,[1] Wenzheng Qin,[1] Mingyan Cai,[1] and Pinghong Zhou[1]

[1]*Endoscopy Centre and Endoscopy Research Institute, Zhongshan Hospital, Fudan University, Shanghai, China*
[2]*Internal Medicine Department, Gastroenterology Division, Faculty of Medicine, Cairo University, Egypt*

Correspondence should be addressed to Mingyan Cai; cai.mingyan@zs-hospital.sh.cn and Pinghong Zhou; zhou.pinghong@zs-hospital.sh.cn

Academic Editor: Maikel P. Peppelenbosch

Background and Aims. Gastric peroral endoscopic myotomy (G-POEM) has been regarded as a novel and minimally invasive therapy for refractory gastroparesis. This study reports the long-term outcomes and possible predictive factors for successful outcomes after G-POEM in an Asian population. *Methods.* This is a retrospective single-centre study of 16 patients who underwent G-POEM for refractory gastroparesis from August 2016 to October 2017. This study included 11 males and 5 females; in addition, 13 patients had postsurgical gastroparesis, and 3 patients had diabetes. The patients included had severe and refractory gastroparesis, as indicated by a Gastroparesis Cardinal Symptom Index (GCSI) score ≥20, and evidence of a delay on gastric emptying scintigraphy (GES). The primary outcome parameter was an assessment of the long-term clinical efficacy of the procedure. The secondary outcome parameter was the detection of possible predictive factors for success and the determination of cut-off values for such predictors. *Results.* Technical success was achieved in 100% of the patients, with a mean procedure time of 45.25±12.96 min. The long-term clinical response was assessed in all patients during a median follow-up of 14.5 months. Clinical success was achieved in 13 (81.25%) patients. There was a significant reduction in the GCSI scores and GES values after the procedure compared to the baseline values, with P values of <0.0001 and 0.012, respectively. Univariate regression analysis showed that the GCSI and GES had significant associations with the future clinical outcomes of the patients, but this finding was not confirmed in multivariate analysis. A GCSI cut-off score of ≤30 had a high sensitivity and a negative predictive value (NPV) of 100% for predicting a successful procedure. GES (half emptying time ≤221.6 min and 2-hour retention ≤78.6%) had a high specificity and a positive predictive value (PPV) of 100%. *Conclusions.* G-POEM is a safe and effective treatment option with a long-term efficacy of 81.6%. GCSI and GES could serve as good predictive measures.

1. Introduction

Gastroparesis is a chronic and debilitating gastric motility disorder with limited effective therapeutic options [1]. This disorder can result in frequent hospitalization and repeated nutrition support interventions. Multiple conditions have been associated with gastroparesis, and most aetiologies are postsurgical, diabetic, or idiopathic [2]. The pathogenesis of delayed gastric emptying is associated with fundus abnormalities, antrum and antroduodenal discoordination, pyloric dysfunction, and abnormal small bowel motility [3]. The pathogenesis of gastroparesis comprises two main components: altered gastric motility and increased pyloric pressure. Currently available medical therapies have limited efficacy and the potential for significant adverse events [4].

A recent innovation of the endoscopic submucosal tunnelling technique is gastric peroral endoscopic myotomy (G-POEM). This technique is emerging as a promising option for the treatment of refractory gastroparesis. In 2013, Khashab et al. [5] reported the first human case in a 27-year-old woman who was diagnosed with insulin-dependent diabetes mellitus at age 17 and was evaluated in the clinic for diabetic gastroparesis. Twelve weeks after the procedure, she remained well with significant improvement in daily symptoms and was

Table 1: Gastroparesis Cardinal Symptom Index (GCSI).

	None	Very mild	Mild	Moderate	Severe	Very severe
Nausea (feeling sick to your stomach as if you were going to vomit or throw up)	0	1	2	3	4	5
Retching (heaving as if to vomit, but nothing comes up)	0	1	2	3	4	5
Vomiting	0	1	2	3	4	5
Stomach fullness	0	1	2	3	4	5
Not able to finish a normal-sized meal	0	1	2	3	4	5
Feeling excessively full after a meal	0	1	2	3	4	5
Loss of appetite	0	1	2	3	4	5
Bloating (feeling like you need to loosen your clothes)	0	1	2	3	4	5
Stomach or belly visibly large	0	1	2	3	4	5

able to tolerate a soft diet appropriately. Since then, several case reports [6, 7] and small case series [8, 9] have been published. Mekaroonkamol et al. [10] reported symptomatic improvement in patients with postinfection, postsurgery, and idiopathic gastroparesis. This technique is starting to attract attention due to its minimally invasive nature and promising initial outcomes. The overall data are still very limited. Thus, we report the long-term outcomes for Asian patients who underwent G-POEM, focusing on the predictive factors of clinical success.

2. Patients and Methods

2.1. Study Design and Inclusion Criteria. This study is a retrospective study that was designed to analyse data from 16 consecutive patients who underwent G-POEM performed by an expert endoscopist for refractory gastroparesis between August 2016 and October 2017 at Zhongshan Hospital. The inclusion criteria were as follows: (1) patients who were older than 18 years old; (2) patients who had gastroparesis based on the presence of symptoms, including postprandial fullness/early satiety, nausea/vomiting, and bloating, and who had a score ≥20 on the Gastroparesis Cardinal Symptom Index (GCSI) (Table 1) and evidence of impairment in gastric emptying scintigraphy (GES) (either a delay in the half emptying time or a retention percentage >60% at 2 hours); and (3) patients who were refractory to conservative treatment, including dietary modification and drug therapy with prokinetics and antiemetics. All patients received conservative treatment and showed minimal response to traditional medical therapy. Medication, such as proton pump inhibitors (PPIs), metoclopramide, mosapride, and domperidone, was given to all patients (100%), and a nasojejunal nutrition tube was placed in five patients (31.3%).

GES was performed using 50 g of bread marked with a nuclear tracer, and patients were scanned in the supine position. However, 2 patients completed GES in a semireclining position to avoid aspiration because they vomited violently after lying down.

The exclusion criteria included patients younger than 18 years old, patients whose endoscopy showed peptic ulcer or gastric outlet obstruction (tumour, fibrosis, etc.), and patients who had GCSI<20, normal GES, or any contraindication to G-POEM or anaesthesia.

The study was approved by the Ethics Committee of Fudan University. Written informed consent was obtained before the endoscopic procedure. Patient demographics and related medical history data (aetiology of gastroparesis, gastroparetic symptoms, GCSI score, results of GES, procedure details (length of tunnel and myotomy, closure method, and procedure time), adverse events, duration of hospital stay, and follow-up (GES and GCSI score)) were evaluated.

2.2. G-POEM Procedure. The G-POEM procedure was performed with single-channel gastroscopy or dual-channel endoscopy (GIF-H260 or GIF-2T240, Olympus). To provide a better view of the submucosal layer, a transparent cap (D-201-11802, Olympus) was attached to the tip. Other equipment included a hybrid knife (T-type, Erbe, Germany), hot biopsy forceps (FD-410LR, Olympus), clips (HX-610-90, HX-600-135, Olympus; ROCC-D-26-195, Micro-Tech, Nanjing, China), an OverStitch suturing device (Apollo Endosurgery, Austin, Texas), and a high-frequency generator (VIO-200, Erbe, Germany).

All patients were treated under general anaesthesia with tracheal intubation. The G-POEM procedure was performed as follows. (a) A submucosal cushion was created by submucosal injection (a mixed solution of 100 ml saline, 1 ml indigo carmine, and 1 ml epinephrine). (b) A mucosal incision was made 5 cm from the pylorus in the greater curvature of the stomach. (c) A submucosal tunnel was created from the mucosal entry to approximately 1 cm over the pylorus. (d) Full-thickness myotomy was performed from 2 to 3 cm proximal to the pylorus to 1 cm beyond the duodenal bulb. (e) After haemostasis, the mucosal entry was closed with metal

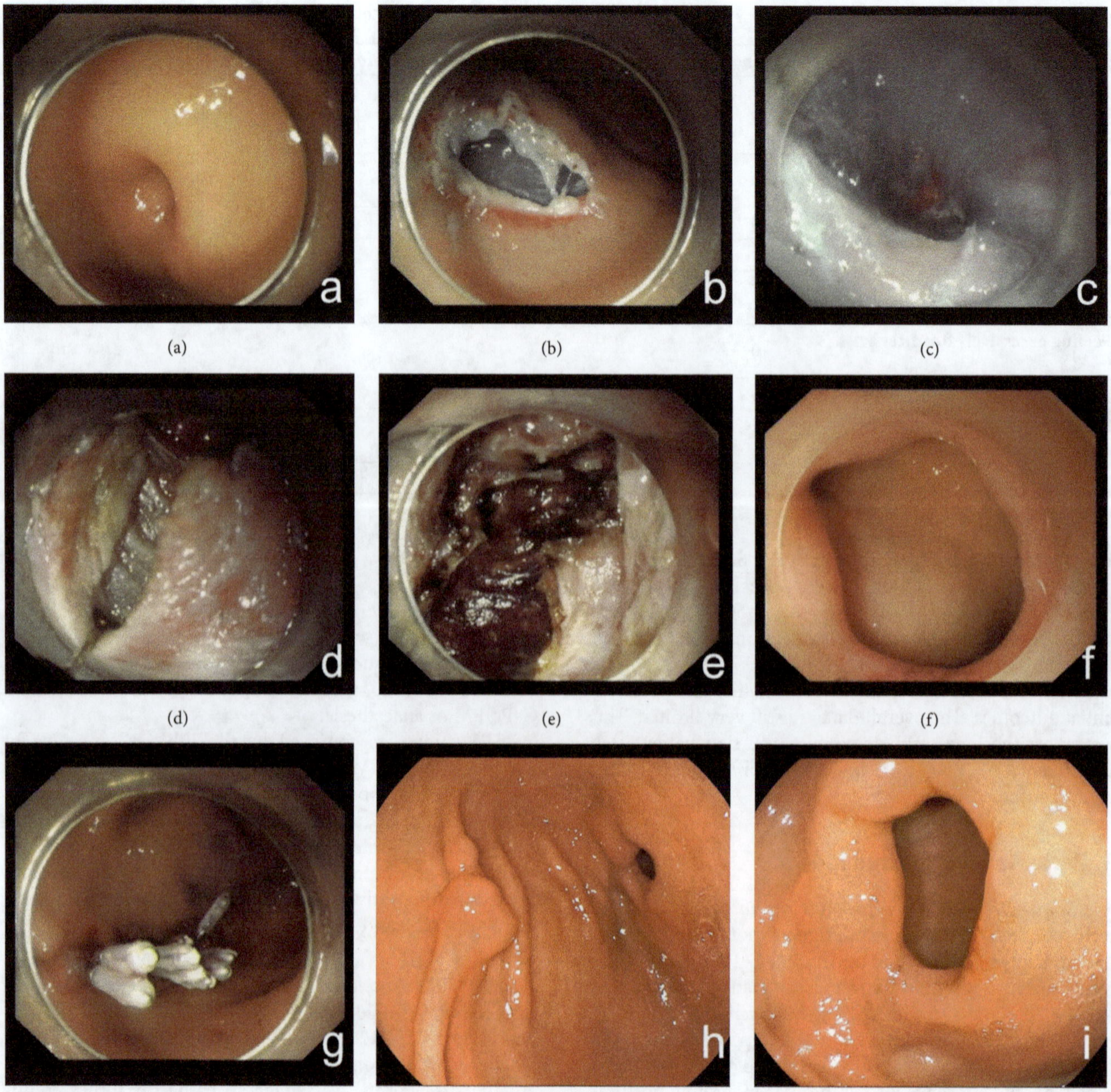

(a) (b) (c)

(d) (e) (f)

(g) (h) (i)

Figure 1: G-POEM procedure: (a) endoscopic view of the narrow pylorus; (b) injection and submucosal incision made 3 to 4 cm from the pylorus in the greater curvature of the antrum; (c) tunnel creation to approximately 2 cm passing over the pylorus; (d)-(e) myotomy of the pyloric and antral muscular layers; (f) endoscopic view of the pylorus after G-POEM; (g) mucosal entry closure by metal clips; (h) mucosal entry scar after 3 months of healing; and (i) endoscopic view of the pylorus after 3 months.

clips or a suturing device (Figure 1). The mucosal incision was closed by metallic clips in thirteen patients (81.2%) and by an endoscopic suture device (OverStitch) in three patients (18.8%). During the procedure, mucosal injury occurred in three patients and was closed completely by metallic clips.

2.3. Perioperative Management. Before the G-POEM procedure, routine blood tests, including complete blood counts and coagulation profiles, and electrocardiography were obtained to evaluate the patient's general condition. PPIs and intravenous antibiotics were administered conventionally to all patients after G-POEM. The patients' abdominal symptoms and signs were carefully monitored during the postoperative period. Patients were discharged on PPIs for two months.

2.4. Follow-Up. Gastric emptying function was assessed by GES in our hospital three months after G-POEM, and

TABLE 2: Demographic features, clinical features, and follow-up.

Age (years, median (range))	63.5 (26-82)
Gender (ratio, male/female)	11/5
Aetiology of gastroparesis	
Postsurgical	13 (81.2%)
Diabetic	3 (18.8%)
Duration of disease before G-POEM (months, median (range))	22 (2-84)
Previous therapy	
PPIs	16 (100%)
Metoclopramide	14 (87.5%)
Nasojejunal nutrition tube	5 (31.3%)
GCSI score (mean (±SD)) before G-POEM	
Nausea	3.37±1.59
Retching	2.56±1.82
Vomiting	3.75±1.61
Stomach fullness	3.13±1.67
Not able to finish a normal-sized meal	4.06±1.18
Feeling excessively full after a meal	3.31±1.54
Loss of appetite	1.94±1.98
Bloating	1.94±1.88
Stomach or belly visibly large	0.19±0.75
Total	24.25±5.47
Gastric emptying scintigraphy before G-POEM	
Half emptying time (min, mean (±SD))	183.20±77.39
Retention at 2 hours (mean (±SD))	69.33±11.46%
Technical success rate	100%
Procedure time (min, mean (±SD))	45.25±12.96
Closure of mucosal incision	
Metal clip	13 (81.2%)
Overstitch	3 (18.8%)
Hospital stay (days, median (range))	6 (4-10)
Intraoperative adverse events	0
Follow-up time (months, median (range))	14.5 (5-19)
Total GCSI score (mean (±SD)) after G-POEM	6.37±6.34
Gastric emptying scintigraphy (n=8) after G-POEM	
Half emptying time (min, mean (±SD))	83.98±34.65
Retention at 2 hours	33.38±18.17%
Long-term clinical remission	13 (81.3%)

G-POEM: gastric per oral endoscopy myotomy, GSCI: Gastroparesis Cardinal Symptom Index.

the patients' symptoms were measured by GCSI after the procedure (at one month, three months, and every 6 months thereafter). The first endoscopic follow-up was arranged within 3 months after G-POEM, and the procedure was repeated annually thereafter to observe wound healing and monitor potential reflux.

2.5. Outcome Parameters. The primary outcome parameter was an assessment of the clinical efficacy of G-POEM, which was defined by symptomatic improvement of the patient and *a significant drop in the GCSI* at least > 50% of the baseline and without the need for further hospitalizations for nutritional support [11].

The secondary outcome parameter was the identification of possible predictive factors for clinical success and the detection of possible cut-off values for such predictive factors.

3. Results

This study included a total of sixteen patients; 11 (68.7%) patients were males, and 5 (31.3%) patients were females. Their ages ranged from 26 to 82 years, with a median age of 63.5 years. Thirteen patients were postsurgical (81.2%), and three patients had diabetes (18.8%). The patients' demographic data and clinical features are shown in Table 2.

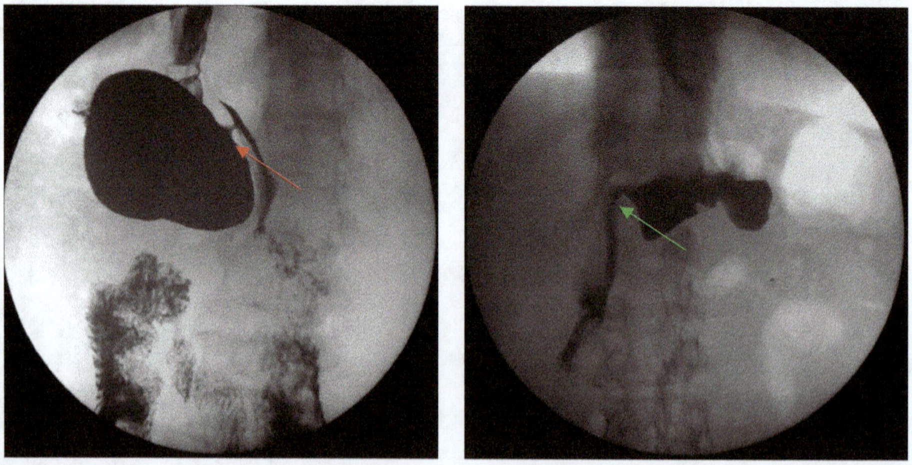

(a) (b)

FIGURE 2: (a) Upper gastrointestinal radiography before G-POEM showing a narrow pyloric canal (shown with a red arrow) in the patient post-subtotal gastrectomy and (b) upper gastrointestinal radiography showing contrast passing freely through the pylorus after G-POEM (shown with a green arrow).

Before the G-POEM procedure, all patients suffered from severe nausea/vomiting, fullness/early satiety and bloating. The GCSI score ranged from 20 to 38, with a mean (±SD) of 24.25 (±5.47). Early satiety, vomiting, and nausea were the top three predominant symptoms, with mean scores of 4.06±1.18, 3.75±1.61, and 3.37±1.59, respectively, as shown in Table 2. Patients who underwent proximal subtotal gastrectomy were recommended for upper gastrointestinal radiography, and a narrow pyloric canal was found in all patients (Figure 2).

The GES half emptying time ranged from 102.2 to 328.9 min, with a mean (±SD) of 183.20±77, while the mean retention time at 2 hours ranged from 60.2% to 92%, with a mean (±SD) of 69.33±11.46%.

The G-POEM procedure was achieved successfully in all patients (100%), with a mean procedure time of 45.25±12.96 min. No severe intraoperative adverse events, including significant bleeding or pneumoperitoneum, occurred. The median hospital stay was 6 days (range: 4-10 days). No procedure-related adverse events, such as mucosal tears, delayed bleeding, or perforation, were observed. Only one patient developed pyloric stenosis secondary to scar formation on the 45th day, and he underwent endoscopic radial incision (ERI).

3.1. The Primary Outcome Parameter. Clinical response was assessed in all patients during a median follow-up of 14.5 months (range: 5-19 months). There were significant decreases in GCSI scores, mean half emptying time and 2-hour retention after G-POEM compared to the baseline values, with *P* values of <0.0001, 0.012, and 0.012, respectively (Table 3).

Thirteen (81.25%) patients showed a substantial long-term clinical improvement in symptoms related to delayed gastric emptying and GCSI scores.

Among the three patients who failed to experience a long-lasting improvement, one patient developed persistent vomiting on the 45th day after the procedure, as mentioned above.

TABLE 3: Patient assessments before and after G-POEM.

	Before G-POEM mean (±SD)	After G-POEM mean (±SD)	*P* value
GCSI	24.25±5.47	6.37±6.34	<0.001
GES			
Half emptying time (min)	183.20±77.39	83.98±34.65	0.012
Retention at 2 hours (%)	69.33±11.46%	33.38±18.17%	0.012

G-POEM: gastric per oral endoscopy myotomy, GSCI: Gastroparesis Cardinal Symptom Index, GES: gastric emptying scintigraphy.

Gastroscopy was performed and revealed pyloric stenosis secondary to scar formation. The patient received a salvage ERI and was discharged successfully after semifluid diet was allowed (Figure 3). The other two patients had suboptimal responses to G-POEM; both patients had a long-standing history of uncontrolled diabetes and were previously diagnosed with diabetic peripheral neuropathy. One patient showed little early response to G-POEM at the first follow-up (three months after the procedure); the GCSI score was 34 before the procedure and 28 after the procedure. The other patient showed marked improvement, with a GCSI score of 22 before the procedure and 10 after the first follow-up, at which he had gained approximately 10 kg in weight. However, he developed worsening of symptoms 7 months after G-POEM, and his GCSI started to increase again, reaching 19. Both patients were readmitted to the hospital for nutritional support.

3.2. The Secondary Outcome Parameter. Univariate regression analysis showed significant positive correlations of GCSI score and GES values with unfavourable future clinical outcomes of the patients (Table 4). The predictive factors identified in the univariate analysis were not confirmed in the multivariate analysis.

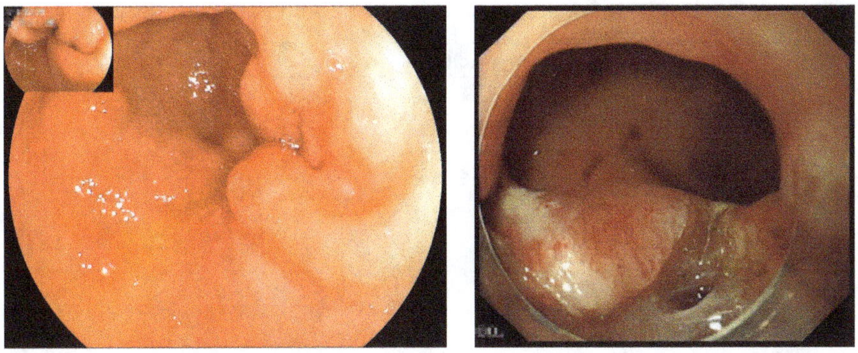

(a) (b)

Figure 3: (a) Endoscopic view of a recurrent patient showing the mucosa near the pylorus shrinking and the scar beneath contracting and (b) pylorus opened widely after endoscopic radial incision.

Table 4: Univariate regression analysis of the clinical outcomes of the patients.

	Coefficient	Odds Ratio	95% CI	*P* value
Age	0.11	1.1168	0.99-1.25	0.017
Disease duration	0.076	1.07	0.93-1.24	0.1255
GCSI	-0.3	0.74	0.54-1.0037	0.0157
Half emptying time	-0.021	0.971	0.95-1.0042	0.059
Retention at 2 hours	-0.204	0.815	0.65-1.008	0.0078

GSCI: Gastroparesis Cardinal Symptom Index.

GCSI scores had a high sensitivity (100%) and specificity (66.7%) at a cut-off value of ≤30 for predicting favourable clinical outcomes in patients (Figure 4). GCSI scores have a high negative predictive value (NPV) of 100% and a positive predictive value (PPV) of 92.86% (Table 5). The box plot showed that GCSI scores in those who achieved clinical success ranged from 20 to 30, with a median of 21 and an interquartile range (IQR) of 4, while the GCSI scores of those who failed to achieve clinical success ranged from 22 to 38, with a median of 34 and an IQR of 8 (Figure 5).

In GES, the half emptying time and the 2-hour retention had high specificity (100%) and sensitivity (84.6%) at cut-off values of <221.6 minutes and 78%, respectively (Figure 6). GES had a high PPV (100%) and an NPV of 59.97% (Table 5). Box plots of the half emptying time and the retention percentage at 2 hours showed ranges from 102.2 to 328.9 min and 60.2% to 92%, respectively, with median values (IQRs) of 185 (64) and 69 (13), respectively, among patients who achieved clinical success. Additionally, among patients who failed to achieve clinical success, these values ranged from 226.4 to 314.8 min and 80 to 92.8%, respectively, with median values (IQRs) of 260.7 (44) and 91.6 (6), respectively (Figure 7). Box plots of the GES including the half emptying time and the retention percentage at 2 hours against GSCI are shown in Figure 8.

4. Discussion

Gastroparesis is a clinical syndrome that is characterized by a delay in gastric emptying in the absence of true mechanical obstruction [12]. Gastric emptying entails interactions among smooth muscle, enteric and extrinsic autonomic nerves, and the interstitial cells of Cajal (ICCs) [13]. The exact pathogenesis of gastroparesis is not fully understood; however, multiple hypotheses have attempted to explain its pathogenesis. Autonomic neuropathy, gastric hypersensitivity, vagal nerve dysfunction impairing pyloric relaxation, loss of expression of neuronal nitric oxide synthase, and loss of ICCs are the most recent and most common hypotheses [14, 15]. Accordingly, the treatment of gastroparesis is usually directed towards targeted pathogenesis. Pharmacotherapy in the form of prokinetics and selective motilin and ghrelin agonists is the mainstay of treatment. However, pharmacotherapy has limited efficacy and undesirable side effects, including some side effects that are irreversible [16]. Gastric electrical stimulation has been reported in several studies [17, 18] and has shown some benefits, especially in relieving nausea/vomiting symptoms; however, the use of this approach is limited by uncontrolled trials and the high cost of surgical devices.

Recent therapeutic options have focused on relieving pylorospasm, which presents with increased pyloric tone and phasic contractions. These therapies include botulinum toxin injection, endoscopic transpyloric stent placement and fixation, and laparoscopic pyloroplasty. Several open-labelled studies on botulinum toxin injection [19–22] observed improvements in gastric emptying and symptoms for several months. However, two randomized double-blind placebo-controlled studies [20, 21] found no specific improvement in symptoms compared with placebo (saline solution injection). Nevertheless, botulinum toxin injection is still regarded as

TABLE 5: Predictive values for successful clinical outcomes in the patients.

	Sensitivity	Specificity	AUC	P value	PPV	NPV
GSCI	100%	66.7%	0.885	0.002	95.3%	100%
Half emptying time (min)	84.6%	100%	0.872	<0.001	100%	59.97%
Retention at 2 hours (%)	84.6%	100%	0.923	<0.001	100%	59.97%

GSCI: Gastroparesis Cardinal Symptom Index.

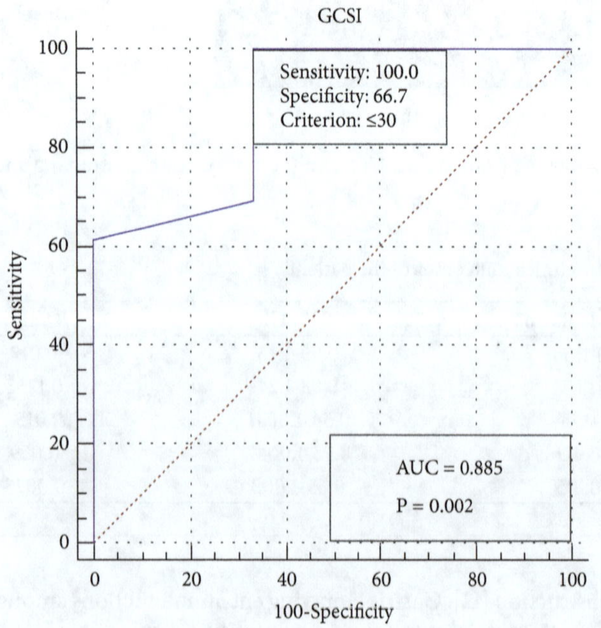

FIGURE 4: Receiver operating characteristic (ROC) curve showing 100% sensitivity and 66.7% specificity of the Gastroparesis Cardinal Symptom Index (GCSI) at a cut-off value ≤30 for predicting the clinical response of the patients.

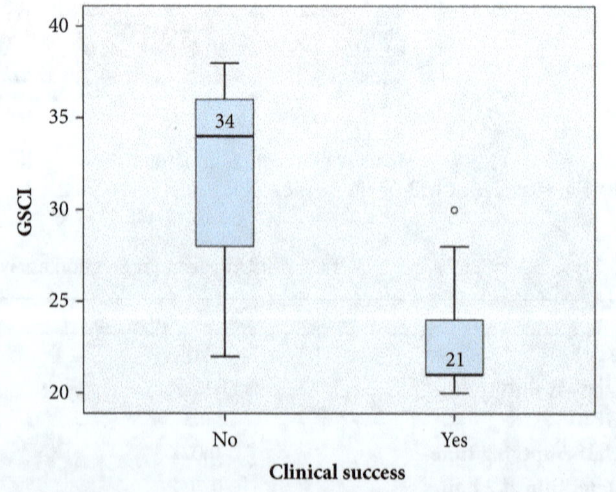

FIGURE 5: Box plot of the Gastroparesis Cardinal Symptom Index (GSCI) among patients who achieved clinical success and patients who did not.

a screening tool for patients who respond to therapies targeting pyloric and antral hypertonicity. Endoscopic transpyloric stent [23] and laparoscopic pyloroplasty [24] are two promising techniques associated with statistically significant reductions in symptoms. A long-term study [25] included 177 patients who underwent laparoscopic pyloroplasty over a period of five years and showed an 86% improvement in GES, with normalization in 77% of patients. Unfortunately, this technique still requires surgical abdominal entry with potential adverse events, including leakage, bleeding, and wound infections.

Building on the concept of relieving pylorospasm, endoscopic pyloromyotomy (G-POEM) evolved and is becoming a potential viable alternative for the treatment of gastroparesis. Herein, we present a series of Asian patients who were treated by this novel technique with encouraging outcomes. The mean procedure time was 45.25±12.96 min, which is consistent with most previous studies [7, 9, 11]. However, Xue et al. [26] stated that the use of fluoroscopic guidance with the placement of an endoclip on the pylorus at the 9 to 11 o'clock position to facilitate identification (a challenging step in G-POEM) significantly shortened the procedure time by approximately 36±13 min.

Technical success was achieved in all patients, and this finding is consistent with the results of many studies that reported the safety of the procedure. Questions remain concerning the efficacy of the procedure. We report an 81.25% clinical success rate with a mean follow-up period of 14.5 months. Gonzalez et al. showed success rates of 79% and 70% for periods of 3 and 6 months, respectively [27]. Additionally, a recent study showed a success rate of 81% with a follow-up of 6 months, which could represent a promising outcome for those patients [28].

In our study, we found that GCSI and GES showed significant improvements before and after procedure. Nevertheless, these parameters could also be used as predictive measures of clinical success after the procedure, with high sensitivity and NPV for the GCSI, which indicates that it is a good negative test at a cut-off value of ≤30. The GES appears to be a good positive test, with a high specificity and PPV for predicting clinical success based on both the half emptying time and the retention at 2 hours. Currently, there are no reliable ways to predict which patients will respond to G-POEM. A recent study that focused on the predictive factors for clinical response found that female gender and diabetes were predictors of failure after G-POEM [27].

The reasons for unresponsiveness remain unclear. The cause of gastroparesis has been investigated, especially in patients with diabetes [29, 30]; however, only 3 diabetic

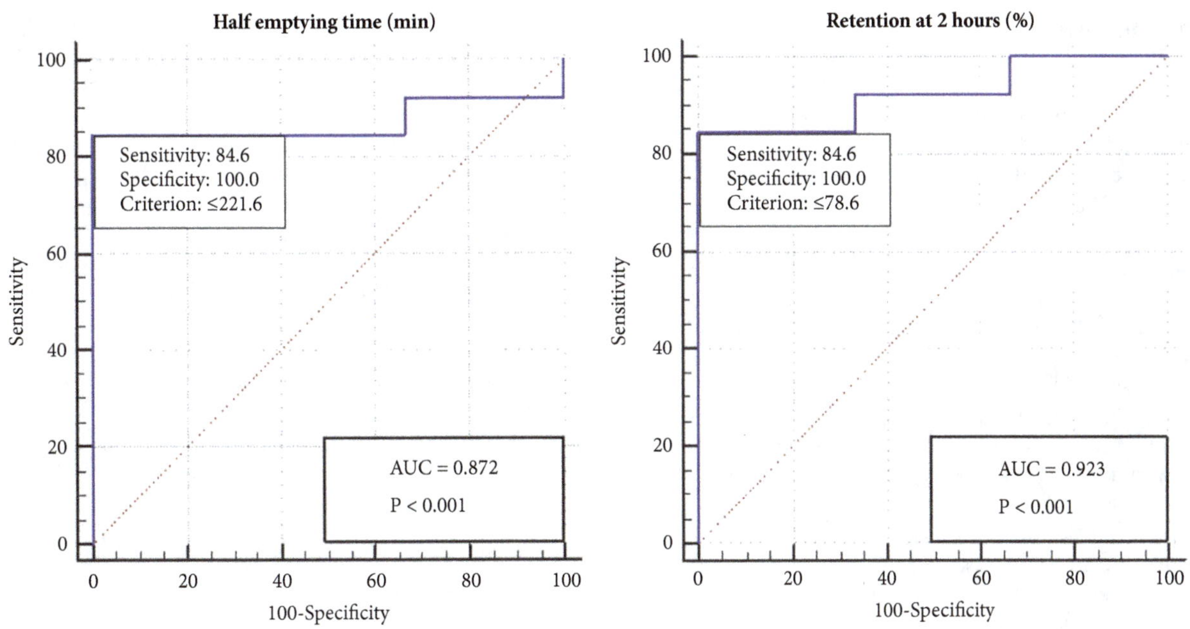

FIGURE 6: Receiver operating characteristic (ROC) curve showing 84.6% sensitivity and 100% specificity of gastric emptying scintigraphy (GES) for predicting the clinical response of the patients.

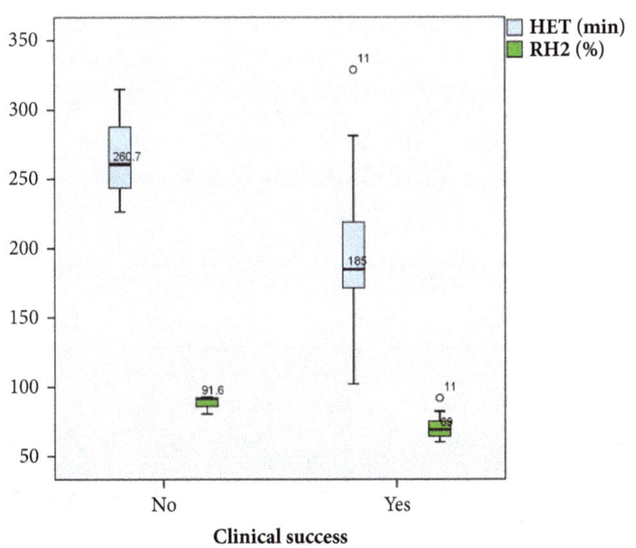

FIGURE 7: Box plot showing the distribution of gastric emptying scintigraphy (GES), including both half emptying time (HET) in minutes and retention percentage at 2 hours (RH2), among patients who achieved clinical success and patients who did not.

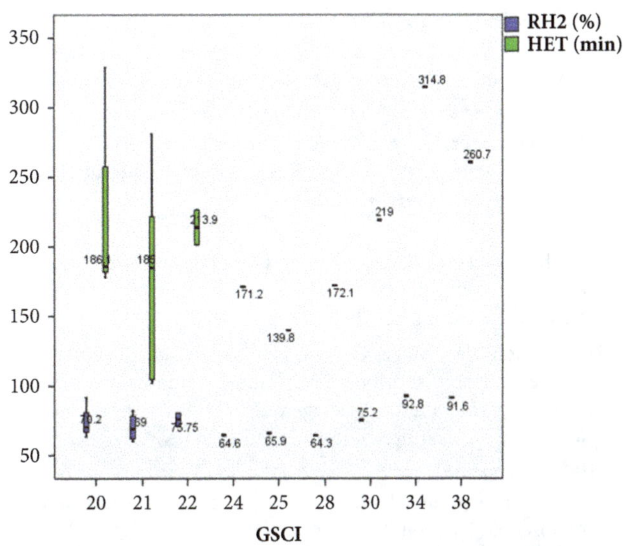

FIGURE 8: Box plot of the gastric emptying scintigraphy (GES) including the half emptying time (HET) and the retention percentage at 2 hours (RH2) against Gastroparesis Cardinal Symptom Index (GSCI).

patients were included in our study, and this number would not lead to clinical significance.

In conclusion, this study presents a promising long-term clinical outcome for G-POEM, with a high technical success rate and few adverse events. GCSI score and GES values could be used as predictors of favourable outcomes. Prospective multicentre randomized controlled trials are still needed to confirm these findings and determine the exact factors that predict patient responsiveness to G-POEM.

Disclosure

Dr. Elkholy shares the co-first authorship with Dr. Jiaxin Xu and Dr. Tianyin Chen.

Authors' Contributions

Jiaxin Xu and Tianyin Chen contributed equally to this work.

Acknowledgments

This study was supported by grants from the National Natural Science Foundation of China (81470811 and 81670483) (Dr. Pinghong Zhou) and the Major Project of the Shanghai Municipal Science and Technology Committee (16411950400 and 14441901500).

References

[1] W. L. Hasler, "Gastroparesis: Symptoms, Evaluation, and Treatment," *Gastroenterology Clinics of North America*, vol. 36, no. 3, pp. 619–647, 2007.

[2] H. P. Parkman, W. L. Hasler, and R. S. Fisher, "American gastroenterological association technical review on the diagnosis and treatment of gastroparesis," *Gastroenterology*, vol. 127, no. 5, pp. 1592–1622, 2004.

[3] J. H. Oh and P. J. Pasricha, "Recent advances in the pathophysiology and treatment of gastroparesis," *Journal of Neurogastroenterology and Motility*, vol. 19, no. 1, pp. 18–24, 2013.

[4] N. Liu and T. Abell, "Gastroparesis updates on pathogenesis and management," *Gut and Liver*, vol. 11, no. 5, pp. 579–589, 2017.

[5] M. A. Khashab, E. Stein, J. O. Clarke et al., "Gastric peroral endoscopic myotomy for refractory gastroparesis: First human endoscopic pyloromyotomy (with video)," *Gastrointestinal Endoscopy*, vol. 78, no. 5, pp. 764–768, 2013.

[6] H. Chung, B. Dallemagne, S. Perretta et al., "Endoscopic pyloromyotomy for postesophagectomy gastric outlet obstruction," *Endoscopy*, vol. 46, no. 1, pp. E345–E346, 2014.

[7] J.-M. Gonzalez, G. Vanbiervliet, V. Vitton et al., "First European human gastric peroral endoscopic myotomy, for treatment of refractory gastroparesis," *Endoscopy*, vol. 47, pp. E135–E136, 2015.

[8] E. Shlomovitz, R. Pescarus, M. A. Cassera et al., "Early human experience with per-oral endoscopic pyloromyotomy (POP)," *Surgical Endoscopy*, vol. 29, no. 3, pp. 543–551, 2014.

[9] J.-M. Gonzalez, V. Lestelle, A. Benezech et al., "Gastric peroral endoscopic myotomy with antropyloromyotomy in the treatment of refractory gastroparesis: clinical experience with follow-up and scintigraphic evaluation (with video)," *Gastrointestinal Endoscopy*, vol. 85, no. 1, pp. 132–139, 2017.

[10] P. Mekaroonkamol, L. Y. Li, S. Dacha et al., "Gastric peroral endoscopic pyloromyotomy (G-POEM) as a salvage therapy for refractory gastroparesis: a case series of different subtypes," *Neurogastroenterology & Motility*, vol. 28, no. 8, pp. 1272–1277, 2016.

[11] M. A. Khashab, S. Ngamruengphong, D. Carr-Locke et al., "Gastric per-oral endoscopic myotomy for refractory gastroparesis: results from the first multicenter study on endoscopic pyloromyotomy (with video)," *Gastrointestinal Endoscopy*, vol. 85, no. 1, pp. 123–128, 2017.

[12] P. Kashyap and G. Farrugia, "Diabetic gastroparesis: What we have learned and had to unlearn in the past 5 years," *Gut*, vol. 59, no. 12, pp. 1716–1726, 2010.

[13] R. H. Hunt, M. Camilleri, S. E. Crowe et al., "The stomach in health and disease," *Gut*, vol. 64, no. 10, pp. 1650–1668, 2015.

[14] C.-L. He, E. E. Soffer, C. D. Ferris, R. M. Walsh, J. H. Szurszewski, and G. Farrugia, "Loss of interstitial cells of Cajal and inhibitory innervation in insulin-dependent diabetes," *Gastroenterology*, vol. 121, no. 2, pp. 427–434, 2001.

[15] Z. Malik, R. Kataria, R. Modayil et al., "Gastric Per Oral Endoscopic Myotomy (G-POEM) for the Treatment of Refractory Gastroparesis: Early Experience," *Digestive Diseases and Sciences*, pp. 1–8, 2018.

[16] M. Camilleri, H. P. Parkman, M. A. Shafi, T. L. Abell, and L. Gerson, "Clinical guideline: management of gastroparesis," *American Journal of Gastroenterology*, vol. 108, no. 1, pp. 18–37, 2013.

[17] F. Brody, S. L. Zettervall, N. G. Richards et al., "Follow-up after gastric electrical stimulation for gastroparesis," *Journal of the American College of Surgeons*, vol. 220, no. 1, pp. 57–63, 2015.

[18] D. S. Keller, H. P. Parkman, D. O. Boucek et al., "Surgical Outcomes After Gastric Electric Stimulator Placement for Refractory Gastroparesis," *Journal of Gastrointestinal Surgery*, vol. 17, no. 4, pp. 620–626, 2013.

[19] R. Coleski, M. A. Anderson, and W. L. Hasler, "Factors associated with symptom response to pyloric injection of botulinum toxin in a large series of gastroparesis patients," *Digestive Diseases and Sciences*, vol. 54, no. 12, pp. 2634–2642, 2009.

[20] F. K. Friedenberg, A. Palit, H. P. Parkman, A. Hanlon, and D. B. Nelson, "Botulinum toxin A for the treatment of delayed gastric emptying," *American Journal of Gastroenterology*, vol. 103, no. 2, pp. 416–423, 2008.

[21] M. Q. Bromer, F. Friedenberg, L. S. Miller, R. S. Fisher, K. Swartz, and H. P. Parkman, "Endoscopic pyloric injection of botulinum toxin A for the treatment of refractory gastroparesis," *Gastrointestinal Endoscopy*, vol. 61, no. 7, pp. 833–839, 2005.

[22] J. Arts, L. Holvoet, P. Caenepeel et al., "Clinical trial: a randomized-controlled crossover study of intrapyloric injection of botulinum toxin in gastroparesis," *Alimentary Pharmacology & Therapeutics*, vol. 26, no. 9, pp. 1251–1258, 2007.

[23] J. O. Clarke, R. Z. Sharaiha, A. Kord Valeshabad, L. A. Lee, A. N. Kalloo, and M. A. Khashab, "Through-the-scope transpyloric stent placement improves symptoms and gastric emptying in patients with gastroparesis," *Endoscopy*, vol. 45, no. 2, pp. E189–E190, 2013.

[24] M. L. Hibbard, C. M. Dunst, and L. L. Swanström, "Laparoscopic and Endoscopic Pyloroplasty for Gastroparesis Results in Sustained Symptom Improvement," *Journal of Gastrointestinal Surgery*, vol. 15, no. 9, pp. 1513–1519, 2011.

[25] A. L. Shada, C. M. Dunst, R. Pescarus et al., "Laparoscopic pyloroplasty is a safe and effective first-line surgical therapy for refractory gastroparesis," *Surgical Endoscopy*, vol. 30, no. 4, pp. 1326–1332, 2016.

[26] H. B. Xue, H. Z. Fan, X. M. Meng et al., "Fluoroscopy-guided gastric peroral endoscopic pyloromyotomy (G-POEM): a more reliable and efficient method for treatment of refractory gastroparesis," *Surgical Endoscopy*, vol. 31, no. 11, pp. 4617–4624, 2017.

[27] J. M. Gonzalez, A. Benezech, V. Vitton, and M. Barthet, "G-POEM with antro-pyloromyotomy for the treatment of refractory gastroparesis: mid-term follow-up and factors predicting outcome," *Alimentary Pharmacology & Therapeutics*, vol. 46, no. 3, pp. 364–370, 2017.

[28] S. Dacha, P. Mekaroonkamol, L. Li et al., "Outcomes and quality-of-life assessment after gastric per-oral endoscopic pyloromyotomy (with video)," *Gastrointestinal Endoscopy*, vol. 86, no. 2, pp. 282–289, 2017.

[29] F. Mearin, M. Camilleri, and J.-R. Malagelada, "Pyloric dysfunction in diabetics with recurrent nausea and vomiting," *Gastroenterology*, vol. 90, no. 6, pp. 1919–1925, 1986.

11

Good Tolerance of Citrate Accumulation due to Plasma Exchange among Patients with Acute-on-Chronic Liver Failure

Yuanji Ma,[1,2] Yan Xu,[1,2] Fang Chen,[1,2] Ying Wang,[1,2] Lang Bai,[1,2] and Hong Tang[1,2]

[1] *Center of Infectious Diseases, West China Hospital of Sichuan University, Chengdu 610041, China*
[2] *Division of Infectious Diseases, State Key Laboratory of Biotherapy, Sichuan University, Chengdu 610041, China*

Correspondence should be addressed to Lang Bai; pangbailang@163.com

Academic Editor: Alessandro Granito

Aim. To assess the tolerance of citrate accumulation due to plasma exchange (PE) among patients with acute-on-chronic liver failure (ACLF). *Methods.* A prospective, observational study was conducted among patients with ACLF who received heparin anticoagulation during PE-centered therapy without filtration and dialysis. Citrate accumulation was defined as the value of total calcium (Ca_{tot}) to ionized calcium (Ca_{ion}) ratio (Ca_{tot}/Ca_{ion}) greater than or equal to 2.5 ($Ca_{tot}/Ca_{ion} \geq 2.5$). *Results.* Fifty-four patients were enrolled. The mean age and MELD score were 50.0 ± 11.3 years old and 25 ± 7, respectively. Thirty-three patients had liver cirrhosis. The total 3-month survival rate was 57.4% (31/54). The mean Ca_{tot}/Ca_{ion} at the time before PE was 2.05 ± 0.14. $Ca_{tot}/Ca_{ion} \geq 2.5$ occurred in 100.0% (54/54) and 29.6% (16/54) of patients with mean Ca_{tot}/Ca_{ion} of 4.34 ± 1.52 and 2.36 ± 0.32 immediately after PE and 1 hour after PE, respectively, and these levels were much higher than those before PE ($p < 0.01$). However, all values returned to lower than 2.5 by the next morning with no difference from those before PE (2.10 ± 0.14 versus 2.05 ± 0.14, $p > 0.05$). Hypocalcemia (ionized calcium) and mild alkalosis were the main metabolic alterations. No symptoms associated with hypocalcemia occurred. *Conclusions.* Citrate accumulation is well tolerated by patients with ACLF who receive PE-centered therapy without filtration and dialysis. This study is regeristed with ChiCTR-OOC-17013618.

1. Introduction

Acute-on-chronic liver failure (ACLF) remains an important cause of mortality. The accumulation of various toxins and inflammatory cytokines leads to life-threatening complications, including renal failure, altered immune response, hepatic coma, and systemic hemodynamic dysfunction, which eventually culminate in multiorgan failure [1, 2]. Current medical therapy involves the management of the precipitating event and treatment of complications until the liver eventually recovers. Removal of toxins improves the capacity of the liver to regenerate, or artificial liver support system (ALSS) therapy can be a bridge to liver transplantation until a suitable organ is available [2–7].

To adequately maintain extracorporeal circulation, heparin or low-molecular-weight heparin anticoagulation is often used in clinical practice, but its side effects such as bleeding and thrombocytopenia threaten the safety of the patient. In recent years, regional citrate anticoagulation (RCA) has become the preferred anticoagulation method in continuous renal replacement therapy (CRRT) for patients with acute kidney injury (AKI) [8]. Several studies have focused on the safety and efficacy of RCA during blood purification for patients with liver failure and have concluded that RCA seems safe and feasible for these patients [9–16]. However, the blood purification techniques used in these studies, including continuous venovenous hemodialysis (CVVHD) [9, 11, 16, 17], sustained low-efficiency dialysis [12], molecular adsorbent recirculating system (MARS) [10, 14, 15], and fractionated plasma separation and adsorption (FPSA; the Prometheus system) [13], contain a dialysis technique that has the ability to remove citrate. Despite partial removal of the

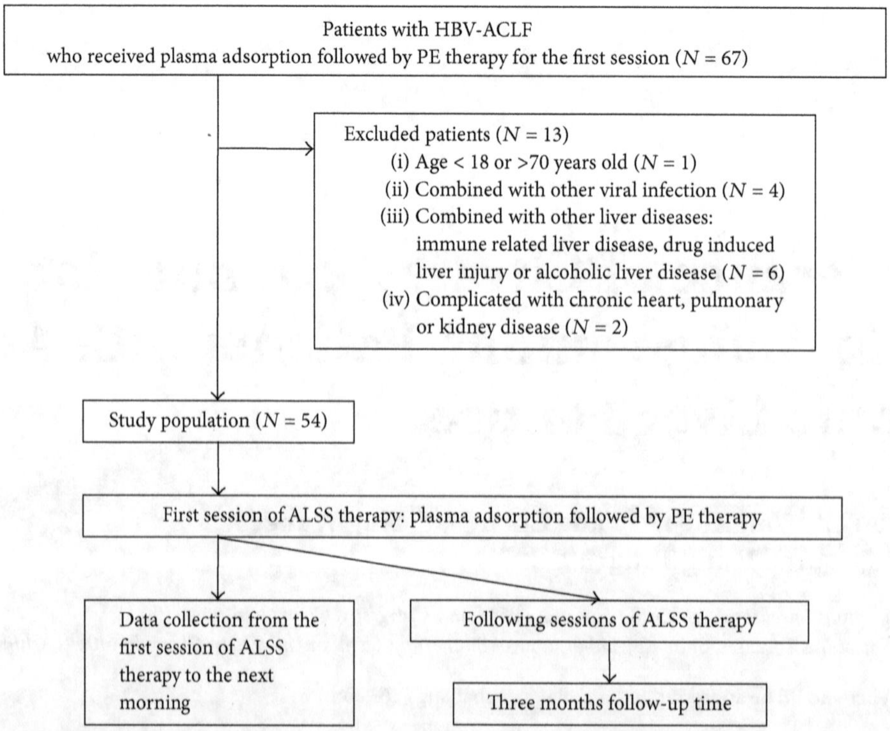

FIGURE 1: Flow diagram of patient selection and study process. PE, plasma exchange; HBV-ACLF, hepatitis B virus-related acute-on-chronic liver failure; ALSS, artificial liver support system.

citrate by the dialyzer as a complex bound with ionized calcium (Ca_{ion}), a certain amount of citrate enters the systemic circulation, which might lead to citrate accumulation, acid-base imbalance, and hypocalcemia and so on [18].

MARS and FPSA have been widely used for liver failure in Western countries during the past 3 decades, while plasma exchange- (PE-) centered ALSS therapy has been widely used in China for nearly the last 2 decades. With the benefit of having no effect on the blood clotting mechanism in vivo, RCA seems safe and feasible in patients with liver failure who received MARS or FPSA [10, 13–15]. However, without dialysis and filtration techniques, it remains uncertain whether RCA is still effective and safe for patients with liver failure and bleeding tendency or active bleeding who received PE-centered ALSS therapy or not.

Although citrate metabolism is severely impaired and the risk of adverse effects is high in patients with acute liver failure who receive PE therapy with frozen plasma containing citrate [19], it might be not necessarily the same as ACLF for there are big differences between acute liver failure and ACLF [20], and, more importantly, two prospective, controlled studies have found that PE plus standard medical therapy versus standard medical therapy alone could improve the short-term prognosis of patients with acute liver failure [4] and patients with ACLF [3]. Thus, we predict that patients with liver failure still have a certain ability to tolerate and metabolize citrate. However, the tolerance of citrate in patients with ACLF has not been studied in detail. Here, we conducted a prospective, observational study to assess the tolerance of citrate accumulation due to PE among patients with hepatitis B virus (HBV) related ACLF (HBV-ACLF) who received PE-centered ALSS therapy but did not receive filtration or dialysis.

2. Materials and Methods

2.1. Study Design and Patients. To assess the tolerance of citrate accumulation due to PE among patients with HBV-ACLF, a prospective, observational study was conducted in the Center of Infectious Diseases, West China Hospital of Sichuan University. Patients with HBV-ACLF who received PE-centered therapy for the first session were recruited from March 1, 2017, to June 31, 2017.

Patients with HBV-ACLF who received plasma adsorption followed by PE for the first session of ALSS therapy (a kind of nonbioartificial liver support system widely used in China) were enrolled (Figure 1). The diagnosis of HBV-ACLF was mainly based on the following criteria: (i) preexisting chronic hepatitis B virus infection; (ii) progressive hyperbilirubinemia, defined as a >50% increase in bilirubin or up to a level of >171 μmol/L within 4 weeks; (iii) prothrombin time activity (PTA) ≤ 40% or international normalized ratio (INR) ≥ 1.5. Patients whose age was less than 18 years or more than 70 years were excluded.

Patients were excluded if they had the following diseases: drug-induced liver injury, immune-related liver disease, alcoholic liver disease, and hyperthyroidism, and patients who were pregnant were also excluded. In addition, patients with HBV-ACLF were excluded if they were complicated with other viral infections (including hepatitis A, C, D, or E virus, cytomegalovirus, herpes simplex virus, or human immunodeficiency virus) or had evidence of chronic heart, pulmonary,

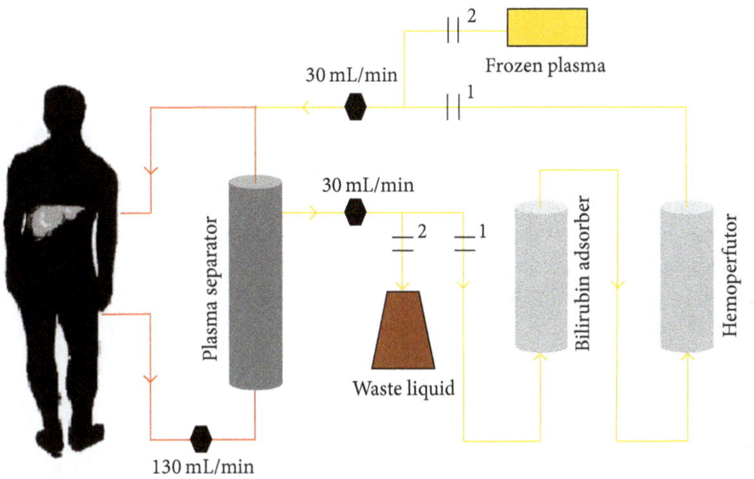

Figure 2: Schematic diagram of the double plasma molecular adsorption system (DPMAS) and plasma exchange (PE). PE (circuit 2) is initiated immediately when DPMAS (circuit 1) is completed in this study.

or kidney diseases. The diagnosis of liver cirrhosis was based on ultrasound and/or computed tomography.

All the patients with HBV-ACLF received standard medication, including antiviral drugs, hepatoprotective agents, and drugs to treat complications. Plasma adsorption followed by PE therapy was performed with heparin anticoagulation. The first session of ALSS therapy was identified as the observational session. Until September 30, 2017, all the patients were followed up for 3 months to identify the status of clinical outcomes.

This study was approved by the Ethics Committee of West China Hospital of Sichuan University. All study components were performed according to the ethical standards laid down in the 1964 Declaration of Helsinki and its later amendments. Written informed consent was obtained from each patient or his/her legal guardian.

2.2. ALSS Therapy, Plasma and Citrate. All the study patients received plasma adsorption therapy for 2 hours followed immediately by PE therapy for nearly an hour.

PE-centered ALSS therapy is widely used in China. The dose recommended by the American Society for Apheresis is 1 to 1.5 total plasma volume [21]. In the past, the dose was usually set to one total plasma volume, which was approximately 5% of body weight (approximately 3,000 mL) [22]. Due to the shortage of plasma in recent years and a retrospective study suggesting that plasma adsorption plus PE therapy could reduce the amount of plasma needed for PE therapy without impairing the therapeutic efficiency [23], plasma adsorption plus PE with half the total plasma volume (approximately 1,500 mL) is now widely used for ALSS therapy in China.

Citrate is a regular anticoagulant element in the blood preservation solution. Every 1000 mL of the blood preservation solution consists of sodium citrate 13.2 g, citrate 4.8 g, and glucose 14.7 g. A single blood bag contains 75 mL blood preservation solution. Frozen plasma was provided by the Chengdu Blood Center affiliated to Chengdu Health and Family Planning Commission. Whole blood was collected and stored in a blood bag, and plasma was separated and stored in another blood bag for clinical use. Each patient received 7 to 8 (7.9 ± 0.3) bags of plasma, and the total amount of plasma was 1,500 to 1,550 ($1,513 \pm 22$) mL. Therefore, the mean dose of citrate was approximately 61.3 mmol and the mean concentration of citrate in frozen plasma was approximately 40.5 mmol/L.

Plasma adsorption was combined with a plasma bilirubin adsorption followed by a plasma hemoperfusion (Figure 2), which is referred to as double plasma molecular adsorption system (DPMAS) in China [24]. The extracorporeal blood lines, plasma separator (MICROPLAS MPS05), plasma bilirubin adsorption column (DX350), and plasma hemoperfutor (HA330-II) were manufactured by B.Braun Diapact CRRT, Bellco S.r.l, Biosun Corporation, and Jafron Biomedical Corporation, respectively.

The treatment parameters were set to postdilution fluid replacement for continuous venovenous hemofiltration (CVVH) with blood flow of 130 mL/min, substitution flow of 1800 mL/h, and ultrafiltration flow of 0 mL/h. Therefore, the total time of PE using 1,500 to 1,550 mL plasma for each patient was 50 to 60 min. Patients received an intravenous injection of heparin sodium with an initial dose of 6,250 U at 5 to 10 minutes before plasma adsorption, and those with suspected coagulation would receive an additional heparin sodium injection with a dose of 3,125 U. Patients received 50 mL of 10% calcium gluconate supplement with a speed of 60 mL/h during PE. At the end of ALSS therapy, all patients received an intravenous injection of protamine sulfate with a dose of 50 mg.

2.3. Data Collection and Laboratory Examination. The death or survival information of patients was obtained from electronic medical records in the hospital and/or telephone follow-up. If the survival information could not be obtained from these 2 ways, we made the assumption that the patient had died by the follow-up time. The data of clinical characteristics and laboratory results were obtained from electronic medical records in the hospital. The severity of liver failure was rated according to the model for end-stage liver disease (MELD) [25].

Venous blood samples from the observational sessions of ALSS therapy were collected at the time before DPMAS (the time before ALSS therapy), before PE (immediately after DPMAS), immediately after PE (the time after ALSS therapy), 1 hour after PE (1 hour after ALSS therapy), and the next morning. All the samples were sent to the Department of Laboratory Medicine, West China Hospital of Sichuan University, for analysis within 30 minutes. Routine blood parameters, biochemical parameters, and coagulation function were measured by automatic analyzers according to standard laboratory procedures at the time before DPMAS, immediately after PE, and the next morning. Blood gas analysis was performed using the COBAS b 123 system (Roche Diagnostics) at the time before PE, immediately after PE, 1 hour after PE, and the next morning.

2.4. Definition. The presence of total calcium (Ca_{tot}) to ionized calcium (Ca_{ion}) ratio (Ca_{tot}/Ca_{ion}) greater than or equal to 2.5 ($Ca_{tot}/Ca_{ion} \geq 2.5$) with or without metabolic acidosis and an enlarged anion gap are the typical manifestations of citrate accumulation. This means that citrate is not being metabolized in a timely manner into bicarbonate, carbon dioxide, and water [9]. Thus, citrate accumulation was defined as $Ca_{tot}/Ca_{ion} \geq 2.5$ in this study [9, 16, 26].

2.5. Statistical Analysis. Quantitative variables were expressed as mean ± standard deviation (SD), and categorical variables as absolute and relative frequencies. One-way ANOVA was performed to calculate differences between quantitative data, while chi-square test or Fisher's exact test was performed to calculate differences between qualitative data. A p value of less than 0.05 was considered to indicate statistical significance. All statistical analyses were performed with SPSS Version 17.0 (SPSS Inc.), and the figures were drawn using GraphPad Prism 6 (GraphPad Software Inc.)

3. Results

3.1. Patients' Characteristics. From March 1, 2017, to June 31, 2017, fifty-four patients with HBV-ACLF who received plasma adsorption followed by PE for the first session of ALSS therapy were enrolled. Of these patients, the mean age was 50.0 ± 11.3 years old, 41 patients were male, 33 patients had a diagnosis of liver cirrhosis, and the mean level of HBV DNA was 3.8 ± 2.2 log IU/mL. The baseline laboratory parameters of patients before the first session of ALSS therapy are summarized in Table 1. The mean levels of total bilirubin, international normalized ratio (INR) of prothrombin time, creatinine, and MELD score were elevated to 408.1 ± 137.1 μmol/L, 2.0 ± 0.6, 101 ± 91 μmol/L, and 25 ± 7, respectively.

Table 1: Baseline laboratory parameters of patients before the first session of ALSS therapy.

Hemoglobin, g/dL	11.1 ± 2.1
Platelets, $\times 10^9$/L	126 ± 76
White blood cells, $\times 10^9$/L	8.2 ± 6.5
INR	2.0 ± 0.6
Total bilirubin, μmol/L	408.1 ± 137.1
Direct bilirubin, μmol/L	307.2 ± 107.9
Alanine transaminase, IU/L	200 ± 232
Aspartate transaminase, IU/L	177 ± 178
Alkaline phosphatase, IU/L	223 ± 320
gamma-Glutamyl transferase, IU/L	141 ± 276
Albumin, g/L	32.1 ± 4.4
Globulin, g/L	28.2 ± 8.2
Total bile acid, μmol/L	290.7 ± 78.6
Creatinine, μmol/L	101 ± 91
Ammonia, mmol/L	76 ± 35
Sodium, mmol/L	133.9 ± 5.3
Potassium, mmol/L	3.4 ± 0.6
Chloride, mmol/L	97.1 ± 6.4
MELD scores	25 ± 7

ALSS, artificial liver support system; MELD, model for end-stage liver disease; INR, international normalized ratio; measurement data are represented as mean ± SD.

3.2. Patient Outcomes. During hospitalization, all the patients with HBV-ACLF received standard medication including antiviral drugs, hepatoprotective agents, and drugs to treat complications. Thirty-seven patients underwent right internal jugular vein catheterization, and the remaining patients right femoral vein catheterization. Patients received a total of 203 sessions of ALSS therapy with a mean number of sessions of 3.8 ± 2.0. The immediate effect of the first session of ALSS therapy is summarized in Table 2.

At the final follow-up on September 30, 2017, all enrolled patients had been discharged. The mean length of hospital stay was 26.0 ± 13.4 days. The survival information was available for all. Four patients received living-donor liver transplantation during hospitalization or the 3-month follow-up period, and then we assumed here that they had died. The occurrences of major complications of liver disease (infection, hemorrhage, hepatorenal syndrome, and hepatic encephalopathy) are summarized in Table 3. The total 3-month survival rate was 57.4% (31/54).

3.3. Alteration in Calcium Status and Safety of Citrate Accumulation. In this study, we used Ca_{tot}/Ca_{ion}, an indicator with the cut-off value of 2.5, to assess whether there was citrate accumulation [9, 16, 26], instead of using citrate concentration to indirectly evaluate the presence of citrate accumulation. Changes of Ca_{tot}, Ca_{ion}, Ca_{tot}/Ca_{ion} and anion gap during and after ALSS therapy are summarized in Table 4 and their trends were shown in Figure 3.

The mean level of Ca_{ion} before PE therapy was 1.05 ± 0.06 mmol/L. Although supplied with 50 mL of 10% calcium gluconate during PE, the mean level of Ca_{ion} decreased noticeably to 0.71 ± 0.16 mmol/L immediately after PE, which was much lower than the level before PE ($p < 0.01$). It is worth noting that the mean level of Ca_{ion} returned to normal levels 1 hour after the ALSS therapy and remained stable until the next morning. Although there was an obviously

TABLE 2: Immediate effect of the first session of ALSS therapy.

	Rate of reduction between pre- and post-ALSS therapy (%)	Rate of reduction between pre-ALSS therapy and the next morning (%)
Hemoglobin	12.1 ± 6.3	3.3 ± 5.9
Platelets	20.0 ± 18.1	17.4 ± 15.3
White blood cells	−7.3 ± 31.6	7.1 ± 21.5
INR	12.7 ± 17.8	9.4 ± 15.2
Total bilirubin	49.1 ± 6.7	14.1 ± 14.8
Direct bilirubin	47.5 ± 7.2	16.8 ± 9.8
Alanine transaminase	36.9 ± 12.2	27.4 ± 13.5
Aspartate transaminase	30.4 ± 57.8	17.1 ± 11.3
Alkaline phosphatase	24.9 ± 33.6	3.2 ± 61.3
gamma-Glutamyl transferase	31.2 ± 14.1	20.0 ± 18.8
Albumin	5.6 ± 7.6	−2.2 ± 8.9
Globulin	13.4 ± 12.3	12.7 ± 8.6
Total bile acid	19.9 ± 14.1	28.5 ± 14.4
Creatinine	7.7 ± 15.4	3.2 ± 16.6
Ammonia	16.3 ± 36.3	−32.5 ± 68.3
Sodium	−3.1 ± 2.5	−1.9 ± 2.4
Potassium	−6.3 ± 10.0	−10.6 ± 14.0
Chloride	−1.2 ± 4.7	−0.3 ± 4.5
MELD score	21.4 ± 13.4	9.2 ± 10.2

ALSS, artificial liver support system; MELD, model for end-stage liver disease; INR, international normalized ratio; measurement data are represented as mean ± SD.

TABLE 3: Disease state during hospitalization and short-term prognosis.

Hospital stay, days	26.0 ± 13.4
Spontaneous bacterial peritonitis, yes/no	30/24
Infection, yes/no	16/38
Hemorrhage, yes/no	7/47
Hepatorenal syndrome, yes/no	12/42
Hepatic encephalopathy, yes/no	15/39
Three-month survival, yes/no*	31/23

ALSS, artificial liver support system. *Four patients received living donor liver transplantation during hospitalization or the 3-month follow-up period, we assume here that they have died. Measurement data are represented as mean ± SD. Enumeration data are represented as frequencies.

lower level of Ca_{ion} during and after ALSS therapy, none of the patients complained about numbness of the mouth and fingers, nor did we observe any twitching of the calf muscles.

Because of calcium supplements, the mean level of Ca_{tot} immediately after PE was much higher than the level before PE (2.90 ± 0.21 mmol/L versus 2.15 ± 0.13 mmol/L, $p < 0.01$), and the mean level of Ca_{tot} 1 hour after PE was much higher than the level before PE (2.52 ± 0.21 mmol/L versus 2.15 ± 0.13 mmol/L, $p < 0.01$). Although the mean level of Ca_{tot} at the next morning was higher than that before PE (2.27 ± 0.14 mmol/L versus 2.15 ± 0.13 mmol/L, $p < 0.01$), it was noticeably decreased from 2.52 ± 0.21 mmol/L at 1 hour after PE ($p < 0.01$), and the level returned to normal next morning.

$Ca_{tot}/Ca_{ion} \geq 2.5$, an indicator of citrate accumulation, did not occur before PE, and the mean value of Ca_{tot}/Ca_{ion} was 2.05 ± 0.14. $Ca_{tot}/Ca_{ion} \geq 2.5$ occurred in 100.0% (54/54) and 29.6% (16/54) of patients immediately after PE and 1 hour after PE, respectively, which were much higher than values before PE ($p < 0.01$). The mean values of Ca_{tot}/Ca_{ion} immediately after PE and 1 hour after PE were 4.34 ± 1.52 and 2.36 ± 0.32, respectively, which were much higher than that before PE ($p < 0.01$). However, the mean value of Ca_{tot}/Ca_{ion} did noticeably decrease 1 hour after PE, and all values returned to lower than 2.5 the next morning. Furthermore, the mean value of Ca_{tot}/Ca_{ion} the next morning was similar to that before PE (2.10 ± 0.14 versus 2.05 ± 0.14, $p > 0.05$).

As shown in Table 4 and Figure 3, the mean level of anion gap had similar trends to the mean value of Ca_{tot}/Ca_{ion}. The mean level of anion gap before PE was 6.2 ± 2.6 mmol/L. The mean level of anion gap was much higher at the time immediately after PE than that before PE (9.8 ± 2.6 mmol/L versus 6.2 ± 2.6 mmol/L, $p < 0.01$). However, the mean level of anion gap returned to the baseline level 1 hour after PE and remained stable the next morning ($p > 0.05$).

3.4. Alterations in Acid-Base Status and Lactate. In the human body, citrate is metabolized into bicarbonate, carbon dioxide, and water. The acid-base status values during and after ALSS therapy are shown in Table 4 and Figure 4.

Although the mean pH immediately after PE was similar to that before PE (7.42 ± 0.04 versus 7.42 ± 0.04, $p > 0.05$), the mean pH noticeably increased 1 hour after PE and the

TABLE 4: Calcium and acid-base status during and after ALSS therapy.

Time	Before PE	Immediately after PE	1 hour after PE	Next morning★
Ca_{tot}, mmol/L	$2.15 \pm 0.13^{\$}$	$2.90 \pm 0.21^{\#\$}$	$2.52 \pm 0.21^{\#\$}$	$2.27 \pm 0.14^{\#}$
Ca_{ion}, mmol/L	1.05 ± 0.06	$0.71 \pm 0.16^{\#\$}$	1.08 ± 0.10	1.08 ± 0.06
Ca_{tot}/Ca_{ion}	2.05 ± 0.14	$4.34 \pm 1.52^{\#\$}$	$2.36 \pm 0.32^{\#\$}$	2.10 ± 0.14
$Ca_{tot}/Ca_{ion} \geq 2.5$, yes/no	0/54	$54/0^{\#\$}$	$16/38^{\#\$}$	0/54
Anion gap, mmol/L	6.2 ± 2.6	$9.8 \pm 2.6^{\#\$}$	6.7 ± 2.3	6.1 ± 1.8
pH	$7.42 \pm 0.04^{\$}$	$7.42 \pm 0.04^{\$}$	$7.47 \pm 0.05^{\#}$	$7.46 \pm 0.04^{\#}$
HCO_3^-, mmol/L	$25.4 \pm 4.6^{\triangle}$	25.8 ± 4.3	26.6 ± 3.9	$27.4 \pm 3.2^{*}$
PCO_2, mmHg	39.5 ± 5.7	40.1 ± 5.6	37.5 ± 7.0	39.4 ± 5.5
Lactate, mmol/L	2.4 ± 0.6	2.5 ± 1.3	2.6 ± 0.8	2.6 ± 0.6

ALSS, artificial liver support system; PE, plasma exchange; Ca_{tot}, total calcium; Ca_{ion}, ionized calcium; Ca_{tot}/Ca_{ion}, total-to-ionized calcium ratio; HCO_3^-, standard bicarbonate; PCO_2, partial pressure of carbon dioxide. ★The interval time between the time after PE therapy and the next morning is 16.5 ± 1.9 hours. Compared with the data at the time before PE, $^{*}p < 0.05$, $^{\#}p < 0.01$, the others, $p > 0.05$. Compared with the data at the next morning, $^{\triangle}p < 0.05$, $^{\$}p < 0.01$, the others, $p > 0.05$. Measurement data are represented as mean ± SD. Enumeration data are represented as frequencies.

TABLE 5: Univariate analysis and multivariate analysis of predictors for citrate accumulation at 1 hour after ALSS therapy.

	Correlation coefficient	p	Regression coefficient	Standard error	p	Odds ratio	95% CI
Gender	0.393	0.003	−2.130	0.938	0.023	0.12	0.02–0.75
Baseline lactate	0.396	0.003	1.710	0.856	0.046	5.53	1.03–29.57
Baseline Ca_{tot}/Ca_{ion}	0.356	0.008	8.632	3.917	0.028	5607.59	2.60–12108390.04
Baseline Ca_{ion}	−0.380	0.005	1.974	8.144	0.809	7.20	0.00–61574425.76
Baseline platelets	−0.368	0.006	0.000	0.006	0.873	1.00	0.99–1.01

ALSS, artificial liver support system; Ca_{tot}, total calcium; Ca_{ion}, ionized calcium; Ca_{tot}/Ca_{ion}, total-to-ionized calcium ratio.

next morning compared with the value before PE (7.47 ± 0.05 versus 7.42 ± 0.04 and 7.46 ± 0.04 versus 7.42 ± 0.04, $p < 0.01$, respectively). However, the mean pH next morning was similar to that 1 hour after PE (7.46 ± 0.04 versus 7.47 ± 0.05, $p > 0.05$).

As shown in Table 4 and Figure 4, the mean level of standard bicarbonate (HCO_3^-) increased during and after ALSS therapy. It was higher the next morning than before and immediately after PE and 1 hour after PE (27.4 ± 3.2 mmol/L versus 25.4 ± 4.6 mmol/L, 27.4 ± 3.2 mmol/L versus 25.8 ± 4.3 mmol/L, and 27.4 ± 3.2 versus 26.6 ± 3.9, $p < 0.05$, resp.). The partial pressure of carbon dioxide (PCO_2) and the lactate level remained stable around the time of ALSS therapy with no difference among the observation time ($p > 0.05$).

3.5. Predictors for Citrate Accumulation. Under normal conditions, citrate's half-life is approximately 5 minutes and citrate is metabolized completely within 30 minutes of discontinuing a citrate infusion [27, 28]. However, $Ca_{tot}/Ca_{ion} \geq 2.5$ occurred in 29.6% (16/54) of our patients 1 hour after PE. Correlation analysis showed that gender ($p = 0.003$), baseline lactate levels ($p = 0.003$), baseline Ca_{tot}/Ca_{ion} ($p = 0.008$), baseline Ca_{ion} ($p = 0.005$), and baseline platelet counts ($p = 0.006$) before the ALSS therapy were all predictors for $Ca_{tot}/Ca_{ion} \geq 2.5$ at 1 hour after PE therapy (Table 5). Multivariate analysis revealed that gender (OR, 0.12; 95% CI, 0.02–0.75; $p = 0.023$), baseline lactate, (OR, 5.53; 95% CI, 1.03–29.57; $p = 0.046$), and baseline Ca_{tot}/Ca_{ion} (OR, 5607.59; 95% CI, 2.60–12108390.04; $p = 0.028$) were the independent predictors for citrate accumulation at 1 hour after PE therapy. The highest AUC value regarding citrate accumulation was observed for serum lactate (AUC, 0.750; 95% CI, 0.601–0.899). An increase in $Ca_{tot}/Ca_{ion} \geq 2.5$ at 1 hour after PE was predicted by the presence of baseline levels of plasma lactate greater than or equal to 2.65 mmol/L (sensitivity 62.5%; specificity 84.2%). The AUC values for gender and baseline Ca_{tot}/Ca_{ion} were 0.684 and 0.725, respectively.

4. Discussion

In this prospective, observational study, we found that citrate accumulation due to PE occurred in all these patients, and it was still present in 29.6% of these patients at 1 hour after PE. However, all of the levels returned to normal the next morning. Hypocalcemia (ionized calcium) and mild metabolic alkalosis due to PE were the main alterations in calcium and acid-base status. An increase in citrate accumulation at 1 hour after PE was predicted by the presence of baseline levels of plasma lactate greater than or equal to 2.65 mmol/L.

The possible occurrence of citrate accumulation is the main issue for patients with liver failure who are receiving citrate anticoagulation. Several studies have focused on the safety and efficacy of RCA for blood purification in patients with liver failure and AKI and found that RCA seems safe and feasible in these patients [9–17]. Despite partial removal of the citrate by the dialyzer, a certain amount of citrate enters the systemic circulation. Citrate accumulation does occur in 2.3% to 23.2% sessions of CRRT for patients with liver failure and AKI [9, 11, 16, 17] and in 21.4% sessions of MARS therapy for patients with liver failure [10]. In our study, citrate was metabolized by the patients themselves,

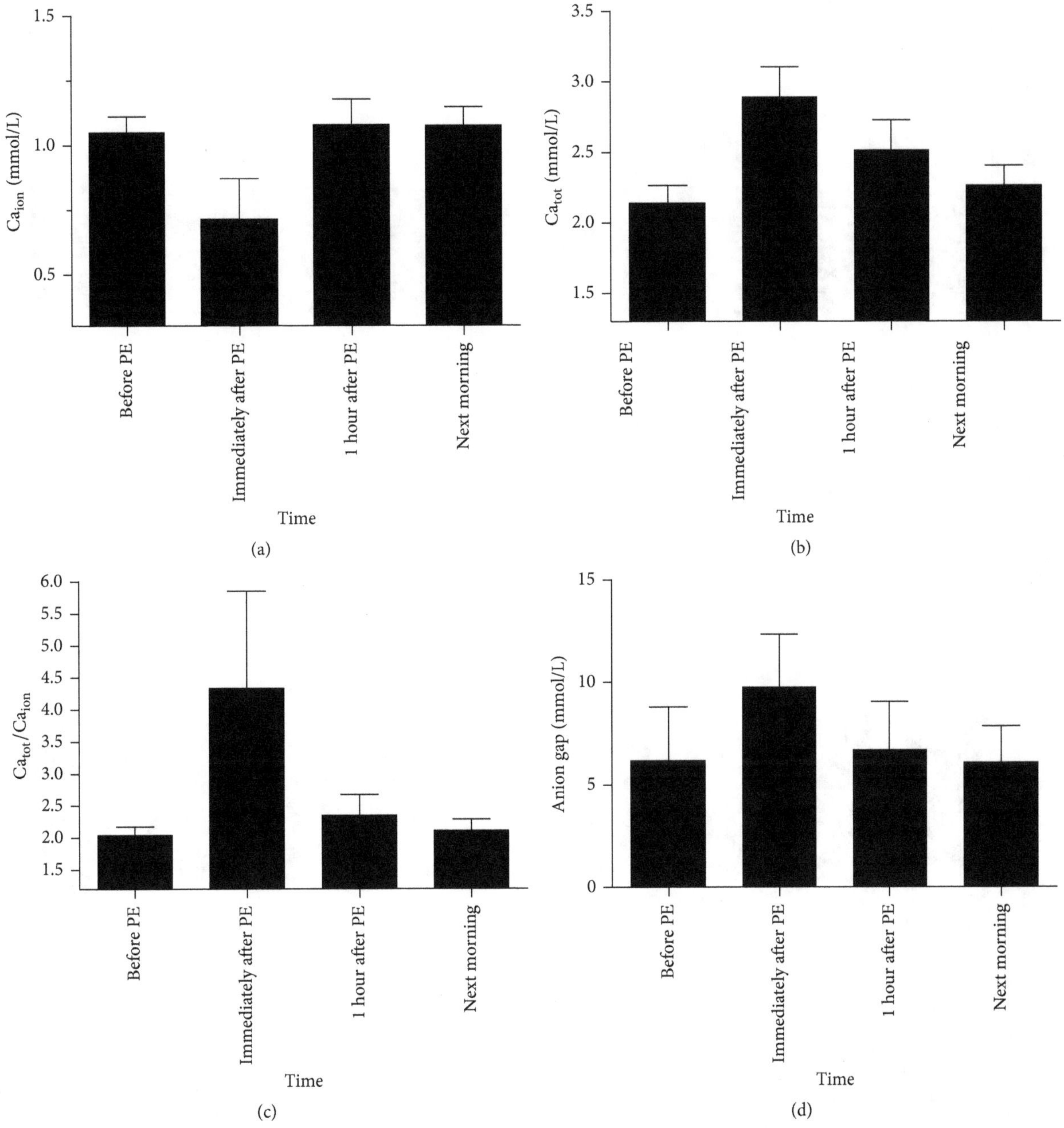

FIGURE 3: Trends of ionized calcium (Ca_{ion}, (a)), total calcium (Ca_{tot}, (b)), total-to-ionized calcium ratio (Ca_{tot}/Ca_{ion}, (c)), and anion gap (d) during and after ALSS therapy for patients with HBV-ACLF.

and citrate accumulation due to PE occurs in all the patients with HBV-ACLF. However, the main acid-base imbalance is mild metabolic alkalosis rather than metabolic acidosis in our study. A similar result was found in a study of patients with cirrhosis, in which the total body clearance of citrate was significantly reduced and the net metabolic changes were quantitatively similar to those in patients with no cirrhosis [29]. Another study of patients with acute liver failure found that citrate metabolism was severely impaired and the risk of adverse effects was high [19]. However, the results from acute liver failure were not necessarily the same as ACLF for there are big differences between them [20]. Our findings suggest that citrate accumulation is well tolerated with good safety among patients with HBV-ACLF, and these patients still have a certain ability to metabolize citrate.

The use of RCA could induce a lower activation of coagulation than both conventional and fractionated heparin, and this lower activation might contribute to an improvement of biocompatibility of extracorporeal circulation [30]. A meta-analysis conducted in adult critically ill patients with AKI who require CRRT reported that RCA is more efficacious in prolonging circuit lifespan and reducing the risk of bleeding with no difference in mortality between the RCA and heparin anticoagulation groups [31]. The benefits mentioned above

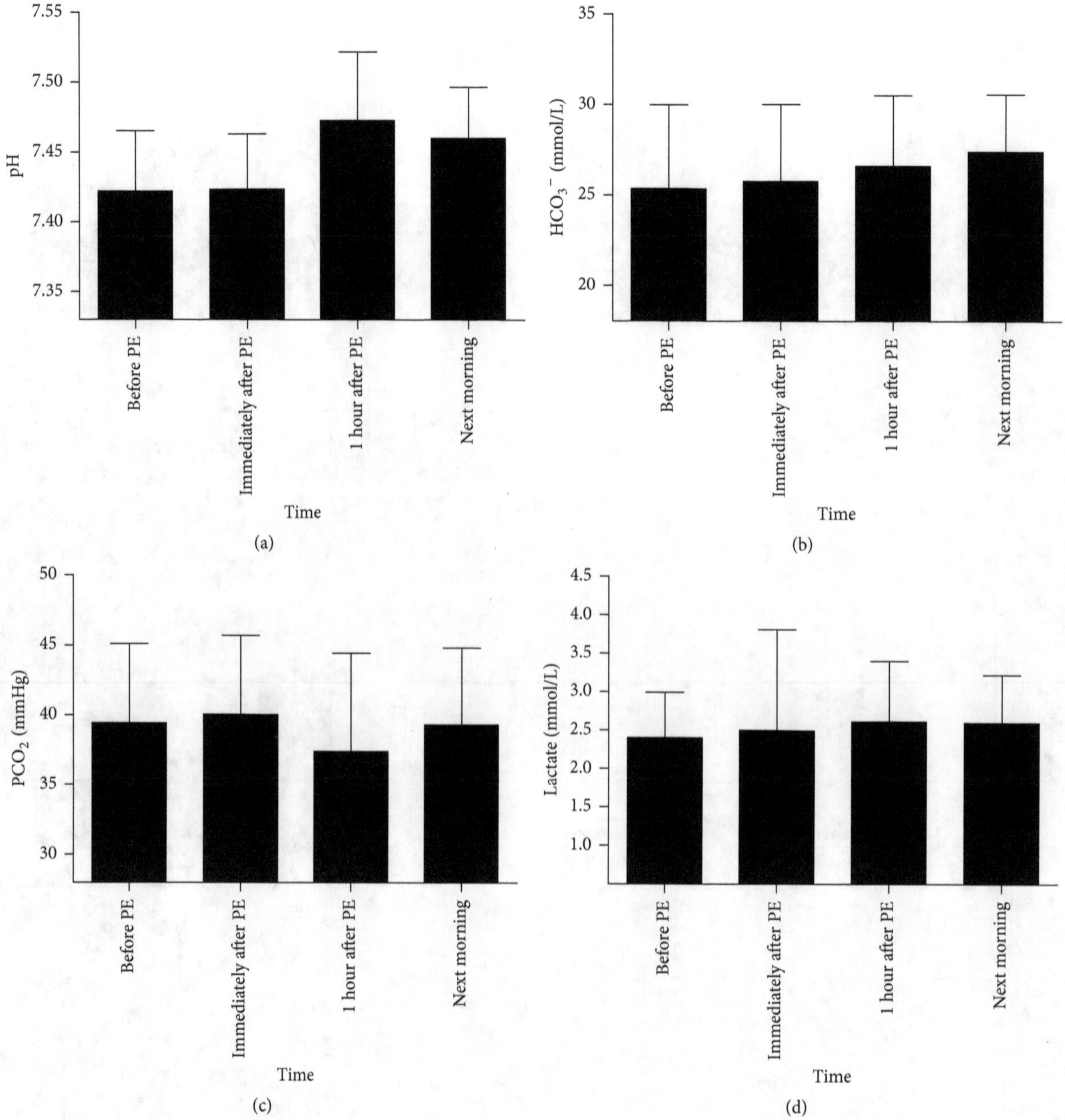

FIGURE 4: Trends of pH (a), standard bicarbonate (HCO_3^- (b)), partial pressure of carbon dioxide (PCO_2 (c)), and lactate (d) during and after ALSS therapy for patients with HBV-ACLF.

and good tolerance to citrate seem to somewhat dispel the idea that RCA is contraindicated in patients with liver failure [32]. We think that RCA might be particularly beneficial in patients with impaired coagulation due to liver failure. A similar study reporting dose adaptation and monitoring of Ca_{ion} has also suggested that RCA is feasible for patients with decompensated cirrhosis [29]. However, further research is needed to assess the safety and efficacy of RCA for PE-centered ALSS therapy in patients with HBV-ACLF who do not receive dialysis and filtration.

In this study, we found that gender, baseline lactate levels, and baseline Ca_{tot}/Ca_{ion} are independent predictors for citrate accumulation at 1 hour after PE therapy. Similar to our findings, 2 studies have reported that standard liver-function parameters show poor predictive capabilities regarding citrate accumulation in patients with cirrhosis and in patients with liver failure and AKI who received CVVHD [9, 29]. In our study, an increase in citrate accumulation at 1 hour after PE is predicted by the presence of baseline plasma lactate levels greater than or equal to 2.65 mmol/L (sensitivity 62.5%; specificity 84.2%). This finding is similar to that in patients with liver failure and AKI who received CVVHD, in which serum lactate levels greater than or equal to 3.4 mmol/L and prothrombin time activity less than or equal to 26% predict an increase in citrate accumulation with high sensitivity (86% for both lactate and prothrombin time activity) and specificity (86% for lactate; 92% for prothrombin time) [9].

Our study has several limitations. First, we used Ca_{tot}/Ca_{ion} instead of direct measurement of plasma citrate concentration to reflect the citrate accumulation. However, citrate metabolism seems not to be restricted to the liver [17], and an upper normal or even toxic level of citrate in the blood is not well established [9]. Being a physiological metabolite, citrate might not be toxic itself but could induce metabolic disorders [9]. Second, we did not directly check the concentration of citrate in frozen plasma. Although we calculated it indirectly by summing up the amount of blood preservation solution the patients used, this might lead to erroneous estimation. Third, we performed blood gas analysis with venous blood samples instead of artery blood samples to reflect acid-base status because of poor clotting function and possible bleeding. However, venous gases are suitable for initial evaluation of acid-base status in critically ill patients [33].

In conclusion, in this prospective, observational study, we found that citrate accumulation due to PE occurred in all the patients with HBV-ACLF who received plasma adsorption and PE but did not receive filtration or dialysis, and it was well tolerated. Further research should be carried out to assess the safety and efficacy of RCA for PE-centered ALSS therapy in patients with HBV-ACLF who do not receive dialysis and filtration.

Authors' Contributions

Yuanji Ma and Yan Xu contributed equally to this work.

Acknowledgments

This work was supported by grants from Research Project of Sichuan Provincial Health and Family Planning Commission (16PJ279).

References

[1] R. Hernaez, E. Solà, R. Moreau, and P. Ginès, "Acute-on-chronic liver failure: an update," *Gut*, vol. 66, no. 3, pp. 541–553, 2017.

[2] S. K. Sarin and A. Choudhury, "Acute-on-chronic liver failure: Terminology, mechanisms and management," *Nature Reviews Gastroenterology & Hepatology*, vol. 13, no. 3, pp. 131–149, 2016.

[3] G. Qin, J.-G. Shao, B. Wang et al., "Artificial liver support system improves short- and long-term outcomes of patients with HBV-associated acute-on-chronic liver failure: a single-center experience," *Medicine*, vol. 93, no. 28, p. e338, 2014.

[4] F. S. Larsen, L. E. Schmidt, C. Bernsmeier et al., "High-volume plasma exchange in patients with acute liver failure: an open randomised controlled trial," *Journal of Hepatology*, vol. 64, no. 1, pp. 69–78, 2016.

[5] A. Vaid, H. Chweich, E. M. Balk, and B. L. Jaber, "Molecular adsorbent recirculating system as artificial support therapy for liver failure: a meta-analysis," *ASAIO Journal*, vol. 58, no. 1, pp. 51–59, 2012.

[6] G. L. He, L. Feng, C. Y. Duan et al., "Meta-analysis of survival with the molecular adsorbent recirculating system for liver failure," *International Journal of Clinical and Experimental Medicine*, vol. 8, no. 10, pp. 17046–17054, 2015.

[7] E. Tsipotis, A. Shuja, and B. L. Jaber, "Albumin dialysis for liver failure: a systematic review," *Advances in Chronic Kidney Disease*, vol. 22, no. 5, pp. 383–390, 2015.

[8] Kidney Disease: Improving Global Outcomes (KDIGO) Acute Kidney Injury Work Group, "KDIGO clinical practice guideline for acute kidney injury," *Kidney International Supplements*, vol. 2, no. 1, pp. 1–138, 2012.

[9] C. Schultheiß, B. Saugel, V. Phillip et al., "Continuous venovenous hemodialysis with regional citrate anticoagulation in patients with liver failure: a prospective observational study," *Critical Care*, vol. 16, no. 4, article R162, 2012.

[10] B. Meijers, W. Laleman, P. Vermeersch, F. Nevens, A. Wilmer, and P. Evenepoel, "A prospective randomized open-label crossover trial of regional citrate anticoagulation vs. anticoagulation free liver dialysis by the molecular adsorbents recirculating system," *Critical Care*, vol. 16, no. 1, article R20, 2012.

[11] T. Slowinski, S. Morgera, M. Joannidis et al., "Safety and efficacy of regional citrate anticoagulation in continuous venovenous hemodialysis in the presence of liver failure: the liver citrate anticoagulation threshold (L-CAT) observational study," *Critical Care*, vol. 19, no. 1, article 349, 2015.

[12] T. Lahmer, M. Messer, S. Rasch et al., "Sustained low-efficiency dialysis with regional citrate anticoagulation in medical intensive care unit patients with liver failure: a prospective study," *Journal of Critical Care*, vol. 30, no. 5, pp. 1096–1100, 2015.

[13] E. Şentürk, F. Esen, P. E. Özcan et al., "The treatment of acute liver failure with fractionated plasma separation and adsorption system: experience in 85 applications," *Journal of Clinical Apheresis*, vol. 25, no. 4, pp. 195–201, 2010.

[14] A. Dyla, W. Mielnicki, J. Bartczak, T. Zawada, and P. Garba, "Effectiveness and safety assessment of citrate anticoagulation during albumin dialysis in comparison to other methods of anticoagulation," *Artificial Organs*, vol. 41, no. 9, pp. 818–826, 2017.

[15] P. Faybik, H. Hetz, G. Mitterer et al., "Regional citrate anticoagulation in patients with liver failure supported by a molecular adsorbent recirculating system," *Critical Care Medicine*, vol. 39, no. 2, pp. 273–279, 2011.

[16] H. U. Meier-Kriesche, J. Gitomer, K. Finkel, and T. DuBose, "Increased total to ionized calcium ratio during continuous venovenous hemodialysis with regional citrate anticoagulation," *Critical Care Medicine*, vol. 29, no. 4, pp. 748–752, 2001.

[17] M. Klingele, T. Stadler, D. Fliser, T. Speer, H. V. Groesdonk, and A. Raddatz, "Long-term continuous renal replacement therapy and anticoagulation with citrate in critically ill patients with severe liver dysfunction," *Critical Care*, vol. 21, no. 1, article 294, 2017.

[18] D. Khadzhynov, C. Schelter, I. Lieker et al., "Incidence and outcome of metabolic disarrangements consistent with citrate accumulation in critically ill patients undergoing continuous venovenous hemodialysis with regional citrate anticoagulation," *Journal of Critical Care*, vol. 29, no. 2, pp. 265–271, 2014.

[19] R. Apsner, M. Schwarzenhofer, K. Derfler, C. Zauner, K. Ratheiser, and A. Kranz, "Impairment of citrate metabolism in

acute hepatic failure," *Wiener Klinische Wochenschrift*, vol. 109, no. 4, pp. 123–127, 1997.

[20] S. K. Sarin, C. K. Kedarisetty, Z. Abbas et al., "Acute-on-chronic liver failure: consensus recommendations of the Asian Pacific Association for the Study of the Liver (APASL) 2014," *Hepatology International*, vol. 8, no. 4, pp. 453–471, 2014.

[21] J. Schwartz, J. L. Winters, A. Padmanabhan et al., "Guidelines on the use of therapeutic apheresis in clinical practice—evidence-based approach from the writing committee of the american society for apheresis: the sixth special issue," *Journal of Clinical Apheresis*, vol. 28, no. 3, pp. 145–284, 2013.

[22] L. J. Li, Y. M. Zhang, X. L. Liu et al., "Artificial liver support system in china: a review over the last 30 years," *Therapeutic Apheresis and Dialysis*, vol. 10, no. 2, pp. 160–167, 2006.

[23] P.-Q. Zhou, S.-P. Zheng, M. Yu, S.-S. He, and Z.-H. Weng, "Prognosis of acute-on-chronic liver failure patients treated with artificial liver support system," *World Journal of Gastroenterology*, vol. 21, no. 32, pp. 9614–9622, 2015.

[24] J. Chen, J. Huang, Y. Chen, Y. Lu, and L. Li, "A clinical study on the treatment of severe hepatitis by a combined artificial liver," *Hepato-Gastroenterology*, vol. 59, no. 119, pp. 2273–2275, 2012.

[25] P. S. Kamath, R. H. Wiesner, M. Malinchoc et al., "A model to predict survival in patients with end-stage liver disease," *Hepatology*, vol. 33, no. 2, pp. 464–470, 2001.

[26] A. Link, M. Klingele, T. Speer et al., "Total-to-ionized calcium ratio predicts mortality in continuous renal replacement therapy with citrate anticoagulation in critically ill patients," *Critical Care*, vol. 16, no. 3, article R97, 2012.

[27] A. G. Schneider, D. Journois, and T. Rimmele, "Complications of regional citrate anticoagulation: accumulation or overload?" *Critical Care*, vol. 21, no. 1, article 281, 2017.

[28] D. J. Kutsogiannis, I. Mayers, W. D. N. Chin, and R. T. N. Gibney, "Regional citrate anticoagulation in continuous venovenous hemodiafiltration," *American Journal of Kidney Diseases*, vol. 35, no. 5, pp. 802–811, 2000.

[29] L. Kramer, E. Bauer, C. Joukhadar et al., "Citrate pharmacokinetics and metabolism in cirrhotic and noncirrhotic critically ill patients," *Critical Care Medicine*, vol. 31, no. 10, pp. 2450–2455, 2003.

[30] R. Hofbauer, D. Moser, M. Frass et al., "Effect of anticoagulation on blood membrane interactions during hemodialysis," *Kidney International*, vol. 56, no. 4, pp. 1578–1583, 1999.

[31] C. Liu, Z. Mao, H. Kang, J. Hu, and F. Zhou, "Regional citrate versus heparin anticoagulation for continuous renal replacement therapy in critically ill patients: a meta-analysis with trial sequential analysis of randomized controlled trials," *Critical Care*, vol. 20, no. 1, article 144, 2016.

[32] S. Patel and J. Wendon, "Regional citrate anticoagulation in patients with liver failure—time for a rethink?" *Critical Care*, vol. 16, no. 5, article 153, 2012.

[33] C. M. Martin and F. Priestap, "Agreement between venous and arterial blood gas analysis of acid-base status in critical care and ward patients: a retrospective cohort study," *Canadian Journal of Anesthesia*, vol. 64, no. 11, pp. 1138–1143, 2017.

12

Alcohol Consumption in Diabetic Patients with Nonalcoholic Fatty Liver Disease

Preya J. Patel,[1,2] David Smith,[3] Jason P. Connor,[4] Leigh U. Horsfall,[1,2] Kelly L. Hayward,[2] Fabrina Hossain,[5] Suzanne Williams,[5] Tracey Johnson,[5] Katherine A. Stuart,[1] Nigel N. Brown,[6] Nivene Saad,[7] Andrew D. Clouston,[2] Katharine M. Irvine,[2,8] Anthony W. Russell,[9,10] Patricia C. Valery,[2,3,9] and Elizabeth E. Powell[1,2]

[1] *Department of Gastroenterology and Hepatology, Princess Alexandra Hospital, Brisbane, QLD, Australia*
[2] *Centre for Liver Disease Research, Translational Research Institute, School of Medicine, The University of Queensland, Brisbane, QLD, Australia*
[3] *QIMR Berghofer Medical Research Institute, Brisbane, QLD, Australia*
[4] *Discipline of Psychiatry, The University of Queensland, Brisbane, QLD, Australia*
[5] *Inala Primary Care, Brisbane, QLD, Australia*
[6] *Pathology Queensland, Brisbane, QLD, Australia*
[7] *Department of Radiology, Princess Alexandra Hospital, Brisbane, QLD, Australia*
[8] *Mater Research, Translational Research Institute, University of Queensland, Brisbane, QLD, Australia*
[9] *School of Clinical Medicine, The University of Queensland, Brisbane, QLD, Australia*
[10] *Department of Diabetes and Endocrinology, Princess Alexandra Hospital, Brisbane, QLD, Australia*

Correspondence should be addressed to Elizabeth E. Powell; e.powell@uq.edu.au

Academic Editor: Tatsuo Kanda

Aim. To examine the association between lifetime alcohol consumption and significant liver disease in type 2 diabetic patients with NAFLD. *Methods.* A cross-sectional study assessing 151 patients with NAFLD at risk of clinically significant liver disease. NAFLD fibrosis severity was classified by transient elastography; liver stiffness measurements ≥8.2 kPa defined significant fibrosis. Lifetime drinking history classified patients into nondrinkers, light drinkers (always ≤20 g/day), and moderate drinkers (any period with intake >20 g/day). *Result.* Compared with lifetime nondrinkers, light and moderate drinkers were more likely to be male ($p = 0.008$) and to be Caucasian ($p = 0.007$) and to have a history of cigarette smoking ($p = 0.000$), obstructive sleep apnea ($p = 0.003$), and self-reported depression ($p = 0.003$). Moderate drinkers required ≥3 hypoglycemic agents to maintain diabetic control ($p = 0.041$) and fibrate medication to lower blood triglyceride levels ($p = 0.044$). Compared to lifetime nondrinkers, light drinkers had 1.79 (95% CI: 0.67–4.82; $p = 0.247$) and moderate drinkers had 0.91 (95% CI: 0.27–3.10; $p = 0.881$) times the odds of having liver stiffness measurements ≥8.2 kPa (adjusted for age, gender, and body mass index). *Conclusions.* In diabetic patients with NAFLD, light or moderate lifetime alcohol consumption was not significantly associated with liver fibrosis. The impact of lifetime alcohol intake on fibrosis progression and diabetic comorbidities, in particular obstructive sleep apnea and hypertriglyceridemia, requires further investigation.

1. Introduction

In people with type 2 diabetes mellitus (T2DM), modest alcohol intake is associated with a lower risk of cardiovascular disease and mortality. Analysis of a large T2DM cohort ($n = 11{,}140$; 30% drinkers) followed up for five years found that, compared with abstainers, moderate alcohol consumption (≤21 and ≤14 standard drinks weekly for men and women, resp.) was associated with a 17% lower risk of cardiovascular events, a 15% lower risk of microvascular complications, and a 13% lower risk of all-cause mortality [1]. These cardiovascular benefits may be a consequence of enhanced insulin sensitivity and favorable effects on inflammation and high-density lipoprotein (HDL) levels [2]. In contrast, higher levels of alcohol intake were associated with increased cardiovascular events and all-cause mortality in a dose-dependent manner [1].

Limited data exist, however, regarding the effect of alcohol use on other diabetic complications. In particular, people with T2DM have a high prevalence of nonalcoholic fatty liver disease (NAFLD), are more likely to develop cirrhosis, and have a 2-3-fold increased risk of mortality from chronic liver disease [3, 4]. It is therefore important to determine whether alcohol intake influences liver disease development or progression in diabetic patients with NAFLD. By definition, a diagnosis of NAFLD requires the exclusion of significant alcohol consumption in patients with steatosis and metabolic risk factors [5]. Population studies have shown a dose-response relationship between the level of alcohol use and the risk of liver injury, with an increase in relative risk observed at approximately 1-2 and 2-3 standard drinks per day for women and men, respectively [6–8]. The effect of modest alcohol intake in patients with NAFLD remains controversial, with some studies suggesting that low-to-moderate alcohol consumption is associated with lesser NAFLD severity [9–11]. However, in these studies, the prevalence of patients with T2DM or metabolic syndrome was relatively low, ranging from 7% to 41% of individuals within each study cohort [9–12].

In diabetic patients with NAFLD who have an increased risk of nonalcoholic steatohepatitis (NASH) and fibrosis, the effect of modest alcohol consumption on fibrosis progression and patient outcomes remains unclear. In order to investigate this, we examined the association between lifetime alcohol consumption and liver stiffness, a noninvasive marker of liver fibrosis, in a cohort of diabetic patients at risk of clinically significant NAFLD. Additionally, we examined the association between alcohol consumption and other comorbidities and medication use.

2. Methods

Consecutive patients with T2DM were offered participation in a cross-sectional study when they attended the Endocrine Clinic at the Princess Alexandra Hospital, Brisbane ($n = 96$), or from primary care practices within the Metro South Hospital and Health Services District ($n = 55$), between October 2015 and November 2016.

2.1. Case Ascertainment/Study Eligibility. Patients were eligible to be included in the study if they had a diagnosis of T2DM defined using standard criteria [13], NAFLD, and an indeterminate or high score on the FIB-4 [14] or NAFLD fibrosis scores [15]. A diagnosis of NAFLD required demonstration of hepatic steatosis by liver ultrasound in the presence of metabolic risk factors and the exclusion of significant alcohol consumption (>20 g/day) within the preceding 5 years, steatosis-inducing drugs, or other chronic liver diseases (including a prior history of alcohol-related liver disease). Patients were excluded if they had stage 5 chronic kidney disease (estimated glomerular filtration rate <15 mL/min), renal replacement therapy, or history of organ transplant. The NAFLD fibrosis and FIB-4 scores have good negative predictive values and can be used clinically to exclude advanced fibrosis in patients who have low scores [16]. The study therefore selectively recruited patients who were more likely to have clinically significant liver disease.

2.2. Study Population. Eligible patients were invited to attend the liver clinic at the Princess Alexandra Hospital, Brisbane, for clinical assessment. Informed written consent was obtained from each patient and the protocol was approved by the Metro South Health and the University of Queensland Human Research Ethics Committees (HREC/15/QPAH/301; UQ2015001047).

2.3. Clinical Data. Data were collected prospectively by the study clinician (PP). Firstly, medical history was obtained during a consultation in the liver clinic. Patients underwent a clinical assessment and were subsequently informed about their diagnosis.

Medical history was obtained using a structured questionnaire. Interview items included self-reported sociodemographic characteristics, history of tobacco or recreational drug use, previously diagnosed liver disease, other medical conditions, and use of medications. Alcohol intake was assessed using a standardized questionnaire and the Alcohol Use Disorders Identification Test [17] (AUDIT). The AUDIT was developed by the World Health Organization and is the most widely used measure of alcohol consumption and alcohol-related problems. The AUDIT-C, consisting of the first three AUDIT questions (how often is alcohol consumed, how many alcoholic drinks are typically drunk in a day, and how often are six or more drinks consumed), provides a standardized continuous measure of alcohol consumption. Alcohol intake within the preceding 5 years was used to define NAFLD, and drinkers consumed <20 g/day. Lifetime drinking history classified patients into nondrinkers (never drinkers), light drinkers (always ≤20 g/day), and moderate drinkers (any period with intake >20 g/day).

Clinical assessment included anthropometric measurements (weight, height, and waist circumference), laboratory tests (routine biochemical, hematological, and serological assays), transient elastography, and liver ultrasound. Metabolic syndrome was defined as central obesity (waist circumference: Europid male ≥94 cm, South Asian male ≥90 cm, female ≥80 cm), plus any two of the following four factors: raised fasting plasma glucose or previously diagnosed type 2 diabetes, raised blood pressure or treatment of previously diagnosed hypertension, raised triglycerides or reduced HDL cholesterol, or specific treatment for these lipid abnormalities [18].

Transient elastography with simultaneous Controlled Attenuation Parameter (CAP) was performed after a 3-hour fast using FibroScan® technology (Echosens, Paris, France) using the standard M or XL probes. Examinations were performed by a trained clinical nurse (with experience in performing more than 250 liver stiffness measurements

(LSM)) and reviewed by a hepatologist (KAS) with extensive FibroScan experience (more than 2000 LSM performed). Recommended standard FibroScan operating procedures were followed along with adherence to criteria for definition of reliable LSM: minimum of 10 valid measurements with a success rate of ≥60% and IQR ≤30% of the final (median) result. The XL probe was used when the skin-capsule depth was ≥2.5 cm. Although optimal liver stiffness cut-off values in NAFLD remain under discussion, for the purposes of this study, we used the following cut-off values: 8.2 kPa for severe fibrosis and 10.5 kPa for the diagnosis of cirrhosis, respectively, for *ruling out* disease with at least 90% sensitivity, as described by Cassinotto et al. [19].

Liver ultrasound was performed by one of the sonographers at the Department of Diagnostic Radiology, Princess Alexandra Hospital, Brisbane, trained in advanced liver imaging. The Princess Alexandra Hospital is the referral center for the state-wide liver transplant service, and over 1650 liver ultrasounds are performed in the department each year. Steatosis was determined by increased hepatic echogenicity and beam attenuation, resulting in the renal cortex appearing relatively hypoechoic to the liver parenchyma, absence of the normal echogenic walls of the portal vein, and poor visualization of the diaphragm and deep portions of the liver [20]. Evidence of cirrhosis or portal hypertension on liver imaging was determined by liver surface nodularity or signs of portal hypertension including portal vein dilatation, splenomegaly, portosystemic collaterals, and ascites.

NAFLD severity was broadly classified by transient elastography and liver ultrasound. Participants were categorized as "no advanced disease" (LSM < 8.2 kPa and no evidence of cirrhosis or portal hypertension on liver imaging) and "clinically significant liver disease" (LSM ≥ 8.2 kPa). Liver biopsy was performed in a subset of the patients (n = 28) for clinical indications, based on increased likelihood of advanced disease or patient interest in participating in clinical therapy trials. Histological changes of NAFLD (steatosis, lobular and portal inflammation, presence of ballooning, Mallory-Denk bodies, and fibrosis) were assessed and scored according to accepted criteria [21, 22].

2.4. Data Analysis. Data analysis was conducted using SPSS (SPSS Inc.) version 24.0 (College Station, TX; StataCorp LP, 2013). Participants' sociodemographic and clinical characteristics were described using frequency distribution and percentage and mean and standard deviation (data normally distributed). Pearson's chi-square tests were used to compare proportions (Fisher's exact test was used when cell counts were less than 5) and one-way ANOVA was used to compare means between groups. All p values were 2-sided and statistical significance was set at alpha = 0.05. Multinomial logistic regression was used to calculate adjusted p values between nondrinkers, light drinkers, and moderate drinkers.

Bivariable logistic regression analysis was used to determine the odds of being categorized as having "clinically significant liver disease" compared to "no advanced disease." Obesity or girth, age, and gender, as variables of clinical relevance, were included in the model. Odds ratios (OR) and 95% confidence interval (CI) were reported.

3. Results

3.1. Study Population and Alcohol Consumption. One hundred and fifty-one "at-risk" patients with T2DM and NAFLD were reviewed in the NAFLD clinic over a 12-month period. Overall, the mean age of subjects was 61 ± 10.3 years and 63.6% were males. The majority of subjects were Caucasian, with a mean body mass index (BMI) of 35.9 ± 8.3 kg/m^2 and mean girth of 120.8 ± 18.6 cm. The cohort included 46 lifetime nondrinkers, 70 light drinkers (never more than 20 g alcohol/day), and 35 moderate drinkers (any prior period of alcohol intake >20 g/day). Moderate drinkers had significantly higher median lifetime alcohol consumption of 66.7 g/week compared with light drinkers (4.8 g/week) and nondrinkers (0 g/week) (p = 0.000) and had a mean of 23.7 (±10.9) years from their period of regular drinking >20 g/day up to the time of enrolment in the study. In validation of the alcohol history-based subgrouping, moderate drinkers had a significantly higher alcohol consumption score and alcohol-related harm score (4) when compared with light drinkers (2) and nondrinkers (0) (p = 0.012 and 0.000, resp.) (Supplementary Table 1 in Supplementary Material available online at https://doi.org/10.1155/2017/7927685). A post hoc analysis demonstrated a significant difference between moderate and light drinkers' alcohol consumption (p = 0.035), further corroborating the alcohol history taken at the time of interview.

3.2. Alcohol Consumption and Clinical/Metabolic Characteristics. The demographic and clinical characteristics of the 151 subjects according to lifetime drinking history are summarized in Table 1. Compared with lifetime nondrinkers, light and moderate drinkers were more likely to be male (p = 0.008) and Caucasian (p = 0.007) and to have a history of cigarette smoking (p = 0.000). Girth and BMI were not significantly different between the three cohorts (p > 0.05). Although there was no significant difference in glycated hemoglobin (HbA1c) or insulin therapy between the three cohorts, significantly more moderate drinkers required ≥3 hypoglycemic agents to maintain diabetic control (p = 0.041), suggesting that moderate drinkers may have worse diabetic control. In particular, a higher proportion of moderate drinkers (49%) were using a glucagon-like peptide type 1 (GLP-1) receptor agonist or a dipeptidyl peptidase-4 (DPP-4) inhibitor, compared to light drinkers (26%) and nondrinkers (20%) (p = 0.027).

Serum triglyceride levels were higher in moderate drinkers (p = 0.033) but this was not statistically significant following adjustment for age and BMI (p = 0.086). Importantly, a higher proportion of moderate drinkers (20%) were taking a fibrate medication to lower blood triglyceride levels, compared to light drinkers (4%) and nondrinkers (11%) (p = 0.044). Serum low-density lipoprotein (LDL) levels were significantly lower in females with a history of moderate alcohol intake (p = 0.045); however, this should be interpreted with caution as the number of females in this subgroup was very small (n = 7) (data not presented). There was no significant difference in HDL levels or use of statin therapy between the three cohorts (p > 0.05).

TABLE 1: Demographic and clinical characteristics of the 151 subjects according to lifetime drinking history.

	Nondrinker (n = 46)	Light drinker (n = 70)	Moderate drinker (n = 35)	Crude p values	Adjusted p values[b]
Age	62.8 ± 10.6	61.2 ± 9.9	58.3 ± 10.4	0.147	0.167
Gender (male)[a]	22 (48)	46 (66)	28 (80)	**0.010**	**0.008**
Ethnicity (Caucasian)[a]	28 (61)	58 (83)	30 (86)	**0.008**	**0.007**
BMI (kg/m^2)					
Male	33.1 ± 7.5	34.5 ± 6.4	36.4 ± 0.2	0.170	0.313[c]
Female	37.3 ± 10.3	39.1 ± 9.1	36.4 ± 8.6	0.519	0.313[c]
Girth (cm)					
Male	115.5 ± 16.3	120.4 ± 16.5	126.2 ± 18.7	0.098	0.173[c]
Female	119.3 ± 20.1	121.7 ± 17.7	111.6 ± 24.9	0.338	0.204[c]
Never smoker[a]	36 (78)	30 (43)	13 (37)	**0.000**	**0.000**
Diabetic "control"					
HbA1c	7.9 ± 1.3	8.0 ± 1.7	8.5 ± 1.6	0.197	0.515
Insulin therapy[a]	23 (50)	32 (46)	22 (63)	0.250	0.239
DPP4/GLP1[a]	9 (20)	18 (26)	17 (49)	**0.012**	**0.027**
Dyslipidemia					
Triglycerides	2.0 ± 1.5	2.0 ± 1.1	2.8 ± 2.1	**0.033**	0.086
Fibrate therapy[d]	5 (11)	3 (4)	7 (20)	**0.037**	**0.044**
Comorbidities					
Ischemic heart disease[a]	10 (22)	20 (29)	13 (37)	0.314	0.300
Obstructive sleep apnea[a]	8 (17)	25 (36)	25 (71)	**0.005**	**0.003**
Depression[a]	22 (48)	25 (35)	25 (71)	**0.003**	**0.003**
Respiratory disease[a]	9 (20)	15 (21)	10 (29)	0.603	0.615
Osteoarthritis[a]	15 (33)	29 (41)	13 (37)	0.629	0.487

Data presented continuously (mean ± standard deviation) and analyzed using one-way ANOVA, unless specified. [a]Data presented categorically (n, %) and analyzed using Pearson's χ^2 test. [b]All p values adjusted for age and BMI unless specified. [c]Adjusted for age. [d]Data presented categorically (n, %) and analyzed using Fisher's exact test.

Interestingly, the prevalence of obstructive sleep apnea (OSA) differed significantly between patients with and without alcohol consumption (p = 0.003). Seventy-one percent of moderate drinkers had a history of obstructive sleep apnea compared to 36% of light drinkers and 17% of nondrinkers. Self-reported depression was also significantly more common in moderate drinkers (71%), compared to light and nondrinkers (35% and 48%, resp.; p = 0.003).

3.3. Alcohol Consumption and NAFLD Fibrosis Severity. LSM met quality criteria in 134 patients. Median LSM was 6.3 kPa with a range from 2.6 to 63.9 kPa and required the use of the XL probe in 83%. Eighty-eight of 134 patients (65.7% of the cohort) had LSM <8.2 kPa, suggesting the absence of severe fibrosis. Liver biopsy was performed in a subset of the patients (n = 28), and an additional 8 patients had liver imaging diagnostic of cirrhosis. Twenty-nine of these 36 patients had liver stiffness measurements ≥8.2 kPa and 23 of these 29 patients (79%) had bridging fibrosis or cirrhosis.

There was no significant difference between those patients with LSM <8.2 kPa or ≥8.2 kPa and their alcohol consumption, dependence, alcohol-related harm, and overall AUDIT score. Compared to male lifetime nondrinkers, the proportion of male light and moderate drinkers with LSM ≥8.2 kPa (24, 35 and 37 per cent, resp.) was not significantly different (p > 0.05). In females, the proportion of patients with LSM ≥ 8.2 kPa was 35% in nondrinkers and 50% in light drinkers. However, none of the 7 female patients with a history of moderate alcohol intake had LSM ≥ 8.2 kPa. Compared to lifetime nondrinkers, light drinkers had 1.79 (95% CI: 0.67–4.82; p = 0.247) and moderate drinkers had 0.91 (95% CI: 0.27–3.10; p = 0.881) times the odds of having LSM ≥ 8.2 (adjusted for age, gender, and BMI).

Similarly, there was no significant difference in biochemical, hematological, or liver imaging parameters between the three patient groups (Table 2).

4. Discussion

Increasing evidence suggests that moderate alcohol consumption (≤30 g/day) reduces the risk of coronary artery disease and other vascular conditions associated with the metabolic syndrome [23–27]. However, the effect of modest alcohol intake on the *liver* component of the metabolic syndrome (NAFLD) and other comorbid conditions remains controversial. Due to the high prevalence of NAFLD and

TABLE 2: Liver stiffness measurements and selected biochemical, hematological, and liver imaging parameters according to lifetime drinking history.

	Nondrinker (n = 46)	Light drinker (n = 70)	Moderate drinker (n = 35)	Crude p value	Adjusted p value[e]
LSM kPa[a]					
All	8.4 ± 8.0	9.8 ± 7.1	10.7 ± 12.5	0.570	0.546
Male	8.7 ± 10.1	8.0 ± 4.8	12.0 ± 13.4	0.226	0.639
Female	8.2 ± 5.1	12.4 ± 9.8	4.6 ± 1.7	0.053	**0.016**
LSM ≥ 8.2 kPa[a]					
All	12 (29)	24 (40)	10 (30)	0.459	0.302
Male	5 (24)	14 (35)	10 (37)	0.584	0.581
Female[b]	7 (35)	10 (50)	0 (0)	0.092	0.132
CAP (dB/m)[a]	322.1 ± 68.5	333.4 ± 54.2	340.6 ± 59.5	0.910	0.492
ALT (IU/ml)	36.4 ± 26.4	38.4 ± 29.5	37.4 ± 15.8	0.909	0.818
AST (IU/ml)	29.0 ± 17.6	28.6 ± 26.1	24.7 ± 11.2	0.606	0.457
GGT (IU/ml)	44.2 ± 42.9	53.6 ± 83.1	47.6 ± 45.4	0.738	0.750
Platelets ($\times 10^9$)	242.0 ± 62.6	229.5 ± 58.7	255.0 ± 45.6	0.095	0.081
Albumin (g/dL)	40.4 ± 2.8	40.6 ± 2.7	41.0 ± 3.4	0.704	0.601
Spleen size (cm)[c]	10.6 ± 2.9	10.4 ± 2.9	9.9 ± 3.1	0.666	0.617
Liver size (cm)[d]	17.3 ± 3.5	17.0 ± 2.3	17.9 ± 3.4	0.501	0.502

Data presented continuously (mean ± standard deviation) and analyzed using one-way ANOVA. Data presented categorically (n, %) and analyzed using Pearson's χ^2 test, unless specified. [a]Smaller cohort of patients as LSM met quality criteria in 134 patients. [b]Data presented categorically (n,%) and analyzed using Fisher's exact test.[c]Spleen size documented in 99 patients. [d]Liver size documented in 94 patients.[e]All p values adjusted for age and BMI unless specified. ALT: alanine aminotransferase; AST: aspartate aminotransferase; GGT: gamma-glutamyl transferase.

increased risk of advanced fibrosis in people with T2DM, determining the effect of light or moderate alcohol intake on liver disease progression in these patients is crucial. The present study indicated that, in diabetic patients at risk of clinically significant NAFLD, light or moderate lifetime alcohol consumption was not associated with a protective effect on liver fibrosis. Of concern, alcohol consumption was associated with an increased prevalence of metabolic comorbidities, specifically hypertriglyceridemia and OSA, and a history of smoking and self-reported depression.

Prior studies examining the relationship between alcohol, obesity, and liver injury have produced conflicting results. In comparison with obesity alone, an earlier cross-sectional study showed that the combination of obesity and heavy alcohol intake (>60 g/day) was associated with a 1.3-fold increased risk for steatosis detected by liver ultrasound [28]. The effects of alcohol intake and body weight on liver enzyme levels were examined in a large US population-based study [29]. Among obese and overweight subjects, alcohol intake of ≥1 and >2 standard drinks per day, respectively, was associated with a higher prevalence of elevated aminotransferase levels in multivariate analyses [29]. In contrast to these data, a number of studies have suggested that low-to-moderate alcohol intake may be associated with a lower risk of obesity-related liver disease [30], possibly due to the beneficial effect of reduced insulin resistance [31]. Among severely obese patients (BMI > 35 kg/m^2) presenting for weight loss surgery, modest alcohol consumption (<200 g/week) was associated with a reduction in NASH, but the effect was not significant after controlling for diabetes or insulin resistance index [31]. In comparison with no alcohol use, self-reported wine consumption up to 10 g/day was associated with a lower prevalence of NAFLD (defined using unexplained serum alanine aminotransferase (ALT) elevation) among participants in the Third National Health and Nutrition Examination Survey [30].

Few studies have examined the effect of modest alcohol consumption in the presence of preexisting NAFLD. Heavy episodic drinking (>60 or 48 g ethanol in males and females, resp., consumed on one occasion at least once a month) was associated with fibrosis progression on repeat liver biopsy or development of end-stage liver disease after a mean of 13.8 years [12]. In contrast, light alcohol consumption (up to 2 drinks per day) was associated with lesser degrees of NAFLD severity in three cross-sectional studies [9–11]. However, in these studies, the prevalence of patients with T2DM or metabolic syndrome was relatively low, ranging from 7% to 41% of the study populations [10–12, 32]. In our cohort of diabetic subjects, light or moderate alcohol consumption was not associated with lesser degrees of NAFLD severity as assessed by liver stiffness, a noninvasive marker of liver fibrosis. Reasons for the lack of liver disease protection in our patient cohort are unclear but may include alcohol-related exacerbation of lipotoxicity, liver inflammation, and oxidative stress in the presence of type 2 diabetes [33].

In our study, fasting serum triglyceride levels were higher in moderate drinkers, and a higher proportion of moderate drinkers (20%) were taking a fibrate medication to lower blood triglyceride levels, compared to light drinkers (4%) and nondrinkers (11%). Although high alcohol intake is known to increase blood triglyceride levels, prior studies of the effect of low-to-moderate alcohol intake on triglycerides have provided variable results [34]. As alcohol can impair lipolysis and raise very-low-density lipoprotein (VLDL) levels [35], alcohol intake in diabetic patients may worsen their predisposition to hypertriglyceridemia. This is a consequence of raised VLDL and increased cholesteryl ester transfer protein activity causing a higher hepatic flow of free fatty acids in combination with a deficiency in lipoprotein lipase activity [35]. Although currently there remain no consensus guidelines regarding appropriate triglyceride levels, this association is of concern as evidence suggests that hypertriglyceridemia independently increases the risk of cardiovascular events [36–38].

We have previously shown a high burden of multimorbidity in diabetic NAFLD patients, with the most common coexisting chronic conditions including ischemic heart disease, obstructive sleep apnea, self-reported depression, respiratory diseases, and osteoarthritis [39]. Our data also demonstrated an association between OSA and alcohol consumption: 71% of moderate drinkers had a history of OSA compared to 36% of light drinkers and 17% of nondrinkers. This is consistent with prior studies demonstrating an association between alcohol use and OSA [40]. Alcohol has been shown to relax the upper airway whilst diminishing the normal arousal response to airway obstruction, resulting in impaired normal breathing with sleep fragmentation and sleep disordered breathing [40]. Similarly, self-reported depression was very prevalent in this patient cohort and was significantly more common in moderate drinkers compared to light and nondrinkers. The high prevalence of depression has been corroborated by a recent meta-analysis, where 30% of T2DM patients reported depression [41]. In particular, elderly patients suffering from depression and alcohol misuse have worse health outcomes, poorer physical and mental health, and a higher mortality rate [42]. Alcohol abuse can also result in unsatisfactory patient control of diabetes and hypertension [42].

Study strengths include the prospective collection of history of alcohol consumption by the study clinician before a diagnosis was established and face-to-face patient interviews to overcome literacy concerns and patient understanding of questions. The downside of using face-to-face interviews is that they may promote social-desirability bias, where patients answer questions in a certain way or feel self-conscious in the presence of an interviewer, thereby inaccurately or incompletely disclosing alcohol consumption. This was a small single-center study and therefore our findings may not be truly representative of the wider population with T2DM and NAFLD. In order to ensure we were assessing the impact of alcohol intake in patients with NAFLD, participants with alcohol intake >20 g/day within 5 years prior to study entry were excluded. However, these exclusion criteria may have led to a selection bias excluding patients in whom moderate ongoing alcohol intake may have been beneficial, resulting in resolution of NAFLD. Although liver biopsy remains the gold standard for the diagnosis and assessment of liver fibrosis, the method of assessing advanced fibrosis used in this study (LSM) is an accepted noninvasive procedure for identification of advanced fibrosis [43].

5. Conclusion

Lifetime alcohol consumption was not significantly associated with liver fibrosis in T2DM patients when assessed by LSM. Of concern, alcohol consumption was associated with an increased prevalence of metabolic comorbidities, specifically hypertriglyceridemia and OSA, and a history of smoking and self-reported depression. This study highlights the importance of taking a detailed alcohol history from patients regarded as "without a history of significant alcohol consumption," as the impact of alcohol on diabetes comorbidities cannot be dismissed and requires further investigation.

Abbreviations

NAFLD: Nonalcoholic fatty liver disease
T2DM: Type 2 diabetes mellitus
HDL: High-density lipoprotein
NASH: Nonalcoholic steatohepatitis
AUDIT: Alcohol Use Disorders Identification Test
CAP: Controlled Attenuation Parameter
LSM: Liver stiffness measurement
OR: Odds ratios
CI: Confidence interval
BMI: Body mass index
HbA1c: Glycated hemoglobin
GLP-1: Glucagon-like peptide type 1
DPP-4: Dipeptidyl peptidase-4
LDL: Low-density lipoprotein
OSA: Obstructive sleep apnea
ALT: Alanine aminotransferase
VLDL: Very-low-density lipoprotein
AST: Aspartate aminotransferase
GGT: Gamma-glutamyl transferase.

Ethical Approval

This study was conducted in accordance with the National Statement on Ethical Conduct in Human Research 2007 (updated May 2015) and was approved by the Human Ethics Committees of Metro South Hospital and Health Service (HREC/15/QPAH/301) and the University of Queensland (UQ2015001047).

Authors' Contributions

Patricia C. Valery and Elizabeth E. Powell have an equal contribution as senior authors.

Acknowledgments

This study was funded by the Pathology Queensland-Study, Education and Research Trust Fund. P. C. Valery was supported by the Australian National Health and Medical

Research Council (Career Development Fellowship no. 1083090).

References

[1] J. I. Blomster, S. Zoungas, J. Chalmers et al., "The relationship between alcohol consumption and vascular complications and mortality in individuals with type 2 diabetes," *Diabetes Care*, vol. 37, no. 5, pp. 1353–1359, 2014.

[2] J. H. O'Keefe, K. A. Bybee, and C. J. Lavie, "Alcohol and Cardiovascular Health. The Razor-Sharp Double-Edged Sword," *Journal of the American College of Cardiology*, vol. 50, no. 11, pp. 1009–1014, 2007.

[3] Q. M. Anstee, G. Targher, and C. P. Day, "Progression of NAFLD to diabetes mellitus, cardiovascular disease or cirrhosis," *Nature Reviews Gastroenterology & Hepatology*, vol. 10, no. 6, pp. 330–344, 2013.

[4] G. Zoppini, U. Fedeli, N. Gennaro, M. Saugo, G. Targher, and E. Bonora, "Mortality from chronic liver diseases in diabetes," *American Journal of Gastroenterology*, vol. 109, no. 7, pp. 1020–1025, 2014.

[5] N. Chalasani, Z. Younossi, J. E. Lavine et al., "The diagnosis and management of non-alcoholic fatty liver disease: practice guideline by the American Association for the Study of Liver Diseases, American College of Gastroenterology, and the American Gastroenterological Association," *American Journal of Gastroenterology*, vol. 107, no. 6, pp. 811–826, 2012.

[6] U. Becker, A. Deis, T. I. A. Sorensen et al., "Prediction of risk of liver disease by alcohol intake, sex, and age: A prospective population study," *Hepatology*, vol. 23, no. 5, pp. 1025–1029, 1996.

[7] NHMRC, "Australian Guidelines To reduce Health Risk from Drinking Alcohol," Commonwealth of Australian, 2009.

[8] J. P. Connor, P. S. Haber, and W. D. Hall, "Alcohol use disorders," *The Lancet*, vol. 387, no. 10022, pp. 988–998, 2016.

[9] H. Hagström, P. Nasr, M. Ekstedt et al., "Low to moderate lifetime alcohol consumption is associated with less advanced stages of fibrosis in non-alcoholic fatty liver disease," *Scandinavian Journal of Gastroenterology*, vol. 52, no. 2, pp. 159–165, 2017.

[10] H. K. Kwon, J. K. Greenson, and H. S. Conjeevaram, "Effect of lifetime alcohol consumption on the histological severity of non-alcoholic fatty liver disease," *Liver International*, vol. 34, no. 1, pp. 129–135, 2014.

[11] W. Dunn, A. J. Sanyal, E. M. Brunt et al., "Modest alcohol consumption is associated with decreased prevalence of steatohepatitis in patients with non-alcoholic fatty liver disease (NAFLD)," *Journal of Hepatology*, vol. 57, no. 2, pp. 384–391, 2012.

[12] M. Ekstedt, L. E. Franzén, M. Holmqvist et al., "Alcohol consumption is associated with progression of hepatic fibrosis in non-alcoholic fatty liver disease," *Scandinavian Journal of Gastroenterology*, vol. 44, no. 3, pp. 366–374, 2009.

[13] World Health Organization IDF, "Definition and Diagnosis of Diabetes Mellitus and Intermediate Hyperglycaemia." Geneva, Switzerland: 1-46.

[14] R. K. Sterling, E. Lissen, N. Clumeck et al., "Development of a simple noninvasive index to predict significant fibrosis in patients with HIV/HCV coinfection," *Hepatology*, vol. 43, no. 6, pp. 1317–1325, 2006.

[15] P. Angulo, J. M. Hui, G. Marchesini et al., "The NAFLD fibrosis score: a noninvasive system that identifies liver fibrosis in patients with NAFLD," *Hepatology*, vol. 45, no. 4, pp. 846–854, 2007.

[16] S. McPherson, S. F. Stewart, E. Henderson, A. D. Burt, and C. P. Day, "Simple non-invasive fibrosis scoring systems can reliably exclude advanced fibrosis in patients with non-alcoholic fatty liver disease," *Gut*, vol. 59, no. 9, pp. 1265–1269, 2010.

[17] J. B. Saunders, O. G. Aasland, T. F. Babor, J. R. de la Fuente, and M. Grant, "Development of the alcohol use disorders identification test (AUDIT): WHO collaborative project on early detection of persons with harmful alcohol consumption II," *Addiction*, vol. 88, no. 6, pp. 791–804, 1993.

[18] K. G. M. M. Alberti, P. Zimmet, and J. Shaw, "Metabolic syndrome—a new world-wide definition. A consensus statement from the International Diabetes Federation," *Diabetic Medicine*, vol. 23, no. 5, pp. 469–480, 2006.

[19] C. Cassinotto, J. Boursier, V. de Lédinghen et al., "Liver stiffness in nonalcoholic fatty liver disease: A comparison of supersonic shear imaging, FibroScan, and ARFI with liver biopsy," *Hepatology*, vol. 63, no. 6, pp. 1817–1827, 2016.

[20] S. Saadeh, Z. M. Younossi, E. M. Remer et al., "The utility of radiological imaging in nonalcoholic fatty liver disease," *Gastroenterology*, vol. 123, no. 3, pp. 745–750, 2002.

[21] D. E. Kleiner, E. M. Brunt, M. van Natta et al., "Design and validation of a histological scoring system for nonalcoholic fatty liver disease," *Hepatology*, vol. 41, no. 6, pp. 1313–1321, 2005.

[22] E. M. Brunt, C. G. Janney, A. M. Di Bisceglie, B. A. Neuschwander-Tetri, and B. R. Bacon, "Nonalcoholic steatohepatitis: a proposal for grading and staging the histological lesions," *American Journal of Gastroenterology*, vol. 94, no. 9, pp. 2467–2474, 1999.

[23] L. L. J. Koppes, J. M. Dekker, H. F. J. Hendriks, L. M. Bouter, and R. J. Heine, "Meta-analysis of the relationship between alcohol consumption and coronary heart disease and mortality in type 2 diabetic patients," *Diabetologia*, vol. 49, no. 4, pp. 648–652, 2006.

[24] L. L. J. Koppes, J. M. Dekker, H. F. J. Hendriks, L. M. Bouter, and R. J. Heine, "Moderate alcohol consumption lowers the risk of type 2 diabetes: a meta-analysis of prospective observational studies," *Diabetes Care*, vol. 28, no. 3, pp. 719–725, 2005.

[25] K. A. Britton, J. M. Gaziano, H. D. Sesso, and L. Djoussé, "Relation of Alcohol Consumption and Coronary Heart Disease in Hypertensive Male Physicians (from the Physicians' Health Study)," *American Journal of Cardiology*, vol. 104, no. 7, pp. 932–935, 2009.

[26] K. J. Mukamal, H. Chung, N. S. Jenny et al., "Alcohol consumption and risk of coronary heart disease in older adults: The cardiovascular health study," *Journal of the American Geriatrics Society*, vol. 54, no. 1, pp. 30–37, 2006.

[27] K. Reynolds, L. B. Lewis, J. D. L. Nolen, G. L. Kinney, B. Sathya, and J. He, "Alcohol Consumption and Risk of Stroke: A Meta-analysis," *Journal of the American Medical Association*, vol. 289, no. 5, pp. 579–588, 2003.

[28] S. Bellentani, G. Saccoccio, F. Masutti et al., "Prevalence of and risk factors for hepatic steatosis in Northern Italy," *Annals of Internal Medicine*, vol. 132, no. 2, pp. 112–117, 2000.

[29] C. E. Ruhl and J. E. Everhart, "Joint effects of body weight and alcohol on elevated serum alanine aminotransferase in the United States population," *Clinical Gastroenterology and Hepatology*, vol. 3, no. 12, pp. 1260–1268, 2005.

[30] W. Dunn, R. Xu, and J. B. Schwimmer, "Modest wine drinking and decreased prevalence of suspected nonalcoholic fatty liver disease," *Hepatology*, vol. 47, no. 6, pp. 1947–1954, 2008.

[31] J. B. Dixon, P. S. Bhathal, and P. E. O'Brien, "Nonalcoholic fatty liver disease: predictors of nonalcoholic steatohepatitis and liver

fibrosis in the severely obese," *Gastroenterology*, vol. 121, no. 1, pp. 91–100, 2001.

[32] E. Hagström, C. Held, R. A. H. Stewart et al., "Growth differentiation factor 15 predicts all-cause morbidity and mortality in stable coronary heart disease," *Clinical Chemistry*, vol. 63, no. 1, pp. 325–333, 2017.

[33] S. Munukutla, G. Pan, M. Deshpande, R. A. Thandavarayan, P. Krishnamurthy, and S. S. Palaniyandi, "Alcohol Toxicity in Diabetes and Its Complications: A Double Trouble?" *Alcoholism: Clinical and Experimental Research*, vol. 40, no. 4, pp. 686–697, 2016.

[34] A. T. Do Rego, B. Klop, E. Birnie et al., "Diurnal triglyceridemia in relation to alcohol intake in men," *Nutrients*, vol. 5, no. 12, pp. 5114–5126, 2013.

[35] G. Yuan, K. Z. Al-Shali, and R. A. Hegele, "Hypertriglyceridemia: its etiology, effects and treatment," *Canadian Medical Association Journal*, vol. 176, no. 8, pp. 1113–1120, 2007.

[36] E. B. Rimm, P. Williams, K. Fosher, M. Criqui, and M. J. Stampfer, "Moderate alcohol intake and lower risk of coronary heart disease: Meta-analysis of effects on lipids and haemostatic factors," *British Medical Journal*, vol. 319, no. 7224, pp. 1523–1528, 1999.

[37] R. Scragg and P. Metcalf, "Do triglycerides explain the U-shaped relation between alcohol and diabetes risk? Results from a cross-sectional survey of alcohol and plasma glucose," *Diabetes Research and Clinical Practice*, vol. 66, no. 2, pp. 147–156, 2004.

[38] J. Kovar and K. Zemankova, "Moderate alcohol consumption and triglyceridemia," *Physiol Res*, vol. 64, supplement 3, pp. S371–S375, 2015.

[39] P. J. Patel, K. L. Hayward, R. Rudra et al., "Multimorbidity and polypharmacy in diabetic patients with NAFLD," *Medicine*, vol. 96, no. 26, p. e6761, 2017.

[40] S. Chakravorty, N. S. Chaudhary, and K. J. Brower, "Alcohol Dependence and Its Relationship With Insomnia and Other Sleep Disorders," *Alcoholism: Clinical and Experimental Research*, vol. 40, no. 11, pp. 2271–2282, 2016.

[41] E. Ivanova, R. J. Burns, S. S. Deschênes, B. Knäuper, and N. Schmitz, "A Longitudinal Investigation of Anxiety and Depressive Symptomatology and Exercise Behaviour Among Adults With Type 2 Diabetes Mellitus," *Canadian Journal of Diabetes*, vol. 41, no. 1, pp. 73–81, 2017.

[42] O. Mowbray, T. Washington, G. Purser, and J. O'Shields, "Problem Drinking and Depression in Older Adults with Multiple Chronic Health Conditions," *Journal of the American Geriatrics Society*, vol. 65, no. 1, pp. 146–152, 2017.

[43] N. Chalasani, Z. Younossi, J. E. Lavine et al., "The diagnosis and management of nonalcoholic fatty liver disease: Practice guidance from the American Association for the Study of Liver Diseases," *Hepatology*.

13

Prevalence of Anxiety and Depression in Patients with Inflammatory Bowel Disease

Glynis Byrne,[1] Greg Rosenfeld,[2] Yvette Leung,[2] Hong Qian,[3] Julia Raudzus,[4] Carlos Nunez,[4] and Brian Bressler[2]

[1]*Department of Medicine, University of British Columbia, Vancouver, BC, Canada*
[2]*Department of Medicine, Division of Gastroenterology, University of British Columbia, Vancouver, BC, Canada*
[3]*Centre for Health Evaluation and Outcome Sciences, University of British Columbia, St. Paul's Hospital, Vancouver, BC, Canada*

[4]*Department of Psychiatry, University of British Columbia, Vancouver, BC, Canada*

Correspondence should be addressed to Brian Bressler; brian_bressler@hotmail.com

Academic Editor: Yousuke Nakai

Background. Inflammatory bowel disease (IBD) patients are not routinely screened for depression and anxiety despite knowledge of an increased prevalence in people with chronic disease and negative effects on quality of life. *Methods.* Prevalence of anxiety and depression was assessed in IBD outpatients through retrospective chart review. The presence of anxiety and/or depression was determined using the Patient Health Questionnaire-9 and Generalized Anxiety Disorder-7 self-report questionnaires or by diagnosis through psychiatric interview. Patient demographics, disease characteristics, and medication information were also collected. Multivariable analysis was used to determine associations between patient factors and depression and anxiety. *Results.* 327 patient charts were reviewed. Rates of depression and anxiety were found to be 25.8% and 21.2%, with 30.3% of patients suffering from depression and/or anxiety. Disease activity was found to be significantly associated with depression and/or anxiety ($p = 0.01$). Females were more likely to have anxiety ($p = 0.01$). *Conclusion.* A significant proportion of IBD patients suffer from depression and/or anxiety. The rates of these mental illnesses would justify screening and referral for psychiatric treatment in clinics treating this population. Patients with active disease are particularly at risk for anxiety and depression.

1. Introduction

The prevalence of depression and anxiety is higher in patients with chronic diseases compared to the general population [1] and having a long term medical illness is a risk factor for depression [2]. There is evidence that inflammatory bowel disease (IBD), which includes Crohn's disease (CD) and ulcerative colitis (UC), is associated with higher rates of anxiety and depression compared to the general population [3] and that depression is associated with decreased quality of life in IBD patients [4]. Research on patients with both chronic disease [5] and IBD [6] reveals that the presence of an anxiety or depressive disorder is associated with poor treatment compliance. In addition, depressive disorders are associated with poorer functioning and higher morbidity and mortality in persons with chronic medical conditions [7]. Provision of treatment for mental disorders may improve long term outcomes, and it is therefore important to identify patients at greater risk of anxiety and depression so that they can be offered the appropriate treatment and support.

In a previous Canadian study, IBD cases were extracted from two nationally representative health surveys and depression rates were examined [8]. Depression was diagnosed using a structured diagnostic interview and cases were identified based on self-report of "a bowel disorder such as Crohn's disease or colitis" that has lasted longer than 6 months and been diagnosed by a health professional. The twelve-month depression rates were found to be 14.7% and 16.3% in the two survey samples for IBD patients, rates that are triple those in the general population. Depression rates were found to be higher among those that were female, single, and younger, had greater pain, and had functional limitations. A limitation of this study was that cases were identified through self-report without any medical record verification, and the nonspecific wording of the self-report question may have resulted in inaccurate reporting of IBD.

The primary aim of this study was to determine the prevalence of anxiety and depression in IBD patients attending a gastroenterology outpatient clinic. A secondary aim was identification of patient characteristics associated with increased rates of these mental disorders.

2. Methods

Prevalence of anxiety and depression was assessed in IBD outpatients attending a gastroenterology clinic associated with a tertiary care academic hospital (St. Paul's Hospital, Vancouver, Canada) from January to July 2016. All consecutive IBD patients attending the outpatient clinic were asked to fill out the Generalized Anxiety Disorder-7 (GAD-7) and Patient Health Questionnaire-9 (PHQ-9) questionnaires at their medical appointments to screen for anxiety and depression. The GAD-7 and PHQ-9 are brief self-report scales used to identify Generalized Anxiety Disorder and depression, respectively. Validated in the primary care setting, the GAD-7 has a sensitivity of 89% and a specificity of 82% [9], and the PHQ-9 has a sensitivity of 88% and a specificity of 88% [10] when using a cut-off of 10 or greater as a positive result. Patients were offered referral to psychiatry if they screened positive for anxiety and/or depression, if they discussed mood symptoms with the gastroenterologist, or if they requested referral. A psychiatric interview was then conducted and a diagnosis or lack thereof of Generalized Anxiety Disorder (GAD) or major depressive disorder (MDD) was recorded.

Information collected from patient charts included gender, age at time of mental health assessment, smoking status, disease duration, disease diagnosis (UC versus CD), Partial Mayo scores (UC patients), Harvey-Bradshaw Index (CD patients), previous surgical resection, disease phenotype according to the Montreal classification scores, c-reactive protein (CRP, a noninvasive marker of inflammation with a sensitivity of 60.7% and a specificity of 75.9% in IBD patients for endoscopic inflammation using a cut-off >0.5 mg/dL [11]), current medications, and past use of a biologic medication. Information regarding current psychiatric treatment (including pharmacotherapy or psychotherapy), the use of psychiatric drugs including antidepressants and anxiolytic medications, and history of past diagnosis of anxiety or depression were recorded. These variables were not formally assessed in gastroenterology appointments and were therefore only reliably assessed in patients who had appointments with psychiatry. Patients were considered to have anxiety and/or depression given they had a positive score (10 or greater) on the GAD-7 and/or PHQ-9 screening questionnaires and/or a diagnosis of anxiety or depression from psychiatric interview after referral to a psychiatrist. Both screening questionnaire administration and psychiatric interview took place between January 2016 and August 2016. Psychiatry evaluated referred patients for current presence of anxiety or depressive disorders at appointments, and a diagnosis was made based on physician assessment. Active disease was defined as a Partial Mayo score greater than 4 or a Harvey-Bradshaw Index greater than 7, both accepted cut-offs to indicate moderate to severe disease for these two disease activity measures [12, 13].

Univariate and multivariable logistic regression was used to determine if associations existed between patient characteristics and depression and anxiety. The following potential risk factors, which were identified a priori, were investigated for association with mental disorders in IBD patients: gender, disease diagnosis, disease activity, perianal disease, current steroid use, current or previous biologics, current age, and disease duration. The results shown in the current manuscript are from complete case analysis. We recognized the missing data issues in the data set and the analyses based on the complete case might be biased. In order to examine the impact of the missing data on the results of the analyses, a multiple imputation using chained equations was applied as a sensitivity analysis. The imputation process was conducted in SAS and replicated 200 times.

3. Results

3.1. Study Population. A total of 327 IBD patients were included in the study, Table 1 describes clinical characteristics associated with our cohort. Disease activity is not formally assessed at each clinic visit; therefore, for some patients a Partial Mayo or Harvey-Bradshaw Index score was not provided or possible to calculate for the time of the mental health assessment. Sufficient information to determine disease activity was available for 170/327 patients in the study, 13% had at least moderately active disease using the Partial Mayo score (UC) and Harvey-Bradshaw Index (CD). Sixty-four percent of those with moderately to severely active disease had CRP lab value, 86% of which had a value over 5 mg/L indicating biochemical confirmation of inflammation.

Past psychiatric history and treatment were not formally assessed in gastroenterology appointments; therefore information regarding psychiatric treatment and diagnosis is presented for patients who attended psychiatric appointments only, as these variables were more consistently assessed via psychiatry. Twenty-two patients attended an appointment with psychiatry; of those patients seven were taking an antidepressant medication, three were also taking benzodiazepines, and one patient was receiving cognitive behavioural therapy. Eleven patients had received psychiatric treatment in the past, two had previously been diagnosed with anxiety alone, five with depression alone, and two with anxiety and depression.

3.2. Prevalence of Anxiety and Depression. The presence or absence of depression could be assessed for 314 patients, anxiety for 322 patients, and depression and/or anxiety for 317 patients; missing data is due to lack of or incomplete questionnaires. Prevalence with 95% confidence intervals (CI) of anxiety was 21.1% (95% CI: 17.0%–25.9%), 25.5% (95% CI: 21.3%–30.9%) for depression, and 30.3% (95% CI 25.5%–35.6%) for depression and/or anxiety. Of the patients who screened positive for depression and/or anxiety and

TABLE 1: Characteristics of the patient population.

Variable	Anxiety and/or depression n = 96	No anxiety or depression n = 231
Age, year (mean, std)	38.57 +/− 13.80	38.78 +/− 14.73
Female sex, n (%)	52 (54.2%)	111 (48.1%)
Smoking status, n (%)		
Nonsmoker	58 (71.6%)	146 (80.2%)
Past smoker	12 (14.8%)	20 (11.0%)
Current smoker	11 (13.6%)	16 (8.8%)
Disease diagnosis, n (%)		
Crohn's disease	38 (39.6%)	86 (37.2%)
Ulcerative colitis	58 (60.4%)	145 (62.8%)
Time since diagnosis, years (mean, std)	11.85 +/− 8.76	10.60 +/− 8.58
Active disease, n (%)	11/41 (26.8%)	11/129 (23.4%)
Elevated CRP, n (%)	20 (36.4%)	34 (25.9%)
Previous surgical resection, n (%)	25 (26.0%)	54 (21.6%)
Perianal disease, n (%)	23 (24.0%)	50 (21.6%)
Steroids, n (%)	3 (3.2%)	8 (3.5%)
Current/previous biologic, n (%)	64 (66.7%)	137 (59.3%)
Depression, n (%)	81 (25.8%)	
Anxiety, n (%)	68 (21.1%)	
Diagnosis via screening questionnaire, n (%)	142 (95%)	
Diagnosis via psychiatric interview, n (%)	7 (5%)	
Current psychiatric treatment, n (%)	7/22 (31.8%)	
Current psychiatric medication, n (%)	7/22 (31.8%)	
Past psychiatric treatment, n (%)	11/22 (50%)	
Past diagnosis anxiety/depression, n (%)	9/22 (40.9%)	

TABLE 2: Multivariable logistic regression analysis of the association between patient demographic and disease characteristics and the presence of depression and/or anxiety.

Variable	Odds ratio (95% CI)	p value
Gender (male)	0.67 (0.31–1.45)	0.31
Disease diagnosis (CD)	0.53 (0.21–1.33)	0.17
Disease activity (active)	4.28 (1.52–12.04)	0.01
Perianal disease	1.28 (0.45–3.62)	0.65
Current steroids	0.73 (0.05–10.6)	0.81
Current or previous biologic use	1.54 (0.62–3.86)	0.35
Current age (year)	0.97 (0.94–1.00)	0.07
Time since diagnosis (year)	1.02 (0.96–1.08)	0.52

accepted referral to a psychiatrist, 18 of 20 patients (90%) with positive PHQ-9 scores had a diagnosis of depression confirmed, and 16 of 19 patients (84%) with positive GAD-7 scores had a diagnosis of anxiety confirmed.

3.3. Factors Associated with Anxiety and Depression. Univariate analysis found that presence of active disease was significantly associated with depression and/or anxiety (OR: 4.14, p value: 0.003), as well as with depression (OR: 4.47, p value: 0.002) and anxiety (OR: 3.37, p value: 0.02). In multivariable analysis, presence of active disease was independently significantly associated with depression and/or anxiety (OR: 4.28, p value: 0.01), as well as with depression (OR: 4.70, p = 0.004) and anxiety (OR: 2.97, p = 0.05). Male gender was protective from development of anxiety (OR: 0.29, p = 0.01). None of the other variables investigated were found to be significantly associated with anxiety or depression. Odds ratios and p values from multivariable analysis of each variable with anxiety and/or depression are described in Table 2.

Disease activity was significantly associated with increased risk of depression and anxiety in IBD patients. Figure 1 shows the percentage of patients with anxiety and/or depression with active disease and those with inactive disease.

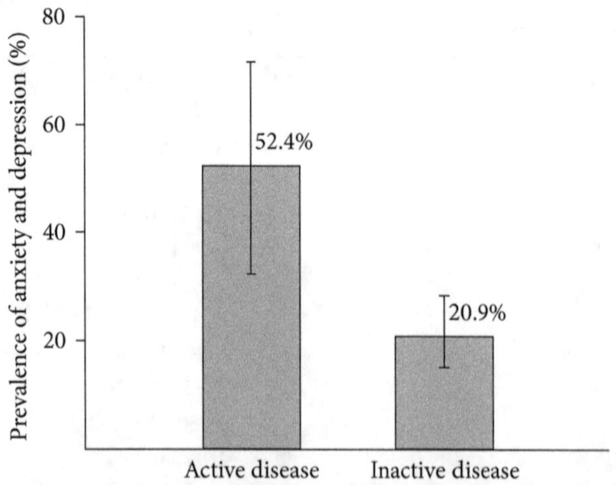

Figure 1: Percentage of patients found to have anxiety and/or depression at present with active and inactive disease. Error bars represent 95% CI.

4. Discussion

4.1. Prevalence of Anxiety and Depression in IBD Patients. The prevalence of anxiety (21.2%) and depression (25.8%) in IBD patients reported in this study is higher than that reported for the general Canadian population. According to the 2013 Statistics Canada Health Survey, the 12-month and lifetime prevalence of depression in the Canadian population were 4.7% and 11.3%, and the 12-month and lifetime prevalence of Generalized Anxiety Disorder were 2.6% and 8.7% [14]. Our results are consistent with findings that patients with long term medical conditions are at increased risk of major depression [2] and with studies that have found the prevalence of anxiety and depression to be higher in IBD patients compared with healthy controls [15–17].

There is variation in the rates of depression and anxiety reported in different studies likely due to differences in populations studied, methods used to assess depression and anxiety, and the period of time within which depression and/or anxiety was assessed (lifetime versus 12 months versus current) [3, 8, 18]. Previous Canadian studies have assessed rates of depression and anxiety in survey samples of self-reported IBD patients [8, 18] and in an IBD patient cohort [19] but none in consecutive patients attending an outpatient clinic. Our study is unique in that it is the first Canadian study to investigate the prevalence of anxiety and depression in consecutive outpatients attending a gastroenterology clinic. Screening for anxiety and depression in consecutive patients may provide a more accurate estimate of the prevalence as this design removes the selection bias introduced when depending on patients to volunteer to be part of a cohort or to reply to a survey. Therefore, our study should provide a more accurate estimate of the point prevalence of anxiety and depression in an outpatient IBD population.

Twelve-month rates of depression reported from two nationally representative surveys with patients identified through self-report of "a bowel disorder such as Crohn's disease or colitis" were 14.7% and 16.3% [8]. Our results show a higher prevalence of depression, likely due to the lack of specificity in the criteria used to diagnose IBD in these survey studies. Another study used survey samples of self-reported IBD patients to assess the prevalence of anxiety and found that IBD patients had 2.18 greater odds of anxiety compared to the general population [18]. Limitations of these studies are that cases of IBD were not verified through medical records, and only 82.6%, 84.7%, and 79.8% of households responded to the surveys, potentially introducing bias due to differences between those who chose to respond and those who did not. It has been observed that those with less education, older age, and greater use of psychopharmaceutical drugs are less likely to participate in survey research [20].

A Canadian cohort study which drew on patients from the University of Manitoba Research Registry found lifetime rates of Generalized Anxiety Disorder (GAD) and major depressive disorder (MDD) in IBD patients to be 13.4% and 27.2% [19]. IBD patients eligible for inclusion in the registry were identified through the database of Manitoba Health. A limitation of this study is that the registry is composed of a subset of IBD patients that may not be representative of all of those living in the community: patients had to be diagnosed within the past 7 years for inclusion and patients needed to agree to participate in the registry, which resulted in only just over half of eligible IBD patients being included. Further, of those eligible in the registry 14% declined to take part in the cohort study and a further 35 of 388 patients initially enrolled were lost throughout the 2-year duration. The characteristics of the patients who agreed and were able to meet the demands of inclusion in the registry and cohort study may vary from those unable or unwilling to participate. Research of nonparticipation in a prospective study on chronic respiratory and cardiovascular diseases found that patients who did not feel well and/or had been admitted to hospital during the last 12 months had lower participation rates [21].

Our study included IBD patients attending a gastroenterology outpatient clinic where all patients are asked to complete the GAD-7 and PHQ-9 questionnaires to limit selection bias. One limitation was that the patient population assessed was drawn from a tertiary IBD clinic; this may result in a patient population with more severe or active IBD, or more comorbidities compared to community samples. Additionally, this study did not include any patients that were currently hospitalized, and because anxiety and depression have been associated with disease flares and inpatient status, prevalence of anxiety and depression may be lower in the population studied compared to inpatient IBD populations [3, 16].

As previously reported in the literature [15, 22], we found that disease activity was significantly associated with increased risk of depression and anxiety in IBD patients. Häuser et al. (2011) [17] found that IBD patients with moderate/severe disease activity had higher rates of depression and anxiety compared to both those with slight disease activity and to an age and sex matched representative sample of the general population. Patients in remission were not at an increased risk of depression and anxiety compared to the general population. We found that prevalence of anxiety and depression did not differ between UC and CD patients, which is consistent with previous research [17]. Female sex was associated with increased risk of anxiety, which has been reported in other studies of patients with IBD [18, 22], as well as in the general population [14, 23].

Variation in methods of psychiatric assessment is likely partially responsible for the variation in reported prevalence of anxiety and depression in IBD patients between studies. Use of screening questionnaires may overestimate rates of depression and anxiety: when patients were assessed using both the DSM-3 criteria and the Hospital Anxiety and Depression Scale (HADS) screening questionnaire rates of psychiatric illness were lower using the DSM criteria [24]. We used the GAD-7 and PHQ-9 screening questionnaires, which have been validated in the primary care setting, to assess anxiety and depression. When using a cut-off of 10 or greater as a positive result for both questionnaires, the GAD-7 has a sensitivity of 89% and a specificity of 82% [9], while the PHQ-9 has a sensitivity of 88% and a specificity of 88% [10]. Some of the symptoms of depression used for screening, such as changes in appetite and fatigue, may overlap with IBD symptoms; therefore, the PHQ-9 may overestimate depression in IBD patients. Assessment of the accuracy of the PHQ-9 screening questionnaire in this population is important. In our study this screening tool seems to be accurate; of those patients who agreed to referral to a psychiatrist, 90% of patients who scored positive on the PHQ-9 had a diagnosis of depression confirmed by psychiatric interview.

The high prevalence of mental disorders we have found in our study is an important problem that requires further attention. A meta-analysis which investigated any correlation between depression and patient compliance in a variety of chronic disease patients (end stage renal disease, angina, cancer, renal transplant, and rheumatoid arthritis) with a variety of interventions (dietary and health behaviour interventions and medications) found that depression was associated with three times greater odds of noncompliance with treatment recommendation [5]. Both depression [25] and presence of psychiatric disorders [6] have been associated with decreased treatment compliance in IBD patients. Adherence to medical treatment in IBD patients is important not only in the short term for preventing flares of disease activity but also to prevent long term complications. Identification and treatment of anxiety and depression in IBD patients may be important in improving treatment adherence and long term patient outcomes. Anxiety and depression in IBD have been shown to contribute to poor health related quality of life (HR-QOL) independent of disease severity [26]. Zhang et al. (2013) [4] examined the role of depression and disease activity as independent factors in predicting HR-QOL. Depression was found to be the most significant predictor of poor HR-QOL in IBD patients, with disease activity being only weakly predictive. Therefore, addressing mental health in patients with IBD may be important in maximizing patient quality of life. Additionally, psychiatric illness in IBD patients has been found to predict high cost outcomes including emergency department visits, IBD-related hospitalizations, and high treatment charges [27]. The potential benefits of mental health treatment, along with the increased prevalence of anxiety and depression in IBD patients, suggest that screening for anxiety and depression in this population would be of value.

5. Conclusion

In summary, our study shows that a significant proportion (30.3%) of IBD outpatients suffer from anxiety and/or depression. The prevalence of anxiety and/or depression found in our study justifies screening and referral for psychiatric treatment in clinics treating this population. The finding that disease severity is associated with increased risk of depression and anxiety suggests that those with active disease may benefit from more intense psychiatric screening.

References

[1] D. M. Clarke and K. C. Currie, "Depression, anxiety and their relationship with chronic diseases: A review of the epidemiology, risk and treatment evidence," *Med. J. Aust*, vol. 190, no. 7, pp. S54–S60, 2009.

[2] S. B. Patten, "Long-term medical conditions and major depression in a Canadian population study at waves 1 and 2," *Journal of Affective Disorders*, vol. 63, no. 1-3, pp. 35–41, 2001.

[3] L. A. Graff, J. R. Walker, and C. N. Bernstein, "Depression and anxiety in iflammatory bowel disease: a review of comorbidity and management," *Inflammatory Bowel Diseases*, vol. 15, no. 7, pp. 1105–1118, 2009.

[4] C. K. Zhang, J. Hewett, J. Hemming et al., "The influence of depression on quality of life in patients with inflammatory bowel disease," *Inflammatory Bowel Diseases*, vol. 19, no. 8, pp. 1732–1739, 2013.

[5] M. R. Dimatteo, H. S. Lepper, and T. W. Croghan, "Depression is a risk factor for noncompliance with medical treatment meta-analysis of the effects of anxiety and depression on patient adherence," *JAMA Internal Medicine*, vol. 160, no. 14, pp. 2101–2107, 2000.

[6] G. Nigro, G. Angelini, S. B. Grosso, G. Caula, and C. Sategna-Guidetti, "Psychiatric predictors of noncompliance in inflammatory bowel disease: Psychiatry and compliance," *Journal of Clinical Gastroenterology*, vol. 32, no. 1, pp. 66–68, 2001.

[7] W. J. Katon, "Epidemiology and treatment of depression in patients with chronic medical illness," *Dialogues Clin. Neurosci*, vol. 13, no. 1, pp. 7–23, 2011.

[8] E. Fuller-Thomson and J. Sulman, "Depression and inflammatory bowel disease: Findings from two nationally representative Canadian surveys," *Inflammatory Bowel Diseases*, vol. 12, no. 8, pp. 697–707, 2006.

[9] R. L. Spitzer, K. Kroenke, J. B. W. Williams, and B. Löwe, "A brief measure for assessing generalized anxiety disorder: the GAD-7," *JAMA Internal Medicine*, vol. 166, no. 10, pp. 1092–1097, 2006.

[10] K. Kroenke, R. L. Spitzer, and J. B. W. Williams, "The PHQ-9: validity of a brief depression severity measure," *Journal of General Internal Medicine*, vol. 16, no. 9, pp. 606–613, 2001.

[11] J. Langhorst, S. Elsenbruch, J. Koelzer, A. Rueffer, A. Michalsen, and G. J. Dobos, "Noninvasive markers in the assessment of intestinal inflammation in inflammatory bowel diseases: performance of fecal lactoferrin, calprotectin, and PMN-elastase, CRP, and clinical indices," *American Journal of Gastroenterology*, vol. 103, no. 1, pp. 162–169, 2008.

[12] F. Nagy, T. Molnár, K. Farkas et al., "P436 Clinical course of ulcerative colitis according to the partial Mayo score based classification during two-year follow-up period: Result from a Hungarian multicenter IBD database," *Journal of Crohn's and Colitis*, vol. 6, p. S183, 2012.

[13] L. Peyrin-Biroulet, J. Panés, W. J. Sandborn et al., "Defining Disease Severity in Inflammatory Bowel Diseases: Current and Future Directions," *Clinical Gastroenterology and Hepatology*, vol. 14, no. 3, pp. 348–354.e17, 2016.

[14] C. Pearson, T. Janz, and J. Ali, "Health at a glance mental and substance use disorders in Canada," *Stat. Canada*, vol. no. 82, pp. 1–8, 2013.

[15] G. Addolorato, E. Capristo, G. F. Stefanini, and G. Gasbarrini, "Inflammatory bowel disease: A study of the association between anxiety and depression, physical morbidity, and nutritional status," *Scandinavian Journal of Gastroenterology*, vol. 32, no. 10, pp. 1013–1021, 1997.

[16] J. R. Goodhand, M. Wahed, J. E. Mawdsley, A. D. Farmer, Q. Aziz, and D. S. Rampton, "Mood disorders in inflammatory bowel disease: relation to diagnosis, disease activity, perceived stress, and other factors," *Inflammatory Bowel Diseases*, vol. 18, no. 12, pp. 2301–2309, 2012.

[17] W. Häuser, K.-H. Janke, B. Klump, and A. Hinz, "Anxiety and depression in patients with inflammatory bowel disease: Comparisons with chronic liver disease patients and the general population," *Inflammatory Bowel Diseases*, vol. 17, no. 2, pp. 621–632, 2011.

[18] E. Fuller-Thomson, R. Lateef, and J. Sulman, "Robust Association between Inflammatory Bowel Disease and Generalized Anxiety Disorder: Findings from a Nationally Representative Canadian Study," *Inflammatory Bowel Diseases*, vol. 21, no. 10, pp. 2341–2348, 2015.

[19] J. R. Walker, J. P. Ediger, L. A. Graff et al., "The Manitoba IBD Cohort study: a population-based study of the prevalence of lifetime and 12-month anxiety and mood disorders," *American Journal of Gastroenterology*, vol. 103, no. 8, pp. 1989–1997, 2008.

[20] K. Korkeila, S. Suominen, J. Ahvenainen et al., "Non-response and related factors in a nation-wide health survey," *European Journal of Epidemiology*, vol. 17, no. 11, pp. 991–999, 2001.

[21] L. Janzon, B. S. Hanson, S.-O. Isacsson, S. E. Lindell, and B. Steen, "Factors influencing participation in health surveys. Results from prospective population study 'Men born in 1914' in Malmo, Sweden," *Journal of Epidemiology and Community Health*, vol. 40, no. 2, pp. 174–177, 1986.

[22] S. Nahon, P. Lahmek, C. Durance et al., "Risk factors of anxiety and depression in inflammatory bowel disease," *Inflammatory Bowel Diseases*, vol. 18, no. 11, pp. 2086–2091, 2012.

[23] C. P. McLean, A. Asnaani, B. T. Litz, and S. G. Hofmann, "Gender differences in anxiety disorders: Prevalence, course of illness, comorbidity and burden of illness," *Journal of Psychiatric Research*, vol. 45, no. 8, pp. 1027–1035, 2011.

[24] H. Andrews, P. Barczak, and R. N. Allan, "Psychiatric illness in patients with inflammatory bowel disease," *Gut*, vol. 28, no. 12, pp. 1600–1604, 1987.

[25] A. Lopez-Sanroman and F. Bermejo, "Review article: How to control and improve adherence to therapy in inflammatory bowel disease," *Alimentary Pharmacology & Therapeutics*, vol. 24, no. 3, pp. 45–49, 2006.

[26] E. Guthrie, J. Jackson, J. Shaffer, D. Thompson, B. Tomenson, and F. Creed, "Psychological disorder and severity of inflammatory bowel disease predict health-related quality of life in ulcerative colitis and Crohn's disease," *American Journal of Gastroenterology*, vol. 97, no. 8, pp. 2–7, 2002.

[27] J. Limsrivilai, R. W. Stidham, S. M. Govani, A. K. Waljee, W. Huang, and P. D. R. Higgins, "Factors That Predict High Health Care Utilization and Costs for Patients With Inflammatory Bowel Diseases," *Clinical Gastroenterology and Hepatology*, vol. 15, no. 3, pp. 385–392, 2017.

14

The use of Biomarkers in Early Diagnostics of Pancreatic Cancer

Lumir Kunovsky,[1,2] Pavla Tesarikova,[3] Zdenek Kala,[2] Radek Kroupa,[1] Petr Kysela,[2] Jiri Dolina,[1] and Jan Trna[1,3]

[1]*Department of Gastroenterology, University Hospital Brno Bohunice, Faculty of Medicine, Masaryk University, Czech Republic*
[2]*Department of Surgery, University Hospital Brno Bohunice, Faculty of Medicine, Masaryk University, Czech Republic*
[3]*Department of Internal Medicine, Hospital Boskovice, Czech Republic*

Correspondence should be addressed to Jan Trna; jan.trna@seznam.cz

Academic Editor: Yousuke Nakai

Pancreatic ductal adenocarcinoma (PDAC) is one of the most lethal solid malignancies with increasing incidence. The poor prognosis is due to the aggressive nature of the tumor, late detection, and the resistance to chemotherapy and radiotherapy. A radical surgery procedure is the only treatment that has been shown to improve the 5-year survival rate to 20-25%. However, the majority of patients (80-85%) are diagnosed with locally advanced or metastatic disease and just 15-20% patients are diagnosed in an early stage allowing them to undergo the potentially curative surgical resection. The early detection of PDAC without the use of invasive methods is challenging and discovery of a cost-effective biomarker with high specificity and sensitivity could significantly improve the treatment and survival in these patients. In this review, we summarize current and newly examined biomarkers in early PDAC detection.

1. Introduction

Pancreatic ductal adenocarcinoma (PDAC) is one of the most lethal solid malignancies with increasing incidence [1] and is the fourth leading cause of cancer-related mortality in the United States and Canada [2–5].

The poor prognosis is due to the aggressive nature of the tumor, late detection, and the resistance to chemotherapy and radiotherapy [6–8]. Unfortunately, compared to other malignancies, there has been little improvement in the survival rate of patients with PDAC in recent decades [9].

The overall 5-year survival rate is approximately about 5% [2, 3, 10]. Most of the patients (80-85%) are diagnosed with locally advanced or metastatic disease. Only 15-20% are diagnosed in an early stage allowing them to undergo surgical resection [1, 11, 12]. Radical surgery has been shown to improve the 5-year survival rate to a 20-25% [12–15].

Differential diagnosis without the use of invasive methods yields difficulties distinguishing between PDAC, benign lesions, or chronic pancreatitis [16].

As shown in Figure 1, most studies and clinical trials have sought to identify an inexpensive, noninvasive, or minimally invasive biomarker with high sensitivity and specificity for PDAC to improve early diagnosis and subsequent treatment [17]. Biomarkers for a PDAC can be classified as diagnostic, prognostic, and predictive. In this article, we will focus on a current view on diagnostic markers for early pancreatic cancer detection. The summary of possible biomarkers can be found in Table 1.

2. CA 19-9

The only routinely used serum marker for PDAC is carbohydrate antigen 19-9 (CA 19-9).

CA19-9 is an isolated form of Lewis antigen, which was first separated in 1979 [1, 18]. Elevation of CA 19-9 signify advanced PDAC and poor prognosis [19, 20]. However, the elevation of CA19-9 can also be caused by many other conditions, including various benign diseases (pancreatitis, cirrhosis, and acute cholangitis) [21, 22] or other malignancies (colorectal cancer, gastric, and uterine cancer) [19]. CA 19-9 is also not expressed in some individuals with a specific Lewis genotype and only 65% of patients with resectable PDAC have elevated serum levels [19, 23]. Due to all this reasons, CA 19-9 is not recommended as a screening marker for PDAC [20].

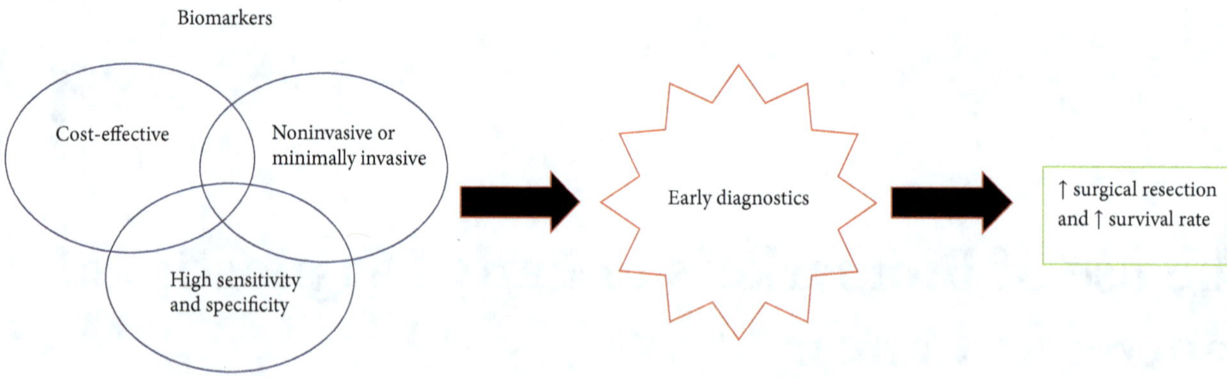

FIGURE 1: Characteristics required for biomarkers of pancreatic cancer.

TABLE 1: Overview of biomarkers of early pancreatic cancer.

Traditional biomarkers	CA 19-9, CEA
Proteomics	CEMIP, C4BPA, IGFBP2, IGFBP3
Metabolites	M2-pyruvate kinase (M2-PK), palmitic acid, glucitol, xylitol, inositol, histidine, proline, sphingomyelin, phosphatidylcholine, isocitrate, ceramide
Antibodies	immunoglobulin G4 (IgG4)
Cytokines	interleukin-1β, interleukin-6, interleukin-8, interleukin-10, vascular endothelial growth factor and transforming growth factor (macrophage inhibitory cytokine-1 [MIC-1])
Noncoding RNAs (ncRNAs)	microRNAs (miRNAs), small ncRNAs (sncRNAs), long ncRNAs (lncRNAs)
Liquid biopsy	circulating tumor cells (CTCs), circulation tumor DNA (ctDNA) and exosomes
Body fluids	detecting biomarkers from saliva, urine, stool or pancreatic juice

Some trials tried to improve the diagnostic value of CA 19-9 by measuring the CA 19-9 antigen on individual proteins or combining CA 19-9 with another cancer marker.

Yue et al. [24] published an article combining measurements of the standard CA 19-9 assay with detection of CA 19-9 on proteins mucin MUC5AC and MUC16; the sensitivity of cancer detection was improved relative to CA 19-9 alone in each sample set, achieving 67-80% sensitivity at 98% specificity.

Many sources confirm a better performance in the diagnosis of PDAC than CEA (carcinoembryonic antigen) measured alone [18, 21]. However, meta-analysis from 2017 showed that a combination of elevated levels CA 19-9 together with CEA (as a vital supplementary to CA19-9) can play an important role in clinical diagnosis of PDAC [25].

Lee et al. (2018) found that combined detection with CA 19-9 and cell migration-inducing hyaluronan binding protein (CEMIP) levels may have the potential to become a new laboratory indicator for the clinical diagnosis of PDAC. CEMIP exists as a newly identified protein involved in hyaluronan degradation and its increased expression has been reported in various cancers. Results suggest that CEMIP proteins were highly expressed in patients with PDAC compared to healthy individuals. Combining the use of CA 19-9 and CEMIP significantly increased the sensitivity and specificity in discriminating not only patients with all stage pancreatic cancer, but also patients with stage I/II pancreatic cancer from healthy individuals [26].

In 2015 Ritchie et al. [27] presented a new biomarker, serum fatty acid metabolite PC-594, that more clearly identified PDAC than did CA 19-9.

In summary, CA19-9 is the only routinely used serum marker of PDAC in clinical practice today. However, its elevation is usually a sign of an advanced disease and it can also be related to a variety of benign and malignant diseases other than PDAC. Thus, future studies should be directed at exploring if CA19-9 in combination with other markers can yield improved sensitivity and specificity.

3. Proteomics

As mentioned above, proteins such as CEMIP can be used for pancreatic cancer detection. Other proteins have been investigated as well. Sogawa et al. [28] demonstrated that the serum C4b-binding protein α-chain (C4BPA) level functions as a potential serum biomarker which distinguishes PDAC from chronic pancreatitis and major gastroenterological cancers, including biliary tract cancer. Yoneyama et al. [29] reported that insulin-like growth factor-binding protein (IGFBP) 2 and IGFBP3 have the ability to discriminate PDAC patients at an early stage from healthy controls. Furthermore, diagnosis of PDAC using the combination of CA19-9, IGFBP2, and IGFBP3 is significantly more effective than CA19-9 alone. This suggests that IGFBP2 and IGFBP3 may serve as compensatory biomarkers for CA19-9.

In summary, proteomics represents a promising area of research with several potentially useful proteins that seem to be able to detect PDAC even at an early stage. Future research is likely to focus on testing the role of various proteins in combination with CA19-9.

4. M2-Pyruvate Kinase (M2-PK)

In 2008 Novotny et al. [30] investigated M2-pyruvate kinase (M2-PK) as a potential tumor marker for distinguishing pancreatic cancer, chronic pancreatitis (ChP), and healthy controls. In group of 132 patients, a higher serum level of M2-PK was found in patients with advanced PDAC. The resulting levels were significantly higher than in patients with early PDAC, ChP, and healthy controls. Unfortunately, the differences between early PDAC and ChP were not found, which makes this marker not suitable for an early PDAC detection.

Joergensen et al. [31] sought to compare the diagnostic utility of M2-PK versus CA 19-9. The sensitivity and specificity of M2-PK were lower compared with CA 19-9 in overall PDAC detection. However, the levels of M2-PK were not affected by cholestasis or Lewis phenotype as is a limitation in the case of CA 19-9.

An additional benefit of M2-PK as a marker includes the finding that M2-PK has been associated with poorer prognosis and survival rate in those diagnosed with PDAC or periampullary malignancy [32, 33].

In summary, M2-PK has been tested as a potential marker for PDAC; unfortunately, findings reflect lower rates of sensitivity and specificity when compared with CA 19-9.

5. Other Metabolomic Biomarkers

Several investigators have identified some metabolomics as promising diagnostic markers for the early detection of PDAC, including palmitic acid, glucitol, xylitol, inositol, and histidine [34, 35].

The recent and largest study conducted to identify a tumor biomarker signature distinguishing PDAC from ChP using a metabolomics approach was published by Mayerle et al. [36] in 2018. They investigated 914 subjects (patients with PDAC, ChP, liver cirrhosis, and healthy cohorts) and identified a metabolic biomarker signature comprising 9 metabolites (histidine, proline, sphingomyelin d18:2, sphingomyelin d17:1, phosphatidylcholine, isocitrate, sphingagine-1-phosphate, pyruvate, and ceramide), which was used in conjunction with CA19-9 to detect PDAC with a much higher diagnostic accuracy than CA19-9 alone.

The list of metabolomics used for detection of early PDAC can be seen in Table 1.

In summary, metabolomic studies appear to represent a promising approach for the detection of PDAC at an early stage, especially when tested as a panel of several markers and in combination with CA19-9.

6. IgG4

High levels of immunoglobulin G4 (IgG4) in blood serum are associated with a group of autoimmune diseases called IgG4-related diseases [37]. The most common clinical manifestation is autoimmune pancreatitis (AIP) [38].

In some patients with PDAC, IgG4 elevation has been reported and it can constitute a differential diagnostic problem between AIP and PDAC. In 2012, Dite et al. [39] found in his group of 81 patients with histologically verified PDAC an elevated serum level of IgG4 (exceeding 135 mg/dl) in 8 patients. Due to this result IgG4 elevation is not suitable as a sole marker to differentiate between PDAC and AIP. However, more than twice elevated serum IgG4 level is considered to be an important diagnostic indicator, as it is present in less than 1% of PDAC patients. Some investigators explored a possible correlation between serum elevated IgG4 and pancreatic cancer. Ngwa et al. [40] reported that approximately 10% of PDAC patients have an elevated IgG4 serum level. Mild elevations in serum IgG4 are unlikely to distinguish AIP from PDAC. Serum IgG4 elevation appears to have no prognostic significance in PDAC and serum IgG4 elevation more than 2 times the upper limit appears to be most commonly associated with AIP.

In contrast to the findings reported above, a 2018 meta-analysis [41] found that serum IgG4 has high specificity and relatively low sensitivity in the differential diagnosis between AIP and pancreatic cancer, and therefore it considers serum IgG4 as useful in distinguishing AIP from PDAC.

In 2016 Liu et al. [42] published a study looking at IgG4-positive plasma cell infiltration in patients with pancreatic cancer and its correlation with the clinicopathologic traits and overall survival of pancreatic cancer. Findings suggest that high-level infiltration of IgG4-positive plasma cells may be an independent predictor for poor overall survival in PDAC patients after curative resection. The study did not investigate a possible IgG4-positive plasma cells infiltration in early diagnostics of PDAC, so this remains unclear and a potential area of further inquiry.

In summary, elevated levels of IgG4 are a typical finding in AIP; however, mild elevation can also be present in PDAC. Levels of IgG4 more than 2 times the upper limit are rare in PDAC and in conjunction with negative CA19-9 are highly suggestive of AIP.

7. Cytokines

In 2016, Yako el al. [2] conducted a systemic review of sixty-five studies analyzing 41 different cytokines in connection with PDAC. Six cytokines (interleukin-1β, interleukin-6, interleukin-8, interleukin-10, vascular endothelial growth factor, and transforming growth factor) were consistently reported to be increased in PDAC by more than four studies. However, the review did not demonstrate sufficient evidence to support individual cytokines as a diagnostic biomarker for PDAC. However, the use of panel of cytokines may be a tool for distinguishing PDAC from other pancreatic benign diseases or healthy controls.

Increased serum levels of macrophage inhibitory cytokine-1 (MIC-1), a distant member of transforming growth beta factor, in PDAC patients compared to those with benign pancreatic diseases and healthy controls were reported in some studies [43, 44]. Additionally, an elevated MIC-1 level has been shown to be related to tumor progression [2, 45].

A 2017 meta-analysis comparing 14 studies with a total of 2826 subjects has demonstrated that serum MIC-1 yields a diagnostic accuracy comparable to CA19-9 for PDAC [46].

Some studies suggest that the lack of diagnostic specificity of MIC-1 may be enhanced using a combination of MIC-1 and CA 19-9 [11, 47].

In summary, testing of cytokine levels may be beneficial in PDAC detection; however, testing of levels of individual cytokines (e.g., MIC-1) was only comparable to CA19-9. Thus, future research may focus on the use of a combined panel of individual cytokines.

8. Noncoding RNAs

Noncoding RNAs (ncRNAs) are divided into two groups according to their lengths, small ncRNAs (sncRNAs) (up to 200 bases), and long ncRNAs (lncRNAs) (over 200 bases) [48, 49].

Micro-RNAs (miRNAs) belong to a noncoding RNA, which do not code for proteins. They are a group of small ncRNAs (approximately 18-25 bases long) that regulate gene expression at the posttranscriptional level, through transcript degradation or translational repression. In recent years, the role of miRNA has increasingly gained attention as a potential marker for many types of cancer, including as a potential biomarker for the early detection of PDAC [11, 48]. For this reason, the miRNA has been isolated and studied from pancreatic tumor tissue, blood samples (serum, plasma), pancreatic juice, stool, urine, and even saliva.

Several studies have reported that miRNAs or panels of miRNAs identified in the plasma or serum of PDAC patients show potential diagnostic value, some of them beyond that of CA19-9 [9, 50–52].

Liu et al. [50] showed miR-1290 as biomarker able to distinguish early PDAC from healthy subjects with better diagnostic performance than CA19-9.

The largest case-control study on miRNA in patients with pancreatic diseases was conducted by Schultz et al. [51], including 409 individuals with PDAC, 25 patients with ChP, and 312 healthy controls. The authors found 9 miRNAs with diagnostic value (after testing more than 700 miRNAs), but this result was not superior to CA19-9.

In a multicenter study, Xu et al. [52] showed that miR-486-5p exhibits diagnostic value in discriminating patients with PDAC from normal subjects or patients with ChP (with a the diagnostic value comparable to CA19-9). Similar results were obtained by Le Large et al. [16], where the diagnostic potential of miR-486-5p for distinguishing PDAC from healthy controls was comparable to CA19-9.

In 2015, Vychytilova-Faltejskova et al. [53] published results showing that expression levels of miR-21, miR-34a, and miR-198 were significantly higher, whereas levels of miR-217 were significantly lower in PDAC, in comparison to healthy controls and patients with ChP.

Several studies found that miR-216 and miR-217 are downregulated in PDAC while miR-143, miR145, miR-146, miR-148, miR-150, miR155, miR-196a, miR-196b, miR-210, miR-222, miR-223, and miR-31 are upregulated in PDAC [17, 54, 55].

Hernandez et al. [6] in 2016 wrote a review article about the current knowledge on miRNA in PDAC and its precursor lesions, concluding that miR-21, miR-155, miR-196, and miR-210 are dysregulated in serum, tumor tissue, cyst fluid, and also stool of PDAC patients. In PanIN and intraductal papillary mucinous neoplasm lesions the miR-21, miR-155, and miR-196 are dysregulated as well and suggest their use as early biomarkers.

In summary, miRNAs appear promising as candidates for biomarkers of early PDAC [49], though additional studies are required for further validation of these findings. Additionally, methodology should be standardized if these approaches are ever to be used in the clinical practice [17, 48].

The use of miRNAs detected from stool, urine, pancreatic juice, and saliva will be discussed in chapter about body fluids below.

LncRNAs are restricted to specific cell types and play a crucial role during tumorigenesis by modulating key pathways at the transcriptional, posttranscriptional, and epigenetic levels [9, 56, 57]. The diagnostic value of circulating lncRNA has been demonstrated in various malignancies, such as prostate cancer, hepatocellular carcinoma, colorectal cancer, and non-small cell lung cancer [9, 58–61].

However, the association between lncRNAs and PDAC has not been well investigated, although some studies suggest they may be promising diagnostic markers. Recent studies have reported dysregulation of lncRNAs in patients with PDAC, such as H19, HOTAIR, HOTTIP, and MALAT-1 [62–65].

In 2016, Wang et al. [66] suggested that increased levels of HOTTIP were found in PDAC tissue and described this as a potential marker. In 2016, Xie at al. [67] showed that salivary HOTAIR and PVT1 distinguished PDAC patients from healthy controls and patients with benign pancreatic tumor with sensitivities and specificities ranging from 60 to 97%.

Although lncRNAs seem to possess a potential diagnostic value for early PDAC, the use of lncRNAs as a noninvasive examination modality in PDAC remains relatively uncommon. Further study on the use of lncRNAs as a potential markers is warranted.

9. Liquid Biopsy

The potential for the use of liquid biopsy in several malignancies (including PDAC) has been investigated, in terms of the possible role of circulating tumor cells (CTCs), circulating tumor DNA (ctDNA), and exosomes.

9.1. Circulating Tumor Cells (CTCs). In 1869, Ashworth first reported the existence of circulating tumor cells (CTCs) [12, 68, 69]. CTCs are cells derived from a primary tumor that have entered the vasculature and circulate within the blood stream looking to seed in distant organs [8, 70]. CTCs appear in extremely low frequencies, approximately 1 CTC per billion blood cells in patients with a malignancy [13], and the identification and isolation in pancreatic cancer have proven difficult thus far [17]. However, several studies have shown that CTCs can enter the bloodstream in the early stages even in the case of PDAC [68, 71, 72].

In a recent trial, Kulemann et al. [73] (using a filtration-based method and KRAS [Kirsten rat sarcoma] mutational analysis) reported that CTCs can be found in most patients with PDAC of any stage (localized, locally advanced, or metastatic). They detected CTCs in 73% of patients with PDAC regardless of tumor stage. CTCs were identified in 3 of 4 patients (detection rate 75%) with early PDAC and were not detected in blood from 9 health donors.

Gao et al. [74] reported sensitivity of 88% and a specificity of 90% in patients of various stages of PDAC using subtraction enrichment and immunostaining-fluorescence in situ hybridization.

In 2016, Ankeny et al. reached a sensitivity of 75% and a specificity of 96,5% in detecting PDAC (also counted in all PDAC stages) using a different technique (microfluidic NanoVelcro CTC chip) [75].

Although CTCs seem promising in the early detection of PDAC [9], more data on the sensitivity and specificity of CTCs is needed [12, 13, 17]. A limitation of the use of CTCs as a liquid biopsy is their relatively low sensitivity, rarity and heterogeneity of CTCs, and a lack of clarity on the most effective method of detection [13, 76]. Therefore, a standardized detection method and large-scale validation are required before clinical application [9].

9.2. Circulating Tumor DNA (ctDNA). Circulating free DNA, also called cell-free DNA (cfDNA), was first reported and verified by two French biochemists (Mandel and Metais) in 1948 [77]. The cfDNA consists of small double-stranded DNA fragments found in blood. In healthy people, most cfDNA is derived from bone marrow and other organs such as the liver [12]. Tumor cells also release fragments of DNA called circulating tumor DNA (ctDNA), which was firstly described in 1989 [78, 79].

The ctDNA represents a variable fraction of cfDNA, accounting for 0.01% to more than 50% of the cfDNA [80]. Due to the presence of cancer-related mutations, ctDNA can be effectively distinguished from normal cfDNA [12, 68].

In pancreatic intraepithelial neoplasms (PanINs) and PDAC, the predominant genetic characteristic is the high rate of KRAS mutations, which is directly correlated with PanINs grade [9, 12]. Due to this high frequency of KRAS mutations in PanINs and PDAC, ctDNA could be potentially used as a biomarker in detecting early PDAC. However, there is some concern regarding specificity, as KRAS mutations are not exclusive to PDAC, but are also present in various types of malignancies and even in ChP [9, 81].

Several research groups have reported that ctDNA could be detected in about 50% of early stage PDAC by digital PCR approaches [82–84].

Bettegowda et al. [84] detected ctDNA in 640 plasma samples of patients with different types and stages of cancers, including 155 PDAC patients, and showed that the detection rate of ctDNA was 48% in patients with localized PDAC. A similar result was obtained by Sausen et al. [83], who reported a ctDNA detection rate of 43% in 51 patients with resectable PDAC.

Based on results published by Tjensvoll et al. [85] ctDNA measurements on KRAS mutations seem to be a marker for monitoring treatment efficacy and PDAC disease progression rather than initial diagnosis. Chen et al. [86] also showed that KRAS mutations in plasma DNA functioned as a strong prognostic factor of survival. Also Marchese et al. [87] found a relatively low sensitivity of KRAS mutations in detecting PDAC. Another current limitation of ctDNA in early PDAC diagnostics seems to be limited consistency in the detection techniques and a lack of technical standardization.

Nevertheless, some investigators have implied that sensitivity and specificity for detection of PDAC can be improved by combining KRAS mutations in blood with an increase in the serum CA19-9 level [79]. For example, Maire et al. [88] reported that the sensitivity and specificity of serum KRAS mutations for the diagnosis of PDAC were 47 and 87%, respectively, whereas the combination of serum KRAS mutations and CA19-9 had a sensitivity and specificity of 98 and 77%, respectively. Moreover, Sefrioui et al. [89] analyzed in his trial a combination of traditional tumor marker CA 19-9 with ctDNA and/or CTCs. The positivity of at least 2 markers was associated with a sensitivity and specificity of 78% and 91%, respectively. As such, CA19-9 in combination with ctDNA and/or CTC analysis may represent an efficient method for diagnosing PDAC.

9.3. Exosomes. Exosomes are small vesicles released from the plasma membrane by almost all cells, including cancer cells that have been shown to play an important role in intercellular communication and tumorigenesis [9]. Exosomes carrying various pathogenic miRNAs, mRNAs, DNA fragments, and proteins play an important role in PDAC progression and can be used for the early detection of PDAC [12, 90, 91].

PDAC-derived exosomes enter the circulation at an early stage of cancer development and therefore are promising biomarkers for the early detection of PDAC. However, the method for isolating PDAC related exosomes should be simplified for use in the clinic. Additionally, more evidence from large-scale validation studies is required prior to clinical application.

In summary, the possible role of liquid biopsy (detection of either circulating tumor cells or circulating tumor DNA or tumor exosomes) in early diagnosis of PDAC is in theory very promising. However, data available thus far appear to be conflicting and the real role is unclear. One of the main limitations is a lack of a standardized detection method. Therefore, large-scale validation studies are necessary before clinical application. Overall, findings suggest that higher diagnostic values of liquid biopsy methods available today can be reached when analyzed in a combination with CA19-9.

10. Body Fluids

Body fluids and excrements such as saliva, urine, stool, or pancreatic juice can be used to detect PDAC; therefore, it is relevant to consider the role of body fluids in determining biomarkers.

The saliva contains almost the same molecules as the serum because of the high blood flow in salivary glands and it is an easy target for diagnosis of PDAC [12]. Exosomes and miRNAs in saliva could discriminate pancreatic cancer and might be potential biomarkers for detecting PDAC [92, 93].

Urine is an ultrafiltrate of plasma and also may contain valuable biomarkers that could assist with PDAC diagnosis [12]. Patients with early PDAC can be accurately detected by a three-protein biomarker panel (REG1A, TFF1, and LYVE1109) [94] and by the protein NGAL108 [95] in urine. In support of this, a 2015 study reported the use of miRNA in urine also for early detection of PDAC [12, 96].

Similarly, in 2014, Yang et al. [97] showed that miRNAs could be extracted and detected from pancreatic juice and stool efficiently and that miR-21, miR-155, and miR-216 in stool have the potential of becoming biomarkers for screening PDAC.

Disadvantage of investigation of pancreatic juice is the need for upper endoscopy to obtain it. Despite this potential limitation, Wang el al. [3] published a promising data as part of his study focused on profiling miRNAs in pancreatic juice. Results indicated a marked difference in the profiles of four circulating miRNAs (miR-205, miR-210, miR-492, and miR-1427) in pancreatic juice collected from patients with PDAC (miRNAs together predicted PDAC with a specificity of 88% and sensitivity of 87%). Inclusion of serum CA19-9 level further increased the sensitivity to 91% and the specificity to 100%.

In summary, several novel markers (e.g., exosomes, miRNAs, and proteomics) investigated for PDAC detection in blood have also been tested in other types of biological material (e.g., saliva, urine, stool, or pancreatic juice). Initial results seem promising; however, in general they do not appear to exceed the results of particular markers in blood. Furthermore, the use of pancreatic juice for the analyses is hampered by need of upper endoscopy.

11. Animal Models

Early pancreatic cancer is not commonly diagnosed in routine clinical practice and the typical inability to detect the disease before it reaches an advanced stage is one of the reasons for the high mortality rate of PDAC [98]. This is a barrier for studies on early diagnosis of PDAC, for example, by clinical trial. Most of the current reviews are actually differential diagnosis studies and thus diagnostic values of the studied biomarkers for early PDAC are somewhat limited. Animal models represent one of the theoretical solutions. Several types of animal models that can replicate the growth process of PDAC from healthy tissue through PanIN lesions to invasive carcinoma have been developed and used in research [99]. Most of the studies focus on detailed analysis of pathophysiological processes throughout the carcinogenesis and testing the effect of therapeutics. Testing of possible biomarkers of early pancreatic cancer in animal models has been studied in smaller extent but with somewhat positive results. Hingorani et al. have shown specific serum proteomic signature in a mouse model of PanINs that was detectable even in mice with very early stage preinvasive lesions and low overall burden of disease [100].

In summary, animal models of PDAC may be useful modality for research, as early pancreatic cancer is not easy to diagnose in clinical practice and studies in humans are therefore hard to conduct. Some knowledge on PDAC biomarkers has been obtained on animal models, which have suggested a distinctive proteomic profile of premalignant lesions and PDAC. Further research directed at applicability to humans is warranted.

12. Conclusion

At present, the only chance of curative treatment for pancreatic cancer is based on prompt diagnosis followed by surgical treatment.

Unfortunately, routine cancer markers (such as CA 19-9) do not seem to be reliable in prediction and detection of early stage of PDAC.

However, there is hope in the area of newly emerging biomarkers of this disease. In particular, the use of combination of these new biomarkers together with traditional CA 19-9 may significantly increase a specificity and sensitivity in early PDAC detection.

While it is hard to predict future development in the field, methods of liquid biopsy, proteomics, metabolomics, and miRNAs appear most promising. The near future probably lies in a carefully selected panel of biomarkers that would allow for earlier diagnosis of PDAC and easier determination of its stage and, ideally, also allow for tailoring of the treatment plan and provide indicator of prognosis/outcome. Therefore, future research inquiries should focus on defining of the precise panel of useful markers and provide clear indications for use in routine daily clinical practice. More research is also vital to identify which of the aforementioned novel markers truly define early PDAC with low risk of metastasizing, as, for example, circulating tumor cells might be the first step in widespread of the disease.

Abbreviations

AIP: Autoimmune pancreatitis
CA 19-9: Carbohydrate antigen 19-9
CEA: Carcinoembryonic antigen
CEMIP: Cell migration-inducing hyaluronan binding protein
C4BPA: C4b-binding protein α-chain
IGFBP2,3: Insulin-like growth factor-binding protein 2,3
ChP: Chronic pancreatitis
M2-PK: M2-pyruvate kinase
MIC-1: Macrophage inhibitory cytokine-1
PDAC: Pancreatic ductal adenocarcinoma
ctDNA: Circulating tumor DNA
cfDNA: Circulating free DNA or also cell-free DNA
CTCs: Circulating tumor cells

IgG4: Immunoglobulin G4
miRNA: Micro-RNA
ncRNA: Noncoding RNA
lncRNA: Long noncoding RNA
KRAS: Kirsten rat sarcoma
PanINs: Pancreatic intraepithelial neoplasms.

References

[1] J. L. Humphris, D. K. Chang, A. L. Johns et al., "The prognostic and predictive value of serum CA19.9 in pancreatic cancer," *Annals of Oncology*, vol. 23, no. 7, Article ID mdr561, pp. 1713–1722, 2012.

[2] Y. Y. Yako, D. Kruger, M. Smith, and M. Brand, "Cytokines as biomarkers of pancreatic ductal adenocarcinoma: A systematic review," *PLoS ONE*, vol. 11, no. 5, 2016.

[3] J. Wang, M. Raimondo, S. Guha et al., "Circulating microRNAs in pancreatic juice as candidate biomarkers of pancreatic cancer," *Journal of Cancer*, vol. 5, no. 8, pp. 696–705, 2014.

[4] R. L. Siegel, K. D. Miller, and A. Jemal, "Cancer statistics, 2018," *CA: A Cancer Journal for Clinicians*, vol. 68, no. 1, pp. 7–30, 2018.

[5] I. S. Yu and W. Y. Cheung, "A Contemporary Review of the Treatment Landscape and the Role of Predictive and Prognostic Biomarkers in Pancreatic Adenocarcinoma," *Canadian Journal of Gastroenterology and Hepatology*, vol. 2018, Article ID 1863535, 10 pages, 2018.

[6] Y. G. Hernandez, "MicroRNA in pancreatic ductal adenocarcinoma and its precursor lesions," *World Journal of Gastrointestinal Oncology*, vol. 8, no. 1, pp. 18–29, 2016.

[7] M. Falasca, M. Kim, and I. Casari, "Pancreatic cancer: Current research and future directions," *Biochimica et Biophysica Acta (BBA) - Reviews on Cancer*, vol. 1865, no. 2, pp. 123–132, 2016.

[8] A. Gharibi, Y. Adamian, and J. A. Kelber, "Cellular and molecular aspects of pancreatic cancer," *Acta Histochemica*, vol. 118, no. 3, pp. 305–316, 2016.

[9] X. Zhang, S. Shi, B. Zhang, Q. Ni, X. Yu, and J. Xu, "Circulating biomarkers for early diagnosis of pancreatic cancer: facts and hopes," *Am J Cancer Res*, vol. 8, no. 3, pp. 332-53, 2018.

[10] T. Conroy, J.-B. Bachet, A. Ayav et al., "Current standards and new innovative approaches for treatment of pancreatic cancer," *European Journal of Cancer*, vol. 57, pp. 10–22, 2016.

[11] S. H. Loosen, U. P. Neumann, C. Trautwein, C. Roderburg, and T. Luedde, "Current and future biomarkers for pancreatic adenocarcinoma," *Tumor Biology*, vol. 39, no. 6, p. 101042831769223, 2017.

[12] B. Zhou, J.-W. Xu, Y.-G. Cheng et al., "Early detection of pancreatic cancer: Where are we now and where are we going?" *International Journal of Cancer*, vol. 141, no. 2, pp. 231–241, 2017.

[13] A. R. Lewis, J. W. Valle, and M. G. McNamara, "Pancreatic cancer: Are "liquid biopsies" ready for prime-time?" *World Journal of Gastroenterology*, vol. 22, no. 32, pp. 7175–7185, 2016.

[14] F. Klein, D. Jacob, M. Bahra et al., "Prognostic factors for long-term survival in patients with ampullary carcinoma: The results of a 15-year observation period after pancreaticoduodenectomy," *HPB Surgery*, vol. 2014, 2014.

[15] L. Kunovsky, Z. Kala, V. Prochazka et al., "Surgical treatment of ampullary adenocarcinoma – single center experience and a review of literature," *Klinicka Onkologie*, vol. 31, no. 1, pp. 46–52, 2018.

[16] T. Y. S. Le Large, L. L. Meijer, M. Mato Prado, G. Kazemier, A. E. Frampton, and E. Giovannetti, "Circulating microRNAs as diagnostic biomarkers for pancreatic cancer," *Expert Review of Molecular Diagnostics*, vol. 15, no. 12, pp. 1525–1529, 2015.

[17] M. Herreros-Villanueva and L. Bujanda, "Non-invasive biomarkers in pancreatic cancer diagnosis: What we need versus what we have," *Annals of Translational Medicine*, vol. 4, no. 7, 2016.

[18] Y. Zhang, J. Yang, H. Li, Y. Wu, H. Zhang, and W. Chen, "Tumor markers CA19-9, CA242 and CEA in the diagnosis of pancreatic cancer: a meta-analysis," *International Journal of Clinical and Experimental Medicine*, vol. 8, no. 7, pp. 11683–11691, 2015.

[19] S. Kaur, M. J. Baine, M. Jain, A. R. Sasson, and S. K. Batra, "Early diagnosis of pancreatic cancer: Challenges and new developments," *Biomarkers in Medicine*, vol. 6, no. 5, pp. 597–612, 2012.

[20] G. Y. Locker, S. Hamilton, J. Harris et al., "ASCO 2006 update of recommendations for the use of tumor markers in gastrointestinal cancer," *Journal of Clinical Oncology*, vol. 24, no. 33, pp. 5313–5327, 2006.

[21] S.-Y. Kau, Y.-M. Shyr, C.-H. Su, C.-W. Wu, and W.-Y. Lui, "Diagnostic and prognostic values of CA 19-9 and CEA in periampullary cancers," *Journal of the American College of Surgeons*, vol. 188, no. 4, pp. 415–420, 1999.

[22] K. S. Goonetilleke and A. K. Siriwardena, "Systematic review of carbohydrate antigen (CA 19-9) as a biochemical marker in the diagnosis of pancreatic cancer," *European Journal of Surgical Oncology*, vol. 33, no. 3, pp. 266–270, 2007.

[23] M. Goggins, "Molecular markers of early pancreatic cancer," *Journal of Clinical Oncology*, vol. 23, no. 20, pp. 4524–4531, 2005.

[24] T. Yue, K. A. Maupin, B. Fallon et al., "Enhanced Discrimination of Malignant from Benign Pancreatic Disease by Measuring the CA 19-9 Antigen on Specific Protein Carriers," *PLoS ONE*, vol. 6, no. 12, p. e29180, 2011.

[25] Q. Meng, S. Shi, C. Liang et al., "Diagnostic and prognostic value of carcinoembryonic antigen in pancreatic cancer: A systematic review and meta-analysis," *OncoTargets and Therapy*, vol. 10, pp. 4591–4598, 2017.

[26] H. S. Lee, C. Y. Jang, S. A. Kim et al., "Combined use of CEMIP and CA 19-9 enhances diagnostic accuracy for pancreatic cancer," *Scientific Reports*, vol. 8, no. 1, 2018.

[27] S. A. Ritchie, B. Chitou, Q. Zheng et al., "Pancreatic cancer serum biomarker PC-594: diagnostic performance and comparison to CA19-9," *World Journal of Gastroenterology*, vol. 21, no. 21, pp. 6604–6612, 2015.

[28] K. Sogawa, S. Takano, F. Iida et al., "Identification of a novel serum biomarker for pancreatic cancer, C4b-binding protein α-chain (C4BPA) by quantitative proteomic analysis using tandem mass tags," *British Journal of Cancer*, vol. 115, no. 8, pp. 949–956, 2016.

[29] T. Yoneyama, S. Ohtsuki, K. Honda et al., "Identification of IGFBP2 and IGFBP3 As Compensatory Biomarkers for CA19-9 in Early-Stage Pancreatic Cancer Using a Combination of Antibody-Based and LC-MS/MS-Based Proteomics," *PLoS ONE*, vol. 11, no. 8, p. e0161009, 2016.

[30] I. Novotný, P. Dítě, M. Dastych et al., "Tumor marker M2-pyruvate-kinase in differential diagnosis of chronic pancreatitis and pancreatic cancer," *Hepato-Gastroenterology*, vol. 55, no. 85, pp. 1475–1477, 2008.

[31] M. T. Joergensen, N. H. H. Heegaard, and O. B. Schaffalitzky De Muckadell, "Comparison of plasma Tu-M2-PK and CA19-9 in pancreatic cancer," *Pancreas*, vol. 39, no. 2, pp. 243–247, 2010.

[32] I. A. Bandara, M. Baltatzis, S. Sanyal, and A. K. Siriwardena, "Evaluation of tumor M2-pyruvate kinase (Tumor M2-PK) as a biomarker for pancreatic cancer," *World Journal of Surgical Oncology*, vol. 16, no. 1, 2018.

[33] K. S. Goonetilleke, J. M. Mason, P. Siriwardana, N. K. King, M. W. France, and A. K. Siriwardena, "Diagnostic and prognostic value of plasma tumor M2 pyruvate kinase in periampullary cancer: Evidence for a novel biological marker of adverse prognosis," *Pancreas*, vol. 34, no. 3, pp. 318–324, 2007.

[34] I. M. Di Gangi, T. Mazza, A. Fontana et al., "Metabolomic profile in pancreatic cancer patients: A consensusbased approach to identify highly discriminating metabolites," *Oncotarget* , vol. 7, no. 5, pp. 5815–5829, 2016.

[35] A. Sakai, M. Suzuki, T. Kobayashi et al., "Pancreatic cancer screening using a multiplatform human serum metabolomics system," *Biomarkers in Medicine*, vol. 10, no. 6, pp. 577–586, 2016.

[36] J. Mayerle, H. Kalthoff, R. Reszka et al., "Metabolic biomarker signature to differentiate pancreatic ductal adenocarcinoma from chronic pancreatitis," *Gut*, vol. 67, no. 1, pp. 128–137, 2018.

[37] T. Kamisawa, Y. Zen, S. Pillai, and J. H. Stone, "IgG4-related disease," *The Lancet*, 2014.

[38] P. A. Hart, Y. Zen, and S. T. Chari, "Recent advances in autoimmune pancreatitis," *Gastroenterology*, 2015.

[39] P. Dítě, I. Novotný, Z. Kala et al., "The serological positivity of immunoglobulin IgG4 in patients with pancreatic carcinoma," *Gastroenterologie a Hepatologie*, vol. 66, no. 3, pp. 187–190, 2012.

[40] T. Ngwa, R. Law, P. Hart, T. C. Smyrk, and S. T. Chari, "Serum IgG4 elevation in pancreatic cancer: diagnostic and prognostic significance and association with autoimmune pancreatitis," *Pancreas*, vol. 44, no. 4, pp. 557–560, 2015.

[41] C. Dai, Q. Cao, M. Jiang, and M.-J. Sun, "Serum Immunoglobulin G4 in Discriminating Autoimmune Pancreatitis from Pancreatic Cancer: A Diagnostic Meta-analysis," *Pancreas*, vol. 47, no. 3, pp. 280–284, 2018.

[42] Q. Liu, Z. Niu, Y. Li et al., "Immunoglobulin G4 (IgG4)-positive plasma cell infiltration is associated with the clinicopathologic traits and prognosis of pancreatic cancer after curative resection," *Cancer Immunology, Immunotherapy*, vol. 65, no. 8, pp. 931–940, 2016.

[43] H. Özkan, S. Demirbaş, M. Ibiş, E. Akbal, and S. Köklü, "Diagnostic validity of serum macrophage inhibitor cytokine and tissue polypeptide-specific antigen in pancreatobiliary diseases," *Pancreatology*, vol. 11, no. 3, pp. 295–300, 2011.

[44] S. Kaur, S. Chakraborty, M. J. Baine et al., "Potentials of Plasma NGAL and MIC-1 as Biomarker(s) in the Diagnosis of Lethal Pancreatic Cancer," *PLoS ONE*, vol. 8, no. 2, p. e55171, 2013.

[45] M. J. Baine, M. Menning, L. M. Smith et al., "Differential gene expression analysis of peripheral blood mononuclear cells reveals novel test for early detection of pancreatic cancer," *Cancer Biomarkers*, vol. 11, no. 1, pp. 1–14, 2011.

[46] Y. Yang, S. Yan, H. Tian, and Y. Bao, "Macrophage inhibitory cytokine-1 versus carbohydrate antigen 19-9 as a biomarker for diagnosis of pancreatic cancer," *Medicine (United States)*, vol. 97, no. 9, 2018.

[47] X. Wang, Y. Li, H. Tian et al., "Macrophage inhibitory cytokine 1 (MIC-1/GDF15) as a novel diagnostic serum biomarker in pancreatic ductal adenocarcinoma," *BMC Cancer*, vol. 14, article 578, 2014.

[48] J.-F. Peng, Y.-Y. Zhuang, F.-T. Huang, and S.-N. Zhang, "Non-coding RNAs and pancreatic cancer," *World Journal of Gastroenterology*, vol. 22, no. 2, pp. 801–814, 2016.

[49] T. Kishikawa, M. Otsuka, M. Ohno, T. Yoshikawa, A. Takata, and K. Koike, "Circulating RNAs as new biomarkers for detecting pancreatic cancer," *World Journal of Gastroenterology*, vol. 21, no. 28, pp. 8527–8540, 2015.

[50] J. Liu, J. Gao, Y. Du et al., "Combination of plasma microRNAs with serum CA19-9 for early detection of pancreatic cancer," *International Journal of Cancer*, vol. 131, no. 3, pp. 683–691, 2012.

[51] N. A. Schultz, C. Dehlendorff, B. V. Jensen et al., "MicroRNA biomarkers in whole blood for detection of pancreatic cancer," *Journal of the American Medical Association*, vol. 311, no. 4, pp. 392–404, 2014.

[52] J. Xu, Z. Cao, and W. Liu, "Plasma miRNAs effectively distinguish patients with pancreatic cancer from controls: a multicenter study," *Annals of Surgery*, 2015.

[53] P. Vychytilova-Faltejskova, I. Kiss, S. Klusova et al., "MiR-21, miR-34a, miR-198 and miR-217 as diagnostic and prognostic biomarkers for chronic pancreatitis and pancreatic ductal adenocarcinoma," *Diagnostic Pathology*, vol. 10, no. 1, article no. 38, 2015.

[54] M. Bloomston, W. L. Frankel, F. Petrocca et al., "MicroRNA expression patterns to differentiate pancreatic adenocarcinoma from normal pancreas and chronic pancreatitis," *Journal of the American Medical Association*, vol. 297, no. 17, pp. 1901–1908, 2007.

[55] N. Hanoun, Y. Delpu, A. A. Suriawinata et al., "The silencing of microRNA 148a production by DNA hypermethylation is an early event in pancreatic carcinogenesis," *Clinical Chemistry*, vol. 56, no. 7, pp. 1107–1118, 2010.

[56] I. Ulitsky and D. P. Bartel, "XLincRNAs: genomics, evolution, and mechanisms," *Cell*, vol. 154, no. 1, pp. 26–46, 2013.

[57] J. J. Quinn and H. Y. Chang, "Unique features of long non-coding RNA biogenesis and function," *Nature Reviews Genetics*, vol. 17, no. 1, pp. 47–62, 2015.

[58] S. Ren, F. Wang, J. Shen et al., "Long non-coding RNA metastasis associated in lung adenocarcinoma transcript 1 derived miniRNA as a novel plasma-based biomarker for diagnosing prostate cancer," *European Journal of Cancer*, vol. 49, no. 13, pp. 2949–2959, 2013.

[59] W. Yuan, Y. Sun, L. Liu, B. Zhou, S. Wang, and D. Gu, "Circulating LncRNAs Serve as Diagnostic Markers for Hepatocellular Carcinoma," *Cellular Physiology and Biochemistry*, pp. 125–132, 2017.

[60] W. Zhao, M. Song, J. Zhang, M. Kuerban, and H. Wang, "Combined identification of long non-coding RNA CCAT1 and HOTAIR in serum as an effective screening for colorectal carcinoma," *International Journal of Clinical and Experimental Pathology*, vol. 8, no. 11, pp. 14131–14140, 2015.

[61] J. Tantai, D. Hu, Y. Yang, and J. Geng, "Erratum to "Combined identification of long non-coding RNA XIST and HIF1A-AS1 in serum as an effective screening for non-small cell lung cancer" [Int J Clin Exp Pathol., 8, 7, (2015), 7887-7895]," *International Journal of Clinical and Experimental Pathology*, vol. 9, no. 3, p. 4157, 2016.

[62] V. Scaiewicz, V. Sorin, Y. Fellig et al., "Use of H19 Gene Regulatory Sequences in DNA-Based Therapy for Pancreatic Cancer," *Journal of Oncology*, vol. 2010, Article ID 178174, 10 pages, 2010.

[63] K. Kim, I. Jutooru, G. Chadalapaka et al., "HOTAIR is a negative prognostic factor and exhibits pro-oncogenic activity in pancreatic cancer," *Oncogene*, vol. 32, no. 13, pp. 1616–1625, 2013.

[64] Z. Fu, C. Chen, Q. Zhou et al., "LncRNA HOTTIP modulates cancer stem cell properties in human pancreatic cancer by regulating HOXA9," *Cancer Letters*, vol. 410, pp. 68–81, 2017.

[65] F. Jiao, H. Hu, C. Yuan et al., "Elevated expression level of long noncoding RNA MALAT-1 facilitates cell growth, migration and invasion in pancreatic cancer," *Oncology Reports*, vol. 32, no. 6, pp. 2485–2492, 2014.

[66] Y. Wang, Z. Li, S. Zheng et al., "Expression profile of long non-coding RNAs in pancreatic cancer and their clinical significance as biomarkers," *Oncotarget* , vol. 6, no. 34, pp. 35684–35698, 2015.

[67] Z. Xie, X. Chen, J. Li et al., "Salivary HOTAIR and PVT1 as novel biomarkers for early pancreatic cancer," *Oncotarget* , vol. 7, no. 18, pp. 25408–25419, 2016.

[68] F. Riva, O. I. Dronov, D. I. Khomenko et al., "Clinical applications of circulating tumor DNA and circulating tumor cells in pancreatic cancer," *Molecular Oncology*, vol. 10, no. 3, pp. 481–493, 2016.

[69] T. R. Ashworth, "A case of cancer in which cells similar to those in the tumours were seen in the blood after death," *The Medical Journal of Australia*, vol. 14, pp. 146–149, 1869.

[70] G. P. Gupta and J. Massagué, "Cancer metastasis: building a framework," *Cell*, vol. 127, no. 4, pp. 679–695, 2006.

[71] A. D. Rhim, E. T. Mirek, N. M. Aiello et al., "EMT and dissemination precede pancreatic tumor formation," *Cell*, vol. 148, no. 1-2, pp. 349–361, 2012.

[72] I. Iwanicki-Caron, P. Basile, E. Toure et al., "Usefulness of Circulating Tumor Cell Detection in Pancreatic Adenocarcinoma Diagnosis," *American Journal of Gastroenterology*, vol. 108, no. 1, pp. 152–155, 2013.

[73] B. Kulemann, M. B. Pitman, A. S. Liss et al., "Circulating tumor cells found in patients with localized and advanced pancreatic cancer," *Pancreas*, vol. 44, no. 4, pp. 547–550, 2015.

[74] Y. Gao, Y. Zhu, Z. Zhang, C. Zhang, X. Huang, and Z. Yuan, "Clinical significance of pancreatic circulating tumor cells using combined negative enrichment and immunostaining-fluorescence in situ hybridization," *Journal of Experimental & Clinical Cancer Research*, vol. 35, no. 1, 2016.

[75] J. S. Ankeny, C. M. Court, S. Hou et al., "Circulating tumour cells as a biomarker for diagnosis and staging in pancreatic cancer," *British Journal of Cancer*, vol. 114, no. 12, pp. 1367–1375, 2016.

[76] T. Imamura, S. Komatsu, D. Ichikawa et al., "Liquid biopsy in patients with pancreatic cancer: Circulating tumor cells and cell-free nucleic acids," *World Journal of Gastroenterology*, vol. 22, no. 25, pp. 5627–5641, 2016.

[77] P. Mandel and P. Metais, "Les acides nucleiques du plasma sanguin chez l'homme," *Comptes rendus des séances de la Société de biologie et de ses filiales*, pp. 142–241, 1948.

[78] M. Stroun, P. Anker, P. Maurice, J. Lyautey, C. Lederrey, and M. Beljanski, "Neoplastic characteristics of the DNA found in the plasma of cancer patients," *Oncology*, vol. 46, no. 5, pp. 318–322, 1989.

[79] E. Takai and S. Yachida, "Circulating tumor DNA as a liquid biopsy target for detection of pancreatic cancer," *World Journal of Gastroenterology*, vol. 22, no. 38, pp. 8480–8488, 2016.

[80] F. Diehl, K. Schmidt, M. A. Choti et al., "Circulating mutant DNA to assess tumor dynamics," *Nature Medicine*, vol. 14, no. 9, pp. 985–990, 2008.

[81] A. Yanagisawa, K. Ohtake, K. Ohashi et al., "Frequent c-Ki-ras Oncogene Activation in Mucous Cell Hyperplasias of Pancreas Suffering from Chronic Inflammation," *Cancer Research*, vol. 53, no. 5, pp. 953-956, 1993.

[82] Y. Gao, Y. Zhu, and Z. Yuan, "Circulating tumor cells and circulating tumor DNA provide new insights into pancreatic cancer," *International Journal of Medical Sciences*, vol. 13, no. 12, pp. 902–913, 2016.

[83] M. Sausen, J. Phallen, V. Adleff et al., "Clinical implications of genomic alterations in the tumour and circulation of pancreatic cancer patients," *Nature Communications*, vol. 6, no. 1, 2015.

[84] C. Bettegowda, M. Sausen, R. Leary et al., "Detection of circulating tumor dna in early and late stage human malignancies," *Neuro-Oncology*, vol. 16, no. suppl 3, pp. iii7–iii7, 2014.

[85] K. Tjensvoll, M. Lapin, T. Buhl et al., "Clinical relevance of circulating KRAS mutated DNA in plasma from patients with advanced pancreatic cancer," *Molecular Oncology*, vol. 10, no. 4, pp. 635–643, 2016.

[86] H. Chen, H. Tu, Z. Q. Meng, Z. Chen, P. Wang, and L. M. Liu, "K-ras mutational status predicts poor prognosis in unresectable pancreatic cancer," *European Journal of Surgical Oncology*, vol. 36, no. 7, pp. 657–662, 2010.

[87] R. Marchese, A. Muleti, S. Brozzetti, O. Gandini, E. Brunetti, and D. French, "Low value of detection of KRAS2 mutations in circulating DNA to differentiate chronic pancreatitis to pancreatic cancer [1]," *British Journal of Cancer*, vol. 90, no. 11, p. 2243, 2004.

[88] F. Maire, S. Micard, P. Hammel et al., "Differential diagnosis between chronic pancreatitis and pancreatic cancer: Value of the detection of KRAS2 mutations in circulating DNA," *British Journal of Cancer*, vol. 87, no. 5, pp. 551–554, 2002.

[89] D. Sefrioui, F. Blanchard, E. Toure et al., "Diagnostic value of CA19.9, circulating tumour DNA and circulating tumour cells in patients with solid pancreatic tumours," *British Journal of Cancer*, vol. 117, no. 7, pp. 1017–1025, 2017.

[90] S. A. Melo, L. B. Luecke, C. Kahlert et al., "Glypican-1 identifies cancer exosomes and detects early pancreatic cancer," *Nature*, 2015.

[91] S. Melo, H. Sugimoto, J. O'Connell et al., "Cancer exosomes perform cell-independent microRNA biogenesis and promote tumorigenesis," *Cancer Cell*, vol. 26, no. 5, pp. 707–721, 2014.

[92] C. Lau, Y. Kim, D. Chia et al., "Role of pancreatic cancer-derived exosomes in salivary biomarker development," *The Journal of Biological Chemistry*, vol. 288, no. 37, pp. 26888–26897, 2013.

[93] M. Humeau, A. Vignolle-Vidoni, F. Sicard et al., "Salivary microRNA in pancreatic cancer patients," *PLoS ONE*, vol. 10, no. 6, 2015.

[94] T. P. Radon, N. J. Massat, R. Jones et al., "Identification of a three-biomarker panel in urine for early detection of pancreatic adenocarcinoma," *Clinical Cancer Research*, vol. 21, no. 15, pp. 3512–3521, 2015.

[95] P. Hogendorf, A. Durczyński, A. Skulimowski, A. Kumor, G. Poznańska, and J. Strzelczyk, "Neutrophil Gelatinase-Associated Lipocalin (NGAL) concentration in urine is superior to CA19-9 and Ca 125 in differentiation of pancreatic mass: Preliminary report," *Cancer Biomarkers*, vol. 16, no. 4, pp. 537–543, 2016.

[96] S. Debernardi, N. J. Massat, T. P. Radon et al., "Noninvasive urinary miRNA biomarkers for early detection of pancreatic adenocarcinoma," *American Journal of Cancer Research*, vol. 5, no. 11, pp. 3455–3466, 2015.

[97] Y. Huo, M. Yang, W. Liu et al., "High expression of DDR1 is associated with the poor prognosis in Chinese patients with pancreatic ductal adenocarcinoma," *Journal of Experimental & Clinical Cancer Research*, vol. 34, no. 1, 2015.

[98] M. J. Veite-Schmahl, A. C. Rivers, D. P. Regan, and M. A. Kennedy, "The Mouse Model of Pancreatic Cancer Atlas (MMPCA) for classification of pancreatic cancer lesions: A large histological investigation of the Ptf1aCre/+;LSL-KrasG12D/+ transgenic mouse model of pancreatic cancer," *PLoS ONE*, vol. 12, no. 11, 2017.

[99] C. Scarlett, J. Weidenhofer, E. Colvin, and D. Bond, "Animal models of pancreatic cancer and their application in clinical research," *Gastrointestinal Cancer : Targets and Therapy*, vol. Volume 6, pp. 31–39, 2016.

[100] S. R. Hingorani, E. F. Petricoin III, A. Maitra et al., "Preinvasive and invasive ductal pancreatic cancer and its early detection in the mouse," *Cancer Cell*, vol. 4, no. 6, pp. 437–450, 2003.

15

Combining Genetic Variants to Improve Risk Prediction for NAFLD and its Progression to Cirrhosis

Umberto Vespasiani-Gentilucci,[1] Chiara Dell'Unto,[1] Antonio De Vincentis,[1] Andrea Baiocchini,[2] Marco Delle Monache,[3] Roberto Cecere,[3] Adriano Maria Pellicelli,[4] Valerio Giannelli,[4] Simone Carotti,[5] Giovanni Galati,[1] Paolo Gallo,[1] Francesco Valentini,[1] Franca Del Nonno,[2] Davide Rosati,[6] Sergio Morini,[5] Raffaele Antonelli-Incalzi,[1] and Antonio Picardi[1]

[1] *Internal Medicine, Geriatrics, and Hepatology Unit, University Campus Bio-Medico, Rome, Italy*
[2] *Laboratory of Pathology of The National Institute for Infectious Diseases, Lazzaro Spallanzani, Rome, Italy*
[3] *Hepatology Outpatient Clinic, Colleferro Hospital, Rome, Italy*
[4] *Liver Disease Unit, San Camillo-Forlanini Hospital, Rome, Italy*
[5] *Laboratory of Microscopic and Ultrastructural Anatomy, CIR, University Campus Bio-Medico, Rome, Italy*
[6] *University La Sapienza of Rome, Rome, Italy*

Correspondence should be addressed to Umberto Vespasiani-Gentilucci; u.vespasiani@unicampus.it

Academic Editor: Mariana V. Machado

Background & Aims. Identifying NAFLD patients at risk of progression is crucial to orient medical care and resources. We aimed to verify if the effects determined by different single nucleotide polymorphisms (SNPs) could add up to multiply the risk of NAFLD and NASH-cirrhosis. *Methods.* Three study populations, that is, patients diagnosed with NASH-cirrhosis or with noncirrhotic NAFLD and healthy controls, were enrolled. PNPLA3 rs738409, TM6SF2 rs58542926, KLF6 rs3750861, SOD2 rs4880, and LPIN1 rs13412852 were genotyped. *Results.* One hundred and seven NASH-cirrhotics, 93 noncirrhotic NAFLD, and 90 controls were enrolled. At least one difference in allele frequency between groups was significant, or nearly significant, for the PNPLA3, TM6SF2, and KLF6 variants ($p < 0.001$, $p < 0.05$, and $p = 0.06$, resp.), and a risk score based on these SNPs was generated. No differences were observed for SOD2 and LPIN1 SNPs. When compared to a score of 0, a score of 1-2 quadrupled, and a score of 3-4 increased 20-fold the risk of noncirrhotic NAFLD; a score of 3-4 quadrupled the risk of NASH-cirrhosis. *Conclusions.* The effects determined by disease-associated variants at different *loci* can add up to multiply the risk of NAFLD and NASH-cirrhosis. Combining different disease-associated variants may represent the way for genetics to keep strength in NAFLD diagnostics.

1. Introduction

Nonalcoholic fatty liver disease (NAFLD) is becoming an epidemic in Western populations, with prevalence ranging from approximately 20% to 30% depending on the country and the different reports [1, 2]. Fortunately, against these alarming numbers, only a minority of NAFLD patients evolve to cirrhosis and eventually to hepatocellular carcinoma (HCC), while the majority of them present a relatively benign disease, usually integrated in a dysmetabolic profile [3]. Identifying those patients at risk of progression would be crucial to orient medical care and economic resources, maximizing the benefits of specific hepatologic follow-up and interventions.

A growing body of evidence is demonstrating that genetic susceptibility plays an important role in NAFLD development and evolution [4]. Indeed, the role of genetic variation in NAFLD, specifically single nucleotide polymorphisms (SNPs), has been the focus of extensive research in the last decade. The nonsynonymous rs738409 C/G variant in patatin-like phospholipase domain containing protein 3 (PNPLA3) is considered the major genetic component of NAFLD [5]. More recently, the nonsynonymous rs58542926 variant located in the transmembrane 6 superfamily member 2 (TM6SF2) gene has emerged as the second genetic determinant of NAFLD in terms of importance [6, 7]. Many other SNPs of different genes involved in lipid metabolism, such as lipin 1 (LPIN1), oxidative stress, such as superoxide dismutase 2 (SOD2), and fibrogenesis, such as Kruppel-like factor 6 (KLF6), have been associated with the severity of liver damage in different studies on NAFLD patients [8–12]. Altogether, it seems reasonable to assume that no single gene variant can suffice to accurately stratify the risk, while the predictive power would be enhanced by analyzing different SNPs or combining their effect in a genetic risk score. A proof of concept that genetic scores may be useful in NAFLD patients has been already given by Nobili et al. in the pediatric population, where a 4-polymorphism risk score was demonstrated to predict nonalcoholic steatohepatitis (NASH) [13]. More recently, the only similar experience in the adult population was obtained in a Mexican series of morbid obese patients undergoing bariatric surgery, where a genetic risk score including 4 SNPs was associated with hepatic triglyceride and cholesterol content [14]. However, to our knowledge, no attempt has been made to verify the capability of a genetic risk score to stratify the risk of NAFLD and of its evolution to cirrhosis.

Based on this background, in the present study, we aimed to verify if combining different SNPs in a genetic score could increase the predictive power for more severe forms of NAFLD in adult patients. To address this, we performed a case-control study in a well-characterized NAFLD population and tested the same SNPs which had been previously assembled to provide the genetic score in the pediatric population [13], plus TM6SF2, which has more recently emerged as a genetic key determinant of NAFLD [6, 7]. A control group representing the general healthy population was also included.

2. Patients and Methods

2.1. Patients. Patients followed at the Hepatology Unit of the University Hospital Campus Bio-Medico of Rome, at the Hepatology outpatient clinic of the Colleferro Hospital (Rome, Italy), and at the Liver Disease Unit of the San Camillo-Forlanini Hospital of Rome and those assessed at the Laboratory of Pathology of the National Institute for Infectious Diseases Lazzaro Spallanzani of Rome and recorded in the respective clinical databases with the diagnosis of NASH cirrhosis were extracted. When reviewing the clinical records for the purpose of the present study, the etiological diagnosis of cirrhosis as post-NASH was considered definite and patients eligible for the study only after having verified that all the other causes of liver disease had been excluded and that at least one of the two criteria was satisfied, (1) histological diagnosis of NASH cirrhosis; (2) clinical diagnosis of cirrhosis in patients with a previous documented history of steatosis (by abdominal ultrasonography, computed tomography scan, or magnetic resonance imaging) and at least one of the following diagnoses precede that of cirrhosis: type-2 diabetes mellitus (T2DM), obesity with a body mass index (BMI) > 30 kg/m^2, and metabolic syndrome. Secondly, the group of patients who had received the diagnosis of noncirrhotic NAFLD (simple steatosis or NASH) by liver biopsy performed at the same Centers was extracted from the clinical databases. Also in this case, it was confirmed that all the other causes of liver disease had been excluded before or after liver biopsy. More specifically, it was verified that none of the patients with NASH cirrhosis and noncirrhotic NAFLD had history of alcoholic intake >20 gr/day if woman and >30 gr/day if man or of use of drugs known to induce liver steatosis. Moreover, it was verified that the following results had been obtained from all the patients: negative anti-hepatitis C virus (anti-HCV) antibodies and hepatitis B surface antigen (HBsAg); anti-nuclear antibodies (ANA) ≤1 : 80 and negative anti-mitochondrial (AMA), anti-smooth muscle (ASMA), and anti-liver and kidney microsomal (anti-LKM) antibodies; normal transferrin saturation and serum levels of ceruloplasmin and alpha-1 antitrypsin. Finally, a third group to represent the general population was recruited among consecutive subjects undergoing general medicine company checkups at the Campus Bio-Medico Hospital. Upper abdomen ultrasonography is among the examination included in every checkup, and ultrasonographic steatosis was considered the only exclusion criterion.

Patients with NASH cirrhosis and noncirrhotic NAFLD individuated according to the aforementioned criteria were contacted and invited to participate to the study, as well as all consecutive subjects attending company checkups. All subjects enrolled in the present study agreed to participate and signed an informed consent. The protocol of the study was approved by the Ethics Committee of the University Campus Bio-Medico of Rome.

2.2. Methods. Epidemiological, anthropometric, and clinical data at the time of cirrhosis diagnosis of liver biopsy or of the medical checkup were collected for patients with NASH cirrhosis and noncirrhotic NAFLD and for subjects of the control group, respectively. All subjects enrolled in the study underwent blood drawing and venous blood was stored at −80° until examination.

2.2.1. PNPLA3 rs738409, TM6SF2 rs58542926, KLF6 rs3750861, SOD2 rs4880, and LPIN1 rs13412852 Genotyping. Genomic DNA was extracted from whole blood using the kit DNA-Sorb-B (Sacace Biotechnologies, Como, Italy), as instructed by the manufacturer. The analysis of the five polymorphisms was done by real-time polymerase chain reaction (rt-PCR) using a commercial kit (FLT PLUS Fatty Liver Test; Orga Bio Human, Rome, Italy), as instructed by the manufacturer. For each SNP, the presence of two TaqMan® allows allelic discrimination (ancestral allele, variant allele, or both).

2.2.2. Hepatic Ultrasonography and Liver Biopsy. Abdominal ultrasound was performed with an Acuson S3000 ultrasound system (Siemens®, Munich, Germany), using both a 1.5–6 MHz curved array probe and a 5.5–18 MHz high frequency linear array probe, the latter for the evaluation of the left liver surface. All patients were studied with subcostal, right intercostal and transaxial epigastric scans, and ultrasonography was operated by a single experienced liver sonographer blinded to the patients' clinical data. Liver was defined bright when abnormally intense, high-level echoes arose from hepatic parenchyma and/or when a liver-kidney difference in echo amplitude was detected [15]. The ultrasonographic diagnosis of liver cirrhosis was suggested, to be clinically confirmed by combination with biochemical ± upper endoscopic ± transient elastographic findings, in the presence of nodular liver surface in the left lobe by the high frequency probe and at least one of the following signs of portal hypertension: splenomegaly, dilatation of the main portal, portal-systemic collaterals, and ascites [16, 17].

Liver biopsy was performed under ultrasonographic guidance, and specimens (at least 1.5 cm in length) were fixed in formalin for evaluation. Tissue sections were stained with hematoxylin and eosin and with Sirius red. Liver biopsies were reviewed by two expert liver pathologists (A. B. and S. C.), who were unaware of clinical and genetic data. Histological cases of NASH cirrhosis were reevaluated in order to confirm diagnosis, while cases of noncirrhotic NAFLD were diagnosed as simple steatosis or NASH [18] and staged according to Kleiner et al. [19].

2.3. Statistical Analysis. Results are reported as mean ± standard deviation (SD), number (%), and OR with 95% confidence intervals (CI), as appropriate. Differences between groups of patients with NASH cirrhosis and noncirrhotic NAFLD and healthy controls were tested using Kruskal-Wallis test for continuous variables and χ^2 test for categorical variables. A genetic score was designed taking into account the PNPLA3, TM6SF2, and KLF6 polymorphisms, and its association with noncirrhotic NAFLD and NASH cirrhosis was estimated by means of logistic regression models. Models were finally adjusted for age, sex, BMI, and diabetes mellitus. A $p < 0.05$ was considered statistically significant. All analyses were carried out with R 3.3.3 for Mac (R Foundation).

3. Results

3.1. Study Population. All subjects included in the present study were of Caucasian race and of Italian nationality. One hundred and seventy-five patients with the diagnosis of NASH cirrhosis were extracted from the four clinical databases. Among these patients, 35 had died, 17 refused to participate to the study, and other 16 were discarded, 12 because they did not meet the aforementioned criteria to be included as NASH cirrhosis cases and 4 because of an excessive alcohol intake. Finally, 107 patients with NASH cirrhosis were enrolled: 39 had received histological diagnosis of NASH cirrhosis; 68 had received the clinical diagnosis of cirrhosis (clinical, biochemical, and ultrasonographic ± upper endoscopic ± transient elastographic findings) and, according to inclusion criteria, had a previous documented history of steatosis (mainly ultrasonographic) together with at least one among T2DM (63 patients), obesity (53 patients), and metabolic syndrome (60 patients) preceding the diagnosis of cirrhosis. One hundred and nineteen patients who had received the histological diagnosis of noncirrhotic NAFLD were extracted from the four clinical databases. Five patients had died, 13 of them refused to participate in the study, and 8 were discarded, 5 because of an excessive alcohol intake and three because not all the alternative etiologies had been excluded. Finally, 93 patients with noncirrhotic NAFLD were enrolled in the study. According to Brunt et al. [18], 15 cases had the criteria for simple steatosis and 78 for NASH, and fibrosis was classified as F0, F1, F2, and F3 in 9, 42, 22, and 20 cases, respectively. One hundred and ten consecutive subjects undergoing general medicine company checkups at the Campus Bio-Medico Hospital were evaluated for enrollment as controls. After having excluded 20 subjects due to the finding of ultrasonographic bright liver, 90 subjects were finally recruited since there were no refusals to participate in the study in this group. These subjects were selected to represent the genetic profile in the general population and, therefore, there were no other exclusion criteria.

3.2. Epidemiologic and Clinical Data and Frequency of the Five Different SNPs Analyzed. As reported in Table 1, while gender distribution was not different between the two groups, patients with NASH cirrhosis were significantly older than those with noncirrhotic NAFLD. This finding was expected and is consistent with the natural history of NAFLD and of every liver disorder, since fibrosis evolves with disease duration. Also mean BMI and the prevalence of T2DM were significantly higher in patients with NASH cirrhosis with respect to those with noncirrhotic NAFLD. Healthy control subjects presented a gender distribution comparable with that in the other two groups, but they were significantly younger and, as expected considering the dysmetabolic background of the NAFLD population, they had a lower BMI and a lower prevalence of T2DM.

The frequency of the PNPLA3 rs738409 minor (G) allele was significantly higher in patients with NASH cirrhosis than in the other two study populations, as well as in noncirrhotic NAFLD patients with respect to healthy controls. Concerning the TM6SF2 rs58542926 polymorphism, an increase of the T allele frequency was observed in patients with NASH cirrhosis with respect to healthy subjects, while the comparisons between the other groups did not yield statistically significant differences. Similarly to the latter, the increase in the frequency of the T allele at the KLF6 rs3750861 *locus* tended to significance when comparing NASH cirrhotics to healthy subjects ($p = 0.06$), while there were no significant differences between the other groups. Finally, the frequencies of the T allele at the SOD2 rs4880 *locus* and that of the T allele at the LPIN1 rs13412852 *locus* did not show any significant difference when comparing the three groups of subjects analyzed in the study.

TABLE 1: Epidemiologic and clinical data and frequency of the PNPLA3 rs738409 G, TM6SF2 rs58542926 T, KLF6 rs3750861 T, SOD2 rs4880 T, and LPIN1 rs13412852 T alleles in the study population, divided according to subgroups.

	All	Healthy Subjects	Noncirrhotic NAFLD	NASH cirrhosis
N	290	90	93	107
Age (years)	54.4 (15.1)	43.1 (11.9)	51.6 (13.2)$^{++}$	66.2 (9.8)$^{++**}$
Sex (male)	53.5%	46.6%	60.2%	53.3%
BMI (Kg/m^2)	28.8 (5.3)	25.2 (4.6)	29.5 (4.1)$^{++}$	31.2 (5.2)$^{++*}$
T2DM	41.6%	7%	45.2%$^{++}$	66.4%$^{++*}$
PNPLA3 G allele frequency	0.46	0.24	0.48^{++}	0.61^{++*}
TM6SF2 T allele frequency	0.11	0.06	0.11	0.14^{+}
KLF6 T allele frequency	0.08	0.06	0.07	0.12
SOD2 T allele frequency	0.5	0.48	0.53	0.49
LPIN1 T allele frequency	0.32	0.35	0.32	0.31

Data are shown as mean (standard deviation) or percentages. $^{+}p < 0.05$ and $^{++}p < 0.001$ versus healthy subjects; $^{*}p < 0.01$ and $^{**}p < 0.001$ versus noncirrhotic NAFLD; NAFLD: nonalcoholic fatty liver disease; NASH: nonalcoholic steatohepatitis; BMI: body mass index; T2DM: type 2 diabetes mellitus; PNPLA3: patatin-like phospholipase domain containing protein 3; TM6SF2: transmembrane 6 superfamily member 2; KLF6: Kruppel-like factor 6; SOD2: superoxide dismutase 2; LPIN1: lipin 1.

Table 3 reports epidemiological, anthropometric, and genetic data concerning the noncirrhotic NAFLD group subdivided into patients with absent/mild (F0-1) and advanced (F2-3) fibrosis. Patients with advanced fibrosis were significantly older, with a higher mean BMI and a higher prevalence of T2DM, with respect to patients with absent/mild fibrosis. Conversely, there were no significant differences in allele frequencies between the two subgroups.

3.3. Genotype Distribution at the PNPLA3 rs738409, TM6SF2 rs58542926, KLF6 rs3750861, LPIN1 rs13412852, and SOD2 rs4880 Loci and Derivation of a Genetic Risk Score. Genotype distribution for the polymorphisms of interest at the five different *loci* are reported in Table 2. Concerning PNPLA3, there was a highly significant shift towards the reduction of CC homozygous and the increase of homozygous for the minor G allele (GG) when passing from healthy controls, through noncirrhotic NAFLD patients, to NASH cirrhotics. To note, the different genotype distribution at the PNPLA3 *locus* was significant when comparing all groups except for NASH cirrhotics with noncirrhotic NAFLD patients (p = 0.06). Genotype distribution for the polymorphisms studied at the TM6SF2 and KLF6 *loci* showed a nonsignificant trend towards the reduction of wild-type CC homozygous and the increase of heterozygous carriers of the polymorphic T allele when moving from healthy controls, through noncirrhotic NAFLD, to NASH cirrhotics. In the case of both TM6SF2 and KLF6, when the CT and TT genotypes were grouped, this trend was even stronger and the difference in genotype distribution between NASH cirrhotics and healthy controls became significant for TM6SF2 but still not significant for KLF6 (p = 0.09). Conversely, there was not virtually any difference between the three groups in genotype distribution for the SOD2 rs4880 and the LPIN1 rs13412852 polymorphisms. Finally, when genotype distributions of noncirrhotic NAFLD patients were compared between those with absent/mild and those with advanced fibrosis, no significant differences were observed (Table 3).

The PNPLA3 rs738409, TM6SF2 rs58542926, and KLF6 rs3750861 polymorphisms were then considered for the development of the genetic risk score. Consistent with previous literature [7, 11] and according to the Akaike information criterion (data not shown) [20], the models with the best fit for the association with the risk of NASH cirrhosis with respect to noncirrhotic NAFLD were additive for the PNPLA3 polymorphism (CC = 0; CG = 1; GG = 2) and dominant for the TM6SF2 and KLF6 polymorphisms (CC = 0; CT and TT = 1). The relative weight to give to each polymorphism in the computation of the genetic score was determined considering the coefficients of a logistic regression analysis for the candidate genes (modelled as mentioned above) and the presence of NASH cirrhosis (PNPLA3: 0.43; TM6SF2: 0.39; KLF6: 0.46), standardized for their mean and rounded at the unit (PNPLA3: 0.43/0.43 = 1; TM6SF2: 0.39/0.43 = 0.91; KLF6: 0.46/0.43 = 1.06). Accordingly, the genetic risk score was then computed as the sum of one point for each single polymorphism, ranging from 0 to 4.

The genetic risk score was significantly higher in noncirrhotic NAFLD patients with respect to healthy subjects [1.3 (0.9) versus 0.8 (0.9), $p < 0.001$] and in NASH cirrhotics [1.7 (1.0)] when compared to noncirrhotic NAFLD (p = 0.005) and to healthy subjects ($p < 0.001$). Figure 1 shows the percentages of healthy subjects, noncirrhotic NAFLD patients, and NASH cirrhotics presenting the different results of the genetic risk score. Nearly 50% of healthy subjects showed a risk score of 0, while their prevalence decreased progressively with the increase of the score. On the other hand, only about 10% of NASH cirrhotics exhibited a score of 0, the majority of them showing a score of 1 or 2, and about 20% a score ≥ 3.

Table 4 reports univariate and multivariate logistic regression analyses in which the genetic risk score was tested for its association with the risk of noncirrhotic NAFLD and of NASH cirrhosis. When expressed linearly, with healthy subjects as reference group, the genetic risk score was significantly associated with a doubling of the risk of noncirrhotic NAFLD and a tripling of the risk of NASH cirrhosis,

Table 2: Comparison of PNPLA3 rs738409, TM6SF2 rs58542926, KLF6 rs3750861, SOD2 rs4880, and LPIN1 rs13412852 polymorphisms prevalence, according to study subgroups.

	Healthy Subjects	Noncirrhotic NAFLD	NASH cirrhosis	p
PNPLA3				
CC	53 (58.9%)	30 (32.3%)$^{++}$	20 (18.7%)$^{++}$	
CG	30 (33.3%)	36 (38.7%)$^{++}$	44 (41.1%)$^{++}$	<0.001
GG	7 (7.8%)	27 (29%)$^{++}$	43 (40.2%)$^{++}$	
TM6SF2				
CC	79 (87.8%)	74 (79.6%)	79 (73.8%)	
CT	11 (12.2%)	17 (18.3%)	27 (25.2%)	0.105
TT	0 (0%)	2 (2.2%)	1 (0.9%)	
TM6SF2 dichotomized				
CC	79 (87.8%)	74 (79.6%)	79 (73.8%)$^{+}$	0.06
CT/TT	11 (12.2%)	19 (20.4%)	28 (26.2%)$^{+}$	
KLF6				
CC	79 (87.8%)	80 (86%)	83 (77.6%)	
CT	11 (12.2%)	13 (14%)	23 (21.5%)	0.224
TT	0 (0%)	0 (0%)	1 (0.9%)	
KLF6 dichotomized				
CC	79 (87.8%)	80 (86%)	83 (77.6%)	0.113
CT/TT	11 (12.2%)	13 (14%)	24 (22.4%)	
SOD2				
CC	26 (28.9%)	20 (21.5%)	30 (28%)	
CT	42 (46.7%)	48 (51.6%)	49 (45.8%)	0.795
TT	22 (24.4%)	25 (26.9%)	28 (26.2%)	
LPIN1				
CC	38 (42.2%)	45 (48.4%)	49 (45.8%)	
CT	41 (45.6%)	37 (39.8%)	50 (46.7%)	0.672
TT	11 (12.2%)	11 (11.8%)	8 (7.5%)	

Data are shown as absolute number and column percentages. p for overall chi-square test. $^{+}p < 0.05$ and $^{++}p < 0.001$ versus healthy subjects; PNPLA3: patatin-like phospholipase domain containing protein 3; TM6SF2: transmembrane 6 superfamily member 2; KLF6: Kruppel-like factor 6; SOD2: superoxide dismutase 2; LPIN1: lipin 1.

both in unadjusted models and in models adjusted for age, sex, BMI, and T2DM. Moreover, with noncirrhotic NAFLD patients as reference group, each point of the score was also associated with an about 50% increased risk of NASH cirrhosis. The results were even more interestingly when the score was expressed categorically. Indeed, when compared to a score of 0, with respect to healthy subjects, a genetic risk score of 1-2 approximately quadrupled and a score of 3-4 increased approximately 20-fold the risk of noncirrhotic NAFLD. Consistently, when compared to a score of 0, with respect to noncirrhotic NAFLD patients, a genetic risk score of 3-4 almost quadrupled the risk of NASH cirrhosis.

4. Discussion

This is the first study aimed to verify if combining the presence of different polymorphisms of risk could increase the predictive power for NAFLD and, mainly, for its evolution to cirrhosis. The present results are proof of concept that the effects determined by disease-associated variants at different *loci* can add up to multiply the risk of NAFLD and of NASH cirrhosis.

A growing body of evidence indicates that NAFLD develops as a result of a complex process in which genetic susceptibility plays an important role [21]. According to the available data, the heritability estimates range from 20% to 70%, depending on the study design, ethnicity, and the methodology applied for diagnostic purposes [4]. In the last decade, extensive research deriving from candidate gene studies and, mostly, from genome-wide association studies and exome-wide association studies, has identified several *loci* associated with disease susceptibility and progression. The firstly recognized and still more significant is certainly the rs738409 SNPs in the PNPLA3 gene, encoding for the isoleucine to methionine substitution at position 148 (I148M). Indeed, the I148M variant has been associated with the degree of hepatic injury and all the histopathological aspects of NAFLD, including the presence of NASH, fibrosis, and development of HCC [5, 22]. More recently, we have reported that the rs738409 PNPLA3 SNP is associated not only generically with NAFLD fibrosis but also specifically with the evolution to NASH cirrhosis [23]. To date, the rs58542926 SNP in the TM6SF2 *locus* should be considered in the second place of importance. The TM6SF2 variant

Table 3: Epidemiological, anthropometric, and genetic data of the noncirrhotic NAFLD group divided into two subgroups according to the degree of fibrosis: absent/mild (F0-F1) and advanced (F2-3).

	F0-1	F2-3	p
N	51	42	
Age (years)	46.7 (13.1)	57.5 (11)	<0.001
Sex (male)	64.7%	54.8%	0.332
BMI (Kg/m^2)	28.5 (3.8)	30.8 (4.2)	0.012
T2DM	31.4%	61.9%	0.006
PNPLA3			
G allele frequency	0.44	0.54	0.203
CC	19 (37.3%)	11 (26.2%)	
CG	19 (37.3%)	17 (40.5%)	0.491
GG	13 (25.5%)	14 (33.3%)	
TM6SF2			
T allele frequency	0.09	0.14	0.375
CC	42 (82.4%)	32 (76.2%)	
CT	9 (17.6%)	8 (19%)	0.278
TT	0 (0%)	2 (4.8%)	
KLF6			
T allele frequency	0.06	0.08	0.781
CC	45 (88.2%)	35 (83.3%)	
CT	6 (11.8%)	7 (16.7%)	0.705
TT	0 (0%)	0 (0%)	
SOD2			
T allele frequency	0.56	0.49	0.395
CC	9 (17.6%)	11 (26.2%)	
CT	27 (52.9%)	21 (50%)	0.58
TT	15 (29.4%)	10 (23.8%)	
LPIN1			
T allele frequency	0.31	0.32	1
CC	26 (51%)	19 (45.2%)	
CT	18 (35.3%)	19 (45.2%)	0.585
TT	7 (13.7%)	4 (9.5%)	
SCORE (linear)	1.2 (0.9)	1.5 (1)	0.139

Data are shown as mean (standard deviation), percentages, or absolute number and column percentages. NAFLD: nonalcoholic fatty liver disease; NASH: nonalcoholic steatohepatitis; BMI: body mass index; T2DM: type 2 diabetes mellitus; PNPLA3: patatin-like phospholipase domain containing protein 3; TM6SF2: transmembrane 6 superfamily member 2; KLF6: Kruppel-like factor 6; SOD2: superoxide dismutase 2; LPIN1: lipin 1.

Table 4: Uni- and multivariable regression models for the association of the genetic score (modelled as numeric or as factor variable) and presence of NASH cirrhosis or noncirrhotic NAFLD.

	NASH cirrhosis versus noncirrhotic NAFLD		Noncirrhotic NAFLD versus healthy controls		NASH cirrhosis versus healthy subjects	
	OR	aOR	OR	aOR	OR	aOR
Score	1.54 (1.14–2.1)	1.51 (1.04–2.22)	2.05 (1.46–2.93)	2.22 (1.40–3.65)	3.01 (2.14–4.38)	3.62 (1.63–9.69)
Score = 0	ref	ref	ref	ref	ref	ref
Score = 1	1.62 (0.69–3.9)	2.07 (0.69–6.45)	3.40 (1.63–7.28)	4.59 (1.74–12.91)	5.50 (2.46–13.00)	15.40 (2.32–149)
Score = 2	2.18 (0.93–5.29)	2.5 (0.84–7.79)	3.33 (1.55–7.36)	4.38 (1.58–13.05)	7.28 (3.24–17.35)	18.54 (2.78–176)
Score = 3	3.83 (1.4–11.14)	3.66 (1.04–13.75)	23.00 (4.01–436.62)	21.98 (2.73–496.88)	88.17 (16.11–1658)	125.37 (4.22–19336)

OR: odds ratio; aOR: adjusted odds ratio. aOR are adjusted for age, sex, BMI, and diabetes mellitus.

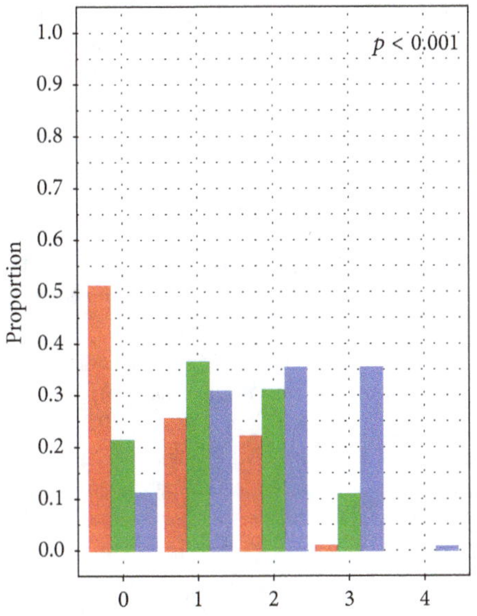

FIGURE 1: Prevalence of different results in the genetic risk score according to the three study populations.

has been associated with steatosis and fibrosis in patients with NAFLD [24, 25]. Actually, the analysis of patients with chronic HCV infection demonstrated that the rs58542926 SNP enhances liver fibrogenesis also in this setting [26], in which the virus and the host can contribute synergistically to the progression of liver disease and atherosclerosis [27].

American and European NAFLD guidelines recognize the disease modifying role of the PNPLA3 variant and of both the PNPLA3 and the TM6SF2 SNPs, respectively, but testing for these genetic variants in routine clinical practice is still not recommended [2, 28], likely because no single variant has demonstrated sufficient discriminative properties.

A pioneering study aimed to combine the effect of different SNPs in a genetic risk score able to predict NASH has been carried out by Nobili et al. in the pediatric population [13]. In adults, a genetic risk score based on 4 different SNPs has been associated with hepatic lipid content in Mexican morbid obese patients [14]. More recently, a significant increase of serum AST activity and trends for increased ALT and GGT activities have been reported with the increment of risk alleles at 3 loci (rs738409 in PNPLA3; rs58542926 in TM6SF2; rs641738 in membrane bound O-acyltransferase containing 7, MBOAT7) in a German population of adult NAFLD patients [29].

Based on this background, we designed this case-control study in a well-characterized NAFLD population from 4 different hepatological tertiary centers from Rome and its province, by recruiting three groups: NASH cirrhotics, noncirrhotic NAFLD, and controls. This subdivision may have the limit to render the noncirrhotic NAFLD population heterogeneous, since it was constituted by patients with both mild (F0-1) and advanced fibrosis (F2-3). Moreover, since NAFLD patients with milder fibrosis are younger than those with more advanced disease, the possibility that they can progress to advanced fibrosis and even cirrhosis in the following years cannot be ruled out. Actually, all the previously relevant studies on this same topic are affected by this same possible bias [v.b.], which can limited only by a fully adjusted statistics, as that applied in our case. Moreover, whatever cut-off is applied for fibrosis in a cross-sectional study, F0 versus F1-4 [30], F0-1 versus F2-4 [31], F0-2 versus F3-4 [32], or F0-3 versus F4, it should be considered completely arbitrary, and it depends on study population composition and on the objectives of the study itself. Here, by enrolling a large cohort of NASH cirrhotics, we specifically aimed to evaluate the risk of progression to cirrhosis, since cirrhotic evolution, together with the incidence of HCC, should be considered the most clinically relevant outcome in the context of liver disease.

In order to avoid the risk of missing cases of early cirrhosis, noncirrhotic NAFLD patients were included rigorously based on the result of a liver biopsy. Conversely, in agreement with previous studies on NASH cirrhosis and NAFLD-related HCC [33], liver histology was not considered an essential requisite for a NASH cirrhotic patient to be included in the study. The validity of the criteria applied for the diagnosis of NASH cirrhosis is reflected in the clinical characteristics of our population of NASH cirrhotics, who present the typical dysmetabolic profile of most severe forms of NAFLD. A group of patients attending the hospital without any disease-oriented reason, that is, those undergoing general medicine checkups, was finally included. Concerning the SNPs to be tested, we decided to include the 4 which had been included in the original pediatric genetic risk score [13], plus the rs58542926 TM6SF2 variant, which has been more recently acquired as a strong disease modifier in the context of NAFLD [6, 7]. Further than the PNPLA3 and the TM6SF2 SNPs, we therefore tested the rs3750861 KLF6, the rs13412852 LPIN1, and the rs4880 SOD2 SNPs, which have demonstrated associations with fibrosis, steatosis and fibrosis, and again fibrosis, respectively, in previous studies on NAFLD patients [8–12].

Epidemiological and anthropometric data confirmed that age, BMI, and T2DM are strong risk factors for NAFLD and for its fibrotic evolution. Concerning genetics, as expectable, the most significant intergroup differences were observed for the PNPLA3 variant. A clear trend towards an increased prevalence of the minor T allele when moving from healthy subjects, through noncirrhotic NAFLD patients, to NASH cirrhotics, was observed also for the TM6SF2 SNP, for which the difference between NASH cirrhotics and healthy controls was actually significant, and for the KLF6 variant, for which the difference between these same two populations was only at the limit of significance. Conversely, concerning the other two SNPs, the frequency of the minor allele in the three different study populations was almost identical. No significant differences in genetics were observed between noncirrhotic NAFLD patients with absent/mild and those with advanced fibrosis, but the limited number in this sub-analysis should be considered. Only the PNPLA3, TM6SF2, and KLF6 SNPs were then selected to constitute the genetic risk score, participating according to the model which best fitted with their association to the risk of NASH cirrhosis. The genetic risk score was significantly associated with the risk of both noncirrhotic NAFLD with healthy subjects as reference group and with the risk of NASH cirrhosis with noncirrhotic NAFLD as reference. The more impressive results were obtained, to our opinion, when the score was expressed categorically; notably, for example, with respect to a score of 0, after adjusting for age, sex, diabetes, and BMI, a score > 2 was associated with about 20-fold increased risk of NAFLD development in healthy subjects and almost 4-fold increased risk of progression to cirrhosis in NAFLD patients.

The strengths of this study are the following: it is carried-out in a well-characterized NAFLD population from hepatological tertiary centers; it includes a control group to represent genetics in the general population; it is the first evident proof of concept that the more the information from genetics the higher possibility to predict the risk of NAFLD and its progression to cirrhosis. This study has also some limitations: it is a case-control study with a transversal design, carrying the possible biases which have been addressed previously; the inclusion of some variants with respect to others which are known to be associated with NAFLD, such as the rs641738 SNP in MBOAT7 [34], can be considered arbitrary. However, it is clear that we did not aim to launch a specific set of variants nor the way to combine them in a genetic risk score; rather, our aim was to give proof of concept that such an approach has a strong logic in the context of NAFLD.

In conclusion, the present study suggests that combining different disease-associated variants may probably represent the way for genetics to keep strength and consent in NAFLD diagnostics. Further studies on larger series are eagerly awaited in order to individuate the best set of variants to be included and the most powerful model and also to verify if combining the best genetic model with clinical predictors would lead to further and meaningful advantages.

Acknowledgments

The authors thank Rita Marini and Barbara Giannetti for their precious technical assistance in laboratory procedures (DNA extraction and genotyping).

References

[1] C. D. Williams, J. Stengel, M. I. Asike et al., "Prevalence of nonalcoholic fatty liver disease and nonalcoholic steatohepatitis among a largely middle-aged population utilizing ultrasound and liver biopsy: a prospective study," *Gastroenterology*, vol. 140, no. 1, pp. 124–131, 2011.

[2] Z. Younossi, Q. M. Anstee, M. Marietti et al., "Global burden of NAFLD and NASH: trends, predictions, risk factors and prevention," *Nature Reviews Gastroenterology & Hepatology*, vol. 15, no. 1, pp. 11–20, 2017.

[3] G. Vernon, A. Baranova, and Z. M. Younossi, "Systematic review: the epidemiology and natural history of non-alcoholic fatty liver disease and non-alcoholic steatohepatitis in adults," *Alimentary Pharmacology & Therapeutics*, vol. 34, no. 3, pp. 274–285, 2011.

[4] S. Sookoian and C. J. Pirola, "Genetic predisposition in nonalcoholic fatty liver disease," *Clinical and Molecular Hepatology*, vol. 23, no. 1, pp. 1–12, 2017.

[5] M. Eslam, L. Valenti, and S. Romeo, "Genetics and epigenetics of NAFLD and NASH: Clinical impact," *Journal of Hepatology*, vol. 68, no. 2, pp. 268–279, 2018.

[6] Q. M. Anstee and C. P. Day, "The genetics of nonalcoholic fatty liver disease: spotlight on *PNPLA3* and *TM6SF2*," *Seminars in Liver Disease*, vol. 35, no. 3, pp. 270–290, 2015.

[7] P. Dongiovanni, S. Petta, C. Maglio et al., "TM6SF2 gene variant disentangles nonalcoholic steatohepatitis from cardiovascular disease," *Hepatology*, 2015.

[8] A. Al-Serri, Q. M. Anstee, L. Valenti et al., "The SOD2 C47T polymorphism influences NAFLD fibrosis severity: evidence from case-control and intra-familial allele association studies," *Journal of Hepatology*, vol. 56, no. 2, pp. 448–454, 2012.

[9] Y.-S. Huang, C.-H. Chang, T.-L. Lin, and C.-L. Perng, "Genetic variations of superoxide dismutase 2 and cytochrome P450 2E1 in non-alcoholic steatohepatitis," *Liver International*, vol. 34, no. 6, pp. 931–936, 2014.

[10] L. Valenti, B. M. Motta, A. Alisi et al., "LPIN1 rs13412852 polymorphism in pediatric nonalcoholic fatty liver disease," *Journal of Pediatric Gastroenterology and Nutrition*, vol. 54, no. 5, pp. 588–593, 2012.

[11] L. Miele, G. Beale, G. Patman et al., "The Kruppel-like factor 6 genotype is associated with fibrosis in nonalcoholic fatty liver disease," *Gastroenterology*, vol. 135, no. 1, pp. 282–291, 2008.

[12] L. P. Bechmann, A. Gastaldelli, D. Vetter et al., "Glucokinase links Krüppel-like factor 6 to the regulation of hepatic insulin sensitivity in nonalcoholic fatty liver disease," *Hepatology*, vol. 55, no. 4, pp. 1083–1093, 2012.

[13] V. Nobili, B. Donati, N. Panera et al., "A 4-polymorphism risk score predicts steatohepatitis in children with nonalcoholic fatty liver disease," *Journal of Pediatric Gastroenterology and Nutrition*, vol. 58, no. 5, pp. 632–636, 2014.

[14] P. León-Mimila, J. Vega-Badillo, R. Gutiérrez-Vidal et al., "A genetic risk score is associated with hepatic triglyceride content and non-alcoholic steatohepatitis in Mexicans with morbid obesity," *Experimental and Molecular Pathology*, vol. 98, no. 2, pp. 178–183, 2015.

[15] S. Ballestri, D. Romagnoli, F. Nascimbeni, G. Francica, and A. Lonardo, "Role of ultrasound in the diagnosis and treatment of nonalcoholic fatty liver disease and its complications," *Expert Review of Gastroenterology & Hepatology*, vol. 9, no. 5, pp. 603–627, 2015.

[16] A. Berzigotti and F. Piscaglia, "Ultrasound in portal hypertension - Part 1," *Ultraschall in der Medizin / European Journal of Ultrasound (UiM/EJU)*, vol. 32, no. 6, pp. 548–571, 2011.

[17] A. Berzigotti, F. Piscaglia, and and the EFSUMB Education and Professional Standards Committee, "Ultrasound in portal hypertension—part 2—and EFSUMB recommendations for the performance and reporting of ultrasound examinations in portal hypertension," *Ultraschall in der Medizin (Stuttgart, Germany : 1980)*, vol. 33, no. 1, pp. -32–31, 2012.

[18] E. M. Brunt, C. G. Janney, A. M. Di Bisceglie, B. A. Neuschwander-Tetri, and B. R. Bacon, "Nonalcoholic steatohepatitis: a proposal for grading and staging the histological

lesions," *American Journal of Gastroenterology*, vol. 94, no. 9, pp. 2467–2474, 1999.

[19] D. E. Kleiner, E. M. Brunt, M. van Natta et al., "Design and validation of a histological scoring system for nonalcoholic fatty liver disease," *Hepatology*, vol. 41, no. 6, pp. 1313–1321, 2005.

[20] K. Burnham and D. Anderson, *Model Selection and Multimodel Inference: A Practical Information-Theoretic Approach*, Springer, New York, NY, USA, 2nd edition, 2002.

[21] E. M. Brunt, V. W. Wong, V. Nobili et al., "Nonalcoholic fatty liver disease," *Nature Reviews Disease Primers*, vol. 1, Article ID 15080, 2015.

[22] M. Krawczyk, P. Portincasa, and F. Lammert, "PNPLA3-associated steatohepatitis: toward a gene-based classification of fatty liver disease," *Seminars in Liver Disease*, vol. 33, no. 4, pp. 369–379, 2013.

[23] U. Vespasiani-Gentilucci, P. Gallo, A. Porcari et al., "The PNPLA3 rs738409 C > G polymorphism is associated with the risk of progression to cirrhosis in NAFLD patients," *Scandinavian Journal of Gastroenterology*, vol. 51, no. 8, pp. 967–973, 2016.

[24] Y.-L. Liu, H. L. Reeves, and A. D. Burt, "TM6SF2 rs58542926 influences hepatic fibrosis progression in patients with non-alcoholic fatty liver disease," *Nature Communications*, vol. 5, article 4309, 2004.

[25] B. K. Koo, S. K. Joo, D. Kim et al., "Additive effects of PNPLA3 and TM6SF2 on the histological severity of non-alcoholic fatty liver disease," *Journal of Gastroenterology and Hepatology*, 2017.

[26] M. Milano, A. Aghemo, R. M. Mancina et al., "Transmembrane 6 Superfamily Member 2 Gene E167K Variant Impacts on Steatosis and Liver Damage in Chronic Hepatitis C Patients," *Hepatology*, vol. 62, no. 1, pp. 111–117, 2015.

[27] U. Vespasiani-Gentilucci, P. Gallo, A. De Vincentis, G. Galati, and A. Picardi, "Hepatitis C virus and metabolic disorder interactions towards liver damage and atherosclerosis," *World Journal of Gastroenterology*, vol. 20, no. 11, pp. 2825–2838, 2014.

[28] European Association for the Study of the Liver (EASL), European Association for the Study of Diabetes (EASD), and European Association for the Study of Obesity (EASO), "EASL-EASD-EASO Clinical Practice Guidelines for the management of non-alcoholic fatty liver disease," *Journal of Hepatology*, vol. 64, no. 6, pp. 1388–1402, 2016.

[29] M. Krawczyk, M. Rau, R. M. Schattenberg et al., "Combined effects of the PNPLA3 rs738409, TM6SF2 rs58542926, and MBOAT7 rs641738 variants on NAFLD severity: A multicenter biopsy-based study1," *Journal of Lipid Research*, vol. 58, no. 1, pp. 247–255, 2017.

[30] E. K. Speliotes, J. L. Butler, C. D. Palmer, B. F. Voight, and J. N. Hirschhorn, "PNPLA3 variants specifically confer increased risk for histologic nonalcoholic fatty liver disease but not metabolic disease," *Hepatology*, vol. 52, no. 3, pp. 904–912, 2010.

[31] L. Valenti, A. Al-Serri, A. K. Daly et al., "Homozygosity for the patatin-like phospholipase-3/adiponutrin i148m polymorphism influences liver fibrosis in patients with nonalcoholic fatty liver disease," *Hepatology*, vol. 51, no. 4, pp. 1209–1217, 2010.

[32] Y. Rotman, C. Koh, J. M. Zmuda, D. E. Kleiner, and T. J. Liang, "The association of genetic variability in patatin-like phospholipase domain-containing protein 3 (PNPLA3) with histological severity of nonalcoholic fatty liver disease," *Hepatology*, vol. 52, no. 3, pp. 894–903, 2010.

[33] Y. L. Liu, G. L. Patman, J. B. S. Leathart et al., "Carriage of the PNPLA3 rs738409 C > G polymorphism confers an increased risk of non-alcoholic fatty liver disease associated hepatocellular carcinoma," *Journal of Hepatology*, vol. 61, no. 1, pp. 75–81, 2014.

[34] R. M. Mancina, P. Dongiovanni, S. Petta et al., "The *MBOAT7-TMC4* variant rs641738 increases risk of nonalcoholic fatty liver disease in individuals of European descent," *Gastroenterology*, vol. 150, no. 5, pp. 1219–1230, 2016.

16

Disability in Patients with Inflammatory Bowel Disease: Correlations with Quality of Life and Patient's Characteristics

Konstantinos Argyriou, Andreas Kapsoritakis, Konstantinos Oikonomou, Anastassios Manolakis, Eirini Tsakiridou, and Spyridon Potamianos

Department of Gastroenterology, University Hospital of Larissa, Mezourlo 1, 41110 Larissa, Greece

Correspondence should be addressed to Konstantinos Argyriou; kosnar2@doctors.org.uk

Academic Editor: Michael Beyak

Background. Inflammatory bowel diseases may cause significant disability. However, little is known regarding the life domains where patients encounter most limitations. *Objectives.* To assess patients' overall disability and determine the life domains where most restrictions were applied. Secondarily, we sought for possible relationships among disability, quality of life (HRQoL), and population characteristics. *Method.* The study lasted for two years (2013–2015) and included 200 patients [52% ulcerative colitis (UC)] from a referral centre. Disability was evaluated using the 36-item version of WHODAS 2.0 questionnaire. The influence of population characteristics on overall disability was assessed with linear regression. *Results.* Crohn's disease (CD) patients showed greater overall disability compared to UC (19.22 versus 15.01, $p = 0.001$), with higher scores in the domains of relationships, life activities, and participation. Disability was negatively associated with HRQoL ($p < 0.001$). Long activity, extensive disease, rural residence, and employment independently influenced the overall disability in both groups. Additionally, significant influence was recorded for lower education in the UC and for operation and celibacy in the CD group. *Conclusions.* CD patients were facing more limitations compared to those with UC, especially in the domains of relationships, activities, and participation. Other than clinical factors, sociodemographic characteristics were also associated with increased disability.

1. Introduction

Inflammatory bowel diseases (IBD), including mainly Crohn's disease (CD) and ulcerative colitis (UC), are chronic relapsing conditions of the gastrointestinal tract [1]. Over their longitudinal course, IBD may cause significant complications and disability to the patients that adversely affect their health related quality of life (HRQoL) [2, 3].

Contrary to progressive and irreversible medical conditions where disability is permanent and clinically recognizable, in relapsing diseases it may be temporary and difficult to address [4]. However, in all cases, disability increases the direct and the indirect cost of living with IBD [5]. Therefore, its prevention should be of particular concern among health care professionals and patient organizations [4, 5].

Until recently, the ability of patients to work was the most commonly used index in the assessment of IBD-related disability. However, working ability is not sufficient to fully cover the working limitations that patients may encounter during the long course of the intestinal disease; let alone the overall disability [5].

Although most disability studies report increased rates of unemployment, sick leave, and disability pension among IBD patients, most patients maintain their ability to work for many years after the initial diagnosis [5–7]. However, recent studies have entered new factors into play. IBD patients have been found to experience significantly more presenteeism (impaired productivity) and absenteeism (loss of working hours) compared to controls, with significant accompanying economic losses not only for the individual but also for the society [8, 9].

The latter shows that IBD represent a high economic burden to society. But, their cost could not be solely confined to economy [10].

Disability is an objective way of understanding the impact of IBD in patients' daily life. However, for many years, most studies were focusing on the subjective estimation of HRQoL when aiming to quantify the experience of living with these diseases [11]. A possible explanation for this shortage was probably the lack of standards not only in the assessment but also in the delimitation of the conceptual framework of disability.

In 2002, the World Health Organization (WHO) set the international standards for the assessment of disability. Including factors of activity and participation to employment as well as attitudes, WHO created the International Classification of Functioning, Disability and Health (ICF) [12].

Based on the concepts of ICF, generic and disease-specific instruments have been developed and become available to be used in the evaluation of disability in IBD [13–15]. Compared to disease-specific tools, generic questionnaires are offered for comparisons across different diseases and cultures. In addition, some generic measures, such as the WHO Disability Assessment Schedule 2.0 (WHODAS 2.0), allow the determination of the domains in patients' daily life where most functional limitations apply [15].

WHODAS 2.0 offers a multidimensional approach to disability. It is available in a short (12-item) and two longer (36-item/full and [12+24]-item/hybrid) versions, with the longer ones to provide additionally a detailed profile of disability. To date, WHODAS 2.0 has been tested in both inflammatory and noninflammatory conditions and has been found to be valid and reliable [15].

A recent study, using the short version of this questionnaire, has examined the prevalence of disability among IBD patients [16]. However, the profile of disability remained mostly unknown.

In our study, we used the 36-item version of WHODAS 2.0 in order not only to assess patients' overall disability but also to determine the domains of their daily life in which IBD patients experienced most restrictions. Secondary outcomes were to find possible relationships among disability, HRQoL, and population's characteristics.

2. Material and Methods

2.1. Patients and Design. The study took place at the University hospital of Larissa which constitutes the sole tertiary referral centre for IBD patients in Central Greece. The study was approved by the Ethics Committee and the Advisory Board of the University Hospital of Larissa (D.N.18484/17-04-2013). All participants provided consensus upon information about the nature, the duration, and the purpose of the study.

During a 2-year period (2013–2015), all consecutive IBD patients from our outpatient clinic and the gastroenterology department (where they have been admitted for an IBD-related cause) were screened for eligibility and entered the study.

Inclusion criteria were the patients to be adults, to be able to read and write Greek fluently, and to have IBD per standard criteria [17]. Patients diagnosed with a major neuropsychiatric disorder or other comorbidities prior to the diagnosis of the intestinal disease as well as those with stoma were excluded from the study, in order to avoid overestimation or underestimation in the assessment of HRQoL and disability.

The data were collected by the same investigator, who was not the treating doctor of the patient, during a personal interview that took place at a time specified by the patient in order to ensure the comfort and the accuracy of the answers. All interviews were held during the follow-up visit of the patients or within two days after admission.

Data collection included a diary card with the characteristics of the population and two measuring instruments for HRQoL and disability.

2.2. Population Characteristics

2.2.1. Sociodemographic Variables. The background information included sex, age, place of residence, marital and employment status, and level of education for each patient.

2.2.2. IBD-Related Variables. The clinical characteristics were as follows:

(i) type, duration, and extension of the intestinal disease,

(ii) activity status (defined as short and long),

(iii) smoking behaviour,

(iv) disease behaviour (defined as complicated disease) in CD patients,

(v) history of previous IBD-related surgeries,

(vi) previous hospitalizations,

(vii) use of biologic agents > 3 months prior to study entry.

Disease activity was assessed by using the clinical indices Harvey-Bradshaw (HB) for CD and Simple Clinical Colitis Activity Index (SCCAI) for UC patients [18, 19]. Short activity referred to the patient's activity status at the time of recruitment. Long active was considered the disease for which activity had been recorded in most of the follow-up visits of the patient over the previous 3 years, based on patient's own medical record. Regarding activity, IBD patients were divided into two categories. Values < 5 in both indices were considered to indicate clinical remission.

2.3. Measuring Instruments

2.3.1. Disability. For the assessment of disability, we used the interviewer-administered 36-item version of the questionnaire WHODAS 2.0. There are two other versions of WHODAS- the brief (12-item) and the hybrid (12+24-item). However, the 36-item (full) version is regarded the most detailed one.

WHODAS 2.0 is a practical, generic tool that can measure health and disability at population level or in clinical practice, without targeting a specific disease. It is available in 14 languages, including the Greek language. Its psychometric properties were subjected to two waves of international testing with the instrument to have been proved valid and reliable.

The full version has 36 questions that relate to the functioning difficulties experienced by the individual during the previous 30 days and captures disability in the following six domains:

(1) Cognition: understanding and communication (6 questions).

(2) Mobility: moving and getting around (5 questions).

(3) Self-care: attending to one's hygiene, dressing, eating, and staying alone (4 questions).

(4) Getting along: interpersonal relationships (5 questions).

(5) Life activities: domestic responsibilities, work, and school (8 questions).

(6) Participation: joining in community activities and social participation (8 questions).

In addition, the final part of the questionnaire includes an optional set of questions in which the responder is called to attribute the difficulties to a particular causative agent and to estimate their impact on his/her everyday life.

The answer to each question follows a 5-point Likert scale with the lowest score to show the smallest difficulty. The total and dimensional scores range from 0 to 100 with the highest score to show greater disability. There are two different ways to compute WHODAS 2.0 summary scores: the simple scoring option, which simply summarises the scores of the items across all domains, and the more complex scoring method, which is called "item-response-theory" (IRT) based scoring. Since simple scoring "is specific to the sample at hand and should not be assumed to be comparable across populations," in our study, we used the complex scoring system which allows a more fine-grained analysis across populations or subpopulations. In complex scoring, summary scores result from standardized SPSS (SYNTAX) algorithms [15].

2.3.2. HRQoL. For the assessment of HRQoL, we used the Greek version of the Inflammatory Bowel Disease Questionnaire (IBDQ) [20]. IBDQ has been widely used in clinical and epidemiological studies [21, 22].

2.4. Statistical Analysis. The study population was divided into two groups according to disease type. Statistical comparisons between the 2 groups were made either with Pearson's chi-square test (for categorical variables), or Mann-Whitney-Wilcoxon test (for continuous variables). Most summary scores in WHODAS 2.0 and IBDQ did not follow the normal distribution. Comparisons between continuous variables were performed with Spearman correlation coefficients. Possible relationships between disability and population's characteristics were evaluated with Mann-Whitney-Wilcoxon test for 2 groups and Kruskal-Wallis test when comparisons involved more than 2 groups.

Factors significantly associated with WHODAS 2.0 summary scores were entered into a linear regression analysis that was performed stepwise (backward elimination of variables).

The level of statistical significance was set at $p < 0.05$. For the statistical analysis, we used the statistical software SPSS 17 for windows.

3. Results

Over the study period, 253 patients were eligible to participate. From the initial population, 33 patients did not wish to participate (due to lack of time) and 20 patients were excluded because of inconclusive answers. Thus, the final population of the study consisted of 200 patients (52% with UC). The majority of the patients (86.5%) were recruited from our IBD clinic while 13.5% were hospitalized.

The sociodemographic and clinical characteristics of the final population are shown in Table 1. As for the population characteristics, no statistical significant differences were found between the excluded patients and the final population.

3.1. Profile and Measurement of Disability among IBD Patients. The majority of IBD patients (61.5% versus 67.7% for those with UC and CD, resp.) replied to the disability questions by comparing their current health status with the period that preceded the appearance of the intestinal disease.

Table 2 shows the mean total and dimensional WHODAS scores of the study population per disease type.

In general, CD patients scored higher compared to those with UC. Apart from cognition, mobility, and self-care, this difference was statistically significant in all other domains. The highest scores were achieved in the domains of relationships, life activities, and participation by both groups.

3.2. Per Domain Analysis. Over the 30 day reference period, the mean number of days that IBD patients had to cut down their usual daily activities was 9.26 ± 4.99 for the UC and 13,1 ± 6.53 for the CD group, respectively ($p = 0{,}001$).

3.2.1. Cognition. In the domain of understanding and communication, 48% of IBD patients estimated that they had experienced difficulties in finding solutions to daily problems.

Between the 2 groups, CD patients encountered difficulties in launching and maintaining a conversation more frequently (33.7% versus 47.9% for UC and CD, resp., $p = 0{,}041$).

No statistically significant differences were found regarding the other domain specific items.

3.2.2. Mobility and Self-Care. No statistically significant differences were found in the domains of mobility and self-care, with the majority (>80%) of IBD patients not reporting any specific restriction.

TABLE 1: Population characteristics.

	Crohn disease ($N = 96$)	Ulcerative colitis ($N = 104$)	
Sex			
Male	46 (47.9)	51 (49)	NS
Females	50 (52.1)	53 (51)	
Age (mean ± sd)	39,2 ± 11.88	42.1 ± 12.9	NS
Residence			
Rural (<4.000 inhabitants)	25 (26)	32 (30.8)	
Semirural (4.000–10.000)	23 (24)	21 (20.2)	NS
Urban (>10.000)	48 (50)	51 (49.0)	
Level of education			
Basic	12 (12.50)	12 (11.5)	
Secondary	52 (54.17)	50 (48.1)	NS
Postsecondary	32 (33.30)	42 (40.4)	
Marital status			
Single	25 (26.1)	40 (38.5)	
Married	63 (65.6)	50 (48.1)	$p = 0.012$
Divorced/widowed	8 (08,3)	14 (13.4)	
Employment status			
Unemployed	20 (20.8)	20 (19.2)	
Part-time employed	21 (21,9)	22 (21.2)	NS
Full-time employed	47 (49.0)	50 (48.1)	
Pensioner	8 (08.3)	12 (11.5)	
Active smoking			
Yes	34 (35.4)	27 (26)	NS
No	62 (64.6)	77 (74)	
Disease duration (mean ± sd in years)	9.11 ± 2.041	9.47 ± 5.14	NS
Short disease activity			
Remission	30 (31.3)	37 (35.6)	
Active	66 (68.7)	67 (64.4)	NS
Long disease activity			
No	68 (70.8)	74 (71.2)	NS
Yes	28 (29.2)	30 (28.8)	
Biologic agents			
No	76 (79.2)	92 (88.5)	NS
Yes	20 (20.8)	12 (11.5)	
IBD-related surgery			
No	82 (85.4)	99 (95.2)	$p = 0.021$
Yes	14 (14.6)	5 (4.8)	
IBD-related previous hospitalization			
No	78 (81.3)	92 (88.5)	NS
Yes	18 (18.8)	12 (11.5)	
Disease location			
Ulcerative colitis			
Proctitis	NA	10 (9.6)	
Up to splenic flexure	NA	35 (33.7)	
Beyond splenic flexure	NA	54 (51.9)	
Pouch	NA	5 (4.8)	

Table 1: Continued.

	Crohn disease ($N = 96$)	Ulcerative colitis ($N = 104$)
Crohn's disease		
Colon	6 (6.3)	NA
Ileum	55 (57.3)	NA
Ileocolonic	35 (36.5)	NA
Complicated disease		NA
Inflammatory	60 (62.5)	NA
Noninflammatory (stenotic-fistulizing-abscessing)	36 (37.5)	NA

NA: non applicable; NS: non significant; $p < 0.05$ statistically significant.

Table 2: Comparison of the total and dimensional summary scores for WHODAS 2.0 between the two patients' groups.

	Ulcerative colitis ($n = 104$) Mean/median (range)	Crohn's disease ($n = 96$) Mean/median (range)	Cohen's r^*	p^{**}
Cognition	6.64/5 (25)	8.59/5 (30)	NC***	NS****
Mobility	3.91/0 (37.50)	4.23/0 (43.75)	NC	NS
Self-care	2.98/0 (40)	3.85/0 (40)	NC	NS
Relationships	29.09/33.33 (58.33)	35.59/41.67 (58.33)	0.26	<0.001
Life activities (domestic tasks)	19.04/20 (90)	25.31/30 (90)	0.20	0.005
Life activities (work/school tasks)	20.24/21.43 (78.57)	26.47/28.57 (78.57)	0.18	<0.001
Participation	24/25 (54.17)	29.95/29.17 (58.33)	0.29	0.030
Overall disability (total score)	15/15.01 (36.79)	18.94/19.22 (40.57)	0.22	0.001

$^*r = 0.1$, 0.3, and 0.5 for small, medium, and large effect size; $^{**}p < 0.05$: statistical significance; ***NC: not calculated; ****NS: no statistical significance.

3.2.3. Getting Along. In the domain of interpersonal relationships, irrespectively of the disease type, more than 70% of the patients were facing difficulties in making new friends and in intimate relationships.

Additionally, the majority of the population experienced functional limitations in sexual life (67.7% for CD versus 64.4% for UC, $p > 0.05$).

Between the 2 groups, CD patients had limitations in getting along with their friends more frequently (76% versus 59.6%, $p = 0{,}014$).

3.2.4. Life Activities. Difficulties in performing the usual work-tasks were encountered by 73.6% of the participants with 55.7% of IBD patients having experienced difficulties in completing all the jobs of their daily schedule.

The majority of IBD patients (>60%) reported that they had worked at a slow pace with those suffering from CD having lost more profits (50% versus 33%, $p = 0.046$).

Similar restrictions applied in the subdomain of domestic activities. Approximately, half of the study population (56% for the CD and 52.8% for the UC group, resp.) encountered functional limitations in the completion of the household tasks.

In addition, compared to the patients with UC, those with CD estimated that they needed more time in order to perform their domestic activities (68.7% versus 37.5%, $p = 0.001$).

3.2.5. Participation. In the domain of participation, difficulties were encountered by the vast majority of the population (>90%).

69.5% of the IBD patients estimated that they had been emotionally affected by their intestinal disease, with a similar proportion of patients (68%) spending time on their health condition and having difficulty in doing things for leisure or pleasure.

Although more than 50% of the UC patients reported to have encountered functional limitation in social participation because of barriers or hindrances from the other people around them, this problem was more prominent among CD patients (52.9% versus 72.9% for UC and CD, resp., $p = 0.004$). Because of others' attitudes, the same group of patients faced also a higher problem of decent living (71% for CD versus 45% for UC, $p = 0.001$).

Between the two groups, a similar proportion of patients perceived IBD as a financial (42.3% for UC versus 47.9% for CD) or as a family problem (40.4% for UC versus 40.6% for CD).

TABLE 3: Relationships between WHODAS 2.0 summary scores and population's characteristics in patients with Crohn's disease.

	WHODAS 2.0							
	Cognition $z/x/r$ p	Mobility $z/x/r$ p	Self-care $z/x/r$ p	Relationships $z/x/r$ p	Life activities (domestic tasks) $z/x/r$ p	Life activities (work) $z/x/r$ p	Participation $z/x/r$ p	Total score $z/x/r$ p
Population characteristics								
Sex	NS	NS	NS	NS	NS	NS	NS	NS
Age	NS	NS	NS	NS	NS	NS	NS	NS
Residence	9.768 0.008	NS	NS	10.815 0.004	6.701 0.035	6.679 0.035	13.876 0.001	14.143 0.001
Education	NS	NS	NS	NS	NS	NS	NS	NS
Marital status	8.155 0.017	NS	NS	10.284 0.006	8.279 0.016	8.143 0.017	10.493 0.005	13,944 0.001
Employment status	21.285 0.001	NS	NS	15.330 0.002	23.843 0.001	8.331 0.040	NS	18.314 0.001
Smoking	NS	NS	NS	NS	NS	NS	NS	NS
Disease duration	NS	NS	NS	NS	NS	NS	NS	NS
Short activity	NS	−2.194 0.028	−2.056 0.040	−3.039 0.002	−2.554 0.011	−2.134 0.033	−2.818 0.005	−3.318 0.001
Long activity	−4.405 0.001	−3.953 0.001	−2.387 0.017	−5.058 0.001	−5.798 0.001	−5.460 0.001	−5.338 0.001	−6.965 0.001
Biologic agents	NS	NS	NS	NS	NS	NS	NS	NS
IBD-related surgery	NS	−4.091 0.001	−2.898 0.004	−2.833 0.005	−3.986 0.001	−2.152 0.031	−3.864 0.001	−4.082 0.001
Previous hospitalization	NS	−4.489 0.001	−3.412 0.001	NS	−2.956 0.003	−3.046 0.002	−3.195 0.001	−3.330 0.001
Disease-location	11.534 0.003	NS	NS	13.972 0.001	NS	NS	8.028 0.018	8,728 0.013
Complicated disease	NS	NS	NS	−1.991 0.046	NS	NS	−2.168 0.030	NS

NS: non statistically significant; $p < 0.05$: statistically significant; $z/x/r$: Mann-Whitney-Wilcoxon test or Kruskal-Wallis test or Spearman correlation coefficients.

3.3. Impact and Severity of Functional Limitations in Daily Life. The impact of the functional limitations on patients' daily life was rated "moderate" by the majority of the study population (62%).

Across domains, the severity of the restrictions was ranging from mild to moderate for the majority of the responders in both patient groups.

3.4. Associations of Disability with HRQoL and Study Variables. The median IBDQ score was 172 and 179.5 for CD and UC patients, with the difference being statistically significant ($p = 0.02$)

Moderate to high negative correlations were found for all summary scores between WHODAS 2.0 and IBDQ ($p < 0.001$).

3.5. Multivariate Analysis. The relationships between disability and population characteristics were examined with univariate analysis. The results are shown in Tables 3 and 4.

All factors significantly associated with disability were entered into linear regression. The results are shown in Tables 5 and 6.

Extensive (defined as disease location beyond the splenic flexure) disease, long activity, rural residence, and full-time employment had an independent influence on the sum score of overall disability in both types of intestinal disease.

Additionally, a statistically significant association with increased disability was found for lower (defined as basic/secondary) education in patients with UC as well as for operations and celibacy (defined as single/divorced) in the CD group.

4. Discussion

In this project, our primary aims were not only the assessment of the IBD-related disability, but also the determination of the profile of the functional limitations that IBD patients experience in their daily life. Secondary outcomes were to

TABLE 4: Relationships between WHODAS 2.0 and population's characteristics in patients with ulcerative colitis.

	WHODAS 2.0							
	Cognition $z/x/r$ p	Mobility $z/x/r$ p	Self-care $z/x/r$ p	Relationships $z/x/r$ p	Life activities (domestic tasks) $z/x/r$ p	Life activities (work) $z/x/r$ p	Participation $z/x/r$ p	Total score $z/x/r$ p
Population characteristics								
Sex	NS	NS	NS	NS	NS	−2.287 0.022	−3.051 0.002	−1.972 0.049
Age	NS	NS	NS	NS	NS	NS	NS	NS
Residence	22.756 0.001	NS	NS	16.288 0.001	12.140 0.002	22.518 0.001	26.318 0.001	25.423 0.001
Education	34.481 0.001	NS	10.312 0.006	30.931 0.001	30.819 0.001	20.511 0.001	21.166 0.001	45.348 0.001
Marital status	21.411 0.001	NS	NS	20.290 0.001	16.652 0.001	14.002 0.001	20.434 0.001	24.073 0.001
Employment status	14.527 0.002	NS	NS	16.075 0.001	16.505 0.001	11.943 0.008	19.037 0.001	24.022 0.001
Smoking	NS	NS	NS	NS	NS	NS	NS	NS
Disease duration	0.310 0.001	NS	NS	0.256 0.009	0.276 0.005	0.256 0.030	0.281 0.004	0.302 0.002
Short activity	−3.698 0.001	NS	NS	−3.954 0.001	−4.061 0.001	−2.386 0.017	−3.717 0.001	−4.037 0.001
Long activity	−2.516 0.012	−4.503 0.001	−2.632 0.008	−3.411 0.001	−3.495 0.001	−3.729 0.001	−4.497 0.001	−4.787 0.001
Biologic agents	NS	−2.673 0.008	NS	NS	NS	NS	NS	NS
IBD-related surgery	−2.574 0.010	NS	NS	−3.468 0.001	−2.770 0.006	−3.052 0.002	−3.323 0.001	−3.475 0.001
Previous hospitalization	NS	−2.085 0.037	NS	NS	NS	−2.059 0.039	NS	−2.164 0.030
Disease-location	22.428 0.001	NS	NS	36.132 0.001	24.567 0.001	9.240 0.026	24.774 0.001	29.824 0.001

NS: nonstatistically significant; $p < 0.05$: statistically significant; $z/x/r$: Mann-Whitney-Wilcoxon test or Kruskal-Wallis test or Spearman correlation coefficients.

search for possible relationships among disability, quality of life, and patients' characteristics. To our knowledge, this is the first study that highlights specific areas of functioning among IBD patients. In Greece, in particular, no previous studies described an individual's profile of the restrictions in functionality in sickness or in health with the 36-item version of WHODAS.

Power analysis indicated that, in order to ensure a power of 0.90 for coefficients as low as 0.25, we needed a total sample size of 164 participants. For comparisons between disease types, we needed at least 200 patients. In order to reduce measurement error, we used highly valid outcome measures.

Our data analysis showed that the level of disability in our population was higher than the one reported in a recent Canadian study [16]. This difference could be attributed to the different characteristics of the study population. In accordance with the same investigators, we observed that CD patients had a higher level of disability compared to those with UC. However, a small to medium effect size was found in the comparisons of all WHODAS 2.0 summary scores between the two patient groups.

The greater restrictions in our patients were recorded in the domains of interpersonal relationships and life activities as well as in the domain of social participation.

Qualitative studies from Europe [23], Australia [24], and Canada [25] suggested that living with IBD affects negatively the interpersonal relationships and the HRQoL of patients. Our findings support these studies. However, contrary to Becker et al. [25], who found that the impact of the intestinal disease on interpersonal relationships is severe, in our study, we found this impact to be mild to moderate for the majority of the population. One possible explanation for this finding is that the Greek IBD patients have strong family support which attenuates the burden of the disease [26]. Therefore, it may indicate how important it is for IBD patients to have a supportive environment in order to cope with the chronic disease.

TABLE 5: Predictors for increased overall disability among population characteristics on the basis of multiple linear regressions in patients with Crohn's disease.

	Adjusted R square	Unstandardized coefficients				95% confidence interval for B		Collinearity statistics
		B	Std Error	t	p	Lower bound	Upper bound	VIF
Long activity	0.703	9.512	1.410	6.744	0.001	6.709	12.314	1.493
IBD-related operations		6.168	1.767	3.491	0.001	2.658	9.679	1.413
Extensive disease (colitis)		−7.934	2.230	−3.558	0.001	−12.364	−3.503	1.058
Place of residence (rural)		3.326	1.336	2.490	0.015	0.672	5.981	1.249
Marital status (celibacy)		3.083	1.173	2.629	0.01	0.752	5.414	1.128
Employment status (full-time job)		5.530	1.140	4.850	0.001	3.265	7.796	1.181

$p < 0.05$: statistically significant.

TABLE 6: Predictors for increased overall disability among population characteristics on the basis of multiple linear regression in patients with ulcerative colitis.

	Adjusted R square	Unstandardized coefficients				95% confidence interval for B		Collinearity statistics
		B	Std Error	t	p	Lower bound	Upper bound	VIF
Long activity	0.700	6.430	1.065	6.036	0.001	4.316	8.545	1.212
Education		6.298	1.126	−5.591	0.001	−8.534	−4.062	1.589
Extensive disease (beyond splenic flexure)		3.023	1.093	2.767	0.007	0.854	5.192	1.550
Place of residence (rural)		3.894	1.063	3.663	0.001	1.784	6.003	1.252
Marital status (celibacy)		NS	NS	NS	NS	NS	NS	NS
Employment status (full-time job)		2.204	0.954	2.311	0.023	0.311	4.097	1.212

NS: nonstatistically significant; $p < 0.05$: statistically significant.

In the domain of interpersonal relationships, the majority of our population has experienced limitations in making new friends, maintaining a friendship and in sex life. Friendship and sexuality can be both negatively affected in IBD with an accompanying negative impact on patients' physical and psychosocial well-being [27, 28]. Patient support groups could be of importance so as to reduce these limitations and improve patients' functionality.

Apart from relationships, IBD interfere with patients' working ability [29–33]. In our study, despite the fact that 85% of the participants maintained their working capacity, the majority admitted having worked at a slow pace and having difficulties in meeting all work commitments with subsequent loss of profits. Our findings are in line with the results of a recent study from the USA which showed increased presenteeism among IBD patients [8]. Presenteeism is an important issue for IBD patients, not only because it highlights the increased indirect cost of living with these diseases, but also because it may reflect patients' ability to cope with the working limitations that are imposed by the intestinal disease [8]. Therefore, its prevention should be of particular concern among health care professionals and organizations in order not only to increase productivity, but also to help our patients adjust to their disease.

Other than productivity at work, similar restrictions of functionality were applied in the performance of domestic tasks, indicating the additional burden that the caregivers often have to bear so as not to interrupt family functioning [34].

In the domain of participation, social activities and leisure have been found to be compromised in our population. These findings are in accordance with other studies [25, 35]. Similarly to our findings, Becker et al. [25] reported a higher impact of IBD on CD patients, attributing the difference to a more pronounced psychological morbidity. However, in our study, the emotional impact of IBD has not been found to differ between groups. A plausible explanation of our findings is that the majority of our patients encountered problems because of barriers and attitudes from the world around them, emphasizing the importance of the environment in the assessment and interpretation of disability.

In all domains of functionality, the severity of the experienced limitations was mild to moderate for the majority of the population. However, these limitations strongly affected patients' quality of life.

In the present study, we found that CD patients had worse quality of life compared to those with UC, with our finding being in accordance with the results of a recent Cypriot study [22]. Taking into account the fact that Greece and Cyprus have the same linguistic but different cultural characteristics, it may be of interest to see whether Cypriot patients experience similar limitations as well.

In regard to the predisposing factors for increased disability in our population, statistically significant associations were found for extensive or long active disease, rural residence, and full-time employment in both patient groups. In addition, statistically significant influence was recorded for lower education in the UC and for operation and marital status in the CD group. Concerning activity, the relationship with disability is easily understandable and not surprising [36, 37]. But for the other parameters, we have not detected corresponding references in literature.

Surprisingly enough, we found that full-time employment was independently associated with increased disability. This finding is opposite to other disability studies [30, 31]. However, it may indicate an attenuated ability of our population to deal with common work-related problems (e.g., fatigue, decreased motivation, and competitiveness) which, in turn, may lead the patients to cut down on their activities and/or to enlarge the restrictions in the other domains of their daily life. Consequently, empowering patients' ability to fight common work-related problems could help IBD patients to improve their overall functionality and/or to prevent disability.

The strength of this study is the use of the full version of the questionnaire WHODAS 2.0. Apart from a multidimensional approach of disability, this version allows researchers not only to make comparisons across different populations and cultures, but also to determine a profile of the functional limitations that an individual experience in his/her daily life.

Considering the potential limitations, we should note the inclusion of patients from a tertiary referral centre. Patients from referral centres are expected to have more severe disease. However, the absence of another IBD-specific healthcare provider in Central Greece has allowed the collection and presentation of data from the majority of IBD patients from our geographical area. Nevertheless, the size of our population was relatively small which precluded us from further subgroup analysis (e.g., to find differences between operated and nonoperated patients or between different treatments) or generalization.

Another potential limitation is the cross-sectional character of our study. However, this type of study allowed us the collection of information about the burden of the intestinal disease several years after the diagnosis and suggested associations that could be used for comparisons in longitudinal studies.

Finally, we note that, in our study, we used a general measurement tool for disability instead of the newly developed disease-specific tools. Apart from the fact that the IBD-specific tools were developed later in the course of our study, their results are not offered for comparisons across different populations; let alone for determining a profile of the functional limitations of IBD patients which was our primary goal. Nevertheless, we believe that a combined approach of overall disability in the future would help researchers to understand in full the various aspects of living with IBD, allowing an evidence-based patient-centred approach in the management of IBD patients.

5. Conclusions

Taking into account the possible limitations of this study, CD patients were found to experience more restrictions in their daily life compared to those with UC, especially in the domains of relationships, activities, and participation. Other than disease related factors, sociodemographic characteristics were found to negatively influence patients' overall disability. Determining the profile of the functional limitations of IBD patients may be of specific value for health care providers and organizations when organizing interventions that aim either to improve or to prevent IBD-related disability.

Acknowledgments

The authors would like to thank Dr Silia Vitoratou, lecturer in applied health statistics, at Kings College London, UK, for the statistical consultation during the analysis in this study and Christine Marou, experienced medical translator, for her language editing services.

References

[1] A. S. Bannaga and C. P. Selinger, "Inflammatory bowel disease and anxiety: links, risks, and challenges faced," *Clinical and Experimental Gastroenterology*, vol. 8, pp. 111–117, 2015.

[2] S. Lönnfors, S. Vermeire, M. Greco, D. Hommes, C. Bell, and L. Avedano, "IBD and health-related quality of life—discovering the true impact," *Journal of Crohn's and Colitis*, vol. 8, no. 10, pp. 1281–1286, 2014.

[3] J.-F. Colombel, "Measuring disability in IBD: the IBD disability index," *Gastroenterology & Hepatology*, vol. 9, no. 5, pp. 300–302, 2013.

[4] T. Bernklev, J. Jahnsen, M. Henriksen et al., "Relationship between sick leave, unemployment, disability, and health-related quality of life in patients with inflammatory bowel disease," *Inflammatory Bowel Diseases*, vol. 12, no. 5, pp. 402–412, 2006.

[5] B. P. Abraham and J. H. Sellin, "Disability in inflammatory bowel disease," *Gastroenterology Clinics of North America*, vol. 41, no. 2, pp. 429–441, 2012.

[6] A. Ramos, X. Calvet, B. Sicilia et al., "IBD-related work disability in the Community: prevalence, severity and predictive factors. A cross-sectional study," *United European Gastroenterology Journal*, vol. 3, no. 4, pp. 335-42, 2015.

[7] M. E. van der Valk, M.-J. J. Mangen, M. Leenders et al., "Risk factors of work disability in patients with inflammatory bowel disease—a Dutch nationwide web-based survey. Work disability in inflammatory bowel disease," *Journal of Crohn's and Colitis*, vol. 8, no. 7, pp. 590–597, 2014.

[8] A. Zand, W. K. Van Deen, E. K. Inserra et al., "Presenteeism in inflammatory bowel diseases: a hidden problem with significant economic impact," *Inflammatory Bowel Diseases*, vol. 21, no. 7, pp. 1623–1630, 2015.

[9] D. Schwartz, D. Greenberg, E. Chernin et al., "P592. Absenteeism and presenteeism amongst Crohn's disease patients: results from a real-world cohort in Israel," *Journal of Crohn's and Colitis*, vol. 10, supplement 1, pp. S400–S400, 2016.

[10] D. T. Rubin, C. A. Siegel, S. V. Kane et al., "Impact of ulcerative colitis from patients' and physicians' perspectives: results from the UC: NORMAL survey," *Inflammatory Bowel Diseases*, vol. 15, no. 4, pp. 581–588, 2009.

[11] S. Ghosh, "Inflammatory bowel disease: appreciating disability and impact of disease," *Canadian Journal of Gastroenterology and Hepatology*, vol. 29, article 66, no. 2, 2015.

[12] "Toward a common language for Functioning, disability and health. ICF," World Health Organization, Geneva, Switzerland 2002 http://www.worldenablenet/escapstats/icfcommon.htm.

[13] C. Gower-Rousseau, H. Sarter, G. Savoye et al., "Validation of the inflammatory bowel disease Disability Index in a population-based cohort," *Gut*, vol. 66, no. 4, pp. 588–596, 2017.

[14] P. B. Allen, M. A. Kamm, L. Peyrin-Biroulet et al., "Development and validation of a patient-reported disability measurement tool for patients with inflammatory bowel disease," *Alimentary Pharmacology & Therapeutics*, vol. 37, no. 4, pp. 438–444, 2013.

[15] T. B. Üstün, N. Kostanjsek, S. Chatterji et al., "Measuring Health and disability: Manual for Disability Assessment Schedule (WHODAS 2.0) World Health Organization," http://www.who.int/classifications/icf/whodasii/en/.

[16] E. Israeli, LA. Graff, I. Clara et al., "Low prevalence of disability among patients with inflammatory bowel diseases a decade after diagnosis," *Clinical Gastroenterology and Hepatology*, vol. 12, no. 8, pp. 1330–1337, 2014.

[17] "Inflammatory bowel disease. World Gastroenterology Organisation Global Guidelines," http://www.worldgastroenterology.org/UserFiles/file/guidelines/inflammatory-bowel-disease-english-2015.pdf.

[18] R. F. Harvey and J. M. Bradshaw, "A simple index of Crohn's-disease activity," *The Lancet*, vol. 1, article 514, no. 8167, 1980.

[19] R. S. Walmsley, R. C. S. Ayres, R. E. Pounder, and R. N. Allan, "A simple clinical colitis activity index," *Gut*, vol. 43, no. 1, pp. 29–32, 1998.

[20] A. G. Pallis, I. G. Vlachonikolis, and I. A. Mouzas, "Quality of life of Greek patients with inflammatory bowel disease. Validation of the Greek translation of the Inflammatory Bowel Disease Questionnaire," *Digestion*, vol. 63, no. 4, pp. 240–246, 2001.

[21] C. J. Hawkey, M. Allez, M. M. Clark et al., "Autologous hematopoetic stem cell transplantation for refractory Crohn disease a randomized clinical trial," *JAMA*, vol. 314, no. 23, pp. 2524–2534, 2015.

[22] M. Tsoukka, E. Jelastopulu, G. Lavranos et al., "Estimation of quality of life in Cypriot patients with inflammatory bowel disease," *World Journal of Gastroenterology*, vol. 23, no. 1, pp. 121–126, 2017.

[23] A.-C. Lesage, H. Hagège, G. Tucat, and J.-P. Gendre, "Results of a national survey on quality of life in inflammatory bowel diseases," *Clinics and Research in Hepatology and Gastroenterology*, vol. 35, no. 2, pp. 117–124, 2011.

[24] K. R. Muller, R. Prosser, P. Bampton, R. Mountifield, and J. M. Andrews, "Female gender and surgery impair relationships, body image, and sexuality in inflammatory bowel disease: patient perceptions," *Inflammatory Bowel Diseases*, vol. 16, no. 4, pp. 657–663, 2010.

[25] H. M. Becker, D. Grigat, S. Ghosh et al., "Living with inflammatory bowel disease: a Crohn's and Colitis Canada survey," *Canadian Journal of Gastroenterology and Hepatology*, vol. 29, no. 2, pp. 77–84, 2015.

[26] N. Viazis, G. Mantzaris, K. Karmiris et al., "Inflammatory bowel disease: Greek patients' perspective on quality of life, information on the disease, work productivity and family support," *Annals of Gastroenterology*, vol. 26, no. 1, pp. 52–58, 2013.

[27] P. Hendy, Y. Inspector, and A. Hart, "Standard medical care, side effects and compliance," in *Psychological Aspects of Inflammatory Bowel Disease: a Biopsychosocial Approach*, pp. 110-111, Routledge. Taylor and Francis Group, 2015.

[28] E. Rosenblatt and S. Kane, "Sex-specific issues in inflammatory bowel disease," *Gastroenterology & Hepatology*, vol. 11, no. 9, pp. 592–601, 2015.

[29] T. Longobardi, P. Jacobs, and C. N. Bernstein, "Work losses related to Inflammatory bowel disease in the United States Folder: results from the National Health interview survey," *The American Journal of Gastroenterology*, vol. 98, pp. 1064–1072, 2003.

[30] M. K. Vester-Andersen, M. V. Prosberg, I. Vind, M. Andersson, T. Jess, and F. Bendtsen, "Low risk of unemployment, sick leave, and work disability among patients with inflammatory bowel disease: a 7-year follow-up study of a danish inception cohort," *Inflammatory Bowel Diseases*, vol. 21, no. 10, pp. 2296–2303, 2015.

[31] B. G. Feagan, M. Bala, S. Yan, A. Olson, and S. Hanauer, "Unemployment and disability in patients with moderately to severely active Crohn's disease," *Journal of Clinical Gastroenterology*, vol. 39, no. 5, pp. 390–395, 2005.

[32] A. G. E. M. De Boer, F. B. Evertsz, P. C. Stokkers et al., "Employment status, difficulties at work and quality of life in inflammatory bowel disease patients," *European Journal of

Gastroenterology and Hepatology, vol. 28, no. 10, pp. 1130–1136, 2016.

[33] M. D. Mandel, A. Bálint, Lovász B. D. et al., "Work disability and productivity loss in patients with inflammatory bowel diseases in Hungary in the era of biologics," *European Journal of Health Economics*, vol. 15, no. Suppl 1, S129 pages, 2014.

[34] K. Argyriou, A. Kapsoritakis, and S. Potamianos, "PTU-098 high levels of emotional and physical distress among family caregivers of individuals with Inflammatory Bowel Disease (IBD)," *Gut*, vol. 63, supplement 1, article A82, 2014.

[35] J. Devlen, K. Beusterien, L. Yen, A. Ahmed, A. S. Cheifetz, and A. C. Moss, "The burden of inflammatory bowel disease: a patient-reported qualitative analysis and development of a conceptual model," *Inflammatory Bowel Diseases*, vol. 20, no. 3, pp. 545–552, 2014.

[36] J. B. Soares, R. Pereira, J. M. Costa et al., "The inflammatory bowel disease-disability index: validation of the Portuguese version according to the COSMIN checklist," *European Journal of Gastroenterology & Hepatology*, vol. 28, no. 10, pp. 1151–1160, Oct 2016.

[37] M. van der Have, H. H. Fidder, M. Leenders et al., "Self-reported disability in patients with inflammatory bowel disease largely determined by disease activity and illness perceptions," *Inflammatory Bowel Diseases*, vol. 21, no. 2, pp. 369–377, 2015.

17

The Effect of Anesthesia on the Immune System in Colorectal Cancer Patients

Yangjie Dang,[1] Xingxing Shi,[1] William Xu,[2] and Mingzhang Zuo[3]

[1]Department of Anesthesiology, Xi'an Children's Hospital, Xi'an, Shaanxi 710032, China
[2]Department of Anesthesiology, Carver College of Medicine, University of Iowa, Iowa City, IA 52246, USA
[3]Department of Anesthesiology, Beijing Hospital, National Center of Gerontology, No. 1 Dahua Road, Dongdan, Beijing 100730, China

Correspondence should be addressed to William Xu; William-xu@uiowa.edu and Mingzhang Zuo; zuomz@163.com

Academic Editor: Yixin E. Yang

Colorectal cancer (CRC) is the key leading cause of high morbidity and mortality worldwide. Surgical excision is the most effective treatment for CRC. However, stress caused by surgery response can destroy the body's immunity and increase the likelihood of cancer dissemination and metastasis. Anesthesia is an effective way to control the stress response, and recent basic and clinical research has shown that anesthesia and related drugs can directly or indirectly affect the immune system of colorectal cancer patients during the perioperative period. Thus, these drugs may affect the prognosis of CRC surgery patients. This review is intended to summarize currently available data regarding the effects of anesthetics and related drugs on perioperative immune function and postoperative recurrence and metastasis in CRC patients. Determining the most suitable anesthesia for patients with CRC is of utmost importance.

1. Introduction

Colorectal cancer (CRC) is the third leading cause of death from cancer worldwide, accounting for approximately 135,430 new cases and 50,260 deaths in the United States in 2017 [1]. The interactions of the colon epithelium microbiome are considered to be important for the formation of colon cancer, and *Enterococcus faecalis* is thought to play an important role in the pathogenesis of CRC [2].

Anesthesia and related drugs can directly or indirectly affect the immune system of patients during the perioperative period and thus affect treatment and prognosis of CRC patients as surgery is currently the most effective treatment for CRC. The 2009 European Society of Anesthesiology (ESA) presented the new concept of "anticancer anesthesia technology" with the intention of identifying the most suitable anesthesia for patients with cancer. Exploring the effects of various anesthetic methods and their related drugs on the immune system of CDC patients continues to be of great significance.

2. Colorectal Cancer and Its Immunological Bases

Tumor generation requires the provision of nutrition in the surrounding microenvironment. Tumors grow and invade and infiltrate surrounding tissues and organs. The tumor microenvironment includes a large number of cells, including immune cells, endothelial cells, and interstitial cells, all of which are involved in the occurrence and development of tumors. Studies have shown that the immunological infiltration of CRC may be clinically related to those cells.

Immune response in the process of tumor development is not just a single factor, but it plays a multifaceted role affecting tumor initiation, growth, progression, and other processes. The immune system regulates and promotes cancer programs, a process known as "immunoediting." There are three phases to this process: elimination, balance, and escape [3].

Although experimental evidence shows that inflammation can also promote the occurrence and development of tumors [2], the immune inflammatory response in colon carcinogenesis requires further study and is still under debate [4]. Some clinical data show that the immune response inhibits the tumor. However, other investigators have concluded that the opposite is true.

2.1. Immune Cells in Colorectal Cancer. Different immune cells play differing roles in the process of cancer: some cells affect its pathogenesis while others contribute to its recurrence.

Macrophages. Macrophages in CRC will appear as infiltration. Known as tumor-infiltrating macrophages, they are important contributors to tumors infiltrating the surrounding tissue. They are derived from peripheral blood mononuclear cells. According to the different functions and characteristics of tumor-infiltrating macrophages, they can be divided into two different subtypes: M1 and M2 [5]. Some cytokines, such as LPS and TNF-α, promote the conversion of classic activated macrophages to the M1 type. The remaining types are classified as M2. M1 is involved in the TH1-type immune response that can kill foreign pathogens and endogenous tumor cells. Glucocorticoids and IL-10 can induce the transformation of tumor-infiltrating macrophages to M2, which mainly causes TH2-type immune response and promotes the occurrence and development of tumors. Both types are involved in the immune response of colon cancer and can be transformed into each other under certain circumstances.

In short, both M1 and M2 participate in the occurrence and outcome of the tumor, and the conversion between the two determines the outcome and prognosis of tumors [6, 7]. Some studies have shown that macrophage infiltration in CRC seems to prefigure a better prognosis [8], since macrophage infiltration may be an important means of fighting against cancer via the regulation of endogenous mechanisms.

NK Cells. Natural killer (NK) cells are immune cells that maintain the defense function of the body. They are involved in antitumor and antiviral infection and immune regulation processes. Both murine [9, 10] and human [11, 12] models have shown that NK cells contribute to preventing tumor and controlling the effects of tumor growth and dissemination. In CRC, it has been reported that extensive infiltration of NK cells in a wide range of tumors can give rise to a better prognosis [13]. Although these studies suggest that NK cells play a beneficial role in tumor control, their specific mechanism of action remains unclear [14]. Therefore, as an important effector cell in innate immunity, NK cells have significant antitumor function and have the potential for positive applications and clinical significance in tumor immunotherapy.

T-Regulatory Cells (Tregs). Tregs, CD25 + regulatory T-cells, can not only prevent human autoimmune diseases, but also help protect against microbial infection and protect the fetus. There are indications that Tregs can indeed prevent human autoimmune diseases [15]. On the one hand, Tregs may control excessive immune response, but on the other hand, such control may also weaken the immune system's effectiveness in eliminating invaders. The most direct application for Tregs is in treating autoimmune diseases by increasing their activity. In addition, reducing the number of Tregs can also reduce tumor-associated immune responses. There is evidence that immune cells constantly monitor the molecular abnormalities that occur when cells become cancerous. To some extent, Tregs interfere with this monitoring and may help to root and grow malignant tumors [16]. On the basis of these studies, it was also found that tumor-associated T-cell-related immune responses are detected in tumor patients [17, 18]. Numerous studies have shown that T-cells infiltrate tumor tissue in patients who are less immunosuppressed. This is considered to be a good prognostic marker [19, 20]. Therefore, modulating the immune response of tumor patients can be an important way to improve the prognosis of patients, but further studies are needed.

2.2. Immune System and Colorectal Cancer. The innate immune response is a nonspecific immune defense already available at birth. This inherent immune response has a wide range of effects, including speed, efficiency, and stability. Innate immunity provides a nonselective rejection to a foreign body's entry into the body of antigens, a protective clearance function. The innate immune system is activated through the recognition of pathogen-associated molecular patterns (PAMPs) by pattern recognition receptors (PRRs) which, in turn, produce a series of cytokines such as interleukins (ILs) and tumor necrosis factor (TNF). The innate immune response initiated by PRRs is important in the shaping of tumor immune microenvironment and tumorigenesis. PRRs are widely expressed in various innate immune cells of the host, such as dendritic cells and mononuclear macrophage NK cells, after which a series of immune responses are initiated. Among various PRRs, Toll-like receptors (TLRs) have attracted much attention and are involved in tumorigenesis through the recognition of the inflammation caused by PAMP. Among these receptors, the inflammasomes formed by the involvement of Nod-like receptors (NLRs) have also received much recent attention, as they have been shown to regulate the immune response and thus to inhibit tumorigenesis [21, 22].

Rakoff-Nahoum et al. [23] studied the dextran sulfate sodium- (DSS-) induced susceptibility to colitis and receptor-interacting protein 2 (RIP2) in TLR4, TLR2, and myeloid differentiation factor (MyD88) knockout mice in 2004. Compared with wild-type (WT) mice, they demonstrated that the MyD88-dependent axis is beneficial. MyD88 is a key linker molecule in the TLR-signaling pathway and plays an important role in the transmission of upstream information and disease development. It is therefore an important mediator of many molecular cascade reactions.

In addition, interleukin-17 (IL-17) is an early promoter of T-cell-induced inflammatory responses and can amplify the inflammatory response by promoting the release of proinflammatory cytokines. The main effector of T-helper interleukin-17-producing cells (Th17 cells) is IL-17. Th17 cells are capable of secreting IL-6 and tumor necrosis factor-α (TNF-α), among others. Subsequently, one study [24] has demonstrated that IL-17 plays a role in the initiation of tumors in IL-17 knockout mice.

At present, the main treatment for CRC is surgery. Therefore, anesthetic management plays a vital role in the prognosis of CRC in the perioperative period.

3. The Effect of Anesthesia on the Immune System in Colorectal Cancer Patients

The immune system mainly includes two subsystems: non-specific immunity and specific immunity. The effect of anesthesia on the immunization of colorectal cancer patients mainly includes the following. (1) Anesthesia affects the number and activity of immune cells: presently, the effects of anesthesia on immunity have been studied on NK cells, B-lymphocytes, T-lymphocytes, macrophages, leukocytes, and erythrocytes. These cells are involved in both nonspecific and specific immune functions. (2) Anesthesia affects the secretion of cytokines. Proinflammatory factors mainly include tumor necrosis factor-a (TNF-α), IL-1, IL-6, and IL-8. The anti-inflammatory factors mainly include IL-10. The levels of interferon-7 (IFN-7), interferon (IFN), TNF-α, and soluble interleukin-2 receptor (sIL-2R) are increased by general anesthesia. (3) Anesthesia affects the biological behavior of tumor cells. The proliferation, migration, and apoptosis are important biological characteristics of tumor cells, which are closely related to tumor growth and metastasis.

3.1. The Effect of Different Anesthesia Methods on Immunization in Colorectal Cancer Patients. A number of scholars have found that, compared to simple general anesthesia, general anesthesia combined with epidural anesthesia or simple spinal anesthesia can reduce the postoperative immunosuppression to varying degrees [25]. Studies on the effects of different anesthesia methods on the long-term survival rate of patients after colon cancer resection suggested that the combined application of epidurals can improve the survival rate of patients without metastasis to 1.46 years postoperatively, but there was no significant difference between the two groups for patients with metastasized tumors [26]. These studies have shown that, compared to general anesthesia, epidural anesthesia, paravertebral block, and other types of regional anesthesia can reduce the inhibition of immune function and improve the prognosis of patients with cancer.

Surgery can cause sympathetic adrenal medulla and hypothalamus-pituitary-adrenal cortical axis excitement based stress response by a variety of factors (pain, blood loss, low temperature, and psychological factors). Many factors produced in the stress response, such as glucocorticoids, catecholamines, and prostaglandin E2 (PGE2), can have an adverse effect on immune function, resulting in immune function inhibition in the perioperative period. Studies have shown that the inhibition of immune function by stress response is caused by inhibition of natural killer cell (NK cell) function. These cells are nonspecific components of cellular immunity. Their effect is not tumor-specific and the major histocompatibility antigen system (MHC) restriction plays an important role in early antitumor immunity. The effect of the stress response on the duration of NK cell activity inhibition is similar to the period of enhanced tumor metastasis [27]. The effect of the stress response on tumor metastasis is achieved by inhibiting the activity of NK cells. Epidural anesthesia can block the pain-conduction pathways, non-pain-conduction pathways, and sympathetic nerve fibers by blocking the spinal nerve root. However, opioid drugs commonly used in general anesthesia only block the pain-conduction pathway [28], indicating that epidural anesthesia can preserve NK cell function. Compared to general anesthesia, epidural anesthesia can better prevent nociceptive irritation transmission to the central nervous system and reduce the body's stress response, which may be beneficial for the prognosis of patients with cancer.

CD4+ T-cells first differentiate into T-helper 0 (TH0) cells after antigen stimulation and continue to differentiate into TH1 or TH2 cells. TH1 or TH2 subgroups secrete different cytokines: TH1 cells mainly secrete interferon-1 (IFN-1), which promotes cellular immunity, while TH2 cells secrete interleukin-4 (IL-4) and are associated with humoral immunity. These cytokines can also promote their own growth and inhibit the growth of other subpopulations. The proportion of IFN-γ IL-4 *in vivo* determines the ratio of TH1/TH2 which, in turn, determines the dominant *in vivo* immune response. Cellular immunity is important in controlling the immune response of the tumor, and thus a reduced TH1/TH2 ratio should be avoided in order to maintain the cell's immune response. Epidural anesthesia, compared to general anesthesia, is able to better preserve the TH1/TH2 ratio and thus can better preserve cellular immune function. Mrakovcic-Sutic et al. found that, in rectal cancer patients with postoperative analgesia, there was a lower inhibitory effect on NK cells than in patients in an intravenous analgesia group [29]. Animal experiments suggested that epidural anesthesia can increase the survival rate of colorectal cancer patients after surgery. The number of lymphocytes, NK cell activity, TH1/TH2 ratio, and tumor metastasis were significantly higher than those of general anesthesia group after spinal anesthesia, indicating that specific regional anesthesia could preserve the function of immune cells. Therefore, general anesthesia combined with epidural anesthesia or simple spinal anesthesia is better than simple general anesthesia in reducing surgery-related immune inhibition by reducing the stress response.

The protective mechanism of local anesthesia technology on immune function is not yet clear; however, there are three possible causes: (1) local anesthesia technology, by blocking the neurotransmitter incoming to the central nervous system, can significantly reduce the pain and surgical stress response; (2) the application of local anesthesia technology can reduce the dosage of opioids; and (3) general anesthesia combined with local anesthesia techniques can reduce the total use of general anesthetic drugs. Epidural anesthesia combined with general anesthesia can reduce the amount of general anesthetics and analgesics, and sustained epidural analgesia can also further reduce the use of opioids after surgery, which may be one of the reasons for reducing the immunosuppressive effects.

However, some scholars still believe that local anesthesia technology cannot protect the immune function and reduce tumor recurrence and metastasis. Gottschalk et al. analyzed the data of 669 colorectal cancer patients undergoing radical surgery and found that the application of epidural analgesia during the perioperative period and a reduced recurrence rate of tumor after surgery are not necessarily linked [30]. The meta-analysis of Conrick-Martin et al. suggests that there was no significant difference between general anesthesia and spinal anesthesia on NK cell function after surgery [31]. The existing clinical research sample size is small, and retrospective studies have inherent bias and other deficiencies. In the future, more multidimensional, prospective, randomized clinical studies will be needed to further explore the linkages and mechanisms between anesthetics and the prognosis of malignant tumors in order to provide safer anesthesia for patients with cancer. For future study, retrospective studies will also require forward-looking large samples.

3.2. The Impact of Anesthesia-Related Drugs on Immunization in Colorectal Cancer Patients

3.2.1. Intravenous Anesthetics. Intravenous anesthesia can maintain a safe, constant concentration of drug treatment during surgery and can reduce the stimulation of surgical trauma. Intravenous anesthesia can also reduce the intraoperative inflammatory response albeit affecting the patient's immune system function. Immune system disorders or inhibition during the perioperative period can cause postoperative complications, especially in cancer patients. Immunosuppression after surgery can accelerate the spread of residual cancer cells and promote a new transfer.

Common opinion is that propofol does not inhibit the immune function. Inada et al. [32] found that propofol produces an antitumor effect by inhibiting cyclooxygenase-2 (COX-2) and prostaglandin E2 (PGE2). Propofol is superior to inhaled anesthetics in postoperative immunoprotection. Propofol can increase the activity of NK cells, inhibit COX-2, prevent PGE2 generation, and protect the immune system function. It can also have a direct biological effect on the tumor. A series of cell culture experiments show that propofol at concentrations commonly used does not inhibit phytohemagglutinin- (PHA-) induced lymphocyte proliferation and does not significantly increase lymphocyte apoptosis. Propofol inhibits immune cells only at concentrations well above clinical concentrations [33–36].

Ketamine, thiophanate, and etomidate increase the chance of tumor retention and metastasis because of the reduced NK cell activity, reduced T-helper cells, and increased T-inhibiting cell viability. Ketamine inhibits NK cell activity due to the activation of alpha and beta adrenergic receptors [37].

Benzodiazepines are one of the most commonly used sedatives in intensive care patients [38]. Midazolam can inhibit the production of IL-2 and IL-8 to produce an immunosuppression effect [39]. Midazolam can inhibit the transcription activity of lipopolysaccharide-induced nuclear factor KB, the activity of TNF-α, the phosphorylation of p38 mitogen kinase, and the formation of peroxides, which can be blocked by peripheral benzodiazepine agonist PKII 195. Midazolam can inhibit neutrophil adhesion and tropism by inhibiting the level of IL-8, thereby reducing immune function [40]. Rapid administration of diazepam will produce a proinflammatory response and improve neutrophil function, but slow and sustained (60 days or longer) administration will inhibit the multinuclear leukocyte function and lead to immune response inhibition [41]. These results show that benzodiazepines have a significant inhibitory effect on innate immunity, but more research is needed on adaptive immunity.

The α2-agonists clonidine and dexmedetomidine can significantly increase tumor cell growth, but the α2-receptor antagonist yohimbine can reverse this effect [42].

3.2.2. Inhaled Anesthetics. Inhaled anesthetics include sevoflurane, halothane, isoflurane, and desflurane. The inhibitory effect of inhaled anesthetics on the immune function has been confirmed by many studies. Guptill et al. found that intravenous anesthesia with propofol and remifentanil is less immunosuppressive than inhaled anesthesia [43]. Inhaled anesthetics have greater immune cell inhibition than intravenous anesthetic drugs. Inhaled anesthetics can produce higher levels of plasma catecholamines and glucocorticoids to inhibit the release of IFN of NK cells in animal models and reduce the number of NK cells, the production of Th cytokines, and the expression of $Foxp_3$ mRNA in the human body [44].

Some studies have shown that halothane inhibits NK cell activity in a dose-dependent manner. *In vitro* experiments show that an increase in halothane concentration is accompanied with a significant reduction of NK cell activity. With an increase in halothane concentration, NK cell activity was significantly reduced in *in vitro* experiments [45].

Other studies have reported that sevoflurane can reduce the invasive ability of colorectal cancer [46].

Fleischmann et al. conducted a follow-up study with 204 colorectal cancer surgery patients and found that the use of nitrous oxide (N_2O) anesthesia does not increase the risk of recurrence of postoperative rectal cancer. However, the mechanism by which inhaled anesthetics affect the immune system remains unknown [47].

3.2.3. Opioid Analgesics. Acute pain is the main cause of the activation of the hypothalamic-pituitary-adrenal axis (HPA axis), the activation of which can cause immunosuppression, decreased NK cell activity, and Th cell imbalance. Opioid is the main analgesic in anesthesia, and now the study found that opioids and tumors have a complex association. The mechanism is unknown and even, to some extent, contradictory.

Opioid itself can directly affect the proliferation, apoptosis, and survival of normal cells and tumor cells. Opioid analgesics have the effect of inhibiting cell and humoral immunity. In isolated experiments, morphine, a commonly used opioid, can inhibit the formation of peroxides and the expression of cytokines. Morphine has also been found to inhibit the function of macrophages and NK cell activity [48].

Morphine regulates tumor cell invasion throughout adhesion, extracellular matrix degradation, and cell migration. An opioid represented by morphine can regulate angiogenesis, promote endothelial cell proliferation and migration, promote angiogenesis, increase vascular permeability, and promote the proliferation of tumor cells in the blood vessels [49].

Another commonly used opioid, fentanyl, exhibited dose-dependent cytotoxicity against NK cells. Forget et al. found that fentanyl was able to inhibit the activity of NK cells in mice [48]. The effect of different doses of fentanyl on human immune function was observed. It was found that the activity of NK cells was reduced in patients with both low and high doses of fentanyl at 24 hours after operation. However, the activity of NK cells in the low-dose group returned to the preoperative level after 48 hours, while NK cell activity in the high-dose group remained low, indicating that the inhibitory effect of fentanyl on NK cells was time- and dose-dependent [49]. However, some studies have suggested that opioids can enhance the immune function by enhancing NK cell activity and the T-cell-mediated immune response. One possible mechanism involves morphine, which can activate the μ receptor and inhibit the release of NF-KB and NO [50, 51].

Sufentanil is a potent opioid analgesic, but it is unclear if it negatively affects the immune function.

Tramadol is a class of weak opioid receptor agonists that play an important role in the current clinical "multimodal analgesia" concept. They exhibit protective effects on cellular immunity in some studies.

3.2.4. Nonsteroidal Anti-Inflammatory Analgesics. Acute and chronic inflammation significantly increases the expression of cyclooxygenase (COX), causing increased prostaglandins, pain, and tumor metastasis rate. Nonsteroidal anti-inflammatory drugs (NSAIDs) have antipyretic, analgesic, anti-inflammatory, and antirheumatic effects. They work by reducing the biosynthesis of prostaglandin (PG) in the local tissue by inhibiting the activity of COX *in vivo*. Because of the strong analgesic effect of nonsteroidal anti-inflammatory drugs, researchers have been concerned in recent years about whether NSAIDs provide immune protection during the perioperative period and about whether or not they relieve the recurrence of tumor metastasis. NSAIDs can improve the immune function of patients and inhibit the recurrence of tumor metastasis. It has been suggested that NSAIDs can be used to reduce pain, reduce opioid dosage, and balance side effects of opioids in patients with radical neoplasm surgery. Animal models suggest that COX inhibitors can prevent tumor growth and metastasis by inhibiting apoptosis and reducing angiogenetic factors and tumor microvessel density. Epidemiological studies have shown that prolonged use of COX inhibitors can reduce the risk of cancer. The use of selective COX inhibitor celecoxib daily can reduce the risk of colorectal cancer by 69% [52]. While encouraging, this conclusion requires further study. In addition to inhibiting the synthesis of PG, NSAIDs also inhibit the release of bradykinin during inflammation, alter lymphocyte responses, and reduce the migration and phagocytosis of granulocytes and monocytes to regulate the immune response [53]. NSAIDs can inhibit the immunosuppression caused by trauma, pain, anesthesia, opioid use, surgery, and so forth to varying degrees [54–56].

We could use COX inhibitors to inhibit PG synthesis in order to slow down tumor progression. Anesthesia and analgesia are associated with the entire perioperative period, although they cannot resolve the issues of tumor spread and tumor residue. However, reducing NK cell activity inhibition and maintaining Th cell balance can improve the immunosuppression caused by surgical stress induced by some anesthesia intervention.

3.2.5. β-Receptor Blockers. The use of beta-blockers can reduce the risk of tumor metastasis by inhibiting the release of catecholamines and the activity of signal transducer and activator of transcription-3 (STAT-3), resulting in reduced NK cell activity inhibition and angiogenesis [57].

3.2.6. Local Anesthetics. Most studies suggest that local anesthetics have antitumor effects and are suitable for anesthesia in patients with cancer. Martinsson found that the clinical concentration of ropivacaine can inhibit colon cancer cell proliferation in dose-dependent *in vitro* experiments [58]. Lucchinetti et al. found that bupivacaine can inhibit mesenchymal stem cell proliferation and negatively regulate tumor formation, metastasis, and cell differentiation [59].

3.3. The Effects of Other Anesthesia Interventions

3.3.1. Heat Preservation. As a stress response, hypothermia activates the sympathetic system and increases glucocorticoid release. A mild temperature (35.5°C) has some effect on cellular immunity, but a moderately low temperature (30°C) will directly inhibit NK cell activity and reduce resistance to tumor metastasis [60]. Therefore, the use of a warm blanket, hot air, infusion of liquid heating, and other measures ensures that patients maintain the appropriate body temperature perioperatively, which can offer protection for the immune function in cancer patients after surgery.

3.3.2. Blood Transfusion. While blood transfusion is an important tool for anesthesiologists during and after operation, perioperative blood use may influence cancer recurrence depending on the patient's nutritional health, anemic status, tumor type, stage and degree of resectability, blood loss, anesthesia type, stress level, and postoperative complications [61–67]. It has been reported that perioperative blood product transfusions, including packed red blood cells, platelets, and fresh frozen plasma, are linked to an increased risk of cancer recurrence in CRC patients [68–72]. Strict control of transfusions should be suggested to avoid unnecessary and excessive blood transfusion.

3.3.3. Mood. Anxiety in patients with cancer is associated with postoperative immunosuppressive levels, and the anesthesiologist can help to relieve the patient's anxiety about surgery and disease by preoperative conversation and medication [73].

Additional Points

Summary. Perioperative factors such as surgical trauma, volatile anesthetics, opioid use, physiological stress, hyperglycemia, hypothermia, blood products transfusion, and mood can cause a significant TH1/TH2 imbalance between the antitumor and protumor environments in the human body and can have a profound effect on the initiation and progression of colon carcinogenesis, colon cancer metastasis, recurrence, response to standard antitumor therapy, and the final clinical outcome. In brief, regional anesthesia is significantly better than general anesthesia in the immune index and in later tumor recurrence and metastasis. General anesthesia combined with regional anesthesia is better than single-use general anesthesia. Most inhaled anesthetics, opioids, local anesthetics, and other intravenous anesthetics can reduce immunity to a certain extent, which sometimes leads to an increased recurrence of malignant tumors. However, tramadol, selective nonsteroidal anti-inflammatory analgesics, and propofol have protective effects on the immune function of the body and can reduce the recurrence and metastasis of the tumor. Therefore, it is important to make a careful anesthesia plan and to select appropriate narcotic drugs for patients with malignant tumors, since these decisions will have a crucial impact on the therapeutic effect and prognosis. In addition, red blood cells, platelets, and FFP transfusion during the perioperative period also directly cause immunosuppression and increase the risk of cancer recurrence in colorectal patients. Hypothermia, hyperglycemia, and even a patient's mood contribute to changes in immunity and clinical outcomes in colorectal cancer perioperatively. Existing clinical research sample sizes are small, and retrospective studies have inherent bias and other deficiencies. In the future, more basic research and large-scale, prospective, randomized clinical studies will be needed to further explore the linkage and mechanisms between anesthetic factors and the prognosis of malignant tumors to provide safer anesthesia for cancer patients.

Disclosure

Yangjie Dang and Xingxing Shi are first authors.

Authors' Contributions

All the authors have sufficiently contributed to this work to merit authorship.

Acknowledgments

This work was supported by the National Natural Science Foundation of China (no. 81774415).

References

[1] R. L. Siegel, K. D. Miller, and A. Jemal, "Cancer statistics," *A Cancer Journal for Clinicians*, vol. 67, no. 1, pp. 7–30, 2017.

[2] M. Jinushi, "Yin and yang of tumor inflammation: how innate immune suppressors shape the tumor microenvironments," *International Journal of Cancer*, vol. 135, no. 6, pp. 1277–1285, 2014.

[3] G. P. Dunn, L. J. Old, and R. D. Schreiber, "The three Es of cancer immunoediting," *Annual Review of Immunology*, vol. 22, pp. 329–360, 2004.

[4] V. Shankaran et al., "IFNgamma and lymphocytes prevent primary tumour development and shape tumour immunogenicity," *Nature*, vol. 410, article 1107, 2001.

[5] S. K. Biswas and A. Mantovani, "Macrophage plasticity and interaction with lymphocyte subsets: cancer as a paradigm," *Nature Immunology*, vol. 11, article 889, 2010.

[6] A. Mantovani and M. Locati, "Tumor-associated macrophages as a paradigm of macrophage plasticity, diversity, and polarization: lessons and open questions," *Arteriosclerosis, Thrombosis, and Vascular Biology*, vol. 33, article 1478, 2013.

[7] P. Allavena, A. Sica, C. Garlanda, and A. Mantovani, "The Yin-Yang of tumor-associated macrophages in neoplastic progression and immune surveillance," *Immunological Reviews*, vol. 222, no. 1, pp. 155–161, 2008.

[8] S. Edin, M. L. Wikberg, J. Rutegard, P. A. Oldenborg, and R. Palmqvist, "Phenotypic skewing of macrophages in vitro by secreted factors from colorectal cancer cells," *PLOS ONE*, vol. 8, Article ID e74982, 2013.

[9] S. Kim, K. Iizuka, H. L. Aguila, I. L. Weissman, and W. M. Yokoyama, "In vivo natural killer cell activities revealed by natural killer cell-deficient mice," *Proceedings of the National Acadamy of Sciences of the United States of America*, vol. 97, article 2731, 2000.

[10] M. J. Smyth, Y. Hayakawa, K. Takeda, and H. Yagita, "New aspects of natural-killer-cell surveillance and therapy of cancer," *Nature Reviews Cancer*, vol. 2, no. 11, pp. 850–861, 2002.

[11] K.-J. Malmberg, Y. T. Bryceson, M. Carlsten et al., "NK cell-mediated targeting of human cancer and possibilities for new means of immunotherapy," *Cancer Immunology, Immunotherapy*, vol. 57, no. 10, pp. 1541–1552, 2008.

[12] E. Carbone, P. Neri, M. Mesuraca et al., "HLA class I, NKG2D, and natural cytotoxicity receptors regulate multiple myeloma cell recognition by natural killer cells," *Blood*, vol. 105, no. 1, pp. 251–258, 2005.

[13] S. Coca, J. Perez-Piqueras, D. Martinez et al., "The prognostic significance of intratumoral natural killer cells in patients with colorectal carcinoma," *Cancer*, vol. 79, no. 12, pp. 2320–2328, 1997.

[14] M. H. Sandel, F. M. Speetjens, A. G. Menon et al., "Natural killer cells infiltrating colorectal cancer and MHC class I expression," *Molecular Immunology*, vol. 42, no. 4, pp. 541–546, 2005.

[15] E. Lazaro et al., "Large granular lymphocyte leukemia: clinical and pathogenic aspects," *La Revue de Médecine Interne*, vol. 34, article 553, 2013.

[16] S. L. Clarke, G. J. Betts, A. Plant et al., "CD4+CD25+FOXP3+ regulatory T cells suppress anti-tumor immune responses in patients with colorectal cancer," *PLoS ONE*, vol. 1, no. 1, article e129, 2006.

[17] D. Nagorsen, U. Keilholz, L. Rivoltini et al., "Natural T-cell response against MHC class I epitopes of epithelial cell adhesion molecule, her-2/neu, and carcinoembryonic antigen in patients with colorectal cancer," *Cancer Research*, vol. 60, no. 17, pp. 4850–4854, 2000.

[18] G. Campi, M. Crosti, G. Consogno et al., "CD4+ T cells from healthy subjects and colon cancer patients recognize a carcinoembryonic antigen-specific immunodominant epitope," *Cancer Research*, vol. 63, no. 23, pp. 8481–8486, 2003.

[19] J. Galon, A. Costes, F. Sanchez-Cabo et al., "Type, density, and location of immune cells within human colorectal tumors predict clinical outcome," *Science*, vol. 313, no. 5795, pp. 1960–1964, 2006.

[20] F. A. Sinicrope, R. L. Rego, S. M. Ansell, K. L. Knutson, N. R. Foster, and D. J. Sargent, "Intraepithelial effector (CD3+)/regulatory (FoxP3+) T-cell ratio predicts a clinical outcome of human colon carcinoma," *Gastroenterology*, vol. 137, no. 4, pp. 1270–1279, 2009.

[21] M. Fukata and M. Arditi, "The role of pattern recognition receptors in intestinal inflammation," *Mucosal Immunology*, vol. 6, no. 3, pp. 451–463, 2013.

[22] E. M. Creagh and L. A. J. O'Neill, "TLRs, NLRs and RLRs: a trinity of pathogen sensors that co-operate in innate immunity," *Trends in Immunology*, vol. 27, no. 8, pp. 352–357, 2006.

[23] S. Rakoff-Nahoum, J. Paglino, F. Eslami-Varzaneh, S. Edberg, and R. Medzhitov, "Recognition of commensal microflora by toll-like receptors is required for intestinal homeostasis," *Cell*, vol. 118, no. 2, pp. 229–241, 2004.

[24] Y. S. Hyun, D. S. Han, A. R. Lee, C. S. Eun, J. Youn, and H.-Y. Kim, "Role of IL-17A in the development of colitis-associated cancer," *Carcinogenesis*, vol. 33, no. 4, pp. 931–936, 2012.

[25] G. Zenonos and J. E. Kim, "A T cell-orchestrated immune response in the adult dorsal spinal cord as a cause of neuropathic pain-like hypersensitivity after peripheral nerve damage: A door to novel therapies?" *Neurosurgery*, vol. 66, no. 4, pp. N24–N25, 2010.

[26] R. Christopherson, K. E. James, M. Tableman, P. Marshall, and F. E. Johnson, "Long-term survival after colon cancer surgery: a variation associated with choice of anesthesia," *Anesthesia and Analgesia*, vol. 107, article 325, 2008.

[27] S. Ben-Eliyahu, G. G. Page, R. Yirmiya, and G. Shakhar, "Evidence that stress and surgical interventions promote tumor development by suppressing natural killer cell activity," *International Journal of Cancer*, vol. 80, no. 6, pp. 880–888, 1999.

[28] S. Liu, R. L. Carpenter, and J. M. Neal, "Epidural anesthesia and analgesia: their role in postoperative outcome," *Anesthesiology*, vol. 82, no. 6, pp. 1474–1506, 1995.

[29] I. Mrakovcic-Sutic, D. Bacic, S. Golubovic, R. Bacic, and M. Marinovic, "Cross-talk between NKT and regulatory T cells (Tregs) in modulation of immune response in patients with colorectal cancer following different pain management techniques," *Collegium Antropologicum*, vol. 35, supplement 2, p. 57, 2011.

[30] A. Gottschalk, J. G. Ford, C. C. Regelin et al., "Association between epidural analgesia and cancer recurrence after colorectal cancer surgery," *Anesthesiology*, vol. 113, no. 1, pp. 27–34, 2010.

[31] I. Conrick-Martin, M. R. Kell, and D. J. Buggy, "Meta-analysis of the effect of central neuraxial regional anesthesia compared with general anesthesia on postoperative natural killer T lymphocyte function," *Journal of Clinical Anesthesia*, vol. 24, no. 1, pp. 3–7, 2012.

[32] T. Inada, Y. Yamanouchi, S. Jomura et al., "Effect of propofol and isoflurane anaesthesia on the immune response to surgery," *Anaesthesia*, vol. 59, no. 10, pp. 954–959, 2004.

[33] E. G. Devlin, R. S. Clarke, R. K. Mirakhur, and T. A. McNeill, "Effect of four i.v. induction agents on T-lymphocyte proliferations to PHA in vitro," *British Journal of Anaesthesia*, vol. 73, p. 315, 1994.

[34] C. E. Schneemilch, T. Hachenberg, S. Ansorge, A. Ittenson, and U. Bank, "Effects of different anaesthetic agents on immune cell function in vitro," *European Journal of Anaesthesiology*, vol. 22, no. 8, pp. 616–623, 2005.

[35] H. K. Song and D. C. Jeong, "The effect of propofol on cytotoxicity and apoptosis of lipopolysaccharide-treated mononuclear cells and lymphocytes," *Anesthesia and Analgesia*, vol. 98, article 1724, 2004.

[36] K.-C. Wu, S.-T. Yang, T.-C. Hsia et al., "Suppression of cell invasion and migration by propofol are involved in down-regulating matrix metalloproteinase-2 and p38 MAPK signaling in A549 human lung adenocarcinoma epithelial cells," *Anticancer Reseach*, vol. 32, no. 11, pp. 4833–4842, 2012.

[37] R. Melamed, S. Bar-Yosef, G. Shakhar, K. Shakhar, and S. Ben-Eliyahu, "Suppression of natural killer cell activity and promotion of tumor metastasis by ketamine, thiopental, and halothane, but not by propofol: mediating mechanisms and prophylactic measures," *Anesthesia & Analgesia*, vol. 97, no. 5, pp. 1331–1339, 2003.

[38] J. Barr and A. Donner, "Optimal intravenous dosing strategies for sedatives and analgesics in the intensive care unit," *Critical Care Clinics*, vol. 11, no. 4, pp. 827–847, 1995.

[39] H. F. Galley, A. M. Dubbels, and N. R. Webster, "The effect of midazolam and propofol on interleukin-8 from human polymorphonuclear leukocytes," *Anesthesia & Analgesia*, vol. 86, no. 6, pp. 1289–1293, 1998.

[40] H. B. Lu, Y. P. Jia, Z. H. Liang, R. Zhou, and J. Q. Zheng, "Effect of continuous infusion of midazolam on immune function in pediatric patients after surgery," *Genetics and Molecular Research*, vol. 14, no. 3, pp. 10007–10014, 2015.

[41] R. D. Sanders, T. Hussell, and M. Maze, "Sedation and immunomodulation," *Critical Care Clinics*, vol. 25, article 551, 2009.

[42] A. Bruzzone, C. P. Piñero, L. F. Castillo et al., "α 2-Adrenoceptor action on cell proliferation and mammary tumour growth in mice," *British Journal of Pharmacology*, vol. 155, no. 4, pp. 494–504, 2008.

[43] V. Guptill, X. Cui, A. Khaibullina et al., "Disruption of the transient receptor potential vanilloid 1 can affect survival, bacterial clearance, and cytokine gene expression during murine sepsis," *Anesthesiology*, vol. 114, no. 5, pp. 1190–1199, 2011.

[44] C. D. M. Griffith and M. B. Kamath, "Effect of halothane and nitrous oxide anaesthesia on natural killer lymphocytes from patients with benign and malignant breast disease," *British Journal of Anaesthesia*, vol. 58, no. 5, pp. 540–543, 1986.

[45] G. M. Woods and D. M. Griffiths, "Reversible inhibition of natural killer cell activity by volatile anaesthetic agents in vitro," *British Journal of Anaesthesia*, vol. 58, pp. 535–539, 1986.

[46] B. Müller-Edenborn, B. Roth-Z'Graggen, K. Bartnicka et al., "Volatile anesthetics reduce invasion of colorectal cancer cells through down-regulation of matrix metalloproteinase-9," *Anesthesiology*, vol. 117, no. 2, pp. 293–301, 2012.

[47] E. Fleischmann, C. Marschalek, K. Schlemitz et al., "Nitrous oxide may not increase the risk of cancer recurrence after colorectal surgery: a follow-up of a randomized controlled trial," *BMC Anesthesiology*, vol. 9, article 1, 2009.

[48] P. Forget, V. Collet, P. Lavand'homme, and M. De Kock, "Does analgesia and condition influence immunity after surgery?

Effects of fentanyl, ketamine and clonidine on natural killer activity at different ages," *European Journal of Anaesthesiology*, vol. 27, no. 3, pp. 233–240, 2010.

[49] B. Beilin, Y. Shavit, J. Hart et al., "Effects of anesthesia based on large versus small doses of fentanyl on natural killer cell cytotoxicity in the perioperative period," *Anesthesia & Analgesia*, vol. 82, no. 3, pp. 492–497, 1996.

[50] M. P. Yeager, M. A. Procopio, J. A. DeLeo, J. L. Arruda, L. Hildebrandt, and A. L. Howell, "Intravenous fentanyl increases natural killer cell cytotoxicity and circulating CD16+ lymphocytes in humans," *Anesthesia and Analgesia*, vol. 94, no. 1, pp. 94–99, 2002.

[51] R. Jacobs, M. Karst, D. Scheinichen et al., "Effects of fentanyl on cellular immune functions in man," *International Journal of Immunopharmacology*, vol. 21, no. 7, pp. 445–454, 1999.

[52] S. A. Ash and D. J. Buggy, "Does regional anaesthesia and analgesia or opioid analgesia influence recurrence after primary cancer surgery? An update of available evidence," *Best Practice and Research: Clinical Anaesthesiology*, vol. 27, no. 4, pp. 441–456, 2013.

[53] P. Forget, M. Berlière, A. van Maanen et al., "Perioperative ketorolac in high risk breast cancer patients. Rationale, feasibility and methodology of a prospective randomized placebo-controlled trial," *Medical Hypotheses*, vol. 81, no. 4, pp. 707–712, 2013.

[54] A. Heaney and D. J. Buggy, "Can anaesthetic and analgesic techniques affect cancer recurrence or metastasis?" *British Journal of Anaesthesia*, vol. 109, supplement 1, p. i17, 2012.

[55] F. M. Shebl, A. W. Hsing, Y. Park et al., "Non-steroidal anti-inflammatory drugs use is associated with reduced risk of inflammation-associated cancers: NIH-AARP study," *PLoS ONE*, vol. 9, no. 12, Article ID e114633, 2014.

[56] D. Wang and R. N. Dubois, "Eicosanoids and cancer," *Nature Reviews Cancer*, vol. 10, pp. 181–193, 2010.

[57] M. Benish, I. Bartal, Y. Goldfarb et al., "Perioperative use of beta-blockers and COX-2 inhibitors may improve immune competence and reduce the risk of tumor metastasis," *Annals of Surgical Oncology*, vol. 15, no. 7, pp. 2042–2052, 2008.

[58] T. Martinsson, "Ropivacaine inhibits serum-induced proliferation of colon adenocarcinoma cells in vitro," *Journal of Pharmacology and Experimental Therapeutics*, vol. 288, p. 660, 1999.

[59] E. Lucchinetti, A. E. Awad, M. Rahman et al., "Antiproliferative effects of local anesthetics on mesenchymal stem cells: potential implications for tumor spreading and wound healing," *Anesthesiology*, vol. 116, no. 4, pp. 841–856, 2012.

[60] A. Gottschalk, S. Sharma, J. Ford, M. E. Durieux, and M. Tiouririne, "The role of the perioperative period in recurrence after cancer surgery," *Anesthesia & Analgesia*, vol. 110, no. 6, pp. 1636–1643, 2010.

[61] I. Q. Molenaar, N. Warnaar, H. Groen, E. M. TenVergert, M. J. H. Slooff, and R. J. Porte, "Efficacy and safety of antifibrinolytic drugs in liver transplantation: a systematic review and meta-analysis," *American Journal of Transplantation*, vol. 7, no. 1, pp. 185–194, 2007.

[62] T. Asahara, K. Katayama, T. Itamoto et al., "Perioperative blood transfusion as a prognostic indicator in patients with hepatocellular carcinoma," *World Journal of Surgery*, vol. 23, no. 7, pp. 676–680, 1999.

[63] C. Miki, E. Ojima, Y. Inoue, Y. Mohri, and M. Kusunoki, "Perioperative allogeneic blood transfusion, the related cytokine response and long-term survival after potentially curative resection of colorectal cancer," *Clinical Oncology*, vol. 18, no. 1, pp. 60–66, 2006.

[64] T. Mynster, I. J. Christensen, F. Moesgaard, and H. J. Nielsen, "Effects of the combination of blood transfusion and postoperative infectious complications on prognosis after surgery for colorectal cancer. Danish RANX05 Colorectal Cancer Study Group," *British Journal of Surgery*, vol. 87, p. 1553, 2000.

[65] H. Shiba, Y. Ishida, S. Wakiyama et al., "Negative impact of blood transfusion on recurrence and prognosis of hepatocellular carcinoma after hepatic resection," *Journal of Gastrointestinal Surgery*, vol. 13, no. 9, pp. 1636–1642, 2009.

[66] F. Harder, U. Laffer, M. Berres, P. Jaggi, and U. Metzger, "Following curative resection of colorectal cancer, portal chemotherapy especially benefits non-transfused patients," *Der Chirurg*, vol. 61, p. 280, 1990.

[67] H. Katoh, K. Yamashita, G. Wang, T. Sato, T. Nakamura, and M. Watanabe, "Anastomotic leakage contributes to the risk for systemicrecurrence in stage II colorectal cancer," *Journal of Gastrointestinal Surgery*, vol. 15, no. 1, pp. 120–129, 2011.

[68] S. Cheslyn-Curtis, L. P. Fielding, R. Hittinger, J. S. Fry, and R. K. Phillips, "Large bowel cancer: the effect of perioperative blood transfusion on outcome," *Annals of the Royal College of Surgeons of England*, vol. 72, article 53, 1990.

[69] P. I. Tartter, "The association of perioperative blood transfusion with colorectal cancer recurrence," *Annals of Surgery*, vol. 216, no. 6, pp. 633–638, 1992.

[70] P. D. Frankish, R. K. mcnee, P. G. Alley, and D. G. Woodfield, "Relation between cancer of the colon and blood transfusion," *British Medical Journal*, vol. 290, no. 6484, p. 1827, 1985.

[71] J. G. A. Houbiers, A. Brand, L. M. G. van de Watering et al., "Randomised controlled trial comparing transfusion of leucocyte-depleted or buffy-coat-depleted blood in surgery for colorectal cancer," *The Lancet*, vol. 344, no. 8922, pp. 573–578, 1994.

[72] O. R. C. Busch, W. C. J. Hop, R. L. Marquet, and J. Jeekel, "The effect of blood transfusions on survival after surgery for colorectal cancer," *European Journal of Cancer*, vol. 31, no. 7-8, pp. 1226–1228, 1995.

[73] M. Herkenham and S. L. Kigar, "Contributions of the adaptive immune system to mood regulation: mechanisms and pathways of neuroimmune interactions," *Progress in Neuro-Psychopharmacology and Biological Psychiatry*, vol. 79, pp. 49–57, 2017.

18

Blood Urea Nitrogen as a Predictor of Severe Acute Pancreatitis based on the Revised Atlanta Criteria: Timing of Measurement and Cutoff Points

Suhan Lin,[1,2] Wandong Hong,[1] Zarrin Basharat,[3] Qipin Wang,[1,2] Jingye Pan,[4] and Mengtao Zhou[5]

[1]*Department of Gastroenterology and Hepatology, The First Affiliated Hospital of Wenzhou Medical University, Wenzhou, Zhejiang, China*
[2]*School of the First Clinical Medical Sciences, Wenzhou Medical University, Wenzhou, Zhejiang, China*
[3]*Microbiology & Biotechnology Research Lab, Department of Environmental Sciences, Fatima Jinnah Women University, Rawalpindi 46000, Pakistan*
[4]*Intensive Care Unit, The First Affiliated Hospital of Wenzhou Medical University, Wenzhou, Zhejiang, China*
[5]*Department of Surgery, The First Affiliated Hospital of Wenzhou Medical University, Wenzhou, Zhejiang, China*

Correspondence should be addressed to Wandong Hong; xhnk-hwd@163.com

Academic Editor: Grigorios I. Leontiadis

Background and Aims. This study evaluated the prognostic accuracy of BUN for severe acute pancreatitis (SAP) and in-hospital mortality (IHM) in terms of the best timing for BUN measurement and the optimal BUN cutoff points. *Methods.* BUN determinants at the time of admission and 24 hrs after hospital admission were recorded and analyzed statistically. The ability of BUN in predicting the SAP and the occurrence of IHM were assessed using the area under the receiver-operating characteristic (ROC) curve. *Results.* For SAP, AUC of BUN at admission and 24 hrs after hospital admission was 0.75 and 0.80, respectively. For IHM in acute pancreatitis, it was 0.86 at admission and 0.84 after 24 hrs of hospital admission, respectively. The optimal cutoff point of BUN 24 hrs after hospital admission for SAP and at admission for IHM was 8.3 mmol/L and 13.3 mmol/L, respectively. *Conclusion.* BUN determination after 24 hrs of hospital admission has high accuracy for prediction of SAP while BUN at initial admission has high accuracy for prediction of IHM.

1. Introduction

Acute pancreatitis (referred to hereafter as AP) is a common clinical condition with variation in severity [1]. In most instances, AP runs a self-limiting and mild course; however, 10–30% of patients might progress to a severe attack, that is, severe acute pancreatitis (SAP) with an in-hospital mortality (IHM) reaching 30% [2, 3]. SAP, representing a paradigm of sterile inflammatory disease, is initiated by acinar cell injury-mediated local inflammation and progresses to the systemic inflammatory response syndrome, accompanied with inevitable multiple organ injury, and eventually leads to multiple organ dysfunction syndrome, which contributes to the main cause of morbidity and mortality in this condition [4]. Moreover, this typical pathological course results in approximately 50% of clinical deaths within the first week [5].

The early risk assessment of patients with AP through reliable methods is necessary to improve the clinical outcomes and reduce the treatment cost and length of hospitalization. A great deal of research has focused on development of approaches for early diagnosis and risk stratification in AP. In addition to the established clinical scores, a variety of single markers have emerged for AP, their measurement being sufficiently fast and cheap to widely enter the clinical routine. The multiparametric scores were essential for clinical trials but had obvious disadvantages that prevent their practical use in daily routine [6].

Blood urea nitrogen (BUN) is an important prognostic marker during the initial 24 hours of hospitalization for measuring SAP and IHM [7–10]. In the literature, there is no consensus on the timing of measurement of BUN for prediction of SAP and IHM during the first 24 hrs of hospitalization [7, 8]. There is also inconsistency in the optimal cutoff points for BUN in terms of predicting IHM of AP [6–8, 11]. In addition, BUN in previous studies was evaluated as a predictor of severe pancreatitis, defined according to the Atlanta criteria but not based on the recent SAP guidelines [12], which limit its use in the current clinical practice. Therefore, the current study aimed to assess the best timings for measurement and the optimal cutoff points of BUN in predicting SAP. This was defined by up-to-date guidelines and IHM in AP.

2. Material and Methods

2.1. Patient Population, Data Collection, and Ethics. Patients aged 18 years or older, admitted with a diagnosis of AP (onset time ≤ 3 days) in the First Affiliated Hospital of Wenzhou Medical University between January 2013 and December 2015, were eligible for study participation. Patients were excluded from participation in case they met any of the following criteria: onset time >3 days (515 cases), not-first-time pancreatitis (194 cases), therapeutic operations (23 cases), organ failure before data collection (including history of cirrhosis/chronic kidney disease with creatinine clearance <40 mL/min/pulmonary disease) (7 cases), malignant gastrointestinal tumors (19 cases), gestation (7 cases), intoxication (5 cases), and merging the above conditions (27 cases).

The following information was collected for each patient: age, gender, Body Mass Index (BMI), etiology, white blood cell (WBC), hemoglobin (Hb), platelet count (PLT), and serum electrolytes (potassium, sodium, and calcium) at admission. BUN and serum creatinine (Scr) were collected at the time of admission and 24 hrs after hospital admission.

This study protocol was approved by the Ethic Committee of the First Affiliated Hospital of Wenzhou Medical University. This study was performed according to the principles expressed in the Declaration of Helsinki and informed consent was obtained from the subjects.

2.2. Definitions and Outcomes. The diagnosis of AP requires two of the following three features in the revised Atlanta criteria [12]: (1) abdominal pain; (2) level of serum lipase or amylase at least three times greater than the upper limit of normal; and (3) characteristic findings of AP on abdominal image. According to the revised Atlanta criteria, SAP is defined as persistent organ failure in patients (organ failure persistent for more than 48 h). According to the modified Marshall Scoring System [13], organ failure includes at least one of the following features: (a) respiratory failure, defined as PaO_2/FiO_2 levels of 300 mmHg or less; (b) renal failure, defined as Scr level of at least 1.9 mg/dl; and (c) shock, defined as systolic blood pressure of less than 90 mmHg and unresponsive to fluid therapy. IHM refers to death occurring from AP or its complications during the initial hospitalization.

The primary endpoint was to assess BUN as predictor of SAP at initial admission and 24 hrs after patient admission. The secondary endpoint was to assess BUN as predictor of IHM at initial admission and 24 hrs after patient admission in the hospital.

2.3. Statistical Analysis. A Shapiro–Wilk test was used to evaluate whether the continuous data was normally distributed. According to the results of the Shapiro–Wilk test, continuous values were expressed by mean ± SD or median and interquartile range. Values were compared using the paired t-test or the Wilcoxon signed-rank test. Categorical values were described by count and proportions and compared by the χ^2 test. P values below 0.05 were considered significant.

Variables in univariate analysis found to be significantly related to SAP were selected as candidates for ROC curve analysis. AUC for BUN as a predictor of SAP and IHM was calculated. A predictor with an AUC above 0.7 was considered useful, while an AUC between 0.8 and 0.9 indicated excellent diagnostic accuracy [14]. To determine the optimal BUN cutoff points for SAP and IHM, Youden Index, sensitivity, specificity, positive predictive value (PPV), and negative predictive value (NPV) were calculated for the different BUN cutoff points. The best Youden Index (sensitivity + specificity – 1) was used to determine the best cutoff points of BUN level to predict SAP and IHM [15, 16].

P values below 0.05 were considered significant. All statistical procedures were performed with Stata 12.0. software.

3. Results

3.1. Patient Characteristics. A total of 671 participants were included in the current study. The median age of the patients was 47 years (range 19–93 years), and 62.44% (n = 419) of patients were males. Biliary disease was the most common cause of the AP (n = 284, 42.32%). 60 (8.94%) patients presented with severe AP symptoms. The median length of the hospital stay was 10 days (interquartile range 7–14 days), with 13 days (interquartile range 7–24 days) for SAP patients. Eleven patients (1.64%) died during hospitalization.

3.2. Univariate Analysis between Patients with or without SAP. Fourteen variables were considered potentially relevant to the severity of AP and tested using univariable analysis. As shown in Table 1, hemoglobin at admission, platelets at admission, WBC at admission, calcium, BUN at admission, BUN 24 hrs after hospital admission, Scr at admission, and Scr after 24 hrs of hospital admission were significantly associated with the severity of AP.

3.3. Prognostic Values of BUN in Predicting SAP. As shown in Figure 1, the AUCs for WBC at admission, platelets at admission, calcium at admission, BUN at admission, BUN after 24 hrs of admission, Scr at admission, and Scr after 24 hrs of admission for the prediction of SAP were 0.59 ± 0.08, 0.61 ± 0.08, 0.74 ± 0.08, 0.75 ± 0.08, 0.80 ± 0.07, 0.68 ± 0.09, and 0.76 ± 0.08, respectively. Both the BUN at admission and BUN after 24 hours of hospitalization were useful predictors of SAP,

Table 1: Univariate analysis of predictive factors of SAP in 671 patients.

Variable	No SAP (n = 611)	SAP (n = 60)	P values
Age (yr)	47 (37, 63)	51.5 (38.5, 66)	0.1441
Male (%)	63.3	53.3	0.1270
Biliary etiology (%)	265 (43.4)	19 (31.7)	
BMI (kg/m^2)	23.5 (21.1, 26.1)	24.2 (22.1, 26.6)	0.1041
WBC (10^9/l)	13.2 (10, 16.77)	15.3 (11.09, 18.365)	0.0185
Hemoglobin (g/l)	144 (129, 158)	149.5 (136, 164.5)	0.0722
Platelet (10^9/l)	198 (233, 160)	172 (209.5, 134)	0.0070
Potassium (mmol/l)	3.98 (3.70, 4.25)	4.02 (3.65, 4.70)	0.1443
Sodium (mmol/l)	139 (141, 136)	137 (142, 133)	0.1390
Calcium (mmol/l)	2.19 (2.28, 2.07)	1.9 (2.195, 1.58)	<0.001
BUN (mmol/l)	4.7 (3.7, 5.9)	7.45 (5.45, 11.95)	<0.001
BUN (24 h) (mmol/l)	4.6 (3.4, 6.2)	9.4 (6.15, 12.35)	<0.001
Scr (umol/L)	64 (54, 76)	82.5 (58, 157.5)	<0.001
Scr (24 h) (umol/L)	63 (52, 77)	92 (66, 206.5)	<0.001

Single continuous variables as median and interquartile range (25th–75th percentiles).

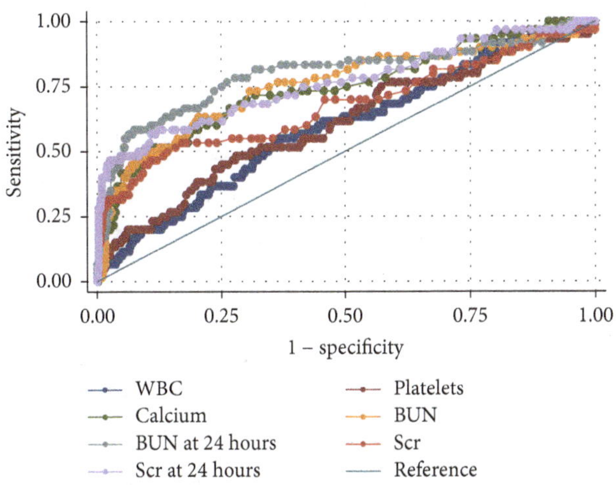

Figure 1: ROC curves for various predictors for SAP. The AUCs were 0.59 ± 0.08, 0.61 ± 0.08, 0.74 ± 0.08, 0.75 ± 0.08, 0.80 ± 0.07, 0.68 ± 0.09, and 0.76 ± 0.08 for WBC at admission, platelets at admission, calcium at admission, BUN at admission, BUN after 24 hrs of hospitalization, Scr at admission, and Scr after 24 hrs of hospitalization, respectively. The ideal AUC was 1.00. The reference line represents AUC of 0.50, based on chance alone.

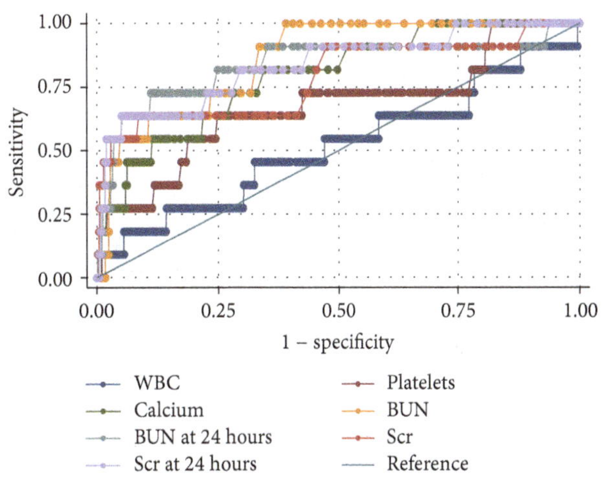

Figure 2: ROC curves for various predictors for IHM. The areas under ROC curves were 0.52 ± 0.20, 0.68 ± 0.19, 0.79 ± 0.13, 0.86 ± 0.09, 0.84 ± 0.16, 0.79 ± 0.175, and 0.84 ± 0.14 for WBC at admission, platelets at admission, calcium at admission, BUN at admission, BUN after 24 hrs of hospitalization, Scr at admission, and Scr after 24 hrs of hospitalization, respectively. The ideal AUC was 1.00. The reference line represents AUC of 0.50, based on chance alone.

with AUC of more than 0.7. In addition, only BUN after 24 hours of hospitalization with an AUC of 0.80 achieved an excellent diagnostic accuracy among single predictors.

Every cutoff point of BUN at admission and after 24 hrs for prediction of SAP was shown in Tables 2 and 3. Based on Youden Index analysis, the optimal BUN cutoff point at admission and after 24 hrs of hospital admission for prediction of SAP was 6.1 mmol/L (17.1 mg/dL) and 8.3 mmol/L (23.2 mg/dL), respectively.

3.4. Prognostic Values of BUN in Predicting IHM of AP. As shown in Figure 2, the AUCs for WBC at admission, platelets at admission, calcium at admission, BUN at admission, BUN after 24 hrs of admission, Scr at admission, and Scr after 24 hrs of admission, for the prediction of SAP, were 0.52 ± 0.20, 0.68 ± 0.19, 0.79 ± 0.13, 0.86 ± 0.09, 0.84 ± 0.16, 0.79 ± 0.175, and 0.84 ± 0.14, respectively. Both the BUN at admission and BUN after 24 hours of hospitalization were excellent predictors of IHM due to AP, with AUC of more than 0.8. In addition, BUN at admission achieved the biggest AUC (0.86) among single predictors of IHM of AP.

Every cutoff point of BUN for prediction of IHM due to AP is shown in Tables 4 and 5. With a cutoff point of 5.2 mmol/L (14.6 mg/dL) at admission and 8.3 mmol/L (23.2 mg/dL) at 24 hrs after hospital admission, BUN achieved the best

TABLE 2: Index of BUN diagnosis for SAP upon patient admission.

BUN (mmol/L)	BUN (mg/dL)	Youden Index	Sensitivity	Specificity	PPV	NPV
5	14	0.343	0.783	0.560	0.149	0.963
6	17	0.388	0.633	0.755	0.202	0.954
6.1	**17.1**	**0.428**	**0.633**	**0.795**	**0.233**	**0.957**
7	20	0.375	0.517	0.858	0.269	0.948
8	22	0.386	0.483	0.903	0.329	0.947
9	25	0.369	0.433	0.936	0.401	0.947
10	28	0.301	0.350	0.951	0.412	0.917
11	31	0.238	0.267	0.971	0.470	0.900
12	34	0.227	0.250	0.977	0.512	0.930

PPV = positive predictive value; NPV = negative predictive value.

TABLE 3: Index of BUN diagnosis for SAP, 24 hrs after hospital admission.

BUN (mmol/L)	BUN (mg/dL)	Youden Index	Sensitivity	Specificity	PPV	NPV
5	14	0.396	0.833	0.563	0.174	0.972
6	17	0.505	0.783	0.722	0.217	0.971
7	20	0.483	0.650	0.833	0.277	0.960
8	22	0.482	0.583	0.899	0.356	0.956
8.3	**23.2**	**0.508**	**0.583**	**0.925**	**0.432**	**0.958**
9	25	0.489	0.550	0.939	0.472	0.955
10	28	0.407	0.450	0.957	0.519	0.947
11	31	0.388	0.417	0.971	0.581	0.947
12	34	0.243	0.267	0.976	0.533	0.931

PPV = positive predictive value; NPV = negative predictive value.

TABLE 4: Index of BUN diagnosis for IHM at initial patient admission in the hospital.

BUN (mmol/L)	BUN (mg/dL)	Youden Index	Sensitivity	Specificity	PPV	NPV
5	14	0.538	1	0.538	0.035	1
5.2	**14.6**	**0.609**	**1**	**0.609**	**0.041**	**1**
6	17	0.454	0.727	0.727	0.043	0.991
7	20	0.462	0.636	0.826	0.058	0.993
8	22	0.513	0.636	0.877	0.077	0.993
9	25	0.457	0.546	0.911	0.079	0.992
10	28	0.478	0.546	0.932	0.117	0.969
11	31	0.411	0.455	0.956	0.148	0.991
12	34	0.419	0.455	0.964	0.172	0.990
13.3	**37.3**	**0.426**	**0.455**	**0.971**	**0.217**	**0.991**
13.9	38.9	0.337	0.364	0.973	0.190	0.989

PPV = positive predictive value; NPV = negative predictive value.

TABLE 5: Index of BUN diagnosis for IHM, after 24 hrs of patient hospitalization.

BUN (mmol/L)	BUN (mg/dL)	Youden Index	Sensitivity	Specificity	PPV	NPV
8	22	0.592	0.727	0.865	0.082	0.995
8.3	**23.2**	**0.616**	**0.727**	**0.889**	**0.099**	**0.995**
9	25	0.541	0.636	0.905	0.104	0.993
10	28	0.566	0.636	0.930	0.132	0.994
11	31	0.582	0.636	0.946	0.163	0.994
12	**34**	**0.508**	**0.546**	**0.962**	**0.205**	**0.989**
13.9	38.9	0.335	0.364	0.971	0.174	0.989
15	42.0	0.247	0.273	0.974	0.150	0.988

PPV = positive predictive value; NPV = negative predictive value.

Youden Index for prediction of IHM. However, these cutoff points result in a very low PPV (only 4% at admission and 9.9% at 24 hrs after hospital admission) for IHM. One may expect to choose another more pragmatic cutoff with a higher PPV for the trade-off of slightly lower NPV (which would still be about 90%) for BUN to predict IHM. Therefore, 13.3 mmol/L (37.3 mg/dL) and 12 mmol/L (34 mg/dL) were selected as the optimal BUN cutoff point at admission and 24 hrs after hospital admission for prediction of IHM in AP.

4. Discussion

The outcomes of the present study prove that (i) both the BUN at admission and that after 24 hrs of hospitalization were useful predictors of SAP, with AUC of more than 0.7. In addition, only BUN after 24 hours of hospitalization with an AUC of 0.80 achieved an excellent diagnostic accuracy among single predictors; (ii) the optimal BUN cutoff point at admission and 24 hrs after hospital admission for prediction of SAP was 6.1 mmol/L (17.1 mg/dL) and 8.3 mmol/L (23.2 mg/dL), respectively; (iii) both BUN at admission and that after 24 hrs of hospitalization were excellent predictors of IHM of AP, with AUC of more than 0.8. In addition, BUN at admission achieved the largest AUC (0.86) among single predictors of IHM of AP; (iv) the optimal cutoff point of BUN at admission and at 24 hrs after hospital admission for prediction of IHM of AP was 13.3 mmol/L (37.3 mg/dL) and 12 mmol/L (34 mg/dL).

There are a lot of grounds, based on which BUN has been selected as useful prognostic/predictor of AP in the literature. First, an ideal prognostic marker should help guide physicians in their approach to accepted interventions such as fluid resuscitation. The BUN at admission/hospitalization might reflect the underlying physiologic state of the patient, including intravascular volume depletion [11] and prerenal azotemia [7]. Therefore, BUN may play an important role in the early assessment of AP [7]. Second, a persistent elevation or subsequent rise in BUN may reflect either a failure to adequately resuscitate patients early in their disease course, deterioration of renal function, or a state of ongoing negative nitrogen balance related to increased protein catabolism induced by AP [17]. Third, it has been suggested that, though without clinical signs of pancreatitis and changes of medical image, the fluctuation of BUN is particularly susceptible to the ischemic injury of pancreas [18]. Besides the influence of pancreatic enzymes, inflammatory factors (such as IL-1β and IL-18) could cause renal dysfunction through cardiac dysfunction, circulatory collapse, hypoperfusion, metabolic acidosis, shock and production of acute respiratory distress syndrome indirectly, and direttissima after SAP induction [19, 20].

Previous study reported that elevated BUN level (more than 25 mg/dl) at admission was associated with increased possibility of developing severe AP defined by Atlanta criteria [21]. It achieved a sensitivity of 27.3%, specificity of 97.7%, positive predictive value of 78.3%, and negative predictive value of 81.3% [21]. To the best of our knowledge, this is the first study to evaluate BUN as predictor of SAP defined by the up-to-date revised Atlanta criteria. Our univariate analysis suggested that there were statistical differences in BUN level both at admission and after 24 hours of admission between patients with or without SAP (Table 1). Every cutoff point of BUN at admission and after 24 hrs for prediction of SAP was evaluated (Tables 2 and 3). Our study noted that BUN after 24 hours of hospitalization had higher AUC than that of BUN at initial admission (Figure 1). With a cutoff of 8.3 mmol/L (23.2 mg/dL), BUN at 24 hours of hospitalization achieved a sensitivity of 0.508, specificity of 0.925, PPV of 0.432, and NPV of 0.958.

The early phase of mortality peak of this dynamic disease usually lasts for the first week, with approximately 50% clinical death occurrence during the first week [5]. Previous studies suggested that elevated BUN and subsequent changes of BUN during the initial 24 hrs of hospitalization are the most valuable independent risk factors for mortality in AP [7–10]. Different studies have proposed different optimal cutoff points of BUN at admission, ranging from 33 mg/dl [6], 25 mg/dl [22], 23 mg/dl [10], and 20 mg/dl [8] to 7.8 mg/dl [7], for prediction of IHM. In one study, the cutoff point of BUN, that is, 7.8 mg/dl, at admission was associated with a corresponding increase in risk of mortality (OR = 2.9) [7]. BUN level in patients at initial admission that declined by 5 mg/dl or more after 24 hrs had a substantially reduced mortality risk (0%–3.2%) [8]. Any rise in BUN level at 24 hours was associated with an OR of 4.3 (CI_{95}, 2.3–7.9%) for death [8]. Our data suggested that both the BUN at admission and BUN at 24 hrs of hospitalization were excellent predictors of IHM of AP. In addition, BUN at admission achieved the largest AUC (i.e., 0.86) among single predictors of IHM of AP (Figure 2). The optimal cutoff point of BUN at admission and at 24 h after hospital admission for prediction of IHM of AP was 13.3 mmol/L (37.3 mg/dL) and 12 mmol/L (34 mg/dL), respectively (Tables 4 and 5). With a cutoff value of 13.3 mmol/L (37.3 mg/dL), BUN at admission achieved a sensitivity of 0.455, specificity of 0.977, PPV of 0.217, and NPV of 0.991. Low mortality might be one of primary reasons why large fluctuations of the optimal cutoff points of BUN exist in most studies, as evidenced by the fact that eleven patients (1.64%) died during hospitalization in the current study.

Multiparametric scores such as APACHE II score and BISAP score are essential for clinical trials but have obvious disadvantages that prevent their practical use in daily routine. APACHE II score is not specific for pancreatitis and time-consuming to be calculated [6]. BISAP score had a moderate diagnostic accuracy in predicting AP [23]. In addition to the established clinical scores, a variety of single markers such as C-reactive protein [24] or interleukin- (IL-) 6 and IL-8 had predictive value [25] and have emerged for AP. However, interleukin- (IL-) 6 and IL-8 cannot be routinely available in the emergency room. C-reactive protein, though easy to check in practice, lacks high specificity [26].

The strength of this study includes adequate sample size which gives significant statistical power. Only patients with short onset time (not more than three days) of AP and having first attack were enrolled, which might help rule out the influence of interferences such as fluid resuscitation on BUN level. It was the first study to evaluate the prognostic value of BUN via up-to-date revised Atlanta criteria of the SAP. However, there were several potential limitations such as the retrospective design which might produce selection bias. The timing of BUN measurement was only available at admission and 24 hrs after hospital admission, which could not let us evaluate the impact of early changes in BUN on prognosis of AP. PPV could not be close to one for this study, even if both sensitivity and specificity were high [27].

In conclusion, BUN was the most valuable independent risk factor for predicting SAP and IHM in AP during the initial 24 hrs of hospitalization. BUN after 24 hrs of hospital admission showed a better prognostic accuracy than BUN at initial admission for SAP. The optimal cutoff point of BUN at 24 hrs after hospital admission was 8.3 mmol/L (23.2 mg/dL). The best timing for BUN measurement for IHM was at admission, whose optimal cutoff point was 13.3 mmol/L (37.3 mg/dL). BUN as a single marker for AP could be useful as it is easy to perform and a cheap marker to predict SAP and IHM, without the need for complex calculations.

Ethical Approval

This study protocol was approved by the Ethic Committee of the First Affiliated Hospital of Wenzhou Medical University. This study was performed according to the principles expressed in the Declaration of Helsinki.

Authors' Contributions

Suhan Lin and Jingye Pan contributed equally to this work. Wandong Hong joined in the design of the study and carried out the studies. Suhan Lin, Wandong Hong, Qipin Wang, Jingye Pan, and Mengtao Zhou participated in data collection. Wandong Hong and Suhan Lin conducted data analysis and drafted the manuscript. Wandong Hong and Zarrin Basharat helped to finalize the manuscript. All of the authors read and approved the manuscript.

References

[1] G. Malleo, E. Mazzon, A. K. Siriwardena, and S. Cuzzocrea, "Role of tumor necrosis factor-α in acute pancreatitis: from biological basis to clinical evidence," *Shock*, vol. 28, no. 2, pp. 130–140, 2007.

[2] R. Talukdar, H. Nechutova, M. Clemens, and S. S. Vege, "Could rising BUN predict the future development of infected pancreatic necrosis?" *Pancreatology*, vol. 13, no. 4, pp. 355–359, 2013.

[3] J. Granger and D. Remick, "Acute pancreatitis: models, markers, and mediators," *Shock*, vol. 24, supplement 1, pp. 45–51, 2005.

[4] Z.-Q. Chen, Y.-Q. Tang, Y. Zhang et al., "Adenoviral transfer of human interleukin-10 gene in lethal pancreatitis," *World Journal of Gastroenterology*, vol. 10, no. 20, pp. 3021–3025, 2004.

[5] A. K. Rustgi, "A historical perspective on clinical advances in pancreatic diseases," *Gastroenterology*, vol. 144, no. 6, pp. 1249–1251, 2013.

[6] M. Faisst, U. F. Wellner, S. Utzolino, U. T. Hopt, and T. Keck, "Elevated blood urea nitrogen is an independent risk factor of prolonged intensive care unit stay due to acute necrotizing pancreatitis," *Journal of Critical Care*, vol. 25, no. 1, pp. 105–111, 2010.

[7] B. U. Wu, R. S. Johannes, X. Sun, D. L. Conwell, and P. A. Banks, "Early changes in blood urea nitrogen predict mortality in acute pancreatitis," *Gastroenterology*, vol. 137, no. 1, pp. 129–135, 2009.

[8] B. U. Wu, O. J. Bakker, G. I. Papachristou et al., "Blood urea nitrogen in the early assessment of acute pancreatitis: an international validation study," *Archives of Internal Medicine*, vol. 171, no. 7, pp. 669–676, 2011.

[9] B. U. Wu, J. Q. Hwang, T. H. Gardner et al., "Lactated Ringer's solution reduces systemic inflammation compared with saline in patients with acute pancreatitis," *Clinical Gastroenterology and Hepatology*, vol. 9, no. 8, pp. 710.e1–717.e1, 2011.

[10] E. Kaya, A. Dervisoglu, and C. Polat, "Evaluation of diagnostic findings and scoring systems in outcome prediction in acute pancreatitis," *World Journal of Gastroenterology*, vol. 13, no. 22, pp. 3090–3094, 2007.

[11] B. U. Wu, R. S. Johannes, X. Sun, Y. Tabak, D. L. Conwell, and P. A. Banks, "The early prediction of mortality in acute pancreatitis: a large population-based study," *Gut*, vol. 57, no. 12, pp. 1698–1703, 2008.

[12] P. A. Banks, T. L. Bollen, C. Dervenis et al., "Classification of acute pancreatitis—2012: revision of the Atlanta classification and definitions by international consensus," *Gut*, vol. 62, no. 1, pp. 102–111, 2013.

[13] J. C. Marshall, D. J. Cook, N. V. Christou, G. R. Bernard, C. L. Sprung, and W. J. Sibbald, "Multiple organ dysfunction score: a reliable descriptor of a complex clinical outcome," *Critical Care Medicine*, vol. 23, no. 10, pp. 1638–1652, 1995.

[14] W.-D. Hong, Q.-H. Zhu, Z.-M. Huang et al., "Predictors of esophageal varices in patients with HBV-related cirrhosis: a retrospective study," *BMC Gastroenterology*, vol. 9, article 11, 2009.

[15] Y.-S. Peng, Y.-C. Chen, Y.-C. Tian et al., "Serum levels of apolipoprotein A-I and high-density lipoprotein can predict organ failure in acute pancreatitis," *Critical Care*, vol. 19, p. 88, 2015.

[16] R. Fluss, D. Faraggi, and B. Reiser, "Estimation of the Youden index and its associated cutoff point," *Biometrical Journal*, vol. 47, no. 4, pp. 458–472, 2005.

[17] R. N. Dickerson, K. L. Vehe, J. L. Mullen, and I. D. Feurer, "Resting energy expenditure in patients with pancreatitis," *Critical Care Medicine*, vol. 19, no. 4, pp. 484–490, 1991.

[18] J. A. Quiros, J. P. Marcin, N. Kuppermann et al., "Elevated serum amylase and lipase in pediatric diabetic ketoacidosis," *Pediatric Critical Care Medicine*, vol. 9, no. 4, pp. 418–422, 2008.

[19] X.-H. Zhang, M.-L. Li, B. Wang, M.-X. Guo, and R.-M. Zhu, "Caspase-1 inhibition alleviates acute renal injury in rats with severe acute pancreatitis," *World Journal of Gastroenterology*, vol. 20, no. 30, pp. 10457–10463, 2014.

[20] D. M. Relles, N. G. Richards, J. P. Bloom et al., "Serum blood urea nitrogen and serum albumin on the first postoperative day predict pancreatic fistula and major complications after pancreaticoduodenectomy," *Journal of Gastrointestinal Surgery*, vol. 17, no. 2, pp. 326–331, 2013.

[21] W. Hong, L. Dong, Q. Huang, W. Wu, J. Wu, and Y. Wang, "Prediction of severe acute pancreatitis using classification and regression tree analysis," *Digestive Diseases and Sciences*, vol. 56, no. 12, pp. 3664–3671, 2011.

[22] T. Ueda, Y. Takeyama, T. Yasuda et al., "Simple scoring system for the prediction of the prognosis of severe acute pancreatitis," *Surgery*, vol. 141, no. 1, pp. 51–58, 2007.

[23] R. Mounzer, C. J. Langmead, B. U. Wu et al., "Comparison of existing clinical scoring systems to predict persistent organ failure in patients with acute pancreatitis," *Gastroenterology*, vol. 142, no. 7, pp. 1476–1482, 2012.

[24] G. I. Papachristou and D. C. Whitcomb, "Inflammatory markers of disease severity in acute pancreatitis," *Clinics in Laboratory Medicine*, vol. 25, no. 1, pp. 17–37, 2005.

[25] N. Pooran, A. Indaram, P. Singh, and S. Bank, "Cytokines (IL-6, IL-8, TNF): early and reliable predictors of severe acute pancreatitis," *Journal of Clinical Gastroenterology*, vol. 37, no. 3, pp. 263–266, 2003.

[26] F. S. Cardoso, L. B. Ricardo, A. M. Oliveira et al., "C-reactive protein prognostic accuracy in acute pancreatitis: timing of measurement and cutoff points," *European Journal of Gastroenterology and Hepatology*, vol. 25, no. 7, pp. 784–789, 2013.

[27] D. G. Altman and J. M. Bland, "Diagnostic tests 2: predictive values," *BMJ*, vol. 309, no. 6947, p. 102, 1994.

19

Alpha-Fetoprotein and Hepatocellular Carcinoma Immunity

Xiaoping Wang[1] **and Qiaoxia Wang**[2]

[1]*Laboratory of Molecular Biology & Pathology, Shaanxi University of Chinese Medicine, Xianyang, Shaanxi 712046, China*

[2]*Department of Infectious Diseases, Xi'an Central Hospital, Xi'an, Shaanxi 710000, China*

Correspondence should be addressed to Xiaoping Wang; wxpphd@aliyun.com

Academic Editor: Maikel P. Peppelenbosch

Hepatocarcinoma is one of the most prevalent gastroenterological cancers in the world with less effective therapy. As an oncofetal antigen and diagnostic marker for liver cancer, alpha-fetoprotein (AFP) possesses a variety of biological functions. Except for its diagnosis in liver cancer, AFP has become a target for liver cancer immunotherapy. Although the immunogenicity of AFP is weak and it could induce the immune escapes through inhibiting the function of dendritic cells, natural killer cells, and T lymphocytes, AFP has attracted more attention in liver cancer immunotherapy. By in vitro modification, the immunogenicity and immune response of AFP could be enhanced. AFP-modified immune cell vaccine or peptide vaccine has displayed the specific antitumor immunity against AFP-positive tumor cells and laid a better foundation for the immunotherapy of liver cancer.

1. Introduction

Hepatocellular carcinoma (HCC) is one of the most common tumors in the world, with a new incidence of up to 600,000 cases per year [1, 2]. This malignancy is becoming more prevalent in Asia because of the high incidences of hepatitis B and C infections [3, 4]. Due to the insidious onset and long incubation period of HCC, patients usually got intermediate or advanced stage with poor prognosis. At present, the treatments of liver cancer mainly rely on surgical resection, liver transplantation, local ablation, chemoembolization, and molecular targeted therapy, but the effects of these strategies are not ideal and the mortality is still high [5, 6]. Therefore, there is an urgent need to develop effective adjuvant therapies that may prolong the life and improve the quality of patients with HCC.

Immunotherapy of HCC could stimulate the identification of specific tumor antigen, inhibit the proliferation of cancer cells, produce memory lymphocytes and prevent recurrence, so the immunotherapy of HCC has attracted more attention in recent years. In this paper, the research progress on the immunotherapy of alpha-fetoprotein (AFP) and HCC is reviewed.

2. Significance of Alpha-Fetoprotein Expression in Hepatocellular Carcinoma

Alpha-fetoprotein is a kind of glycoprotein, derived from embryonic endoderm tissue cells. AFP content in fetal serum is high and gradually decreases to the level of adults after birth. The low content of AFP in the adult blood is mainly due to the loss of the ability to synthesize AFP in mature hepatocytes. When transformed, the liver cancer cells can regain the ability to synthesize AFP. Besides liver cancer, malignant tumors from stomach, pancreas, and reproductive system are often accompanied by a small amount of increased AFP. In general, AFP is produced only at low levels after birth; however, majority of human HCC overexpress high level of AFP in eastern populations [6, 7]. Therefore, the HCC patients with AFP negative or weak positive in serum is usually consistent with the characteristics of high differentiated cancers [6, 7].

Combining detection of AFP with new diagnostic markers increases the sensitivity and specificity to diagnose HCC. For instance, combination of AFP and lens culinaris lectin detection resulted in increased specificity and sensitivity in diagnosing HCC [8, 9]. With the progress of clinical laboratory techniques, the new liver biomarkers have displayed important roles in the diagnosis of liver cancer. Abnormal prothrombin des-γ-carboxy prothrombin (DCP) and alpha-L-fucosidase (AFU) are available in diagnosing AFP-negative HCC [10, 11]. Combining AFP-L3 with Golgi protein 73, the diagnostic sensitivity was 94%, specificity was 93.1%, and the accuracy rate of diagnosis was 93.3% in HCC patients, greatly improving the early diagnosis rate of liver cancer [12, 13].

In addition to being an oncofetal antigen and diagnostic marker for liver cancer, AFP possesses a variety of biological functions, such as transport function similar to the class of albumin family, transporting metal ions, drugs, bilirubin, and steroids [1–4].

3. AFP and Immune Escape Mechanism of Hepatocellular Carcinoma

Liver cancer cells can modify their own surface antigen and change the microenvironment around the tumor lesion to implement their immune escape. Exogenous AFP can not only promote the proliferation of hepatocellular carcinoma cells and the formation of tumor blood vessels, but also enhance the antiapoptosis effect of cancer cells [14–18]. Thus, AFP plays an important role in the development and progression of liver cancer. Cellular immunity is the main immune mechanism of anticancer [19]. Dendritic cells, natural killer cells, and T lymphocytes are involved in immune surveillance [19]. It is confirmed that AFP could affect the three important immune cells to exert their antitumor effects [14, 15].

DC cells own the function of high uptake, processing and presenting antigen, which are the only antigen-presenting cells (APC) directly activating naive T cells. AFP can inhibit the maturation and induce apoptosis of DC cells, so that cancer cells could escape the immune surveillance. Researches demonstrated that when peripheral blood mononuclear cells were cultured in normal umbilical cord blood AFP (nAFP) and tumor derived AFP (tAFP) separately, the phenotype and function of DC cells were altered. Tumor derived AFP could significantly inhibit the differentiation of DCs, and the DC cells restricted by tAFP still maintained the immature mononuclear cell-like morphology [20]. Moreover, the DCs apoptosis index and Caspase-3 expression were significantly increased after AFP treatment [20, 21]. In addition to the increased expression of Caspase-3, p38 mitogen-activated protein kinase (MARK) expression was also increased in DC cells [20, 21]. When AFP was incubated with DCs from human peripheral blood, the cells were found to express Caspase-3 and p38-MARK, which would induce apoptosis and inhibit the maturation of DC cells, thus resulting in the immune escape of cancer cells [21, 22].

NK cell is an important component of the innate immune system, which is the first line of defense against infections and tumors. NK cells could express a variety of surface receptors, including activating receptors (NKG2D, NKp30, NKp44, NKp46) and inhibitory receptors (KIR2DL3/CD158b). When recognizing the tumor cells, the expression of activating receptors increases and the expression of inhibitory receptors decreases, which lead to the enhancement of the antitumor effects. IL-12 is able to stimulate the expression of NKG-2D on the surface of NK cells and improve the toxic effect of NK cells. After binding to its ligand, NKG2D activates NK cells and exerts an immune response [23]. Therefore, when the mice loaded with liver cancer cells were vaccinated with IL-12, it was found that the expression of activating receptors of NK cells increased while inhibitory receptors decreased, and IFN-γ content elevated, thus suppressing the tumor growth [22]. The function of NK cells could also be affected by AFP. AFP does not directly damage the function of NK cells, but through inhibiting the maturation of DC cells, DC cells reduce the secretion of the amount of IL-12, then indirectly inhibiting NK cells [24, 25].

DCs could activate AFP-specific T cells significantly in vitro and in vivo. The main mechanism is the specific upregulation of IL-2, IFN-γ, TNF-α, granzyme, and perforin and downregulation of IL-10, which suppresses the immune function [34]. $CD4^+$ T cells as T helper lymphocytes can assist $CD8^+$ cytotoxic T cells (CTLs) to exert cytotoxic effect. AFP-specific $CD4^+$ T and $CD8^+$ T cells kill the cancer cells mainly relying on the granzyme and perforin pathways without affecting the Fas/Fasl pathways [25, 34]. Although AFP is expected to play a certain role in antitumor immunity, it is still useless to stimulate the immune cells and produce substantial effects on cancer cells due to its weak immunogenicity. On the contrary, AFP contributes to the promotion of the change of $CD4^+$ T and $CD8^+$ T cell proportion and leads to tumor immune escape [33, 35]. Researchers measured $CD4^+$ T (Treg cells) in HCC patients, chronic hepatitis B patients, and healthy population and found that the quantity of Treg cells was high in the peripheral blood of HCC patients, which could inhibit antitumor immune responses and affect the function of $CD8^+$ T lymphocytes [33, 35]. By multiple ways suppressing the immune cells, HCC cells are able to escape immune surveillance and continue to grow in the body, showed as Figure 1, Box 1.

4. Role of AFP in Hepatocellular Carcinoma Immunity

AFP plays an important role in the regulation of cell proliferation, which may be mediated by receptor, signal transportation, and gene expression. Some studies have indicated that AFP is mainly present on the cell surface or inside the cytoplasm, and AFP in the cytoplasm is mediated by the endocytosis of the receptor into the cell [36]. In the AFP-positive tissue, AFP receptor (AFPR) is also positive, while in normal tissue or AFP-negative tissue, AFPR is also negative, indicating that the expression of AFP receptors in the cells is associated with AFP [36]. The promotion of tumor proliferation of AFP/AFPR is dependent on the CAMP-PKA pathway and the induction of Ca^{2+} influx [37]. AFP/AFPR brings about Ca^{2+} influx, so the intracellular Ca^{2+} increases, then the intracellular CAMP correspondingly rises, enhancing protease A activity, prompting DNA synthesis, and achieving the purpose of tumor cell proliferation [37].

The activation of immune response requires enhancing the ability of antigen-presenting cell uptake, processing and presenting antigen, so that T lymphocytes could be activated

Promotion of cancer cell proliferation mediated by the binding of AFP receptors (AFPR), the activation of PI3K/AKT signal pathway, the stimulation of oncogene protein, and the dysfunction of PTEN antioncogene protein [26–32].
Promotion of tumor invasion and metastasis via upregulating expression of metastasis-related proteins, such as keratin 19 (K19), epithelial cell adhesion molecule (EpCAM), matrix metalloproteinase 2/9 (MMP2/9), and CXC chemokine receptor 4 (CXCR4) [26, 27, 33].
Promotion of tumor angiogenesis by increasing expression of vascular endothelial growth factor (VEGF), vascular endothelial growth factor receptor 2 (VEGFR-2), and matrix metalloproteinases-2/9 (MMP2/9) [16, 26].
Antitumor apoptosis by blocking the Fas/FasL, caspase-3, and PI3K/AKT signaling pathways of tumor [13, 14, 16, 19, 27–29].
Escaping from immune surveillance via triggering the Fas/FasL interaction between tumor cells and lymphocytes; inhibiting the maturation and inducing apoptosis of DC cells; reducing the secretion of the amount of IL-12 from DC cells, thus indirectly inhibiting NK cell; promoting the change of $CD4^+$ T and $CD8^+$ T cell proportion; and enhancing the quantity of Treg cells [20–25, 33–35].

Box 1: The mechanisms of AFP promoting cancer cell proliferation.

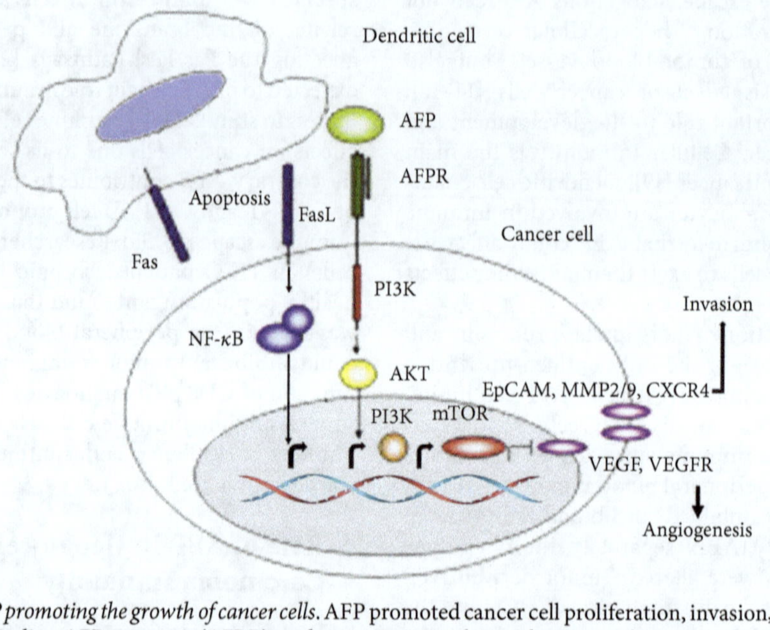

FIGURE 1: *Mechanisms of AFP promoting the growth of cancer cells.* AFP promoted cancer cell proliferation, invasion, and metastasis by inducing apoptosis of immune cells, binding AFP receptors (AFPR), and activating signal transduction pathways.

and the immune response is elicited [38]. Since AFP promotes the proliferation of liver cancer, it could be a new target for the immune therapy of liver cancer. However, despite exposure to high plasma levels of AFP during hepatocellular carcinoma development, only low immunity is mounted against the protein [36, 37]. How to overcome the immune tolerance of AFP is the key point of antitumor immunity. Studies have dissected the immunodominant epitopes of AFP in order to effectively use this protein for immunotherapy of AFP expressing tumors [39–41]. Researches confirmed that these identified epitope peptides could be recognized by the T cells *in vitro* and generated AFP-specific CTLs [39, 40]. Some epitopes of AFP have been found to be recognized by the major histocompatibility complex (MHC) class I or II molecular of APC cells [41]. When presented to $CD8^+$ T or $CD4^+$ T lymphocytes, the epitopes activated specific CTLs to secret high levels of TNF-α and IFN-γ and stimulated specific immune response against hepatocellular carcinoma [41, 42]. DC cells modified by the hAFP peptide (137–145) could successfully induce the peripheral blood mononuclear cells to be specific CTLs, and the immune response was better than that of the intact hAFP alone [43, 44]. Thus, AFP could be a promising candidate for immunotherapy. In this way, we may overcome the immune tolerance of AFP and eliminate the cancer cells.

Tumor immunity has the advantages of high efficiency and low toxicity, whose purpose is to start or restart the immune response independently and continuously and avoid the damage of autologous tissue cells. At present, clinical studies have confirmed that immunotherapy can improve the prognosis of patients with HCC [43]. It was found that when DC cells were incubated with AFP and IL-12, specific

Biomarker for HCC in clinical diagnosis, the evaluation of response to therapy, and the surveillance for tumor recurrence [5–12].
DNA vaccine constructed by the whole or partial AFP gene alone or fused with cytokines or modulation adjuvant such as GM-CSF, IL-2, and HSP70. [57–68].
Protein vaccine established via the whole or partial AFP protein alone or cross-linked with cytokines or modulation adjuvant and so forth [47, 49, 50].
Peptide vaccine recombined by AFP epitope peptides alone or combined with cytokines or modulation adjuvant and so forth [44–47, 49, 50, 67].
DC cell vaccine activated by pulsed with AFP protein or epitope peptides alone or combined with other TAAs, cytokines, or modulation adjuvant and so forth [45–48, 69–73].

Box 2: AFP and tumor immunity.

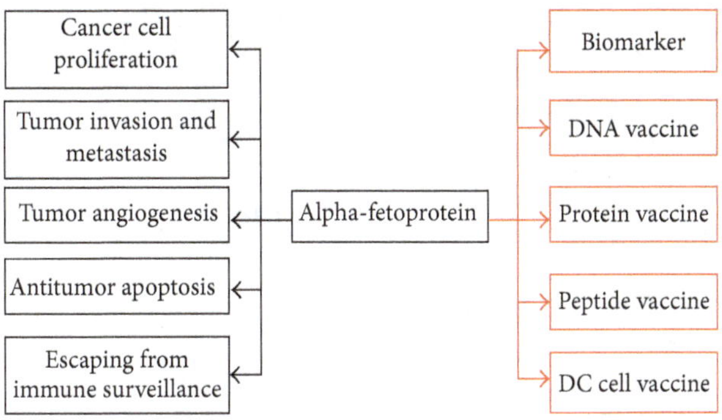

FIGURE 2: *AFP-a sword with two blades.* As an oncofetal antigen and diagnostic marker for liver cancer, AFP is a sword with two blades. AFP promoted tumor proliferation, invasion, angiogenesis, and escaping from immune surveillance, which could be an ideal target for immunotherapy. On the other side, AFP-modified DNA, protein, peptide vaccine, or DC cell vaccine displayed the specific antitumor immunity against AFP-positive liver cancers.

T lymphocytes were activated, resulting in a large number of IL-12 and TNF produced, and specifically attacking HCC cells. The study indicated that DC cells activated by AFP could be made for DC vaccine to induce specific immune effect [45–48]. Research found that the combination of the "internal immune adjuvant" heat shock protein 70 (HSP70) with AFP, forming a HSP70-AFP complex, enhanced AFP immunogenicity and stimulated the immune system to exert its effect [49, 50]. Heat shock protein has the property of "molecular chaperone," which can help the protein fold, transportation, repair, and degrade. Heat shock protein 70 can present antigen, activate the immune cells, and promote the transformation of Th0 cells to Th1. The tumor HSP70 may combine with a variety of tumor antigen peptides and present multiple antigen epitopes to T cells. HSP70 could activate stronger DC cells response and gain a large amount of cytokine release from the polyclonal T cells [51–53]. Studies have verified that the C-terminal of the HSP70 has immunogenicity and can stimulate the immune cells to produce chemokines, which is able to induce DC mature [51, 52]. The N-terminal of HSP70 plays an important role in presenting antigen peptide. The HSP70 presents antigen to APC cells by HSP70-peptide complexes, then activating CTLs by the interaction with MHC-class I molecules, promoting DC cells and macrophages to secrete inflammatory cytokines, upregulating $CD8^+$ T cells and IFN-γ content, and lowering the concentration of TGF-β1 [52].

5. Application of AFP in the Immunotherapy of Hepatocellular Carcinoma

Liver cancer vaccine aims to make use of HCC cells or antigen to induce the specific immune response, achieving the purpose of prevention and treatment of liver cancer. AFP as a tumor-associated antigen can promote the development of cancer and affect the expression of oncogene through the change of cAMP and Ca^{2+} concentration via binding with the cell membrane receptor [37]. Researches indicated that blocking AFP could inhibit the proliferation of hepatoma cells and induce apoptosis of cancer cells [54–56]. Therefore, AFP has become a new target for the treatment of liver cancer (Figure 2, Box 2).

Recently, there has been an increase in the development of therapeutic vaccines, which are expected to target specific tumor-antigens and boost the host's immune system. Thus, therapeutic vaccines can be considered for the treatment of HCC because about 70% of HCC patients express high levels of the alpha-fetoprotein (AFP), which can serve as a target for immunotherapy [3, 4]. However, because of the suppressing of cellular immunity and the immunologic tolerance of AFP, current treatments targeting AFP are generally weak and do not provide reliable antitumor protection [5]. A number of therapeutic approaches have been described to improve preexisting antitumor immunity, including recombinant plasmid DNA, chimeric virus-like particles, viral or bacterial vectors expressing AFP proteins, and adoptive transfer of tumor-specific T cells [57–62]. However, therapeutic vaccination is limited due to the low response of the immune system to AFP antigen. Therefore, there is a need to boost the host's immune response against AFP by improving the immunogenicity of AFP.

Polypeptide vaccine has the characteristics of immune response, safety, and easy production. At present, antivirus, anticancer, antimalaria, contraception, and other peptide vaccines are under clinical trials [62, 69–72, 74, 75]. In the immunotherapy of HCC, DC vaccine has showed good application prospects because of its specific and effective immune response in vivo. Current researches have focused on how to enhance the antigen-presenting function of DC cells and exert its strong ability to kill HCC cells [45–48]. Researches showed that DC cells stimulated with zoledronic acid could make T cells secrete large amounts of interferon and enhance the cytotoxic effects on CTLs [72]; DC cells separated from the patients with HCC were cocultured with IL-2 and GM-CSF for 2 days, and then implanting the DC cells through arterial catheter to the patients could make the serum produce a large number of IL-9, IL-15, and TNF, prolonging life in patients with HCC [69, 70, 72]. Clinical observation suggested that DC cells loaded with AFP showed good safety and tolerability for patients [69, 70]. The ability of CTLs induced by AFP antigen epitope polypeptide vaccine was stronger than that of oligopeptide vaccine, specially attacking AFP-positive tumor cells [71]. Recently, research found that DCs produced high levels of IFN-γ and TNF-α when pulsed with tumor-associated antigens (TAAs) and the percentage of regulatory T cells (Tregs) decreased in patients after DC-CTLs therapy [73], which may be a strategy to elicit effective immune response by combining AFP with other TAAs. Due to the weak immunogenicity, heat shock protein as a kind of "molecular chaperone" and "immune adjuvant" has attracted more attention. Most liver cancer cells express a high level of AFP and HSPs in the cytoplasm and HSPs could transport cytoplasm AFP to the cell membrane and release AFP antigen to serum [71, 72], which indicates that AFP could be an ideal target for immune attack. In a previous study, we introduced HSP70 and several AFP peptides into a eukaryotic expression vector and then injected the recombinant vector into mice. As a result, the recombinant vaccine encoding AFP and HSP70 produced effective AFP-specific T cell response and effectively suppressed the growth of tumor cells, eliciting robust protective immunity against AFP-positive tumors in vivo [73]. Consistent with the findings further researches have also confirmed that conjugating HSP70 to AFP antigen could improve the potency of AFP fusion vaccines [49, 50, 63–68]. In recent years, we developed a series of potential therapeutic proteins or peptide vaccines HSP70-AFP, HSP70-AFP-P, and gp96-AFP-P; the recombinant vaccine can induce specific antitumor immunity against AFP-positive tumor cells [49, 50, 67]. Most of all, a novel therapeutic vaccine, HSP70-P/AFP-P, was constructed to enhance the immunogenicity of AFP by conjugating AFP epitope peptide with the HSP70 functional peptide via peptide synthesis. The results verified that vaccination of mice with the novel HSP70-P/AFP-P vaccine mounted strong natural killer cell and $CD8^+$ T cell responses, inducing a protective effect against AFP-producing tumors in mice [68]. A systemic meta-analysis indicated that cellular immunotherapy was a feasible adjuvant treatment that could be beneficial for the improvement of short-term response and long-term survival of HCC patients after minimally invasive treatment [76]. Recently, clinical trials showed that nivolumab, a programmed cell death protein-1 (PD-1) immune checkpoint inhibitor, produced durable objective responses for treatment of HCC, indicating the possibility of combining nivolumab with AFP to suppress the proliferation of cancer cells [77]. However, the potential to revert an advanced HCC is a long way, which makes immunotherapy a very attractive adjuvant therapeutic option to be combined with other established treatments such as resection, transplantation, TACE, sorafenib/regorafenib, or nivolumab for the therapeutic design.

6. Summary

AFP plays an important role in the development of hepatocellular carcinoma, which can serve as a target for immunotherapy of HCC. Although the current application of immunotherapy for HCC is still on trial, immunotherapy has achieved certain effect in the treatment of liver cancer. With the rapid progress of research, immunotherapy as an important strategy is expected to bring a great prospect for HCC in the future.

Acknowledgments

This work is supported by Scientific Research Program Funded by Shaanxi University of Chinese Medicine and Shaanxi Provincial Education Department (nos. 2007JK233, 2009xj02, 2010JK484, and 14JS025), the Scientific Research Program of Shaanxi Administration of Traditional Chinese Medicine (nos. 15-SCJH001 and JCPT001), and the Natural Science Basic Research Plan in Shaanxi Province of China (nos. 2016JM8023 and 2016JM8150).

References

[1] J. G. Chen and S. W. Zhang, "Liver cancer epidemic in China: past, present and future," *Seminars in Cancer Biology*, vol. 21, no. 1, pp. 59–69, 2010.

[2] A. Obed, A. Bashir, and A. Jarrad, "Rapid virological response after early treatment with a combined therapy of ledipasvir and sofosbuvir in HCV genotype 4 after living donor liver transplantation in a HCC downstaged patient: Case report and review of the literature," *American Journal of Case Reports*, vol. 17, pp. 672–675, 2016.

[3] J. Bruix, G. J. Gores, and V. Mazzaferro, "Hepatocellular carcinoma: clinical frontiers and perspectives," *Gut*, vol. 63, no. 5, pp. 844–855, 2014.

[4] R. Wong and C. Frenette, "Updates in the management of hepatocellular carcinoma," *Journal of Gastroenterology and Hepatology*, vol. 7, no. 1, pp. 16–24, 2011.

[5] G. J. Mizejewski, "Does alpha-fetoprotein contribute to the mortality and morbidity of human hepatocellular carcinoma? A commentary," *Journal of Hepatocellular Carcinoma*, vol. Volume 3, pp. 37–40, 2016.

[6] F. Gao, H. K. Zhu, and Y. B. Zhu, "Predictive value of tumor markers in patients with recurrent hepatocellular carcinoma in different vascular invasion pattern," vol. 15, pp. 371–377, 2016.

[7] M.-A. Buendia and C. Neuveut, "Hepatocellular carcinoma," *Cold Spring Harbor Perspectives in Medicine*, vol. 5, no. 2, Article ID a021444, 2015.

[8] H. Toyoda, T. Kumada, T. Tada et al., "Clinical utility of highly sensitive Lens culinaris agglutinin-reactive alpha-fetoprotein in hepatocellular carcinoma patients with alpha-fetoprotein <20 ng/mL," *Cancer Science*, vol. 102, no. 5, pp. 1025–1031, 2011.

[9] J. Li, T. Gao, S. Gu, J. Zhi, J. Yang, and G. Li, "An electrochemical biosensor for the assay of alpha-fetoprotein-L3 with practical applications," *Biosensors and Bioelectronics*, vol. 87, pp. 352–357, 2017.

[10] Y. J. Yoon, K. Han, and D. Y. Kim, "Role of serum prothrombin induced by vitamin K absence or antagonist-II in the early detection of hepatocellular carcinoma in patients with chronic hepatitis B virus infection," *Scandinavian Journal of Gastroenterology*, vol. 44, no. 7, pp. 861–866, 2009.

[11] P. Stefaniuk, J. Cianciara, and A. Wiercinska-Drapalo, "Present and future possibilities for early diagnosis of hepatocellular carcinoma," *World Journal of Gastroenterology*, vol. 16, no. 4, pp. 418–424, 2010.

[12] Z. Zhang, Y. Zhang, Y. Wang, L. Xu, and W. Xu, "Alpha-fetoprotein-L3 and Golgi protein 73 may serve as candidate biomarkers for diagnosing alpha-fetoprotein-negative hepatocellular carcinoma," *OncoTargets and Therapy*, vol. 9, pp. 123–129, 2015.

[13] M. Dai, X. Chen, X. Liu et al., "Diagnostic value of the combination of golgi protein 73 and alpha-fetoprotein in hepatocellular carcinoma: A meta-analysis," *PLoS ONE*, vol. 10, no. 10, Article ID e0140067, 2015.

[14] M. Zhu, Y. Lu, W. Li et al., "Hepatitis B virus X protein driven alpha fetoprotein expression to promote malignant behaviors of normal liver cells and hepatoma cells," *Journal of Cancer*, vol. 7, no. 8, pp. 935–946, 2016.

[15] W. Meng, B. Bai, and Z. Bai, "The immunosuppression role of alpha-fetoprotein in human hepatocellular carcinoma," *Discovery Medicine*, vol. 21, no. 118, pp. 489–494, 2016.

[16] W. Meng, X. Li, Z. Bai et al., "Silencing alpha-fetoprotein inhibits VEGF and MMP-2/9 production in human hepatocellular carcinoma cell," *PLoS ONE*, vol. 9, no. 2, Article ID e90660, 2014.

[17] M. Li, H. Li, C. Li et al., "Alpha fetoprotein is a novel protein-binding partner for caspase-3 and blocks the apoptotic signaling pathway in human hepatoma cells," *International Journal of Cancer*, vol. 124, no. 12, pp. 2845–2854, 2009.

[18] W. Song, C. Song, and Y. Chen, "Polysaccharide-induced apoptosis in H22 cells through G2/M arrest and BCL2/BAX caspase-activated Fas pathway," *Cellular and Molecular Biolology (Noisy-le-grand)*, vol. 61, no. 7, pp. 88–95, 2015.

[19] N. Schmidt, C. Neumann-Haefelin, and R. Thimme, "Cellular immune responses to hepatocellular carcinoma: Lessons for immunotherapy," *Digestive Diseases*, vol. 30, no. 5, pp. 483–491, 2012.

[20] A. D. Pardee, J. Shi, and L. H. Butterfield, "Tumor-derived α-fetoprotein impairs the differentiation and T cell stimulatory activity of human dendritic cells," *The Journal of Immunology*, vol. 193, no. 11, pp. 5723–5732, 2014.

[21] S. Trompezinski, C. Migdal, M. Tailhardat et al., "Characterization of early events involved in human dendritic cell maturation induced by sensitizers: Cross talk between MAPK signalling pathways," *Toxicology and Applied Pharmacology*, vol. 230, no. 3, pp. 397–406, 2008.

[22] A. Vogt, E. Sievers, V. Lukacs-Kornek et al., "Improving immunotherapy of hepatocellular carcinoma (HCC) using dendritic cells (DC) engineered to express IL-12 in vivo," *Liver International*, vol. 34, no. 3, pp. 447–461, 2014.

[23] M. Yamamoto, T. Tatsumi, T. Miyagi et al., "α-Fetoprotein impairs activation of natural killer cells by inhibiting the function of dendritic cells," *Clinical & Experimental Immunology*, vol. 165, no. 2, pp. 211–219, 2011.

[24] N. Guerra, Y. X. Tan, N. T. Joncker et al., "NKG2D-Deficient Mice Are Defective in Tumor Surveillance in Models of Spontaneous Malignancy," *Immunity*, vol. 28, no. 4, pp. 571–580, 2008.

[25] Y. Liu, Y.-R. Wang, G.-H. Ding et al., "JAK2 inhibitor combined with DC-activated AFP-specific T-cells enhances antitumor function in a Fas/FasL signal-independent pathway," *OncoTargets and Therapy*, vol. 9, pp. 4425–4433, 2016.

[26] M.-S. Li, P.-F. Li, Q. Chen, G.-G. Du, and G. Li, "Alpha-fetoprotein stimulated the expression of some oncogenes in human hepatocellular carcinoma Bel 7402 cells," *World Journal of Gastroenterology*, vol. 10, no. 6, pp. 819–824, 2004.

[27] M. Li, H. Li, C. Li et al., "Alpha-fetoprotein: a new member of intracellular signal molecules in regulation of the PI3K/AKT signaling in human hepatoma cell lines," *International Journal of Cancer*, vol. 128, no. 3, pp. 524–532, 2011.

[28] M. Zhu, J. Guo, H. Xia et al., "Alpha-fetoprotein activates AKT/mTOR signaling to promote CXCR4 expression and migration of hepatoma cells," *Oncoscience*, vol. 2, no. 1, pp. 59–70, 2015.

[29] Y. Lu, M. Zhu, W. Li et al., "Alpha fetoprotein plays a critical role in promoting metastasis of hepatocellular carcinoma cells," *Journal of Cellular and Molecular Medicine*, vol. 20, no. 3, pp. 549–558, 2016.

[30] R. Yamaguchi, H. Yano, A. Iemura, S. Ogasawara, M. Haramaki, and M. Kojiro, "Expression of vascular endothelial growth factor in human hepatocellular carcinoma," *Hepatology*, vol. 28, no. 1, pp. 68–77, 1998.

[31] M. Li, X. Liu, S. Zhou, P. Li, and G. Li, "Effects of alpha fetoprotein on escape of Bel 7402 cells from attack of lymphocytes," *BMC Cancer*, vol. 5, article no. 96, 2005.

[32] L. Zhang, T. He, H. Cui, Y. Wang, C. Huang, and F. Han, "Effects of AFP gene silencing on apoptosis and proliferation of a hepatocellular carcinoma cell line.," *Discovery Medicine*, vol. 14, no. 75, pp. 115–124, 2012.

[33] K.-J. Chen, L. Zhou, H.-Y. Xie, T.-E. Ahmed, X.-W. Feng, and S.-S. Zheng, "Intratumoral regulatory T cells alone or in combination with cytotoxic T cells predict prognosis of hepatocellular carcinoma after resection," *Medical Oncology*, vol. 29, no. 3, pp. 1817–1826, 2012.

[34] S. M. Bray, L. Vujanovic, and L. H. Butterfield, "Dendritic cell-based vaccines positively impact natural killer and regulatory T cells in hepatocellular carcinoma patients," *Clinical and Developmental Immunology*, vol. 2011, Article ID 249281, 2011.

[35] Q. Gao, S.-J. Qiu, J. Fan et al., "Intratumoral balance of regulatory and cytotoxic T cells is associated with prognosis

of hepatocellular carcinoma after resection," *Journal of Clinical Oncology*, vol. 25, no. 18, pp. 2586–2593, 2007.

[36] P. Li, S.-S. Wang, H. Liu et al., "Elevated serum alpha fetoprotein levels promote pathological progression of hepatocellular carcinoma," *World Journal of Gastroenterology*, vol. 17, no. 41, pp. 4563–4571, 2011.

[37] M.-S. Li, P.-F. Li, S.-P. He, G.-G. Du, and G. Li, "The promoting molecular mechanism of alpha-fetoprotein on the growth of human hepatoma Bel7402 cell line," *World Journal of Gastroenterology*, vol. 8, no. 3, pp. 469–475, 2002.

[38] I. Mellman, G. Coukos, and G. Dranoff, "Cancer immunotherapy comes of age," *Nature*, vol. 480, no. 7378, pp. 480–489, 2011.

[39] L. H. Butterfield, A. Koh, W. Meng et al., "Generation of human T-cell responses to an HLA-A2.1-restricted peptide epitope derived from alpha-fetoprotein," *Cancer research*, vol. 59, no. 13, pp. 3134–3142, 1999.

[40] W. S. Meng, L. H. Butterfield, A. Ribas et al., "Fine specificity analysis of an HLA-A2.1-restricted immunodominant T cell epitope derived from human α-fetoprotein," *Molecular Immunology*, vol. 37, no. 16, pp. 943–950, 2001.

[41] L. H. Butterfield, W. S. Meng, A. Koh et al., "T Cell Responses to HLA-A*0201-Restricted Peptides Derived from Human Fetoprotein," *The Journal of Immunology*, vol. 166, no. 8, pp. 5300–5308, 2001.

[42] K. Hiroishi, J. Eguchi, T. Baba et al., "Strong $CD8^+$ T-cell responses against tumor-associated antigens prolong the recurrence-free interval after tumor treatment in patients with hepatocellular carcinoma," *Journal of Gastroenterology*, vol. 45, no. 4, pp. 451–458, 2010.

[43] J.-H. Lee, Y. Lee, M. Lee et al., "A phase I/IIa study of adjuvant immunotherapy with tumour antigen-pulsed dendritic cells in patients with hepatocellular carcinoma," *British Journal of Cancer*, vol. 113, no. 12, pp. 1666–1676, 2015.

[44] J.-Y. Yang, X. Li, L. Gao, Z.-H. Teng, and W.-C. Liu, "Co-transfection of dendritic cells with AFP and IL-2 genes enhances the induction of tumor antigen-specific antitumor immunity," *Experimental and Therapeutic Medicine*, vol. 4, no. 4, pp. 655–660, 2012.

[45] J.-Y. Yang, D.-Y. Cao, Y. Xue, Z.-C. Yu, and W.-C. Liu, "Improvement of dendritic-based vaccine efficacy against hepatitis B virus-related hepatocellular carcinoma by two tumor-associated antigen gene-infected dendritic cells," *Human Immunology*, vol. 71, no. 3, pp. 255–262, 2010.

[46] L. H. Butterfield, "Recent advances in immunotherapy for hepatocellular cancer," *Swiss Medical Weekly*, vol. 137, no. 5-6, pp. 83–90, 2007.

[47] Y. Liu, S. Daley, V. N. Evdokimova, D. D. Zdobinski, D. M. Potter, and L. H. Butterfield, "Hierarchy of α fetoprotein (AFP)-specific T cell responses in subjects with AFP-positive hepatocellular cancer," *The Journal of Immunology*, vol. 177, no. 1, pp. 712–721, 2006.

[48] A. D. Pardee, H. Yano, A. M. Weinstein et al., "Route of antigen delivery impacts the immunostimulatory activity of dendritic cell-based vaccines for hepatocellular carcinoma," *Journal for ImmunoTherapy of Cancer*, vol. 3, no. 1, article no. 32, 2015.

[49] Z. Li, X. P. Wang, H. P. Lin et al., "Anti-tumor immunity elicited by cross-linking vaccine heat shock protein 72 and alpha-fetoprotein epitope peptide," *Neoplasma*, vol. 62, no. 5, pp. 713–721, 2015.

[50] X.-P. Wang, H.-P. Lin, Q.-X. Wang, and Y. Gu, "Specific antitumor immunity induced by cross-linking complex heat shock protein 72 and alpha-fetoprotein," *Cancer Biotherapy and Radiopharmaceuticals*, vol. 27, no. 3, pp. 189–197, 2012.

[51] H. Wang, F. Feng, X.-P. Wang et al., "Dendritic cells pulsed with Hsp70 and HBxAg induce specific antitumor immune responses in hepatitis B virus-associated hepatocellular carcinoma," *Molecular Medicine Reports*, vol. 13, no. 2, pp. 1077–1082, 2016.

[52] D. S. Wheeler, K. E. Dunsmore, A. G. Denenberg, L. Muething, S. E. Poynter, and H. R. Wong, "Biological activity of truncated C-terminus human heat shock protein 72," *Immunology Letters*, vol. 135, no. 1-2, pp. 173–179, 2011.

[53] M. Shevtsov and G. Multhoff, "Heat shock protein-Peptide and HSP-based immunotherapies for the treatment of cancer," *Frontiers in Immunology*, vol. 7, article no. 171, 2016.

[54] T.-M. Hung, R.-H. Hu, C.-M. Ho et al., "Downregulation of alpha-fetoprotein expression by LHX4: A critical role in hepatocarcinogenesis," *Carcinogenesis*, vol. 32, no. 12, Article ID bgr219, pp. 1815–1823, 2011.

[55] H. Tang, X.-Y. Tang, M. Liu, and X. Li, "Targeting alpha-fetoprotein represses the proliferation of hepatoma cells via regulation of the cell cycle," *Clinica Chimica Acta*, vol. 394, no. 1-2, pp. 81–88, 2008.

[56] S.-H. Ma, G. G. Chen, J. Yip, and P. B. S. Lai, "Therapeutic effect of α-fetoprotein promoter-mediated tBid and chemotherapeutic agents on orthotopic liver tumor in mice," *Gene Therapy*, vol. 17, no. 7, pp. 905–912, 2010.

[57] A. Saeki, K. Nakao, Y. Nagayama et al., "Diverse efficacy of vaccination therapy using the α-fetoprotein gene against mouse hepatocellular carcinoma," *International Journal of Molecular Medicine*, 2004.

[58] C. F. Grimm, D. Ortmann, L. Mohr et al., "Mouse α-fetoprotein-specific DNA-based immunotherapy of hepatocellular carcinoma leads to tumor regression mice," *Gastroenterology*, vol. 119, no. 4, pp. 1104–1112, 2000.

[59] P. Hanke, M. Serwe, F. Dombrowski, T. Sauerbruch, and W. H. Caselmann, "DNA vaccination with AFP-encoding plasmid DNA prevents growth of subcutaneous AFP-expressing tumors and does not interfere with liver regeneration in mice," *Cancer Gene Therapy*, vol. 9, no. 4, pp. 346–355, 2002.

[60] W. S. Meng, L. H. Butterfield, A. Ribas et al., "α-fetoprotein-specific tumor immunity induced by plasmid prime-adenovirus boost genetic vaccination," *Cancer Research*, vol. 61, no. 24, pp. 8782–8786, 2001.

[61] F. Ghasemi, S. Rostami, M. Ghayour-Mobarhan, and Z. Meshkat, "Current progress in the development of therapeutic vaccines for chronic hepatitis B virus infection," *Iranian Journal of Basic Medical Sciences*, vol. 19, no. 7, pp. 692–704, 2016.

[62] M. Hirayama and Y. Nishimura, "The present status and future prospects of peptide-based cancer vaccines," *International Immunology*, vol. 28, no. 7, pp. 319–328, 2016.

[63] X. Wang, Y. Zhou, X. Ying, L. Guo, Y. Zhao, and Y. Fang, "Interaction between heat shock protein 72 and α-fetoprotein in human hepatocellular carcinomas," *Clinica Chimica Acta*, vol. 379, no. 1-2, pp. 158–162, 2007.

[64] X. Wang, Q. Wang, H. Lin, S. Li, L. Sun, and Y. Yang, "HSP72 and gp96 in gastroenterological cancers," *Clinica Chimica Acta*, vol. 417, pp. 73–79, 2013.

[65] X.-P. Wang, G.-Z. Liu, A.-L. Song, H.-Y. Li, and Y. Liu, "Anti-tumor immunity induced by DNA vaccine encoding alpha-fetoprotein/heat shock protein 70," *World Journal of Gastroenterology*, vol. 10, no. 21, pp. 3197–3200, 2004.

[66] Y.-H. Lan, Y.-G. Li, Z.-W. Liang et al., "A DNA vaccine against chimeric AFP enhanced by HSP70 suppresses growth of hepatocellular carcinoma," *Cancer Immunology, Immunotherapy*, vol. 56, no. 7, pp. 1009–1016, 2007.

[67] X.-P. Wang, Q.-X. Wang, H.-P. Lin, Y.-L. Wang, and Y. Yang, "Glycoprotein 96 and α-fetoprotein cross-linking complexes elicited specific antitumor immunity," *Cancer Biotherapy and Radiopharmaceuticals*, vol. 28, no. 5, pp. 406–414, 2013.

[68] X.-P. Wang, Q.-X. Wang, H.-P. Lin, B. Xu, Q. Zhao, and K. Chen, "Recombinant heat shock protein 70 functional peptide and alpha-fetoprotein epitope peptide vaccine elicits specific antitumor immunity," *Oncotarget* , vol. 7, no. 44, pp. 71274–71284, 2016.

[69] Y. Nakamoto, E. Mizukoshi, M. Kitahara et al., "Prolonged recurrence-free survival following OK432-stimulated dendritic cell transfer into hepatocellular carcinoma during transarterial embolization," *Clinical & Experimental Immunology*, vol. 163, no. 2, pp. 165–177, 2011.

[70] F. Tada, M. Abe, M. Hirooka et al., "Phase I/II study of immunotherapy using tumor antigen-pulsed dendritic cells in patients with hepatocellular carcinoma," *International Journal of Oncology*, vol. 41, no. 5, pp. 1601–1609, 2012.

[71] L. H. Butterfield, A. Ribas, W. S. Meng et al., "Tcell responses to HLA-A*0201 immunodominant peptides derived from alpha-fetoprotein in patients with hepatocellular cancer," *Clinical Cancer Research*, vol. 9, no. 16, part 1, pp. 5902–5908, 2003.

[72] L. H. Butterfield, A. Ribas, V. B. Dissette et al., "A phase I/II trial testing immunization of hepatocellular carcinoma patients with dendritic cells pulsed with four α-fetoprotein peptides," *Clinical Cancer Research*, vol. 12, no. 9, pp. 2817–2825, 2006.

[73] Y. Wang, X. Yang, Y. Yu et al., " Immunotherapy of patient with hepatocellular carcinoma using cytotoxic T lymphocytes ," *Journal of Cancer*, vol. 9, no. 2, pp. 275–287, 2018.

[74] M. R. Hollingdale and M. Sedegah, "Development of whole sporozoite malaria vaccines," *Expert Review of Vaccines*, vol. 16, no. 1, pp. 45–54, 2017.

[75] F. Cabillic, O. Toutirais, V. Lavoué et al., "Aminobisphosphonate-pretreated dendritic cells trigger successful Vγ9Vδ2 T cell amplification for immunotherapy in advanced cancer patients," *Cancer Immunology, Immunotherapy*, vol. 59, no. 11, pp. 1611–1619, 2010.

[76] M. Ding, Y. Wang, J. Chi et al., "Is adjuvant cellular immunotherapy essential after TACE-predominant minimally-invasive treatment for hepatocellular carcinoma? A systematic meta-analysis of studies including 1774 patients," *PLoS ONE*, vol. 11, no. 12, Article ID e0168798, 2016.

[77] A. B. El-Khoueiry, B. Sangro, T. Yau et al., "Nivolumab in patients with advanced hepatocellular carcinoma (CheckMate 040): an open-label, non-comparative, phase 1/2 dose escalation and expansion trial," *The Lancet*, vol. 389, no. 10088, pp. 2492–2502, 2017.

20

Metastatic Colorectal Cancer in the Era of Personalized Medicine: A More Tailored Approach to Systemic Therapy

Irene S. Yu[1] **and Winson Y. Cheung**[2]

[1] *University of British Columbia, Vancouver, Canada*
[2] *University of Calgary, Calgary, Canada*

Correspondence should be addressed to Winson Y. Cheung; winson.cheung@ahs.ca

Academic Editor: Maikel P. Peppelenbosch

Colorectal cancer is the second most common malignancy diagnosed in Canada. Despite declining incidence and mortality rates in recent years, there is still a significant number of cases that are metastatic at presentation. Fluoropyrimidine-based chemotherapy was the backbone of colorectal cancer treatment, but the addition of irinotecan and oxaliplatin to form combination regimens has significantly improved overall survival. In the past decade, the development of novel biologic agents including therapies directed against vascular endothelial growth factor and epidermal growth factor receptor has further altered the landscape of metastatic colorectal cancer treatment. However, clinical trials have demonstrated that not all patients respond to these therapies similarly and consideration must be given to individual patient- and tumor-related factors. A more tailored and biomarker driven approach to treatment selection can optimize outcomes and avoid unnecessary adverse effects. In this review article, we offer a comprehensive overview of the panel of clinical- and tumor-associated characteristics that influence treatment decisions in metastatic colorectal cancer and how this sets the foundation for a more personalized treatment strategy in oncology.

1. Introduction

Colorectal cancer (CRC) is the second most common malignancy in Canada with an estimated 26,800 new cases per year [1]. Approximately one-fifth of CRC cases are metastatic at the time of diagnosis [2]; a small proportion of these are potential candidates for curative metastasectomy or conversion therapy, but these are usually applicable to those with liver- or lung-limited metastases only. The remainder of metastatic CRC (mCRC) patients pursue systemic treatments, which have evolved significantly over the past 10 to 15 years. With best supportive care (BSC) alone, median overall survival (mOS) is approximately five months [3]. In the modern era of combination chemotherapy and newer biologic agents, overall survival can be extended to 2 years and longer [4]. There are growing efforts to personalize the treatment of mCRC so that appropriate subsets of patients are selected for specific therapies, with the goal of maximizing response and avoiding exposure to adverse effects. In this article, we summarize the most recent evidence on tumor- and patient-related factors that should be considered when selecting treatment options for patients with mCRC.

2. Evolution of Metastatic Colorectal Cancer Treatment

2.1. Chemotherapy Backbone. In the 1990s, 5-FU/leucovorin was the standard of care for treatment of mCRC, which resulted in mOS of up to 12 months [5, 6]. In 2000, Saltz et al. showed that the addition of irinotecan (IFL regimen) extended mOS by an additional 2 months when compared to 5-FU/leucovorin alone (14.8 versus 12.6 months, p=0.04) [7]. Subsequently, the Intergroup N9741 trial demonstrated superiority of FOLFOX over IFL, with mOS reaching close to 20 months (19.5 versus 15.0 months, p=0.0001) [8]. Due to the unfavourable toxicity profile of IFL, the FOLFIRI regimen was developed and found to have comparable survival outcomes to FOLFOX as evidenced in the GERCOR and GOIM trials [9, 10]. Thus, FOLFOX and FOLFIRI emerged as the new standard first-line chemotherapy options for the treatment of mCRC.

2.2. Addition of Biologic Agents. The development of biologic agents, namely, inhibitors of vascular endothelial growth factor (VEGF) and epidermal growth factor receptor (EGFR), began to further alter the landscape of mCRC treatment. The AVF 2107 study showed that the addition of bevacizumab to IFL resulted in significantly longer mOS (20.3 versus 15.6 months, p<0.001) [11]. The Intergroup N9741 trial was published in the same year and prompted many clinicians to add bevacizumab to the FOLFOX chemotherapy backbone. A pooled analysis by Hurwitz et al. confirmed that bevacizumab plus chemotherapy compared to chemotherapy alone resulted in modest improvements in mOS (18.7 versus 16.1 months, p=0.0003) and median progression free survival (mPFS) (8.8 versus 6.4 months, p<0.0001) [12]. The PRIME study showed that panitumumab, when added to FOLFOX, increased mPFS (9.6 versus 8.0 months, p=0.02) with a trend towards improved mOS (23.9 versus 19.7 months, p=0.072) in patients with KRAS wild-type (WT) tumors [13]. The addition of cetuximab to FOLFIRI yielded similar results in the CRYSTAL study, with longer mPFS (9.9 versus 8.4 months, p=0.0012) and mOS (23.5 versus 20.0 months, p=0.0093) [14]. Because of these previous studies, first-line therapy at the present time typically consists of either FOLFIRI or FOLFOX in combination with a biologic agent that targets either VEGF or EGFR.

More recently, further treatment options have been approved by the FDA, including aflibercept, ramucirumab, and regorafenib. These agents all work via antiangiogenesis mechanisms; they are generally reserved for use in the second line or later settings and provide only modest survival benefits of approximately 6 weeks [15–17]. Trifluridine-tipiracil (TAS-102) is an oral chemotherapy agent that was recently evaluated in the RECOURSE study among patients who were considered refractory or intolerant to conventional chemotherapy and biologic agents. The administration of TAS-102 was associated with a two-month prolongation in mOS (7.1 versus 5.3 months, p<0.001) [18]. This drug is already available for use in some Western countries. However, there is limited evidence thus far to guide clinicians on how best to select patients for these therapies or how best to sequence these available treatments. Predictive markers are greatly needed and represent an area of active research.

3. KRAS Status: Predicting Response to Anti-EGFR Agents

KRAS, also known as Kirsten Rat Sarcoma Viral oncogene homolog, is a gene located on human chromosome 12 that encodes for the KRAS protein, a GTP/GDP-binding protein involved in intracellular signal transduction in the EGFR pathway [19]. Activating KRAS mutations have been described in multiple malignancies, with downstream effects that include cell proliferation, antiapoptosis, and angiogenesis. KRAS mutations are found in more than 40% of CRC cases [20, 21], with point mutations involving exon 2 (codons 12 and 13) comprising about 95% of mutations [22]. However, more than 5,000 different KRAS mutations have been described in CRC tumors in the literature and the significance of these variants are less clear.

Cetuximab (Erbitux) is a recombinant human-mouse chimeric monoclonal antibody initially approved in 2004 for the treatment of EGFR-expressing mCRC tumors. It works via competitively binding to the extracellular domain of EGFR, to block phosphorylation and activation of downstream kinases. Early studies evaluated the role of anti-EGFR agents as add-on therapies when progression or intolerance to standard chemotherapy occurred. In the initial study by Cunningham et al., 329 irinotecan-refractory mCRC patients were randomized to cetuximab plus irinotecan versus cetuximab alone [23]. Response rates (22.9% versus 10.8%, p=0.007) and time to progression (4.1 versus 1.5 months, p<0.001) were significantly higher in the combination group, although mOS did not reach significance (8.6 versus 6.9 months, p=0.48). The benefit of cetuximab monotherapy was confirmed in the CO.17 trial by Jonker et al., which enrolled 572 pretreated patients and randomized them to receive either cetuximab or best supportive care (BSC) [24]. Cetuximab was associated with an improvement in PFS (HR 0.68, 95% CI 0.57 to 0.80, p<0.001) and OS (HR 0.77, 95% CI 0.64-0.92, p=0.005). Median survival was 6.1 months for the cetuximab group compared to 4.6 months for BSC.

Importantly, retrospective studies began to report an association between KRAS-WT status and EGFR therapy responsiveness [25, 26]. Karapetis et al. examined for KRAS exon 2 activating mutations in tumor samples from the CO.17 trial and found the benefit of cetuximab was restricted to the KRAS-WT group only [20]. With cetuximab, KRAS-WT patients experienced better mOS (9.5 versus 4.8 months, HR 0.55, 95% 0.41-0.74, p<0.001) and mPFS (3.7 versus 1.9 months, HR 0.40, 95% CI 0.30-0.54, p<0.001) compared to BSC. The KRAS-mutant (MT) cohort did not benefit from cetuximab with regard to PFS (HR 0.99, p=0.96) and OS (HR 0.98, p=0.89).

The role of cetuximab as part of first-line therapy was evaluated by Van Cutsem et al. in the CRYSTAL study [27]. A total of 1198 patients were randomized to compare FOLFIRI versus FOLFIRI plus cetuximab. A subsequent analysis had KRAS status available for 89% of patients from the original study. For KRAS-WT patients, FOLFIRI plus cetuximab significantly prolonged mOS (23.5 versus 20.0 months, HR 0.796, p=0.0093) and mPFS (9.9 versus 8.4 months, HR 0.696, p=0.0012) compared to FOLFIRI alone [14]. This benefit with cetuximab was not seen in KRAS-MT tumors in relation to PFS or OS.

Panitumumab (Vectibix) is a recombinant fully human monoclonal antibody approved in 2006 for EGFR-expressing mCRC after failing conventional chemotherapy regimens. Van Cutsem et al. randomized 463 patients who had progressed on standard chemotherapy to panitumumab versus BSC [28]. Panitumumab significantly prolonged PFS (HR 0.54, 95% CI 0.44-0.66, p<0.0001) but did not affect OS (HR 1.00, 95% 0.82 to 122). Amado et al. reanalyzed the data after obtaining KRAS status in 92% of the tumor samples [21]. Similar to cetuximab, panitumumab efficacy was restricted to KRAS-WT tumors. Treatment effect of panitumumab on PFS was significantly greater in the KRAS-WT (HR 0.45, 95% CI 0.34-0.59) compared to the KRAS-MT group (HR 0.99, 95% 0.73-1.36). Furthermore, 17% and 34% of the KRAS-WT group showed partial response and stable disease, respectively. In contrast, 0% and 12% in the KRAS-MT group experienced partial response and stable disease.

Panitumumab was further studied in the first-line setting in combination with chemotherapy. In the PRIME study, panitumumab was added to FOLFOX. KRAS results were available for 93% of the study participants. In the KRAS-WT cohort, panitumumab plus FOLFOX improved mPFS compared to FOLFOX alone (9.6 versus 8.0 months, HR 0.80, 95% CI 0.66-0.97, p=0.02) with a nonsignificant increase in OS [13]. In contrast, the KRAS-MT group had significantly reduced PFS (HR 1.29, 95% CI 1.04-1.62, p=0.02) and a trend towards worse mOS (15.5 versus 19.3 months, HR 1.24, 95% CI 0.98-1.57, p=0.068) with combination therapy versus FOLFOX alone. In a follow-up extension study, mOS reached significance at a median follow-up of 80 weeks, favoring panitumumab/FOLFOX for KRAS-WT tumors (HR=0.83, 95% CI 0.70-0.98, p=0.03) [29].

Most studies have focused on testing for KRAS mutations in exon 2, but KRAS-MT status in exon 2 alone does not consistently imply lack of response to anti-EGFR agents. Literature has suggested that other RAS mutations may also predict resistance to cetuximab and panitumumab [30, 31], including other exons of KRAS and NRAS. This has been reflected in the American Society of Clinical Oncology (ASCO) recommendations, which suggest the need for extended RAS testing prior to starting anti-EGFR therapy [32]. Recently, the FDA approved an extended RAS panel which detects 56 specific mutations in exons 2, 3, and 4 of both KRAS and NRAS genes. With respect to the optimal tissue used for testing, samples from the primary tumor and the metastatic site have shown good concordance for KRAS mutations, but evidence does not support reliable concordance rates for lymph node metastases or recurrent tumors [33, 34]. The recent development of circulating tumor DNA tests, or liquid biopsies, for the detection of KRAS mutants has shown variable concordance rates. Thus, these methods require further validation prior to widespread adoption and implementation [35, 36].

4. Impact of Primary Tumor Sidedness

It is known that tumors originating from different areas of the colon have distinct clinical and molecular characteristics. From an embryonic standpoint, the midgut gives rise to the right colon whereas the hindgut transforms into the left colon. This has epidemiological, pathological, and prognostic implications, but there has been emerging evidence to indicate that right- and left-sided tumors should also be treated differently. Most studies define left-sided (LS) tumors as those affecting the splenic flexure and areas distal to it, including the rectum [37], whereas right-sided (RS) tumors are proximal to the splenic flexure. Approximately two-thirds of CRC occur on the left side, with the remaining one-third affecting the right side [38]. RS cancers generally affect older patients and females, and the disease tends to be more advanced, poorly differentiated, and of mucinous pathology [39–41]. These RS (or proximal) tumors are also more likely to be associated with microsatellite instability, RAS/BRAF mutations, and CpG island methylator phenotype (CIMP)-high status [42]. In contrast, LS (or distal) tumors tend to carry frequent chromosomal instability and EGFR amplification. With respect to prognostication, RS tumors are associated with worse outcomes. A recent meta-analysis by Petrelli et al. looked at 1.4 million patients to determine the prognostic role of LS versus RS primary CRC localization; LS tumor location was associated with lower risk of death (HR 0.82, 95% CI 0.79-0.84, p<0.001) independent of disease stage [43].

New studies have reported that primary tumor localization (PTL) impacts specific treatment recommendations in the metastatic setting, specifically applicable to KRAS-WT patients [44, 45]. Holch et al. performed a meta-analysis and included 13 first-line trials to assess the prognostic and predictive role of RS versus LS CRC [46]. RS cancers were documented in 27% of cases, which is comparable to that reported in the literature. From a prognostic perspective, RS tumors were associated with worse PFS (HR 1.28, 95% CI 1.20-1.37, p<0.0001) and OS (HR 1.54, 95% CI 1.43-1.65, p<0.0001). The CRYSTAL and PRIME studies were analyzed together to see if PTL correlated with anti-EGFR therapy responsiveness. OS (HR 0.69, 95% CI 0.58-0.83, p<0.0001) and PFS (HR 0.65, 95% CI 0.54-0.79, p<0.0001) were significantly improved with first-line anti-EGFR therapy in the RAS-WT LS group, but not the RAS-WT RS cohort (OS HR 0.96, 95% CI 0.68-1.35, p=0.802 and PFS HR 0.82, 95% CI 0.57-1.19, p=0.307). Analysis of CALGB/SWOG 80405, FIRE-3, and PEAK studies evaluated the impact of both anti-EGFR and anti-VEGF agents. Similarly, LS tumors were associated with significantly improved OS (HR 0.71, 95% CI 0.58-0.85, p=0.0003) and a trend towards better PFS (HR 0.86, 95% CI 0.73-1.02, p=0.084) when treated with anti-EGFR therapy. Conversely, RS cancers were associated with significantly improved PFS (HR 1.53, 95% CI 1.16-2.01, p=0.003) and a trend towards improved OS (HR 1.3, 95% CI 0.97-1.74, p=0.081) with anti-VEGF agents.

These findings have altered practice with clinicians generally recommending the use of an anti-EGFR agent plus chemotherapy in the first-line setting in patients presenting with LS tumors that are RAS-WT, rather than bevacizumab. For RS tumors, there is a preference for bevacizumab combined with chemotherapy. We anticipate that major guidelines will be updated in the near future which will incorporate the use of PTL as a predictive marker for selecting therapy.

5. Microsatellite Instability: Its Role with Immunotherapy Agents

Microsatellite instability (MSI) results from a deficient mismatch repair system (dMMR), which is responsible for correcting nucleotide base mispairings that occur during DNA replication. The most commonly affected mismatch proteins include MLH1, MSH2, MSH6, and PMS2. MSI-high (MSI-H) status is present in 15% of CRC cases, with approximately 12% as sporadic cases and the remainder associated with Lynch

Syndrome [47]. MSI-H tumors harbor excessive mutations and can generate "neoantigens" which can serve as a target for immunotherapy agents [48].

Pembrolizumab is an IgG4 monoclonal antibody against programmed death (PD-1) and was evaluated by Le et al. in a phase II study in which 53 mCRC patients with dMMR and proficient MMR (pMMR) were treated with pembrolizumab [49, 50]. Disease control rate, defined as complete response, partial response and stable disease, was seen in 89% (25/28) and 16% (4/25) in the dMMR and pMMR groups, respectively. Median PFS and OS were not reached for dMMR patients and were 2.4 and 6 months for pMMR cohort, respectively. The CheckMate 142 phase II trial assessed the efficacy of nivolumab, another PD-1 immune checkpoint inhibitor [51]. Overman et al. reported that of the 74 heavily pretreated patients, 31% (23/74) of patients had a documented objective response and 69% (51/74) achieved disease control > 12 weeks. Median duration of response has not been reached in the most recent publication, and 8 patients had disease response lasting greater than one year. Both pembrolizumab and nivolumab appear to provide durable benefit to responders.

Despite the small size of these studies, the FDA has approved pembrolizumab and nivolumab for use in MSI-H mCRC that has progressed on chemotherapy. This is reflected in the most recent National Comprehensive Cancer Network (NCCN) guidelines for metastatic MSI-H CRC [52]. However, the widespread use of these immunotherapy agents is currently limited because the number of metastatic cases that are MSI-H is low [53]. Further exploration into other pathologic and genetic factors beyond MSI status as predictive factors is required. We also await results from the phase III KEYNOTE-177 study that is examining the use of first-line pembrolizumab versus investigator's choice of chemotherapy in MSI-H mCRC patients [54].

6. BRAF: Prognostic and Possible Predictive Factor

The BRAF gene is located on human chromosome 7 and encodes the BRAF protein, also known as serine/threonine-protein kinase B-Raf. It is a member of the Raf family of protein kinases involved in cellular signal transduction, downstream of KRAS. Activating BRAF mutations mostly occur in codon 600 and is known as the V600E mutation; this is found in < 10% of sporadic CRC cases [55]. There is strong evidence for its use as a prognostic factor compared to its predictive value, although data are emerging with respect to predicting response to anti-EGFR therapy.

Tran et al. identified 524 mCRC patients with known BRAF status and evaluated the impact of BRAF mutation on prognosis [56]. BRAF mutants (BRAF-MT) were significantly associated with poorer survival with mOS of 10.4 versus 34.6 months (p<0.001). The BRAF-MT group was more often linked to RS tumors and microsatellite instability. BRAF mutants also displayed a distinct pattern of metastatic spread with higher rates of peritoneal and distant lymph node involvement. Subsequent analyses of phase III trials have confirmed that BRAF-MT are indicators of worse prognosis [14, 57]. In a pooled analysis by Venderbosch et al., greater than 3000 patient samples were examined [58]. Patients with BRAF-MT status had worse PFS (HR 1.34, 95% CI 1.17-1.54) and OS (HR 1.91, 95% CI 1.66-2.19) when compared to their BRAF-WT counterpart.

There is growing evidence that tumors harboring the BRAF V600E mutation are not as likely to respond to anti-EGFR therapies, although studies have been conflicting. A meta-analysis by Pietrantonio et al. evaluated both cetuximab and panitumumab in both first and nonfirst-line settings; the addition of EGFR agents did not increase the benefit of standard therapy in the BRAF-MT group [59]. PFS (HR 0.88, 95% CI 0.67-1.14, p=0.33) and OS (HR 0.91, 95% CI 0.62-1.34, p=0.63) were not significantly different compared to the control group. Conversely, Rowland et al. also conducted a meta-analysis of 8 trials and found longer OS in BRAF-WT patients with the use of anti-eGFR therapy (HR 0.81, 95% 0.70-0.95) which was not seen in BRAF-MT patients. However, the test for interaction was not statistically significant, so the authors concluded that the observation may have been secondary to chance and there is presently insufficient evidence to show that BRAF-MT cancers respond differently to anti-EGFR agents [60].

Despite the variable results, the ESMO guidelines have recommended against using cetuximab or panitumumab in patients harboring a BRAF V600E mutation [61]. Studies are underway to evaluate whether the addition of a BRAF inhibitor (e.g., vemurafenib) can help improve outcomes in BRAF-MT patients when used in combination with anti-EGFR therapy [62].

7. Elderly Population

Approximately 60% of CRC are diagnosed in patients who are aged greater than 65 years [1], with a median age of diagnosis of 67 years among all cases. The proportion of older adults has been steadily increasing over the past few decades and it is expected to comprise one-quarter of the North American population by 2036 [63]. Hence it is also anticipated that the number of mCRC cases in the elderly will increase in the near future. This subset of the population has special considerations, yet historically they have been underrepresented in most clinical trials, with only one-third of clinical trial participants aged ≥ 65 years [64]. In recent years, there has been increasing recognition of the need to place more emphasis on geriatric oncology in order to address the impending increase in cancer burden in this population.

With aging, there is decline in the function of critical organs. Changes to liver and renal physiology may slow drug metabolism and elimination, which can increase treatment toxicities through variable pharmacokinetics and pharmacodynamics; bone marrow reserve also diminishes and older adults are more susceptible to chemotherapy-related cytopenias [65]. The presence of significant comorbidities also increases with age; hypertension and diabetes are the most common ailments in an observational study of newly diagnosed cancer patients [66]. This not only impacts the overall frailty status of the individual, but also has implications for some of the systemic agents that are commonly utilized in mCRC.

Chronological age does not correlate well with functional status and oncologists often utilize other tools to assess functional status. In 2005, the International Society of Geriatric Oncology (SIOG) published recommendations on the use of geriatric assessments [67], but their use in practice has been limited because they are usually very resource-intensive. Geriatric assessments refer to multidisciplinary evaluations that include multiple domains, consisting of an examination of a patient's functional status, psychological health, polypharmacy, comorbidities, nutrition, social support, and cognition. Because adoption of full geriatric assessments has been variable, SIOG subsequently released an updated review of 17 shorter screening tools commonly used in older cancer patients [68], and the consensus statement deemed that the G8 tool was the most robust. Thus, it was recommended as a possible initial screening tool to identify patients in need of further evaluation by full geriatric assessments. Of note, the Eastern Cooperative Oncology Group (ECOG) and Karnofsky Performance Status (KPS) assessments are also commonly used by oncologists in the adult population, but their utility in the elderly is questionable. In one study, with ECOG score of 1 as the cut-off, the sensitivity and specificity were 94% and 55% respectively for predicting fitness for treatment in the elderly [69]. Likewise, KPS was compared to geriatric assessments in two studies, and showed extreme variability in sensitivity and specificity, ranging from 29-78% and 44-91%, respectively, for a KPS cut-off value of < 80 [69, 70]. Unfortunately, there is a lack of standardization for geriatric assessments. Moreover, insufficient personnel and resources in a busy clinical practice may limit the widespread acceptance of their use. In general, use of a screening tool is currently suggested and if abnormal, a more comprehensive geriatric assessment is still recommended.

For fit elderly patients, treatment of mCRC generally mirrors that of younger adults with first-line doublet chemotherapy (FOLFOX or FOLFIRI) with or without a biologic agent. Multiple studies have suggested that use of fluoropyrimidine-oxaliplatin-containing regimens in the elderly results in similar mOS, mPFS, and response rates when compared to the younger population [71–73], although findings across studies have not always been consistent. One study by Arkenau et al. showed that mOS was significantly shorter in those > 70 (18.8 versus 14.4 months, p=0.013) which persisted in their multivariate analysis that adjusted for comorbidities and other confounders [72]. Cen et al. performed a population based study with over 46,000 older patients and found that oxaliplatin-containing regimens have higher incidences of adverse effects, including nausea, neutropenia, and neuropathy when compared to 5-FU alone [74]. With respect to FOLFIRI, evidence is also discordant but it appears to suggest comparable safety and efficacy in older and younger patients [75–77].

In moderately fit patients, it is reasonable to treat with a fluoropyrimidine (5-FU preferably) with bevacizumab based on available literature. The MRC FOCUS2 trial showed that 5-FU plus oxaliplatin resulted in a trend for better mPFS (5.8 versus 4.5 months, p=0.07) compared to 5-FU alone [78]. This trial was initiated at 80% of standard dosing, with the option of escalating the dose if the patient tolerated initial treatment. Based on the FFCD 2001-02 trial, investigators proposed trying infusional 5-FU based therapy alone as the addition of irinotecan did not significantly increase PFS or OS [77]. The AVEX trial by Cunningham et al. was a phase III trial which enrolled patients > 70 years only [79]. Patients received either bevacizumab plus capecitabine or capecitabine alone; the combination resulted in longer mPFS (9.1 versus 5.1 months, p<0.0001). However, one caveat is that capecitabine was associated with more treatment-related adverse effects versus short-term infusional 5-FU, despite the convenience of oral dosing. Bevacizumab must also be prescribed with caution as the risk of arterial thromboembolism is high in elderly patients, and clinicians should avoid its use in those with recent myocardial infarction, cerebrovascular accident, or severe uncontrolled hypertension.

For elderly patients with poor functional status, options include single agent fluoropyrimidine with 5-FU or capecitabine or an anti-EGFR inhibitor if they are KRAS-WT. In a retrospective analysis, Crosara Teixeira et al. examined the effects of chemotherapy on those with poor functional status (i.e., ECOG 3/4) [80]. When stratified by ECOG status, chemotherapy led to nonsignificant survival gain (6.8 versus 2.3 months, p=0.13) but sample size was limited with only 240 patients. For those with better performance status (i.e., ECOG 2), a pooled study of 9 trials by Sargent et al. showed that ECOG 2 patients derived similar benefit compared to those with ECOG 0/1, but there were more adverse effects and higher 60-day mortality (2.8 versus 12%, p<0.0001) in those with worse ECOG status [81]. However, the 5-FU bolus was typically omitted and the "stop and go" approach was also adopted by clinicians.

8. Diabetes: Special Considerations

Diabetes mellitus (DM) is a growing problem, with an estimated 10 million Canadians living with prediabetes or diabetes [82]. The prevalence is expected to increase by over 40% by 2025. DM itself is considered a moderate risk factor for CRC, with an estimated relative risk of 1.38 and 1.20 for colon and rectal malignancies, respectively, when compared to nondiabetics [83]. At this time, however, there are no specific surveillance recommendations for this particular group. Nevertheless, special considerations must be taken when treating mCRC patients who also have coexisting DM, as there are implications for their systemic treatment.

Up to 50% of diabetic patients have evidence of peripheral neuropathy [84], most typically manifesting as "stocking-glove" sensory loss affecting the longer axons preferentially. Thus, the use of oxaliplatin as a part of FOLFOX must be considered carefully. Oxaliplatin is associated with two distinct neurotoxicity syndromes, including acute neurotoxicity and chronic cumulative sensory neuropathy. The mechanism for the latter is hypothesized to be the entry of oxaliplatin into the dorsal root ganglion, leading to the apoptosis of neurons [85]. However, there has been conflicting evidence on the influence of DM on the incidence on oxaliplatin-induced neurotoxicity. In a retrospective pooled analysis of both adjuvant and metastatic CRC cases, Ramanathan et al. examined whether the diagnosis of DM affected the incidence and severity of peripheral neuropathy after oxaliplatin [86]. A total of 1587 patients were included and 8.5% had DM at baseline prior to oxaliplatin therapy; patients with preexisting peripheral neuropathy greater than grade 1 were excluded from the study. Overall, the incidence of grade 1, 2, and 3 peripheral neuropathy for patients with and without DM were similar (46.7% versus 45.0%; 26.7% versus 28.6%; 12.6% versus 13.0%, respectively). The authors therefore concluded that the presence of DM was not associated with an increased risk of peripheral neuropathy. Conversely, Ottaiano et al. examined 102 stage II/III CRC patients treated with capecitabine and oxaliplatin (CAPOX) adjuvant therapy and found a significant association between DM and the occurrence of chronic neurotoxicity (47.3% DM patients versus 1.2% non-DM patients, $p<0.0001$), but this study was limited by a small sample size (n=19 for DM) and the duration of chronic neuropathy was not clearly defined [87].

Studies have shown that the long-term effect of oxaliplatin on peripheral neuropathy is dose-related, with persistent neuropathy seen in 10-15% of patients after a cumulative dose greater than 780-850 mg/m2 [88]. In a retrospective study by Uwah et al., the presence of DM did not impact the severity of oxaliplatin-induced peripheral neuropathy but data suggested that DM patients may develop the complication at a lower mean cumulative dose of oxaliplatin compared to those without DM (388 mg/m2 versus 610 mg/m2) [89]. Furthermore, the time for 50% of patients to develop neuropathy was earlier for the DM group compared to the non-DM group (5th versus 8th cycle, $p=0.35$), although this was not statistically significant.

Individuals with DM may also experience frequent diarrhea, described in up to one-quarter of diabetics. This may be related to multiple mechanisms, including disordered motility due to diabetic autonomic neuropathy and/or diabetic medications such as metformin. There are limited data on the risk of diarrhea in DM patients receiving treatment for CRC. A cohort study by Meyerhardt et al. evaluated the impact of DM on chemotherapy-associated toxicity in stage II/III CRC and found that DM patients have an increase risk of treatment-related diarrhea when compared to non-DM individuals [90]. Hence, clinicians must educate patients about the risks of irinotecan, which frequently causes diarrhea.

One aspect that may be neglected while caring for CRC patients with DM is the risk of side effects from premedications, specifically dexamethasone which is commonly included as an antiemetic prior to and after receiving chemotherapy. Glucocorticoids affect glucose homeostasis via downregulation of glucose transporters in skeletal muscle, increased hepatic production of glucose, inhibition of insulin binding to its receptors on cellular surfaces, and decreased insulin secretion from islet cells [91]. Therefore, DM patients may experience high blood glucose levels when taking dexamethasone. Nonetheless, there are currently no guidelines supporting modified antiemetics for DM patients. In practice, oncologists should ask patients to monitor for hyperglycemia and adjust their antidiabetic medications accordingly, if required.

Overall, published literature does not appear to endorse a different treatment approach for CRC patients with or without DM [92]. The most concerning clinical issue is peripheral neuropathy, but based on limited data, preexisting DM does not appear to affect the incidence or severity of oxaliplatin-induced neuropathy. There is a suggestion that it may occur with lower cumulative doses and with fewer cycles. For the time being, clinicians should be particularly cognizant of this toxicity in their DM patients, and may need to discontinue oxaliplatin at an earlier point in the treatment trajectory in order to prevent long-term debilitating effects.

9. Screening and Surveillance Strategies

The most common strategies utilized in colorectal cancer screening include guaiac-based fecal occult blood test (FOBT), fecal immunochemical test (FIT), endoscopy, and CT colonography. Major guidelines vary slightly in their recommendations, but screening is generally recommended in those with average risk between the age of 50 to 75 years using FIT or an endoscopic procedure [93, 94]. Clinically, the FIT test is rapidly replacing the use of FOBT with the capability to detect human-specific globin. In a large meta-analysis by Wieten et al., the use of FIT was associated with less interval colorectal cancer diagnosed after a negative test compared to FOBT (pooled incidence rates of 20 versus 34 per 100,000 person-years) [95]. The optimal interval between time from a positive fecal test to colonoscopy is unclear, but a large cohort study of over 70,000 patients with positive test results showed that a delay beyond 10 months led to a higher risk of stage IV disease (OR 2.71, 95% CI 1.06-6.89) [96]. This risk was not seen in those who underwent a colonoscopy between 7 to 9 months after a positive fecal test. Thus, these data support a timely referral for endoscopic examination of the colon after a positive FIT test.

In those patients who are cured of their colon cancer, approximately 30% of stage I-III and up to 65% of stage IV patients will recur [97]. The recent COLOFOL trial showed that low intensity surveillance (CEA and CT scans at 12 and 36 months only) in over 2,500 patients with resected stage II and II disease was comparable to conventional surveillance strategies, in terms of frequency of recurrence detection, 5-year survival, and cancer-specific mortality [98]. Currently, most guidelines recommend CEA every 3 to 6 months along with a CT annually for the first 3 to 5 years [97]. With the emerging data, it is anticipated that these may be updated to reflect less frequent testing. For resected stage IV disease, ESMO and NCCN guidelines recommend more intensive imaging, with CT scans every 3 to 6 months for 2 to 3 years [52, 99]; given the heterogeneity of this population, surveillance is often individualized in practice.

10. Future Directions

As interest in the use of predictive clinical and genetic biomarkers continues to increase, human epidermal growth factor 2 (HER2) presents as an attractive target for further development. The HER2 oncogene encodes for a transmembrane glycoprotein receptor, which has a critical role in intracellular signal transduction pathways involved in cell growth, cell differentiation, and angiogenesis [100]. Its role in the pathogenesis of breast cancer is well-established and the success of trastuzumab has significantly impacted the treatment of HER2-positive breast cancer [101]. A small proportion of CRC also overexpresses HER2, which can be detected through immunohistochemical staining, in situ hybridization for gene amplification, or polymerase chain reaction for RNA overexpression. In the phase II HERACLES trial, 914 KRAS-WT mCRC patients were screened for HER2 positivity; 48 (5%) patients were identified as HER2+ and 27 patients were eligible to receive trastuzumab and lapatinib. After a median follow-up of 94 weeks, 30% (8/27) patients had an objective response and 44% (12/27) achieved stable disease [102]. In the recent phase IIa multiple basket MyPathway study, trastuzumab and pertuzumab achieved 38% (14/37, 95% CI 0.23-0.55) objective response rates [103]. It is anticipated that further studies will attempt to clarify the promising role of HER2+ targeted agents, although widespread use may be limited by the small proportion of mCRC that overexpress the oncogene.

There is significant interest in looking at different targets involved in the mitogen-activated protein kinase (MAPK) pathway, which is responsible for regulating fundamental cellular processes such as growth, proliferation, differentiation, migration and apoptosis [104]. The pathway consists of multiple signalling molecules including RAS, RAF, MEK, and ERK; abnormalities along this pathway play a critical role in oncogenesis and hence present as potential targets for therapy. It was hypothesized that MEK inhibitors may work in synergy with PD-L1 inhibitors by upregulating MHC class 1 expression to increase antigen presentation on the surface of tumor cells for recognition by T cells [105]. The MEK inhibitor cobimetinib was studied in combination with the PD-L1 inhibitor atezolizumab in the phase III trial IMblaze370 consisting of 363 metastatic colorectal cancer patients, 91.7% of whom had MSS or MSI-low tumors [106]. However, it did not meet its primary endpoint for OS when comparing it versus regorafenib (8.9 versus 8.5 months, HR 1.0, 95% CI 0.73-1.38). There is an ongoing phase II study of BRAF/MEK inhibition in combination with PD-L1 blockade in BRAF V600E mutants, which can provide insight into another subset of this population [107].

Results are more promising for BRAF/MEK inhibitors in combination with anti-EGFR therapy in the treatment of BRAF V600E mutated cases. The combination of BRAF/MEK inhibitors have been shown to extend PFS and OS in BRAF-mutated metastatic melanoma [108] but melanoma cells express low levels of EGFR activity. The benefit of utilizing BRAF inhibitors does not apply to colorectal cancer due to the rapid feedback activation of EGFR [109]. The phase III BEACON trial is currently recruiting 640 patients to study the efficacy of combination BRAF inhibitor encorafenib, MEK inhibitor binimetinib and anti-EGFR agent cetuximab. Safety lead-in results were presented at GI ASCO, which included 30 patients with an overall response rate of 41%, with tumor regression observed in all but one patient [110]. Updated data at ESMO showed PFS of 8 months, with OS not yet reached [111]. Subsequently, the FDA has granted breakthrough therapy designation for the triplet therapy.

11. Conclusion

As the second most common malignancy in the developed world, the burden of CRC will continue to grow, especially with the aging population. Despite the implementation of routine CRC screening at the population level, a substantial proportion of CRC are still diagnosed at the metastatic stage. Fortunately, there has been significant progress in the development of new targeted therapies in the past decade. When used as monotherapy or in combination with preexisting chemotherapy, improvements in survival have been achieved. Currently, one of the most pressing issues is finding more effective ways to leverage these advances by selecting the right patients for the right therapy at the right time. Tailoring existing therapies based on tumor sidedness, KRAS, MSI, or BRAF status as well as individualizing treatments for elderly or DM patients represent our current efforts to provide more personalized care in oncology. However, these likely reflect only initial steps and more work is clearly warranted on furthering our understanding on additional clinical and pathological characteristics that can be used to personalize treatment in CRC.

References

[1] Canadian Cancer Society's Advisory Committee on Cancer Statistics, Canadian Cancer Statistics 2017, Canadian Cancer Society, Toronto, Canada.

[2] National Cancer Institute Surveillance, Epidemiology, and End Results program, "Cancer Stat Facts: Colorectal Cancer," https://seer.cancer.gov/statfacts/html/colorect.html, (retrieved March 1, 2018).

[3] W. Scheithauer, H. Rosen, G.-V. Kornek, C. Sebesta, and D. Depisch, "Randomised comparison of combination chemotherapy plus supportive care with supportive care alone in patients with metastatic colorectal cancer," *British Medical Journal*, vol. 306, no. 6880, pp. 752–755, 1993.

[4] V. Heinemann, L. F. von Weikersthal, T. Decker et al., "Folfiri plus cetuximab versus folfiri plus bevacizumab as first-line treatment for patients with metastatic colorectal cancer (fire-3): a randomised, open-label, phase 3 trial," *The Lancet Oncology*, vol. 15, pp. 1065–1075, 2014.

[5] M. A. Poon, M. J. O'Connell, C. G. Moertel et al., "Biochemical modulation of fluorouracil: Evidence of significant improvement of survival and quality of life in patients with advanced colorectal carcinoma," *Journal of Clinical Oncology*, vol. 7, no. 10, pp. 1407–1418, 1989.

[6] N. Petrelli, H. O. Douglas Jr., L. Herrera et al., "The modulation of fluorouracil with leucovorin in metastatic colorectal carcinoma: A prospective randomized phase III trial," *Journal of Clinical Oncology*, vol. 7, no. 10, pp. 1419–1426, 1989.

[7] L. B. Saltz, J. V. Cox, C. Blanke et al., "Irinotecan plus fluorouracil and leucovorin for metastatic colorectal cancer," *The New England Journal of Medicine*, vol. 343, no. 13, pp. 905–914, 2000.

[8] R. M. Goldberg, D. J. Sargent, R. F. Morton et al., "A randomized controlled trial of fluorouracil plus leucovorin, irinotecan, and oxaliplatin combinations in patients with previously untreated metastatic colorectal cancer," *Journal of Clinical Oncology*, vol. 22, no. 1, pp. 23–30, 2004.

[9] C. Tournigand, T. André, E. Achille et al., "FOLFIRI followed by FOLFOX6 or the reverse sequence in advanced colorectal cancer: a randomized GERCOR study," *Journal of Clinical Oncology*, vol. 22, no. 2, pp. 229–237, 2004.

[10] G. Colucci, V. Gebbia, G. Paoletti et al., "Phase III randomized trial of FOLFIRI versus FOLFOX4 in the treatment of advanced colorectal cancer: a Multicenter Study of the Gruppo Oncologico Dell'Italia Meridionale," *Journal of Clinical Oncology*, vol. 23, no. 22, pp. 4866–4875, 2005.

[11] H. Hurwitz, L. Fehrenbacher, W. Novotny et al., "Bevacizumab plus irinotecan, fluorouracil, and leucovorin for metastatic colorectal cancer," *The New England Journal of Medicine*, vol. 350, no. 23, pp. 2335–2342, 2004.

[12] H. I. Hurwitz, N. C. Tebbutt, F. Kabbinavar et al., "Efficacy and safety of bevacizumab in metastatic colorectal cancer: Pooled analysis from seven randomized controlled trials," *The Oncologist*, vol. 18, no. 9, pp. 1004–1012, 2013.

[13] J.-Y. Douillard, S. Siena, J. Cassidy et al., "Randomized, phase III trial of panitumumab with infusional fluorouracil, leucovorin, and oxaliplatin (FOLFOX4) versus FOLFOX4 alone as first-line treatment in patients with previously untreated metastatic colorectal cancer: the prime study," *Journal of Clinical Oncology*, vol. 28, no. 31, pp. 4697–4705, 2010.

[14] E. Van Cutsem, C.-H. Köhne, I. Láng et al., "Cetuximab plus irinotecan, fluorouracil, and leucovorin as first-line treatment for metastatic colorectal cancer: updated analysis of overall survival according to tumor KRAS and BRAF mutation status," *Journal of Clinical Oncology*, vol. 29, no. 15, pp. 2011–2019, 2011.

[15] E. van Cutsem, J. Tabernero, R. Lakomy et al., "Addition of aflibercept to fluorouracil, leucovorin, and irinotecan improves survival in a phase III randomized trial in patients with metastatic colorectal cancer previously treated with an oxaliplatin-based regimen," *Journal of Clinical Oncology*, vol. 30, no. 28, pp. 3499–3506, 2012.

[16] J. Tabernero, T. Yoshino, A. L. Cohn et al., "Ramucirumab versus placebo in combination with second-line FOLFIRI in patients with metastatic colorectal carcinoma that progressed during or after first-line therapy with bevacizumab, oxaliplatin, and a fluoropyrimidine (RAISE): a randomised, double-blind, multicentre, phase 3 study," *The Lancet Oncology*, vol. 16, no. 5, pp. 499–508, 2015.

[17] A. Grothey, E. Van Cutsem, A. Sobrero et al., "Regorafenib monotherapy for previously treated metastatic colorectal cancer (CORRECT): an international, multicentre, randomised, placebo-controlled, phase 3 trial," *The Lancet*, vol. 381, no. 9863, pp. 303–312, 2013.

[18] R. J. Mayer, E. Van Cutsem, A. Falcone et al., "Randomized trial of TAS-102 for refractory metastatic colorectal cancer," *The New England Journal of Medicine*, vol. 372, no. 20, pp. 1909–1919, 2015.

[19] S. Jančík, J. Drábek, D. Radzioch, and M. Hajdúch, "Clinical relevance of KRAS in human cancers," *Journal of Biomedicine and Biotechnology*, vol. 2010, Article ID 150960, 13 pages, 2010.

[20] C. S. Karapetis, S. Khambata-Ford, D. J. Jonker et al., "K-ras mutations and benefit from cetuximab in advanced colorectal cancer," *The New England Journal of Medicine*, vol. 359, no. 17, pp. 1757–1765, 2008.

[21] R. G. Amado, M. Wolf, M. Peeters et al., "Wild-type KRAS is required for panitumumab efficacy in patients with metastatic colorectal cancer," *Journal of Clinical Oncology*, vol. 26, no. 10, pp. 1626–1634, 2008.

[22] C. Tan and X. Du, "KRAS mutation testing in metastatic colorectal cancer," *World Journal of Gastroenterology*, vol. 18, no. 37, pp. 5171–5180, 2012.

[23] D. Cunningham, Y. Humblet, S. Siena et al., "Cetuximab monotherapy and cetuximab plus irinotecan in irinotecan-refractory metastatic colorectal cancer," *The New England Journal of Medicine*, vol. 351, no. 4, pp. 337–345, 2004.

[24] D. J. Jonker, C. J. O'Callaghan, C. S. Karapetis et al., "Cetuximab for the treatment of colorectal cancer," *The New England Journal of Medicine*, vol. 357, no. 20, pp. 2040–2048, 2007.

[25] F. di Fiore, F. Blanchard, F. Charbonnier et al., "Clinical relevance of KRAS mutation detection in metastatic colorectal cancer treated by Cetuximab plus chemotherapy," *British Journal of Cancer*, vol. 96, no. 8, pp. 1166–1169, 2007.

[26] A. Lièvre, J.-B. Bachet, V. Boige et al., "KRAS mutations as an independent prognostic factor in patients with advanced colorectal cancer treated with Cetuximab," *Journal of Clinical Oncology*, vol. 26, no. 3, pp. 374–379, 2008.

[27] E. van Cutsem, C.-H. Köhne, E. Hitre et al., "Cetuximab and chemotherapy as initial treatment for metastatic colorectal cancer," *The New England Journal of Medicine*, vol. 360, no. 14, pp. 1408–1417, 2009.

[28] E. Van Cutsem, M. Peeters, S. Siena et al., "Open-label phase III trial of panitumumab plus best supportive care compared with best supportive care alone in patients with chemotherapy-refractory metastatic colorectal cancer," *Journal of Clinical Oncology*, vol. 25, no. 13, pp. 1658–1664, 2007.

[29] J.-Y. Douillard, S. Siena, J. Cassidy et al., "Final results from PRIME: randomized phase III study of panitumumab with FOLFOX4 for first-line treatment of metastatic colorectal cancer," *Annals of Oncology*, vol. 25, no. 7, pp. 1346–1355, 2014.

[30] M. J. Sorich, M. D. Wiese, A. Rowland, G. Kichenadasse, R. A. McKinnon, and C. S. Karapetis, "Extended RAS mutations and anti-EGFR monoclonal antibody survival benefit in metastatic colorectal cancer: a meta-analysis of randomized, controlled trials," *Annals of Oncology*, vol. 26, no. 1, pp. 13–21, 2015.

[31] M. Peeters, K. S. Oliner, T. J. Price et al., "Analysis of KRAS/NRAS mutations in a phase III study of panitumumab with FOLFIRI compared with FOLFIRI alone as second-line treatment for metastatic colorectal cancer," *Clinical Cancer Research*, vol. 21, no. 24, pp. 5469–5479, 2015.

[32] C. J. Allegra, R. B. Rumble, S. R. Hamilton et al., "Extended *RAS* gene mutation testing in metastatic colorectal carcinoma to predict response to anti-epidermal growth factor receptor monoclonal antibody therapy: American Society of Clinical Oncology Provisional Clinical Opinion Update 2015," *Journal of Clinical Oncology*, vol. 34, no. 2, pp. 179–185, 2016.

[33] C.-B. Han, F. Li, J.-T. Ma, and H.-W. Zou, "Concordant KRAS mutations in primary and metastatic colorectal cancer tissue specimens: A meta-analysis and systematic review," *Cancer Investigation*, vol. 30, no. 10, pp. 741–747, 2012.

[34] K. H. Lee, J. S. Kim, C. S. Lee, and J. Y. Kim, "KRAS discordance between primary and recurrent tumors after radical resection of colorectal cancers," *Journal of Surgical Oncology*, vol. 111, no. 8, pp. 1059–1064, 2015.

[35] J. Grasselli, E. Elez, G. Caratù et al., "Concordance of blood- and tumor-based detection of RAS mutations to guide anti-EGFR therapy in metastatic colorectal cancer," *Annals of Oncology*, vol. 28, no. 6, pp. 1294–1301, 2017.

[36] N. Normanno, R. Esposito Abate, M. Lambiase et al., "RAS testing of liquid biopsy correlates with the outcome of metastatic colorectal cancer patients treated with first-line FOLFIRI plus cetuximab in the CAPRI-GOIM trial," *Annals of Oncology*, vol. 29, no. 1, pp. 112–118, 2018.

[37] A. P. Venook, "Right-sided vs left-sided colorectal cancer," *Clinical Advances in Hematology Oncology*, vol. 15, no. 1, pp. 1–3, 2017.

[38] R. Meza, J. Jeon, A. G. Renehan, and E. G. Luebeck, "Colorectal cancer incidence trends in the United States and United Kingdom: Evidence of right- to left-sided biological gradients with implications for screening," *Cancer Research*, vol. 70, no. 13, pp. 5419–5429, 2010.

[39] S. L. Saltzstein and C. A. Behling, "Age and time as factors in the left-to-right shift of the subsite of colorectal adenocarcinoma: A study of 213,383 cases from the California Cancer Registry," *Journal of Clinical Gastroenterology*, vol. 41, no. 2, pp. 173–177, 2007.

[40] A. G. M. T. Powell, R. Wallace, R. F. Mckee et al., "The relationship between tumour site, clinicopathological characteristics and cancer-specific survival in patients undergoing surgery for colorectal cancer," *Colorectal Disease*, vol. 14, no. 12, pp. 1493–1499, 2012.

[41] F. Benedix, R. Kube, F. Meyer, U. Schmidt, I. Gastinger, and H. Lippert, "Comparison of 17,641 patients with right- and left-sided colon cancer: Differences in epidemiology, perioperative course, histology, and survival," *Diseases of the Colon & Rectum*, vol. 53, no. 1, pp. 57–64, 2010.

[42] E. Missiaglia, B. Jacobs, G. D'Ario et al., "Distal and proximal colon cancers differ in terms of molecular, pathological, and clinical features," *Annals of Oncology*, vol. 25, no. 10, pp. 1995–2001, 2014.

[43] F. Petrelli, G. Tomasello, K. Borgonovo et al., "Prognostic survival associated with left-sided vs right-sided colon cancer a systematic review and meta-analysis," *JAMA Oncology*, vol. 3, no. 2, pp. 211–219, 2017.

[44] S. Y. Brulé, D. J. Jonker, C. S. Karapetis et al., "Location of colon cancer (right-sided versus left-sided) as a prognostic factor and a predictor of benefit from cetuximab in NCIC CO.17," *European Journal of Cancer*, vol. 51, no. 11, pp. 1405–1414, 2015.

[45] S. Tejpar, S. Stintzing, F. Ciardiello et al., "Prognostic and predictive relevance of primary tumor location in patients with ras wild-type metastatic colorectal cancer retrospective analyses of the CRYSTAL and FIRE-3 trials," *JAMA Oncology*, vol. 3, no. 2, pp. 194–201, 2017.

[46] J. W. Holch, I. Ricard, S. Stintzing, D. P. Modest, and V. Heinemann, "The relevance of primary tumour location in patients with metastatic colorectal cancer: A meta-analysis of first-line clinical trials," *European Journal of Cancer*, vol. 70, pp. 87–98, 2017.

[47] C. R. Boland and A. Goel, "Microsatellite instability in colorectal cancer," *Gastroenterology*, vol. 138, no. 6, pp. 2073–2087, 2010.

[48] C. Granier, E. De Guillebon, C. Blanc et al., "Mechanisms of action and rationale for the use of checkpoint inhibitors in cancer," *ESMO Open*, vol. 2, no. 2, 2017.

[49] D. T. Le, J. N. Uram, H. Wang et al., "Programmed death-1 blockade in mismatch repair deficient colorectal cancer," *Journal of Clinical Oncology*, vol. 34, no. 15, pp. 103-103, 2016.

[50] D. T. Le, J. N. Uram, H. Wang et al., "PD-1 blockade in tumors with mismatch-repair deficiency," *The New England Journal of Medicine*, vol. 372, no. 26, pp. 2509–2520, 2015.

[51] M. J. Overman, R. McDermott, J. L. Leach et al., "Nivolumab in patients with metastatic DNA mismatch repair-deficient or microsatellite instability-high colorectal cancer (CheckMate 142): An open-label, multicentre, phase 2 study," *The Lancet Oncology*, vol. 18, no. 9, pp. 1182–1191, 2017.

[52] The NCCN Clinical Practice Guidelines in Oncology, "Colon Cancer, Version 3.2018," https://www.nccn.org/professionals/physician_gls/pdf/colon.pdf, (retrieved October 15, 2018). (retrieved October 15, 2018).

[53] P. Boland and W. Ma, "Immunotherapy for colorectal cancer," *Cancers* , vol. 9, no. 5, p. 50, 2017.

[54] U. S. National Library of Medicine, "Study of Pembrolizumab (MK-3475) vs Standard Therapy in Participants With Microsatellite Instability-High (MSI-H) or Mismatch Repair Deficient (dMMR) Stage IV Colorectal Carcinoma (MK-3475-177/KEYNOTE-177)," https://clinicaltrials.gov/ct2/show/NCT02563002 (retrieved March 10, 2018).

[55] D. Barras, "BRAF mutation in colorectal cancer: an update," *Biomarkers in Cancer*, vol. 7, pp. 9–12, 2015.

[56] B. Tran, S. Kopetz, J. Tie et al., "Impact of BRAF mutation and microsatellite instability on the pattern of metastatic spread and prognosis in metastatic colorectal cancer," *Cancer*, vol. 117, no. 20, pp. 4623–4632, 2011.

[57] T. S. Maughan, R. A. Adams, C. G. Smith et al., "Addition of cetuximab to oxaliplatin-based first-line combination chemotherapy for treatment of advanced colorectal cancer: results of the randomised phase 3 MRC COIN trial," *The Lancet*, vol. 377, no. 9783, pp. 2103–2114, 2011.

[58] S. Venderbosch, I. D. Nagtegaal, T. S. Maughan et al., "Mismatch repair status and BRAF mutation status in metastatic colorectal cancer patients: a pooled analysis of the CAIRO, CAIRO2, COIN, and FOCUS studies," *Clinical Cancer Research*, vol. 20, no. 20, pp. 5322–5330, 2014.

[59] F. Pietrantonio, F. Petrelli, A. Coinu et al., "Predictive role of BRAF mutations in patients with advanced colorectal cancer receiving cetuximab and panitumumab: A meta-analysis," *European Journal of Cancer*, vol. 51, no. 5, article no. 9390, pp. 587–594, 2015.

[60] A. Rowland, M. M. Dias, M. D. Wiese et al., "Meta-analysis of BRAF mutation as a predictive biomarker of benefit from anti-EGFR monoclonal antibody therapy for RAS wild-type metastatic colorectal cancer," *British Journal of Cancer*, vol. 112, no. 12, pp. 1888–1894, 2015.

[61] E. Van Cutsem, A. Cervantes, R. Adam et al., "ESMO consensus guidelines for the management of patients with metastatic colorectal cancer," *Annals of Oncology*, vol. 27, no. 8, pp. 1386–1422, 2016.

[62] S. Kopetz, S. L. McDonough, H. Lenz et al., "Randomized trial of irinotecan and cetuximab with or without vemurafenib in BRAF-mutant metastatic colorectal cancer (SWOG S1406)," *Journal of Clinical Oncology*, vol. 35, no. 15, pp. 3505-3505, 2017.

[63] Statistics Canada, "An Aging Population,"https://www.statcan.gc.ca/pub/11-402-x/2010000/chap/pop/pop02-eng.htm, (retrieved March 2, 2018).

[64] L. Talarico, G. Chen, and R. Pazdur, "Enrollment of elderly patients in clinical trials for cancer drug registration: A 7-year experience by the US Food and Drug Administration," *Journal of Clinical Oncology*, vol. 22, no. 22, pp. 4626–4631, 2004.

[65] B. Given and C. W. Given, "Older adults and cancer treatment," *Cancer*, vol. 113, no. 12, pp. 3505–3511, 2008.

[66] J. F. Piccirillo, A. Vlahiotis, L. B. Barrett, K. L. Flood, E. L. Spitznagel, and E. W. Steyerberg, "The changing prevalence of comorbidity across the age spectrum," *Critical Review in Oncology/Hematology*, vol. 67, no. 2, pp. 124–132, 2008.

[67] M. Extermann, M. Aapro, R. Bernabei et al., "Use of comprehensive geriatric assessment in older cancer patients: recommendations from the task force on CGA of the International Society of Geriatric Oncology (SIOG)," *Critical Review in Oncology/Hematology*, vol. 55, no. 3, pp. 241–252, 2005.

[68] L. Decoster, K. Van Puyvelde, S. Mohile et al., "Screening tools for multidimensional health problems warranting a geriatric assessment in older cancer patients: An update on SIOG recommendations," *Annals of Oncology*, vol. 26, no. 2, pp. 288–300, 2015.

[69] C. Owusu, S. M. Koroukian, M. Schluchter, P. Bakaki, and N. A. Berger, "Screening older cancer patients for a Comprehensive Geriatric Assessment: A comparison of three instruments," *Journal of Geriatric Oncology*, vol. 2, no. 2, pp. 121–129, 2011.

[70] S. Luce, S. De Breucker, A. Van Gossum et al., "How to identify older patients with cancer who should benefit from comprehensive geriatric assessment?" *Journal of Geriatric Oncology*, vol. 3, no. 4, pp. 351–358, 2012.

[71] J. Sastre, E. Aranda, B. Massutí et al., "Elderly patients with advanced colorectal cancer derive similar benefit without excessive toxicity after first-line chemotherapy with oxaliplatin-based combinations: Comparative outcomes from the 03-TTD-01 phase III study," *Critical Review in Oncology/Hematology*, vol. 70, no. 2, pp. 134–144, 2009.

[72] H.-T. Arkenau, U. Graeven, S. Kubicka et al., "Oxaliplatin in combination with 5-fluorouracil/leucovorin or capecitabine in elderly patients with metastatic colorectal cancer," *Clinical Colorectal Cancer*, vol. 7, no. 1, pp. 60–64, 2008.

[73] A. Figer, N. Perez-Staub, E. Carola et al., "FOLFOX in patients aged between 76 and 80 years with metastatic colorectal cancer: An exploratory cohort of the OPTIMOX1 study," *Cancer*, vol. 110, no. 12, pp. 2666–2671, 2007.

[74] P. Cen, C. Liu, and X. L. Du, "Comparison of toxicity profiles of fluorouracil versus oxaliplatin regimens in a large population-based cohort of elderly patients with colorectal cancer," *Annals of Oncology*, vol. 23, no. 6, pp. 1503–1511, 2012.

[75] J. Souglakos, A. Pallis, S. Kakolyris et al., "Combination of irinotecan (CPT-11) plus 5-fluorouracil and leucovorin (FOLFIRI regimen) as first line treatment for elderly patients with metastatic colorectal cancer: A phase II trial," *Oncology*, vol. 69, no. 5, pp. 384–390, 2005.

[76] E. François, J.-F. Berdah, E. Chamorey et al., "Use of the folinic acid/5-fluorouracil/irinotecan (FOLFIRI 1) regimen in elderly patients as a first-line treatment for metastatic colorectal cancer: A Phase II study," *Cancer Chemotherapy and Pharmacology*, vol. 62, no. 6, pp. 931–936, 2008.

[77] T. Aparicio, S. Lavau-Denes, J. M. Phelip et al., "Randomized phase III trial in elderly patients comparing LV5FU2 with or without irinotecan for first-line treatment of metastatic colorectal cancer (FFCD 2001-02)," *Annals of Oncology*, vol. 27, no. 1, pp. 121–127, 2016.

[78] M. T. Seymour, L. C. Thompson, H. S. Wasan et al., "Chemotherapy options in elderly and frail patients with metastatic colorectal cancer (MRC FOCUS2): An open-label, randomised factorial trial," *The Lancet*, vol. 377, no. 9779, pp. 1749–1759, 2011.

[79] D. Cunningham, I. Lang, E. Marcuello et al., "Bevacizumab plus capecitabine versus capecitabine alone in elderly patients with previously untreated metastatic colorectal cancer (AVEX): an open-label, randomised phase 3 trial," *The Lancet Oncology*, vol. 14, no. 11, pp. 1077–1085, 2013.

[80] M. Crosara Teixeira, D. F. Marques, A. C. Ferrari et al., "The effects of palliative chemotherapy in metastatic colorectal cancer patients with an ecog performance status of 3 and 4," *Clinical Colorectal Cancer*, vol. 14, no. 1, pp. 52–57, 2015.

[81] D. J. Sargent, C. H. Köhne, H. K. Sanoff et al., "Pooled safety and efficacy analysis examining the effect of performance status on outcomes in nine first-line treatment trials using individual data from patients with metastatic colorectal cancer," *Journal of Clinical Oncology*, vol. 27, no. 12, pp. 1948–1955, 2009.

[82] Diabetes Canada, "Diabetes Statistics in Canada," http://www.diabetes.ca/how-you-can-help/advocate/why-federal-leader-ship-is-essential/diabetes-statistics-in-canada, (retrieved March 2, 2018).

[83] H. Yuhara, C. Steinmaus, S. E. Cohen, D. A. Corley, Y. Tei, and P. A. Buffler, "Is diabetes mellitus an independent risk factor for colon cancer and rectal cancer?" *American Journal of Gastroenterology*, vol. 106, no. 11, pp. 1911–1921, 2011.

[84] A. M. Aring, D. E. Jones, and J. M. Falko, "Evaluation and prevention of diabetic neuropathy," *American Family Physician*, vol. 71, no. 11, pp. 2123–2128, 2005.

[85] L. E. Ta, L. Espeset, J. Podratz, and A. J. Windebank, "Neurotoxicity of oxaliplatin and cisplatin for dorsal root ganglion neurons correlates with platinum-DNA binding," *NeuroToxicology*, vol. 27, no. 6, pp. 992–1002, 2006.

[86] R. K. Ramanathan, M. L. Rothenberg, A. de Gramont et al., "Incidence and evolution of oxaliplatin-induced peripheral sensory neuropathy in diabetic patients with colorectal cancer: a pooled analysis of three phase III studies," *Annals of Oncology*, vol. 21, no. 4, pp. 754–758, 2010.

[87] A. Ottaiano, A. Nappi, S. Tafuto et al., "Diabetes and body mass index are associated with neuropathy and prognosis in colon cancer patients treated with capecitabine and oxaliplatin adjuvant chemotherapy," *Oncology*, vol. 90, no. 1, pp. 36–42, 2016.

[88] M. W. Saif and J. Reardon, "Management of oxaliplatin-induced peripheral neuropathy," *Therapeutics and Clinical Risk Management*, vol. 1, no. 4, pp. 249–258, 2005.

[89] A. N. Uwah, J. Ackler, J. C. Leighton Jr., S. Pomerantz, and W. Tester, "The effect of diabetes on oxaliplatin-induced peripheral neuropathy," *Clinical Colorectal Cancer*, vol. 11, no. 4, pp. 275–279, 2012.

[90] J. A. Meyerhardt, P. J. Catalano, D. G. Haller et al., "Impact of diabetes mellitus on outcomes in patients with colon cancer," *Journal of Clinical Oncology*, vol. 21, no. 3, pp. 433–440, 2003.

[91] A. Rafacho, H. Ortsäter, A. Nadal, and I. Quesada, "Glucocorticoid treatment and endocrine pancreas function: implications for glucose homeostasis, insulin resistance and diabetes," *Journal of Endocrinology*, vol. 223, no. 3, pp. R49–R62, 2014.

[92] A. Iyengar, H. T. Gold, J. Nicholson, and D. J. Becker, "Association of diabetes with colorectal cancer treatment and outcomes," *Journal of Clinical Oncology*, vol. 35, no. 15, 2017.

[93] The NCCN Clinical Practice Guidelines in Oncology, "Colorectal Cancer Screening, Version 1.2018," (retrieved October 15, 2018).

[94] A. M. Wolf, E. T. Fontham, T. R. Church et al., "Colorectal cancer screening for average-risk adults: 2018 guideline update from the American Cancer Society," *CA: A Cancer Journal for Clinicians*, vol. 68, no. 4, pp. 250–281, 2018.

[95] E. Wieten, E. H. Schreuders, E. J. Grobbee et al., "Incidence of faecal occult blood test interval cancers in population-based colorectal cancer screening: a systematic review and meta-analysis," *Gut*, 2018.

[96] D. A. Corley, C. D. Jensen, V. P. Quinn et al., "Association between time to colonoscopy after a positive fecal test result and risk of colorectal cancer and cancer stage at diagnosis," *Journal of the American Medical Association*, vol. 317, no. 16, pp. 1631–1641, 2017.

[97] E. P. Van Der Stok, M. C. W. Spaander, D. J. Grünhagen, C. Verhoef, and E. J. Kuipers, "Surveillance after curative treatment for colorectal cancer," *Nature Reviews Clinical Oncology*, vol. 14, no. 5, pp. 297–315, 2017.

[98] P. Wille-Jørgensen, I. Syk, K. Smedh et al., "Effect of more vs less frequent follow-up testing on overall and colorectal cancer–specific mortality in patients with stage II or III colorectal cancer," *Journal of the American Medical Association*, vol. 319, no. 20, pp. 2095–2103, 2018.

[99] E. Van Cutsem, A. Cervantes, B. Nordlinger, D. Arnold, and The ESMO Guidelines Working Group, "Metastatic colorectal cancer: ESMO clinical practice guidelines for diagnosis, treatment and follow-up," *Annals of Oncology*, vol. 25, pp. iii1–iii9, 2014.

[100] M. M. Moasser, "The oncogene HER2: its signaling and transforming functions and its role in human cancer pathogenesis," *Oncogene*, vol. 26, no. 45, pp. 6469–6487, 2007.

[101] M. J. Piccart-Gebhart, M. Procter, B. Leyland-Jones et al., "Trastuzumab after adjuvant chemotherapy in HER2-positive breast cancer," *The New England Journal of Medicine*, vol. 353, no. 16, pp. 1659–1672, 2005.

[102] A. Sartore-Bianchi, L. Trusolino, C. Martino et al., "Dual-targeted therapy with trastuzumab and lapatinib in treatment-refractory, KRAS codon 12/13 wild-type, HER2-positive metastatic colorectal cancer (HERACLES): a proof-of-concept, multicentre, open-label, phase 2 trial," *The Lancet Oncology*, vol. 17, no. 6, pp. 738–746, 2016.

[103] J. D. Hainsworth, F. Meric-Bernstam, C. Swanton et al., "Targeted therapy for advanced solid tumors on the basis of molecular profiles: Results from mypathway, an open-label, phase IIA multiple basket study," *Journal of Clinical Oncology*, vol. 36, no. 6, pp. 536–542, 2018.

[104] A. S. Dhillon, S. Hagan, O. Rath, and W. Kolch, "MAP kinase signalling pathways in cancer," *Oncogene*, vol. 26, no. 22, pp. 3279–3290, 2007.

[105] E. J. Brea, C. Y. Oh, E. Manchado et al., "Kinase regulation of human MHC class i molecule expression on cancer cells," *Cancer Immunology Research*, vol. 4, no. 11, pp. 936–947, 2016.

[106] J. Bendell, F. Ciardiello, J. Tabernero et al., "Efficacy and safety results from IMblaze370, a randomised Phase III study comparing atezolizumab+cobimetinib and atezolizumab monotherapy vs regorafenib in chemotherapy-refractory metastatic colorectal cancer," *Annals of Oncology*, vol. 29, supplement 5, 2018.

[107] ClinicalTrials.gov, "Dabrafenib + Trametinib + PDR001 in Colorectal Cancer," https://clinicaltrials.gov/ct2/show/NCT03668431, (retrieved October 15, 2018).

[108] G. V. Long, D. Stroyakovskiy, H. Gogas et al., "Combined BRAF and MEK inhibition versus BRAF inhibition alone in melanoma," *The New England Journal of Medicine*, vol. 371, no. 20, pp. 1877–1888, 2014.

[109] A. Prahallad, C. Sun, S. Huang et al., "Unresponsiveness of colon cancer to BRAF(V600E) inhibition through feedback activation of EGFR," *Nature*, vol. 483, no. 7387, pp. 100–104, 2012.

[110] E. Van Cutsem, P. Cuyle, and S. Huijberts, "BEACON CRC study safety lead-in (SLI) in patients with BRAFV600E metastatic colorectal cancer (mCRC): Efficacy and tumor markers," *Journal of Clinical Oncology*, vol. 36, no. 4, 2018.

[111] E. Van Cutsem, P. Cuyle, S. Huijberts et al., "BEACON CRC study safety lead-in: Assessment of the BRAF inhibitor encorafenib + MEK inhibitor binimetinib + anti–epidermal growth factor receptor antibody cetuximab for BRAFV600E metastatic colorectal cancer," *Annals of Oncology*, vol. 29, supplement 5, 2018.

21

Short-Term Outcome of Patients with Cirrhosis and Concurrent Portal Cavernoma Presenting with Acute Variceal Bleeding

Xuefeng Luo, Wanqin Wang, Xiaoli Fan, Ying Zhao, Xiaoze Wang, Jinlin Yang, and Li Yang

Department of Gastroenterology and Hepatology, West China Hospital, Sichuan University, Chengdu, China

Correspondence should be addressed to Li Yang; yangli_hx@scu.edu.cn

Academic Editor: Andrea Mancuso

Background and Aim. The outcome of cirrhotic patients with main portal vein occlusion and portal cavernoma after the first episode of acute variceal bleeding (AVB) is unknown. We compared short-term outcomes after AVB in cirrhotic patients with and without portal cavernoma. *Methods.* Between January 2009 and September 2014, 28 patients with cirrhosis and portal cavernoma presenting with the first occurrence of AVB and 56 age-, sex-, and Child-Pugh score-matched cirrhotic patients without portal cavernoma were included. The primary endpoints were 5-day treatment failure and 6-week mortality. *Results.* The 5-day treatment failure rate was higher in the cavernoma group than in the control group (32.1% versus 12.5%; $p = 0.031$). The 6-week mortality rate did not differ between the cavernoma and control group (25% versus 12.5%, $p = 0.137$). Multivariable Cox proportional hazard regression analyses revealed that 5-day treatment failure (HR = 1.223, 95% CI = 1.082 to 1.384; $p = 0.001$) independently predicted 6-week mortality. *Conclusions.* Cirrhotic patients with AVB and portal cavernoma have worse short-term prognosis than patients without portal cavernoma. The 5-day treatment failure was an independent risk factor for 6-week mortality in patients with cirrhosis and portal cavernoma.

1. Introduction

Acute variceal bleeding (AVB) remains one of the most dangerous complications of portal hypertension and is associated with significant morbidity and mortality in patients with cirrhosis [1]. Despite the advances in AVB management, 6-week mortality still remains high and is related to the severity of the underlying cirrhosis, hepatic venous pressure gradient (HVPG), and the presence of portal vein thrombosis [1–5].

With the increased frequency of liver imaging modalities, portal vein thrombosis (PVT) is increasingly identified in the setting of liver cirrhosis. The estimated prevalence of PVT in these patients varies from 5 to 26% [6, 7]. The chronic PVT may result in main portal vein occlusion and cavernous transformation, while the obstructed portal vein is replaced by a network of hepatopetal vessels [8]. The presence of portal cavernoma negatively affects the prognosis of these patients because of the resultant further increases in portal hypertension, with an increased risk of variceal bleeding, and, furthermore, the extension of PVT may increase the risk of perioperative morbidity and mortality or exclude patients from liver transplantation [9, 10].

The effect of main portal vein occlusion and cavernous transformation on the short-term outcomes of patients with cirrhosis and AVB has not been previously described. The aim of the present study was to evaluate the short-term outcomes of patients with cirrhosis and concurrent main portal vein occlusion and portal cavernoma admitted due to the first episode of AVB in a retrospective matched study.

2. Materials and Methods

2.1. Study Cohort. This retrospective cohort study included consecutive patients with cirrhosis, admitted to West China Hospital (a 4800-bed tertiary medical center in China) from January 2009 to September 2014, with the first episode of AVB and portal cavernoma. Liver cirrhosis was diagnosed by liver biopsy and/or clinical and imaging findings. For each identified patient, 2 patients with cirrhosis and the first episode of AVB without the presence of PVT, admitted during the same period, were matched for age, sex, and Child-Pugh score. Patients with hepatocellular carcinoma were excluded. This study was approved by the Institutional Review Board of West China Hospital.

2.2. Treatments. Vasoactive drugs (somatostatin) were administered to every patient as soon as possible after gastrointestinal bleeding and before endoscopic examination. Endoscopic treatment was performed in patients diagnosed with bleeding from gastroesophageal varices on endoscopy. Endoscopic variceal banding and endoscopic glue injection were used as the primary therapies for bleeding from esophageal or gastric varices, respectively.

2.3. Data Collection and Definition. Complete baseline data were collected through electronic medical records. These data included demographic information, etiology of liver cirrhosis, and basic laboratory information including regular blood tests, hepatic and renal function tests, prothrombin time, international normalized ratio (INR), Child-Pugh score and Model for End-Stage Liver Diseases (MELD) scores, imaging findings on color Doppler ultrasound, contrast-enhanced computed tomography (CT) and magnetic resonance imaging (MRI), and information about the treatments, including endoscopic therapy, surgery, and use of β-blockers.

The diagnosis of portal cavernoma was based on contrast-enhanced CT or MRI, in which the main portal vein was completely obstructed and replaced by fibrous tissue with the development of a hepatopetal network of periportal collateral veins. The time frame for an acute bleeding episode was 120 h (5 days). Five-day treatment failure was defined as uncontrolled index variceal bleeding, rebleeding, or death within 5 days. In particular, we defined the control of active variceal bleeding as a lack of hematemesis; the hemoglobin (Hb) level was stable without requiring blood transfusions or hemodynamic stability for 24 h after drug therapy and endoscopic treatment. Early rebleeding was defined by any of the following events, whichever occurred first: fresh hematemesis or NG aspiration of 100 ml of fresh blood 2 h after the start of vasoactive drugs alone or in combination with endoscopic therapy; development of hypovolemic shock; or a 3 g decrease in Hb (9% drop of Ht) within any 24 h period if no transfusion is administered [11].

2.4. Statistical Analysis. Quantitative variables were expressed as the mean ± standard deviation, and Student's t-test was performed to assess the difference between variables. Qualitative variables were expressed as frequencies and were analyzed using Pearson's $\chi 2$ test or Fisher's exact test. The cumulative incidence of 6-week mortality rate was estimated using the Kaplan–Meier method and compared using the log-rank test. Independent predictors with a p value < 0.05 in univariate analysis were included in the multivariate analyses. Multivariate analyses were performed using Cox regression analysis. Individual variables already included in the Child-Pugh score or MELD score were not considered separately. The risks estimated from the Cox regression models were expressed as hazard ratios (HRs) with their respective 95% confidence intervals (CIs). A two-tailed p value of <0.05 was considered statistically significant. Statistical analysis was performed using SPSS for windows (version 19.0; SPSS, Chicago, IL).

3. Results

3.1. Characteristics of the Cohorts. Twenty-eight patients with cirrhosis and concurrent portal cavernoma presenting with the first episode of AVB were admitted in our hospital during the period of the study. Fifty-six age-, sex-, and Child-Pugh score-matched patients with cirrhosis who experienced the first incident of AVB without PVT were selected from the overall population of patients during the same time period. Overall, a total of 84 patients were enrolled in the study.

The clinical and laboratory characteristics of the cohort are summarized in Table 1. The most common etiology for liver cirrhosis was Hepatitis B Virus infection (60%) followed by alcoholic liver disease (13%). The mean Child-Pugh and MELD score at the time of hospital admission were 8.1 ± 1.9 and 15.8 ± 5.4, respectively. Bleeding originated from esophageal varices in 22 patients (78.6%), from gastric varices in 2 patients (7.1%), and from unknown site in 4 (14.3%) in the cavernoma group. Source of bleeding was esophageal varices in 40 patients (71.4%), gastric varices in 10 patients (17.9%), and unknown in 6 (10.7%) in the control group. These two groups had comparable clinical and laboratory data, except for the higher platelet level, more incidences of ascites and previous splenectomy in the cavernoma group.

3.2. 5-Day Treatment Failure. Table 2 shows the main outcomes of the cohort of patients. Failure to control the index-bleeding episode occurred in 5 cases in the cavernoma group and in 3 cases in the control group. The frequency of index bleeding was not controlled successfully by initial therapy and did not differ significantly between the cavernoma group and the control group (17.9% versus 5.4%, $p = 0.066$). In the cavernoma group, 2 patients were treated with balloon tamponade as a rescue therapy. One patient died of massive bleeding before further intervention could be performed, and 2 patients received pharmacological therapy alone. All 3 patients in the control group underwent transjugular intrahepatic portosystemic shunt (TIPS) as a salvage therapy.

Of the 67 patients in whom index bleeding was controlled successfully without rescue therapy, 6 (9.0%) patients rebled from varices within the first 5 days of their hospital admission. However, the rate of recurrent variceal bleeding did not differ significantly between these two groups (14.3% versus 3.6%, $p = 0.072$). Five patients (3 in the cavernoma group and 2 in the control group) died within the 5-day treatment period.

Ultimately, 5-day treatment failure occurred in 9 out of 28 patients (32.1%) in the cavernoma group and in 7 out of 56 patients (12.5%) in the control group. The rate of 5-day treatment failure was higher in the cavernoma group compared with the control group ($p = 0.031$). Among all of the subjects, no significant independent predictor of 5-day

TABLE 1: Demographics and clinical characteristics at admission.

Characteristic	The cavernoma group (n = 28)	The control group (n = 56)	p value
Age, years	53.1 ± 11.9	53.3 ± 11.8	0.487
Sex, male, %	19/9	38/18	1
Cause of liver disease, n			0.580
Chronic HBV infection	19	31	
Chronic HCV infection	0	2	
Alcohol	3	9	
others	6	14	
Hemoglobin, g/L	79.6 ± 23.9	73.2 ± 23.5	0.242
Platelet, 1000/mm3	121.7 ± 101.9	84.7 ± 57.1	0.036
WBC	5.3 ± 3.1	9.1 ± 11.3	0.091
Creatinine, μmol/L	70.0 ± 20.4	76.4 ± 20.9	0.962
ALT, IU/L	30.3 ± 19.7	41.0 ± 56.2	0.330
AST, IU/L	48.6 ± 30.3	57.2 ± 92.9	0.633
Bilirubin, μmol/L	35.9 ± 38.3	26.1 ± 22.9	0.149
Albumin, g/L	29.7 ± 7.0	30.5 ± 5.8	0.554
INR	1.3 ± 0.4	1.4 ± 0.4	0.455
Ascites, n (%)	24 (85.7%)	33 (58.9%)	0.013
Encephalopathy, n (%)	1 (3.6%)	1 (1.7%)	0.613
Child-Pugh grade, n (%)			0.447
A	4	14	
B	18	34	
C	6	8	
Child score	7.36 ± 2.14	7.96 ± 1.76	0.439
MELD score	15.43 ± 5.3	16.46 ± 5.4	0.851
Heart rate, beats/min	84 ± 13	83 ± 15	0.983
Systolic blood pressure, mmHg	109 ± 20	112 ± 18	0.530
Infection, n (%)	7 (25%)	12 (20.7%)	0.712
Splenectomy, n (%)	10 (35.7%)	9 (15.5%)	0.043

Abbreviations. HBV, hepatitis B virus; HCV, hepatitis C virus; WBC, white blood cell; ALT, alanine aminotransferase; AST, aspartate aminotransferase.

TABLE 2: Summary of efficacy measurements during the 5-day period.

	The cavernoma group (n = 28)	The control group (n = 56)	p value
5-day treatment failure, n (%)	9 (32.1%)	7 (12.5%)	0.031
Failure to control acute bleeding, n (%)	5 (17.9%)	3 (5.4%)	0.066
Early rebleeding in 5 days, n (%)	4 (14.3%)	2 (3.6%)	0.072
5-day mortality, n (%)	3 (10.7%)	2 (3.6%)	0.192

treatment failure was identified using univariate regression and Cox proportional hazard modeling.

3.3. 6-Week Mortality. The overall 6-week mortality after AVB was 16.7% (n = 14) in the entire series, with 35.7% (n = 5) occurring within five days. The cumulative mortality rate did not differ between the cavernoma and control group (25% versus 12.5%, p = 0.137, Figure 1). Causes of death were uncontrolled or reported as relapsing bleeding (n = 7), liver failure (n = 5), sepsis (n = 1), and unknown (n = 1). The multivariable Cox proportional hazard regression analysis identified 5-day treatment failure (HR = 1.223, 95% CI = 1.082 to 1.384; p = 0.001) as the only independent predictor of 6-week mortality.

4. Discussion

Hemorrhage from gastroesophageal varices represents one of the most feared complications in the natural history of cirrhosis and is associated with significant morbidity and mortality [1, 3]. Our study was specifically designed to assess the short-term outcomes of cirrhotic patients with concurrent main portal vein occlusion and portal cavernoma presenting with the first episode of AVB. We found that the presence of portal cavernoma was associated with worse 5-day treatment failure in these patients.

The results of our study confirmed that PVT increased the risk of 5-day treatment failure in patients with AVB [2, 12]. In 2003, D'Amico and de Franchis evaluated the short-term

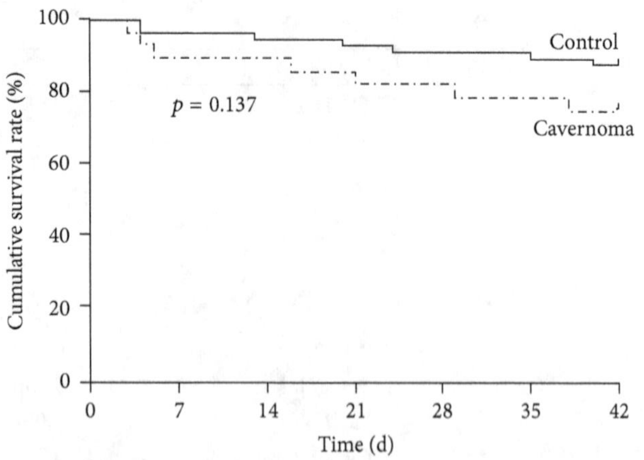

FIGURE 1: Kaplan–Meier estimates of 6-week survival in cirrhotic patients with portal cavernoma and active variceal bleeding.

outcomes and risk factors of 185 patients with liver cirrhosis and AVB retrospectively. They reported that the presence of PVT was an independent predictor for 5-day failure (for any sources of bleeding: OR = 3.19, 95% CI: 1.53–6.67, p = 0.002; for variceal bleeding: OR = 3.06, 95% CI: 1.39–6.68, p = 0.005) [2]. Another Italian study performed in 2012 enrolled 185 patients of whom 32 patients (17.3%) had PVT and demonstrated that the presence of PVT was associated with negative short-term outcomes [12]. This finding was potentially attributed to the higher portal venous pressure due to main portal vein occlusion, which makes the patients more susceptible to both initial medical/endoscopic therapy failure and early rebleeding. However, liver perfusion was decreased to a great extent, and further hepatic decompensation may occur.

TIPS used to be considered as a rescue treatment when bleeding was not controlled by less invasive endoscopic treatment and/or pharmacological therapy [3]. However, there is growing evidence for the support of early TIPS within 72 h (ideally < 24 h) in selected patients at a high risk of treatment failure [e.g., HVPG ≥ 20 mmHg, Child-Pugh C < 14 points, or Child-Pugh B with active bleeding] [13, 14]. All 3 patients who failed the initial therapy in the control group underwent TIPS as a rescue treatment and survived. In contrast, none of the patients in the cavernoma group could benefit from early placement of TIPS due to the complete obstruction of the main portal vein and lack of larger portal-portal collateral vein. The limitations of the treatment options demonstrated negative effects on the outcomes of the patient.

Currently, the effect of PVT on the prognosis of cirrhosis is debatable [7]. Luca et al., in their series of 42 patients with cirrhosis and partial PVT, revealed that liver function at diagnosis was the only independent predictor of survival and hepatic decompensation, instead of progression or regression of PVT [15]. Similarly, Maruyama and his colleagues found that the incidence of variceal bleeding did not differ statistically between patients with PVT compared to patients without PVT, as well as the survival rate [16]. Finally, a very recent prospective study, performed by Nery et al., enrolled 1,243 adults (863 Child A patients and 380 Child B patients) with cirrhosis but without PVT [17]. They found that the 5-year cumulative incidence of PVT was 10.7%, and PVT was mostly partial and varied overtime. In addition, there was no relationship between the development of PVT and the progression of liver disease, which was consistent with the findings obtained in previous reports [17].

Importantly, whether PVT affects the treatment effect and patients' survival in cirrhosis is associated with the degree and extension of PVT, as well as the severity of the underlying liver disease. In a study by Luca et al., which included 42 patients with cirrhosis and PVT, only 9 patients (21.4%) had grade 4 (≥76% of vessel lumen) thrombosis, 5 (11.9%) patients had large esophageal varices, and 12 (28.6%) patients experienced gastroesophageal variceal bleeding [15]. Over the 11-year study period, PVT developed in 28% (42/150) of patients with cirrhosis, and 11 patients (26.2%) suffered from complete portal vein obstruction [16]. Furthermore, 183 out of 1243 patients (16.3%) had grade ≥2 esophageal varices in a study by Nery et al. [17]. In the present series, all patients in the cavernoma group were admitted due to AVB. Unlike previous reports with a relatively high rate of spontaneous thrombosis improvement (45–47.5%), the possibility of spontaneous recanalization of the occluded main portal vein is very low [15, 16]. In addition, the mean MELD score (15.8) of our cohorts appeared to be higher than previous reports (12.1 from Luca, 10.2 in patients without PVT, and 10.6 in patients with PVT from Maruyama, resp.).

To the best of our knowledge, this is the first study to focus on the effect of portal cavernoma on the short-term outcomes of patients with cirrhosis and the first episode of AVB. The optimal management of AVB in patients with cirrhosis and portal cavernoma was difficult to establish due to the scarcity of the clinical trial data. This group of patients is usually excluded from clinical trials, and bleeding is particularly difficult to control because TIPS is often not applicable.

The major limitation of our study is the relatively small sample size and its retrospective design; therefore, bias may exist. The definition of portal cavernoma varied between different studies. Only patients with complete occluded main portal vein and the presence of portal-portal collateral vessels were included in the present study which influenced the number of patients for analysis greatly. We are aware that a prospective, large sample size trial may provide more convincing evidence on this subject. Unfortunately, only 28 patients with cirrhosis and portal cavernoma who presented with the first episode of AVB were identified during the study period in our hospital, which is one of the largest single-site hospitals in the world.

In conclusion, our data indicate that portal cavernoma in cirrhotic patients suffering from the first episode of AVB is associated with higher 5-day treatment failure. However, 6-week mortality did not significantly differ between the cavernoma and control groups. Long-term outcomes of patients with cirrhosis and portal cavernoma need further evaluation.

Acknowledgments

This work was supported by grants from National Natural Science Foundation of China (81570554 and 81501566) and Health and Family Planning Commission of Sichuan Province (150162). The present study has been accepted as an abstract poster in the 17th Congress of Gastroenterology China.

References

[1] D. Tripathi, A. J. Stanley, P. C. Hayes et al., "UK guidelines on the management of variceal haemorrhage in cirrhotic patients," *Gut*, vol. 64, no. 11, pp. 1680–1704, 2015.

[2] G. D'Amico and R. de Franchis, "Upper digestive bleeding in cirrhosis. Post-therapeutic outcome and prognostic indicators," *Hepatology*, vol. 38, no. 3, pp. 599–612, 2003.

[3] G. Garcia-Tsao and J. Bosch, "Management of varices and variceal hemorrhage in cirrhosis," *The New England Journal of Medicine*, vol. 362, no. 9, pp. 778–832, 2010.

[4] E. Moitinho, A. Escorsell, J.-C. Bandi et al., "Prognostic value of early measurements of portal pressure in acute variceal bleeding," *Gastroenterology*, vol. 117, no. 3, pp. 626–631, 1999.

[5] S. K. Sarin, A. Kumar, P. W. Angus et al., "Diagnosis and management of acute variceal bleeding: Asian Pacific Association for study of the Liver recommendations," *Hepatology International*, vol. 5, no. 2, pp. 607–624, 2011.

[6] C. Francoz, D. Valla, and F. Durand, "Portal vein thrombosis, cirrhosis, and liver transplantation," *Journal of Hepatology*, vol. 57, no. 1, pp. 203–212, 2012.

[7] E. A. Tsochatzis, M. Senzolo, G. Germani, A. Gatt, and A. K. Burroughs, "Systematic review: Portal vein thrombosis in cirrhosis," *Alimentary Pharmacology & Therapeutics*, vol. 31, no. 3, pp. 366–374, 2010.

[8] L. D. DeLeve, D.-C. Valla, and G. Garcia-Tsao, "Vascular disorders of the liver," *Hepatology*, vol. 49, no. 5, pp. 1729–1764, 2009.

[9] A. P. Ramos, C. P. H. Reigada, E. C. Ataíde et al., "Portal Vein Thrombosis and Liver Transplantation: Long Term," *Transplantation Proceedings*, vol. 42, no. 2, pp. 498–501, 2010.

[10] K. I. Rodríguez-Castro, R. J. Porte, E. Nadal, G. Germani, P. Burra, and M. Senzolo, "Management of nonneoplastic portal vein thrombosis in the setting of liver transplantation: a systematic review," *Transplantation*, vol. 94, no. 11, pp. 1145–1153, 2012.

[11] R. de Franchis, "Revising consensus in portal hypertension: report of the Baveno V consensus workshop on methodology of diagnosis and therapy in portal hypertension," *Journal of Hepatology*, vol. 53, no. 4, pp. 762–768, 2010.

[12] L. Amitrano, M. A. Guardascione, F. Manguso et al., "The effectiveness of current acute variceal bleed treatments in unselected cirrhotic patients: refining short-term prognosis and risk factors," *American Journal of Gastroenterology*, vol. 107, no. 12, pp. 1872–1878, 2012.

[13] J. C. García-Pagán, K. Caca, C. Bureau et al., "Early use of TIPS in patients with cirrhosis and variceal bleeding," *The New England Journal of Medicine*, vol. 362, no. 25, pp. 2370–2379, 2010.

[14] A. Monescillo, F. Martínez-Lagares, L. Ruiz-Del-Arbol et al., "Influence of portal hypertension and its early decompression by TIPS placement on the outcome of variceal bleeding," *Hepatology*, vol. 40, no. 4, pp. 793–801, 2004.

[15] A. Luca, S. Caruso, M. Milazzo et al., "Natural course of extrahepatic nonmalignant partial portal vein thrombosis in patients with cirrhosis," *Radiology*, vol. 265, no. 1, pp. 124–132, 2012.

[16] H. Maruyama, H. Okugawa, M. Takahashi, and O. Yokosuka, "De novo portal vein thrombosis in virus-related cirrhosis: predictive factors and long-term outcomes," *American Journal of Gastroenterology*, vol. 108, no. 4, pp. 568–574, 2013.

[17] F. Nery, S. Chevret, B. Condat et al., "Causes and consequences of portal vein thrombosis in 1,243 patients with cirrhosis: results of a longitudinal study," *Hepatology*, vol. 61, no. 2, pp. 660–667, 2015.

22

The Effects of Synbiotic "*Bifidobacterium lactis* B94 plus Inulin" Addition on Standard Triple Therapy of *Helicobacter pylori* Eradication in Children

Gonca Handan Ustundag,[1] Halime Altuntas,[2] Yasemin Dilek Soysal,[1] and Furuzan Kokturk[3]

[1]*Faculty of Medicine, Department of Pediatric Gastroenterology, Hepatology and Nutrition, Bulent Ecevit University, Zonguldak, Turkey*
[2]*Faculty of Medicine, Department of Pediatrics, Bulent Ecevit University, Zonguldak, Turkey*
[3]*Faculty of Medicine, Department of Biostatistics, Bulent Ecevit University, Zonguldak, Turkey*

Correspondence should be addressed to Gonca Handan Ustundag; gonnazyuc@yahoo.com

Academic Editor: Maikel P. Peppelenbosch

Aim. The aim of this study is to evaluate the effects of the synbiotic *Bifidobacterium lactis* B94 plus inulin addition to the standard triple therapy on *Helicobacter pylori (H. pylori)* infection eradication rates. *Methods*. Children aged 6–16 years who had biopsy proven *H. pylori* infection were randomly classified into two groups. The first group received the standard triple therapy consisting of amoxicillin + clarithromycin + omeprazole. The second group was treated with the standard triple therapy and *Bifidobacterium lactis* B94 (5×10^9 CFU/dose) plus inulin (900 mg) for 14 days, concurrently. Eradication was determined by ^{14}C-urea breath test 4–6 weeks after therapy discontinuation. *Results*. From a total of 69 *H. pylori* infected children (F/M = 36/33; mean ± SD = 11.2 ± 3.0 years), eradication was achieved in 20/34 participants in the standard therapy group and 27/35 participants in the synbiotic group. The eradication rates were not significantly different between the standard therapy and the synbiotic groups [intent-to-treat, 58.8% and 77.1%, resp., $p = 0.16$; per-protocol, 64.5% and 81.8%, resp., $p = 0.19$]. There was no difference between the groups in terms of symptom relief ($p = 0.193$). The reported side effects were ignorable. *Conclusion*. Considering the eradication rates, synbiotic addition to therapy showed no superiority over the standard triple therapy conducted alone. This trial is registered with NCT03165253.

1. Introduction

Helicobacter pylori (H. pylori) infection is one of the most common chronic bacterial diseases worldwide with an estimated prevalence of more than 50% in adults [1, 2]. Studies in Turkish patients reported that 70–80% of adults and 30–56% of children are infected with *H. pylori* [3–5]. In Western populations, *H. pylori* prevalence is low in children; however, it is still a problem as immigrants from countries where *H. pylori* is endemic constitute a risk group and a reservoir for the infection [6]. If left untreated, it can cause chronic gastritis, peptic ulcer, gastric adenocarcinomas [7], and mucosa-associated lymphoid tissue (MALT) lymphomas [8]. Fortunately, *H. pylori* associated gastric cancer has not been reported in pediatric age group, but MALT lymphomas have been described in a few *H. pylori* infected children [9–11]. In an adult study, early eradication of *H. pylori* has been associated with a sixfold reduction in the recurrence of peptic ulcers as well as a twofold to threefold reduction in the risk of gastric carcinoma [12]. Since *H. pylori* is mostly acquired in childhood, it is important to eradicate the infection in children as well. As stated in Kyoto global consensus report on *H. pylori* gastritis, "the maximum benefit of *H. pylori* eradication is obtained if it is done while the mucosal damage has not progressed beyond the nonatrophic stage" [13]. Further advantages of eradication of the infection in adolescents and young adults are also stated as reduction or prevention of the transmission of the infection to others and especially to their children [13].

Current guidelines recommend eradication of *H. pylori* infection in symptomatic children especially with peptic ulcer disease and with a family history of gastric carcinoma [14, 15]. The standard triple therapy that consists of a proton pump inhibitor and a combination of two antimicrobial agents, amoxicillin and either clarithromycin or an imidazole, for at least 7–14 days, is the main regimen used in both children and adults [14, 16] However, the success rate of this regimen declined from 80 to 96% in the previous years to 60–70% today [17–20]. Sequential therapy or bismuth salts based triple therapies are also mentioned as first-line treatments [14]. With so many different options but far from ideal eradication rates, it is hard to say which treatment is the best for children. Therefore, alternative therapies are still being searched.

Adjuvant treatment with probiotics, prebiotics, and/or synbiotics may be promising options. Probiotics are defined as "living microorganisms that are beneficial to the health of the host when consumed at adequate amounts" [21]. Prebiotics are indigestible foods that enhance the growth or activity of beneficial probiotic bacteria in the gut [22]. Synbiotics are the combination of probiotics and prebiotics, which can work synergistically. In vitro studies demonstrated inhibitory activity of certain probiotic strains against *H. pylori* bacteria [23, 24]. Furthermore, there are randomized controlled trials (RCT) demonstrating favorable outcomes of probiotic addition to *H. pylori* eradication treatments [25–28]. They are believed to increase patient compliance by reducing the side effects such as antibiotic-associated diarrhea [26, 28–30]. Most studies in this area are mainly designed by using a single probiotic strain or a combination of strains. To our knowledge, there are currently a few studies assessing the effects of synbiotics on *H. pylori* eradication [30–32].

In our study, we aimed to investigate the effects of the synbiotic *Bifidobacterium lactis (B. lactis)* B94 plus inulin addition to standard triple therapy in terms of eradication rates, relief of symptoms, and patient compliance.

2. Materials and Methods

The study was conducted between June 2011 and June 2012 in the pediatric gastroenterology clinic of Bulent Ecevit University Faculty of Medicine, Zonguldak, Turkey. The study population consisted of 69 children aged 6–16 years who were investigated by a standard esophagogastroduodenoscopy (EGD) for gastrointestinal symptoms, those suggesting an organic disease such as chronic abdominal pain, unexplained nausea and/or vomiting, severe regurgitation, gastrointestinal bleeding, unexplained weight loss, or chronic diarrhea. Written informed consent was obtained from the parents. The study was approved by the Scientific Research Ethics Committee of the Bulent Ecevit University (Protocol number, 2011-10-08/03).

Patients who were treated for *H. pylori* infection previously, who used an antimicrobial agent, bismuth, a nonsteroid anti-inflammatory drug, or any form of gastric acid suppressor during the eight weeks prior the EGD, or who had history of major gastrointestinal surgery, chronic renal, or hepatic disease and who were known to have drug allergy were excluded from the study.

The patients underwent a standard EGD and biopsies from stomach and duodenum were taken at least two per site. Endoscopic findings such as antral hyperemia, antral nodularity, and peptic ulcer were noted. The biopsy specimens were evaluated by the same pathologist at the Department of Medical Pathology, Bulent Ecevit University Faculty of Medicine. Children who were found to have *H. pylori* infection proven by histopathological examination were randomly assigned to two groups in a double blind manner using a prepared randomization list. Each patient was given a number. Patients in the standard triple therapy group were treated with amoxicillin 50 mg/kg/d and clarithromycin 15 mg/kg/d twice daily for 14 days and omeprazole (OMP) 1 mg/kg/d once daily for a month. The synbiotic group received the same standard triple therapy and *Bifidobacterium lactis* B94 (5×10^9 CFU/dose) plus 900 mg of inulin (Maflor sachet, Mamsel, Turkey) given a single dose for 14 days concurrently. Required amount of drugs for both treatment groups was prescribed. A detailed chart explaining the usage of drugs and a form to record the changes in symptoms and the side effects related to treatment (nausea, vomiting, diarrhea, and abdominal or epigastric pain) were given to the patients and/or their parents. The patients were called for follow-up 4–6 weeks after the cessation of OMP treatment. Then, they were assessed for relief of symptoms and ^{14}C-urea breath test (^{14}C-UBT) was scheduled. Negative ^{14}C-UBT was considered as eradication.

3. Statistical Analysis

Statistical analysis was performed with SPSS 19.0 software (SPSS Inc., Chicago, IL, USA). Distribution of data was determined by Shapiro-Wilk test. Continuous variables were expressed as mean ± std. deviation, categorical variables as frequency and percent. Continuous variables were compared with the independent sample t-test or Mann–Whitney U test for two groups. Categorical variables were compared using Pearson's Chi-square test or Fisher Exact Chi-square test. The eradication rates were determined using both the intent-to-treat (ITT) and per-protocol (PP) analyses. p value of less than 0.05 was considered statistically significant for all tests.

4. Results

Sixty-nine patients with *H. pylori* infection were randomly assigned to the standard therapy group ($n = 34$) and synbiotic group ($n = 35$) (Figure 1). The demographic characteristics of patients were similar between the groups (Table 1). The most frequent complaint was abdominal pain in both groups (87% in the standard therapy group and 97% in the synbiotic group, $p = 0.19$). It was mainly described as epigastric pain by 40.7% of patients in the standard therapy group and 43.8% of patients in the synbiotic group ($p = 0.09$). The second frequent complaint was nausea in 64.5% and 60.6%

TABLE 1: Demographic characteristics and endoscopic findings of study groups.

	Standard therapy	Synbiotic	
Patient characteristics	$n = 34$	$n = 35$	p
Age (year)	11.2 ± 3.1	11.2 ± 2.9	0.97
Sex (female/male)	0.88	1.35	0.55
Height (cm)	145.5 ± 3.0	147.2 ± 3.3	0.71
Weight (kg)	40.9 ± 3.0	42.5 ± 2.5	0.39
Endoscopic findings	$n = 31$	$n = 33$	p
Antral hyperemia	26 (83.9%)	28 (84.8%)	
Antral nodularity	4 (12.9%)	4 (12.1%)	0.99
Antral ulcer	1 (3.2 %)	1 (3%)	
Normal duodenum	22 (71%)	27 (81.8%)	
Duodenitis	5 (16.1%)	4 (12.1%)	0.69
Duodenal ulcer	4 (12.9%)	2 (6.1%)	

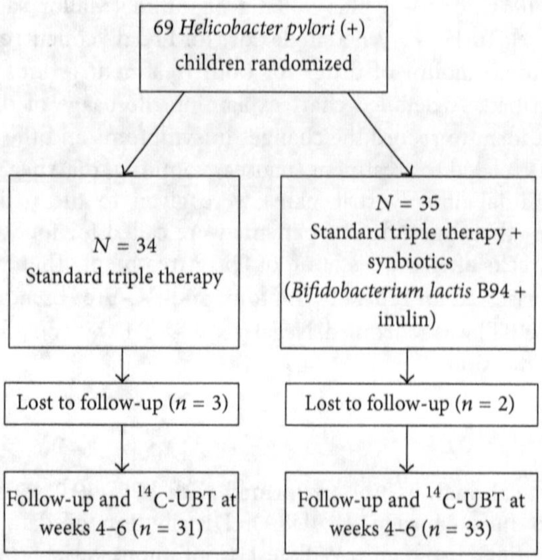

FIGURE 1: Flow diagram of the patients' progression through the study. ^{14}C-UBT: carbon-14 labelled urea breath test.

of patients in the standard therapy and synbiotic groups, respectively ($p = 0.9$). A total of 5 children dropped out the study, since they did not present to the follow-up (Table 2). All the other patients completed the treatment as prescribed. Patients were reassessed at follow-up 4–6 six weeks after the end of OMP treatment.

None of the patients in each group experienced a side effect that would require termination of the treatment. Only one patient complained of increased abdominal pain in the standard therapy group, and one patient had a new onset of diarrhea during the antibiotherapy in the synbiotic group. In the standard therapy group, there was no change of symptoms in 4 patients (12.9%), while a slight relief of symptoms in 11 patients (35.5%) and a marked relief of symptoms in 16 patients (51.6%) were observed. In the synbiotic group, no change of symptoms was reported by 1 patient (3%),

TABLE 2: The eradication success in study groups.

Status	Standard therapy (n)	Synbiotic (n)
Eradication	20	27
Failed eradication	11	6
Missing data	3	2
Total	34	35

TABLE 3: The eradication rates in study groups.

Analyses	Standard therapy	Synbiotic	p
ITT	56.8% (20/34)	77.1% (27/35)	0.16
PP	64.5% (20/31)	81.8% (27/33)	0.19

whereas a slight relief of symptoms and a marked relief of symptoms were reported by 7 patients (21.2%) and by 25 patients (75.8%), respectively. Although, the symptoms were much more improved in the synbiotic group, the difference was not statistically significant between the groups ($p = 0.09$).

H. pylori eradication was confirmed by ^{14}C-UBT. The eradication rates in both the synbiotic and the standard therapy groups were evaluated using ITT and PP analyses (Table 3). Eradication rates did not differ significantly between the groups ($p = 0.16$ and $p = 0.19$, by ITT and PP analyses, resp.).

5. Discussion

In recent years the efficacy of *H. pylori* eradication treatments has fallen below an acceptable level of 80%, mainly due to antimicrobial resistance and inadequate patient compliance [16]. As no new drug has been developed for *H. pylori* eradication, clinical trials have focused on different combinations of known drugs and adjuvant therapy. Probiotics are thought to be beneficial in *H. pylori* infection in two ways: (1) some strains may have a direct effect on the pathogen and inhibit its growth. (2) Some strains may reduce antibiotic-associated side effects and improve compliance to therapy. Moreover, pre- and probiotic supplementation may have immunomodulatory effects on the hosts as experimental studies demonstrated their anti-inflammatory effects in chronic inflammatory diseases like asthma, topical allergies, and inflammatory bowel disease [33, 34].

In vitro studies and animal models have demonstrated inhibitory effects of several probiotic species especially *Lactobacilli* and *Bifidobacterium* on *H. pylori* colonization and growth [23, 24]. This effect is achieved by the production of organic acids, autolysins, mucin, and bacteriocins and/or by the binding of some specific strains to the same glycolipid receptors as *H. pylori* [23, 24, 35–38]. The preclinical studies have supported the possibility of using probiotics in the treatment of *H. pylori* infections in clinical settings.

Several studies evaluated the effects of probiotics as monotherapy in asymptomatic children infected with *H. pylori* [31, 39]. Gotteland et al. demonstrated that children receiving *Saccharomyces boulardii (S. boulardii)* and inulin (a synbiotic) had a significant decrease in ^{13}C-UBTs [31]. In 12% of the participants, the infection was even eradicated by the regular intake of this synbiotic [31]. Similarly, Cruchet et al. treated *H. pylori* infected asymptomatic children for one month with live *Lactobacillus johnsonii* La 1 and showed significant changes [39]. In summary, specific probiotic strains as mentioned above probably lower the bacterial load in the gastric mucosa but not completely eradicate the bacteria. Considering that a certain percentage of the patients had achieved eradication even with monotherapy, we have planned the current study assuming that we would get better results by combining a synbiotic with standard therapy.

To date, several systematic reviews and meta-analyses have been published about the effects of probiotic supplementation to standard treatment regimens of *H. pylori* infection in both children and adults [40, 41]. The systematic review and meta-analysis by Szajewska et al. evaluated the effects of *S. boulardii* supplementation to eradication therapy [40]. Eleven RCTs involving 2200 patients were included in the review. The eradication rates were found to be significantly higher (80% versus 71%) in participants taking *S. boulardii.* Also, overall adverse effects were lower in the probiotic group compared to the control group, and particularly the risk of diarrhea and nausea was reduced [40]. The recent meta-analysis by Lau et al. included thirty RCTs involving more than 4000 patients, both children and adults [41]. They examined the impact of probiotic supplementation on standard triple therapy and concluded that the addition of probiotics increased eradication rates ($p < 0.001$). Moreover, the risk of diarrhea, nausea, vomiting, and epigastric pain was also found to be reduced. In conclusion, generally the authors suggested that the eradication rates improved, and the frequency of adverse effects was reduced. However, the results should be interpreted cautiously, since collecting data on different strains in meta-analysis may be misleading.

In our study, we evaluated the effects of a synbiotic "*B. lactis* B94 and inulin" addition to standard triple therapy in symptomatic children. Although, the eradication rate seemed to be higher in the synbiotic group, the difference was not statistically significant (ITT, $p = 0.16$, and PP, $p = 0.19$). To our knowledge, there are only two reports that used the same synbiotic treatment in *H. pylori* eradication [30, 32]. Similar to our results, Islek et al. could not find a positive effect of this symbiotic treatment on eradication rates in *H. pylori* infected children [30]. However, there was a notable decrease on the occurrence of side effects in the synbiotic group which was interpreted as an indirect positive effect on eradication success [30]. On the other hand, the study by Çekin et al. revealed significantly higher *H. pylori* eradication rates with sequential treatment and *B. lactis* B94 [32]. Furthermore, they have demonstrated lower diarrhea rates and higher treatment compliance in patients receiving *B. lactis* B94 [32]. Inconsistent with these studies, the patients in our study did not report any side effects that would require discontinuation of therapy. Another recent study by Shafagi et al. also investigated the effectiveness of a multistrain synbiotic combination in adult patients taking quadruple therapy [42]. The eradication rates were higher in the synbiotic group based on ITT analysis (92.1% versus 63.2%, $p < 0.05$) [42]. No significant difference was noted between the groups in terms of side effects. However, a considerable number of patients (14/38) were lost to follow-up in the placebo group, mostly due to noncompliance [42]. The results of this study also showed that compliance is a key factor in eradication success. Indeed, compliance to therapy was not a major problem in our study as none of the patients in both groups had an intolerable side effect. The improvement in dyspeptic symptoms was higher in the synbiotic group, although not statistically significant. However, we did not use an objective symptom scale for this evaluation.

The limitations of our study can be listed as follows: (1) *H. pylori* culture and antibiotic susceptibility tests were not done. (2) *Bifidobacterium* colonization in the feces was not evaluated. (3) The sample size was relatively small.

6. Conclusion

The results of our study demonstrated that the addition of *B. lactis* B94 (5×10^9 CFU/dose) plus inulin once daily to standard triple therapy showed no superiority on the eradication rates compared to the standard triple therapy given alone. There are currently a limited number of RCTs in pediatric age group conducted with a diversity of probiotic strains, and the results are conflicting with each other. Thus, it is hard to conclude which probiotic/synbiotic is effective in *H. pylori* eradication, at which doses and duration, and with which antimicrobial regimen. Further large-scale RCTs are needed to clarify these points.

Authors' Contributions

Gonca Handan Ustundag and Halime Altuntas designed the research study, collected and analyzed the data, and wrote the manuscript. Yasemin Dilek Soysal helped in manuscript writing and reviewed the data analysis. Furuzan Kokturk contributed to study design and performed the statistical analysis of the data. All authors approved the final version of the manuscript.

Acknowledgments

This paper has been proofread by Fatma Tanrıverdi-Köksal, a member of the Bulent Ecevit University Article Proofreading and Editing Office.

References

[1] S. Suerbaum and P. Michetti, "*Helicobacter pylori* infection," *The New England Journal of Medicine*, vol. 347, no. 15, pp. 1175–1186, 2002.

[2] L. M. Brown, "Helicobacter pylori: epidemiology and routes of transmission," *Epidemiologic Reviews*, vol. 22, no. 2, pp. 283–297, 2000.

[3] D. Us and G. Hasçelik, "Seroprevalence of Helicobacter pylori infection in an asymptomatic Turkish population," *Journal of Infection*, vol. 37, no. 2, pp. 148–150, 1998.

[4] F. Gurakan, N. Kocak, and A. Yuce, "Helicobacter pylori serology in childhood," *TheTurkish Journal of Pediatrics*, vol. 38, no. 3, pp. 329–334, 1996.

[5] A. Özen, D. Ertem, and E. Pehlivanoglu, "Natural history and symptomatology of Helicobacter pylori in childhood and factors determining the epidemiology of infection," *Journal of Pediatric Gastroenterology and Nutrition*, vol. 42, no. 4, pp. 398–404, 2006.

[6] W. J. Den Hollander, I. L. Holster, B. Van Gilst et al., "Intergenerational reduction in Helicobacter pylori prevalence is similar between different ethnic groups living in a Western city," *Gut*, vol. 64, no. 8, pp. 1200–1208, 2015.

[7] J. Parsonnet, G. D. Friedman, D. P. Vandersteen et al., "*Helicobacter pylori* infection and the risk of gastric carcinoma," *The New England Journal of Medicine*, vol. 325, no. 16, pp. 1127–1131, 1991.

[8] S. Eidt, M. Stolte, and R. Fischer, "Helicobacter pylori gastritis and primary gastric non-Hodgkin's lymphomas," *Journal of Clinical Pathology*, vol. 47, no. 5, pp. 436–439, 1994.

[9] M. Moschovi, D. Menegas, K. Stefanaki, C. Van-Vliet Constantinidou, and F. Tzortzatou-Stathopoulou, "Primary gastric Burkitt lymphoma in childhood: Associated with Helicobacter pylori?" *Medical and Pediatric Oncology*, vol. 41, no. 5, pp. 444–447, 2003.

[10] S. Kurugoglu, I. Mihmanli, T. Celkan, H. Aki, H. Aksoy, and U. Korman, "Radiological features in paediatric primary gastric MALT lymphoma and association with Helicobacter pylori," *Pediatric Radiology*, vol. 32, no. 2, pp. 82–87, 2002.

[11] S. S. Al Furaikh, "Remission of high-grade B-cell lymphoma in a pediatric patient following Helicobacter pylori eradication," *Pediatrics International*, vol. 53, no. 1, pp. 105–107, 2011.

[12] I. F. N. Hung and B. C. Y. Wong, "Assessing the risks and benefits of treating Helicobacter pylori infection," *Therapeutic Advances in Gastroenterology*, vol. 2, no. 3, pp. 141–147, 2009.

[13] K. Sugano, J. Tack, E. J. Kuipers et al., "Kyoto global consensus report on *Helicobacter pylori* gastritis," *Gut*, vol. 64, no. 9, pp. 1353–1367, 2015.

[14] S. Koletzko, N. L. Jones, K. J. Goodman et al., "Evidence-based guidelines from ESPGHAN and NASPGHAN for *Helicobacter pylori* infection in children," *Journal of Pediatric Gastroenterology and Nutrition*, vol. 53, no. 2, pp. 230–243, 2011.

[15] B. Drumm, S. Koletzko, and G. Oderda, "Helicobacter pylori infection in children: A consensus statement," *Journal of Pediatric Gastroenterology and Nutrition*, vol. 30, no. 2, pp. 207–213, 2000.

[16] P. Malfertheiner, F. Megraud, C. A. O'Morain et al., "Management of *Helicobacter pylori* infection—the Maastricht IV/ Florence consensus report," *Gut*, vol. 61, no. 5, pp. 646–664, 2012.

[17] R.-K. Vilaichone, V. Mahachai, and D. Y. Graham, "Helicobacter pylori Diagnosis and Management," *Gastroenterology Clinics of North America*, vol. 35, no. 2, pp. 229–247, 2006.

[18] A. Kadayifci, H. Buyukhatipoglu, M. C. Savas, and I. Simsek, "Eradication of *Helicobacter pylori* with triple therapy: an epidemiologic analysis of trends in Turkey over 10 years," *Clinical Therapeutics*, vol. 28, no. 11, pp. 1960–1966, 2006.

[19] G. Oderda, P. Shcherbakov, P. Bontems et al., "Results from the Pediatric European Register for Treatment of Helicobacter pylori (PERTH)," *Helicobacter*, vol. 12, no. 2, pp. 150–156, 2007.

[20] G. Kutluk, E. Tutar, A. Bayrak et al., "Sequential therapy versus standard triple therapy for Helicobacter pylori eradication in children: Any advantage in clarithromycin-resistant strains?" *European Journal of Gastroenterology and Hepatology*, vol. 26, no. 11, pp. 1202–1208, 2014.

[21] C. Hill, F. Guarner, G. Reid et al., "Expert consensus document: the International Scientific Association for Probiotics and Prebiotics consensus statement on the scope and appropriate use of the term probiotic," *Nature Reviews Gastroenterology & Hepatology*, vol. 11, no. 8, pp. 506–514, 2014.

[22] M. Roberfroid, "Prebiotics: the concept revisited," *The Journal of Nutrition*, vol. 137, supplement 2, no. 3, pp. 830S–837S, 2007.

[23] S. J. Bhatia, N. Kochar, P. Abraham, N. G. Nair, and A. P. Mehta, "Lactobacillius acidophilus inhibits growth of Campylobacter pylori in vitro," *Journal of Clinical Microbiology*, vol. 27, no. 10, pp. 2328–2330, 1989.

[24] G. L. Lorca, T. Wadström, G. Font de Valdez, and Å. Ljungh, "Lactobacillus acidophilus autolysins inhibit Helicobacter pylori in vitro," *Current Microbiology*, vol. 42, no. 1, pp. 39–44, 2001.

[25] J. Sýkora, K. Valečková, J. Amlerová et al., "Effects of a specially designed fermented milk product containing probiotic *Lactobacillus casei* DN-114 001 and the eradication of *H. pylori* in children: a prospective randomized double-blind study," *Journal of Clinical Gastroenterology*, vol. 39, no. 8, pp. 692–698, 2005.

[26] V. Hurduc, D. Plesca, D. Dragomir, M. Sajin, and Y. Vandenplas, "A randomized, open trial evaluating the effect of Saccharomyces boulardii on the eradication rate of Helicobacter pylori infection in children," *Acta Paediatrica, International Journal of Paediatrics*, vol. 98, no. 1, pp. 127–131, 2009.

[27] S. Tolone, V. Pellino, G. Vitaliti, A. Lanzafame, and C. Tolone, "Evaluation of Helicobacter Pylori eradication in pediatric patients by triple therapy plus lactoferrin and probiotics compared to triple therapy alone," *Italian Journal of Pediatrics*, vol. 38, no. 1, article no. 63, 2012.

[28] K. Ahmad, F. Fatemeh, N. Mehri, and S. Mayram, "Probiotics for the treatment of pediatric *Helicobacter pylori* infection: a randomized double blind clinical trial," *Iranian Journal of Pediatrics*, vol. 23, no. 1, pp. 79–84, 2013.

[29] E. Lionetti, V. L. Miniello, S. P. Castellaneta et al., "*Lactobacillus reuteri* therapy to reduce side-effects during anti-*Helicobacter pylori* treatment in children: a randomized placebo controlled trial," *Alimentary Pharmacology and Therapeutics*, vol. 24, no. 10, pp. 1461–1468, 2006.

[30] A. Islek, E. Sayar, A. Yilmaz, and R. Artan, "*Bifidobacterium lactis* B94 plus inulin for treatment of *Helicobacter pylori* infection in children: does it increase eradication rate and patient compliance?" *Acta Gastro-Enterologica Belgica*, vol. 78, no. 3, pp. 282–286, 2015.

[31] M. Gotteland, L. Poliak, S. Cruchet, and O. Brunser, "Effect of regular ingestion of Saccharomyces boulardii plus inulin or Lactobacillus acidophilus LB in children colonized by Helicobacter pylori," *Acta Paediatrica, International Journal of Paediatrics*, vol. 94, no. 12, pp. 1747–1751, 2005.

[32] A. H. Çekin, Y. Şahintürk, F. Akbay Harmandar, S. Uyar, B. O. Yolcular, and Y. Çekin, "Use of probiotics as an adjuvant to sequential *H. pylori* eradication therapy: impact on eradication rates, treatment resistance, treatment-related side effects, and patient compliance," *Turkish Journal of Gastroenterology*, vol. 28, pp. 3–11, 2017.

[33] M. P. Peppelenbosch and C. V. Ferreira, "Immunology of pre- and probiotic supplementation," *British Journal of Nutrition*, vol. 101, no. 1, pp. 2–4, 2009.

[34] A. Sarkar and S. Mandal, "Bifidobacteria—Insight into clinical outcomes and mechanisms of its probiotic action," *Microbiological Research*, vol. 192, pp. 159–171, 2016.

[35] P. Hütt, J. Shchepetova, K. Lõivukene, T. Kullisaar, and M. Mikelsaar, "Antagonistic activity of probiotic lactobacilli and bifidobacteria against entero- and uropathogens," *Journal of Applied Microbiology*, vol. 100, no. 6, pp. 1324–1332, 2006.

[36] A. Gomi, N. Harima-Mizusawa, H. Shibahara-Sone, M. Kano, K. Miyazaki, and F. Ishikawa, "Effect of Bifidobacterium bifidum BF-1 on gastric protection and mucin production in an acute gastric injury rat model," *Journal of Dairy Science*, vol. 96, no. 2, pp. 832–837, 2013.

[37] T. Mukai, T. Asasaka, E. Sato, K. Mori, M. Matsumoto, and H. Ohori, "Inhibition of binding of *Helicobacter pylori*to the glycolipid receptors by probiotic *Lactobacillus reuteri*," *FEMS Immunology and Medical Microbiology*, vol. 32, no. 2, pp. 105–110, 2002.

[38] M. Gotteland, O. Brunser, and S. Cruchet, "Systematic review: are probiotics useful in controlling gastric colonization by Helicobacter pylori?" *Alimentary Pharmacology and Therapeutics*, vol. 23, no. 8, pp. 1077–1086, 2006.

[39] S. Cruchet, M. C. Obregon, G. Salazar, E. Diaz, and M. Gotteland, "Effect of the ingestion of a dietary product containing *Lactobacillus johnsonii* La1 on *Helicobacter pylori* colonization in children," *Nutrition*, vol. 19, no. 9, pp. 716–721, 2003.

[40] H. Szajewska, A. Horvath, and M. Kołodziej, "Systematic review with meta-analysis: Saccharomyces boulardii supplementation and eradication of Helicobacter pylori infection," *Alimentary Pharmacology and Therapeutics*, vol. 41, no. 12, pp. 1237–1245, 2015.

[41] C. S. M. Lau, A. Ward, and R. S. Chamberlain, "Probiotics improve the efficacy of standard triple therapy in the eradication of Helicobacter pylori: A meta-analysis," *Infection and Drug Resistance*, vol. 9, pp. 275–289, 2016.

[42] A. Shafaghi, A. Pourkazemi, M. Khosravani et al., "The Effect of probiotic plus prebiotic supplementation on the tolerance and efficacy of *Helicobacter pylori* eradication quadruple therapy: a randomized prospective double blind controlled trial," *Middle East Journal of Digestive Diseases*, vol. 8, no. 3, pp. 179–188, 2016.

23

Recognition of Lynch Syndrome Amongst Newly Diagnosed Colorectal Cancers at St. Paul's Hospital

Steven Pi,[1] Estello Nap-Hill,[2] Jennifer Telford,[3] and Robert Enns[3]

[1]*Department of Medicine, University of British Columbia Faculty of Medicine, Vancouver, BC, Canada*
[2]*Pacific Gastroenterology Associates, Vancouver, BC, Canada*
[3]*Department of Gastroenterology, Division of Gastroenterology, St. Paul's Hospital, Vancouver, BC, Canada*

Correspondence should be addressed to Robert Enns; rob.enns@ubc.ca

Academic Editor: Maikel P. Peppelenbosch

Background. Lynch Syndrome (LS) is the most common cause of inherited colorectal cancer (CRC). In British Columbia, most centres still use clinical criteria (Amsterdam II, Revised Bethesda, or the BC Cancer Agency's criteria) to determine who should undergo further first-line testing in the form of microsatellite instability or immunohistochemistry staining. Given the limitations with this strategy, LS is thought to be underrecognized. *Objective.* To investigate whether LS is truly underrecognized when compared to the reported prevalence. *Methods.* A retrospective chart review of all CRC cases diagnosed at St. Paul's Hospital from 2010 to 2013 was conducted. *Results.* 246 patients met inclusion criteria. 76% (83/109) with a family history of malignancy were unable to recall the specific malignancy or age of diagnosis. 18% (43/235) were only asked about a history of gastrointestinal related malignancy and 26% (65/246) met at least one of the three criteria but only 21% (13/63) received further investigation. Only 1.6% (4/246) had LS compared to the reported prevalence of 2–5% of all CRC cases. *Conclusion.* This data supports our hypothesis that LS is underrecognized. Issues at the patient, physician, and systems level need to be evaluated to determine where the limitations preventing appropriate testing are occurring.

1. Introduction

Lynch Syndrome is the most common cause of inherited colorectal cancer (CRC), estimated to account for 2–5% of all CRC cases [1]. This autosomal dominant disorder is the result of a loss-of-function mutation in one of the DNA mismatch repair genes (*MLH1*, *MSH2*, *MSH6*, or *PMS2*). The presence of these mutations identifies the syndrome. Consequently, the inability to repair mismatched DNA ultimately leads to an increased risk of both colonic and extracolonic malignancies [1]. Depending on which gene is affected, patients may have an increased risk of endometrial, ovarian, upper urologic tract, gastric, small bowel, biliary/pancreatic, brain, and/or sebaceous gland malignancies. Identification of patients with Lynch Syndrome is essential because intensive cancer screening and prophylactic surgery have been shown to reduce incidence and mortality of both colonic [2] and extracolonic malignancies [3]. In addition, early identification permits directed genetic counselling for relevant family members.

Numerous strategies exist to identify patients at risk for Lynch Syndrome. These include clinical criteria such as the Amsterdam II or Revised Bethesda Guidelines (Table 1), prediction models such as PREMM or MMRPredict, or tumour testing in the form of microsatellite instability (MSI) or immunohistochemistry (IHC) staining. In British Columbia, most centres will utilize the clinical criteria strategy to identify which patients should undergo further tumour testing in the form of microsatellite instability testing or immunohistochemistry staining. Traditionally, these clinical criteria include the Amsterdam II criteria and Revised Bethesda Guidelines; however the Hereditary Cancer Program (HCP) under the BC Cancer Agency has also developed its own criteria (Table 1) which has been shown to have a higher sensitivity and positive predictive value when compared to the Amsterdam II and Revised Bethesda Guidelines [4]. Patients referred to the HCP receive an appointment with an oncologist and geneticist and for further diagnostic testing such as MSI testing, IHC staining, and germline mutation

TABLE 1: Amsterdam II, Revised Bethesda Guidelines, and HCP Referral Criteria.

Amsterdam Criteria II
Requiring three or more relatives with Lynch-associated cancer* in addition to the following
(1) One affected patient should be a first-degree relative of the other two
(2) Two or more successive generations are affected
(3) One or more affected relatives received diagnosis at age younger than 50 years
(4) FAP is excluded. Tumours should be verified by pathological examination
**Endometrial, stomach, ovarian, pancreas, ureter, and renal pelvis*
Revised Bethesda Guidelines
(1) CRC diagnosed in a patient who is younger than 50 years of age
(2) Presence of synchronous, metachronous CRC, or other Lynch-associated tumours
(3) CRC diagnosed in a patient who is younger than 60 years of age, with the presence of tumour infiltrating lymphocytes, Crohn's-like lymphocytic reaction, mucinous/signet-ring differentiation, or medullary growth pattern
(4) CRC diagnosed in a patient with one or more first-degree relatives with a Lynch-associated tumour, with at least one of the cancers being diagnosed at age younger than 50 years
(5) CRC diagnosed in a patient with two or more first- or second-degree relatives with Lynch-associated tumours, regardless of age
HCP Criteria [6]
Any of the following
(1) Personal history of CRC diagnosed at age ≤ 40
(2) Personal history of Lynch syndrome related cancer at any age with IHC-deficient/MSI-H results
(3) Personal history of 2 Lynch syndrome related cancer diagnoses, including at least 1 colorectal cancer and a cancer diagnosed at age ≤ 50
(4) Family history that includes
(a) a close relative with personal history as above OR
(b) 2 first-degree relatives with a Lynch syndrome related cancer, both diagnosed at age ≤ 50 and including at least 1 diagnosis of CRC OR
(c) 3 or more Lynch syndrome related cancers, involving more than 1 generation, at least 1 case of CRC, and at least 1 case diagnosed at age ≤ 50.

testing, if necessary [5]. If these tests ultimately reveal a genetic mutation in the Lynch Syndrome associated genes then a diagnosis is made. Despite its ongoing use, a number of limitations exist for utilizing the clinical criteria approach to identify those who should undergo further testing for Lynch Syndrome. First, the patient must be aware of the exact age of diagnosis for any malignancy in their first- or second-degree relatives. Second, the consulting physician must complete a detailed past medical and family history of all malignancies in their first- and second-degree relatives. Third, the consulting physician must be aware of the above-mentioned criteria and when a referral to the Cancer Agency for further investigation would be appropriate. If any of these factors are missing, a diagnosis of Lynch Syndrome could be missed.

Due to these limitations, Lynch Syndrome is thought to be underrecognized at centres in British Columbia, such as St. Paul's Hospital (SPH), which utilize the clinical criteria approach. Of note, SPH is a major referral centre for colorectal cancers for the Province of British Columbia. This could lead to significant consequences, as a missed diagnosis could potentially lead to further malignancy that may have otherwise been preventable in either the patient or their family. The purpose of this study is to investigate whether Lynch Syndrome is truly underrecognized when compared to the reported prevalence and, if so, identifying what factors may be contributing to this.

2. Materials and Methods

2.1. Database. Patients were initially extracted using the St. Paul's Hospital Department of Pathology's database. A search for the string "adenocarcinoma" was run on all rectal, sigmoid, descending, transverse, ascending, and cecal biopsies between January 1, 2010, and December 31, 2013. These patients were then subsequently identified using the Pacific Gastroenterology Associates Electronic Medical Record to obtain further clinical information as outlined below.

2.2. Inclusion/Exclusion Criteria. Included in this study were patients referred to and seen by the St. Paul's Hospital gastroenterologists that had a pathologic diagnosis of CRC on endoscopic or surgical biopsy between Jan 1, 2010, and Dec 31, 2013. Our population of interest was nonurgent patients in the outpatient setting, as we assume that this would be the ideal setting for the consulting physician to complete a thorough family history and give consideration to investigating for Lynch Syndrome. Of note is that St. Paul's Hospital is a major referral centre for colorectal cancers for the Province of British Columbia.

Excluded in this study were patients seen in the Emergency Department, inpatients at St. Paul's Hospital, or patients in whom an urgent assessment was indicated (e.g., radiographic evidence suggestive of colorectal cancer or palpable rectal mass). Similarly, patients with known colorectal cancer who were referred to gastroenterology solely for a procedure (e.g., endoscopic ultrasound for staging of a known colorectal cancer) were excluded as these patients would also be less likely to receive a thorough family history. Patients with known IBD were excluded as the pathologic findings on their colon cancer could potentially confound the high-risk pathologic findings in the Revised Bethesda Criteria (i.e., Crohn's-like lymphocytic reaction). Patients were also excluded if they were enrolled under the Colon Check Pilot (CCP), the pilot program of the current British Columbia Colon Screening Program, as their screening and management were protocoled differently from the standard of care during that period of time.

2.3. Ethics. Providence Health Care Institutional Approval for ethics was obtained on July 7, 2016, REB number: H16-00881.

2.4. Data Extraction. Patients meeting inclusion criteria had the following data extracted: (1) full name; (2) year of birth; (3) sex; (4) provincial health number; (5) age of diagnosis of colon cancer; (6) indication for colonoscopy; (7) pathology report of colorectal cancer, including staging; (8) location of colorectal cancer on diagnostic and subsequent endoscopies or surgeries; (9) past medical history of previous cancers and, if so, which type and age of the respective diagnosis; (10) family history of previous cancers and, if so, which relatives, type, and age of respective diagnosis; (11) IHC/MSI results for patients/family members.

2.5. Data Analysis. Each patient had their extracted data analyzed to see if any of the Amsterdam II, Revised Bethesda, or Hereditary Cancer Program criteria were met (Figure 1). Those who met any of the criteria were then assessed to see if they had received any form of further investigation for Lynch Syndrome in the form of either a referral to the Hereditary Cancer Program, MSI testing, or IHC staining. Those with positive results yielding a diagnosis of Lynch Syndrome were then used to calculate the proportion of Lynch Syndrome amongst newly diagnosed colorectal cancers at St. Paul's Hospital. This proportion was then compared to the reported baseline prevalence of 2–5% (BCCA 2012) to determine whether or not Lynch Syndrome is underrecognized. Two-tailed *t*-tests and chi-square testing were used to calculate statistical significance between the population who received further investigation and all patients included in the study.

2.6. Confidentiality. Data was stored on an encrypted password protected Excel 2012 spreadsheet. Each subject was assigned a unique identifier. Data was extracted respective to each unique identifier with no identifying information on the data spreadsheet.

3. Results

3.1. Excluded Patients. 592 patients were identified after searching the pathology database (Figure 1) with the following patients excluded: 129 patients were inpatients or seen in the Emergency Department; 72 patients were not seen by the gastroenterologists (with empty EMR charts, not showing up for consultation, etc.); 47 patients with CRC were referred for reasons other than colonoscopy, for example, staging of a known rectal malignancy via endoscopic ultrasound. 44 patients were seen for highly suspected malignancy, for example, colonic mass on imaging or a suspicious rectal mass on exam. 19 patients were under the CCP; 17 patients were seen outside the period of inclusion; 12 patients had known IBD; 6 patients did not have CRC.

Table 2: Summary of data from chart reviews.

Consultations	*N*
Consultations available	242
Age of diagnosis	242
≥60	174
50–59	48
40–49	18
30–39	1
<30	1
Past medical hx	242
Positive hx of any malignancy	39
Negative hx of any malignancy	203
Family hx	235
Positive family hx of malignancy	109
Negative family hx of malignancy	83
Negative family hx of GI malignancy	43
Full consultations not available	4
Total consultations attempted for review	246
Pathology reports	*N*
Pathology reports available	244
Age ≥ 60	176
Age < 60	66
Tumour infiltrating lymphocytes	3
Crohn's-like lymphocytic reaction	0
Mucinous/signet ring differentiation	1
Medullary growth pattern	0
Other	62
Full pathology report unavailable	2
Total pathology reports attempted for review	246
Colonoscopy and OR notes	*N*
Colonoscopy and/or OR notes available	246
Synchronous lesions	7
Metachronous lesions	7
Neither synchronous or metachronous	228
Full colonoscopy and/or OR notes unavailable	0
Total colonoscopy and OR notes attempted for review	246

3.2. Patient Recollection of Family History of Malignancy. There were a total of 246 patients who met the inclusion criteria for this study (Table 2). Four patients had an incompletely documented initial consult; however information about these patients was obtainable through subsequent progress notes and was thus included in the study. 44% (109 of 246 patients)

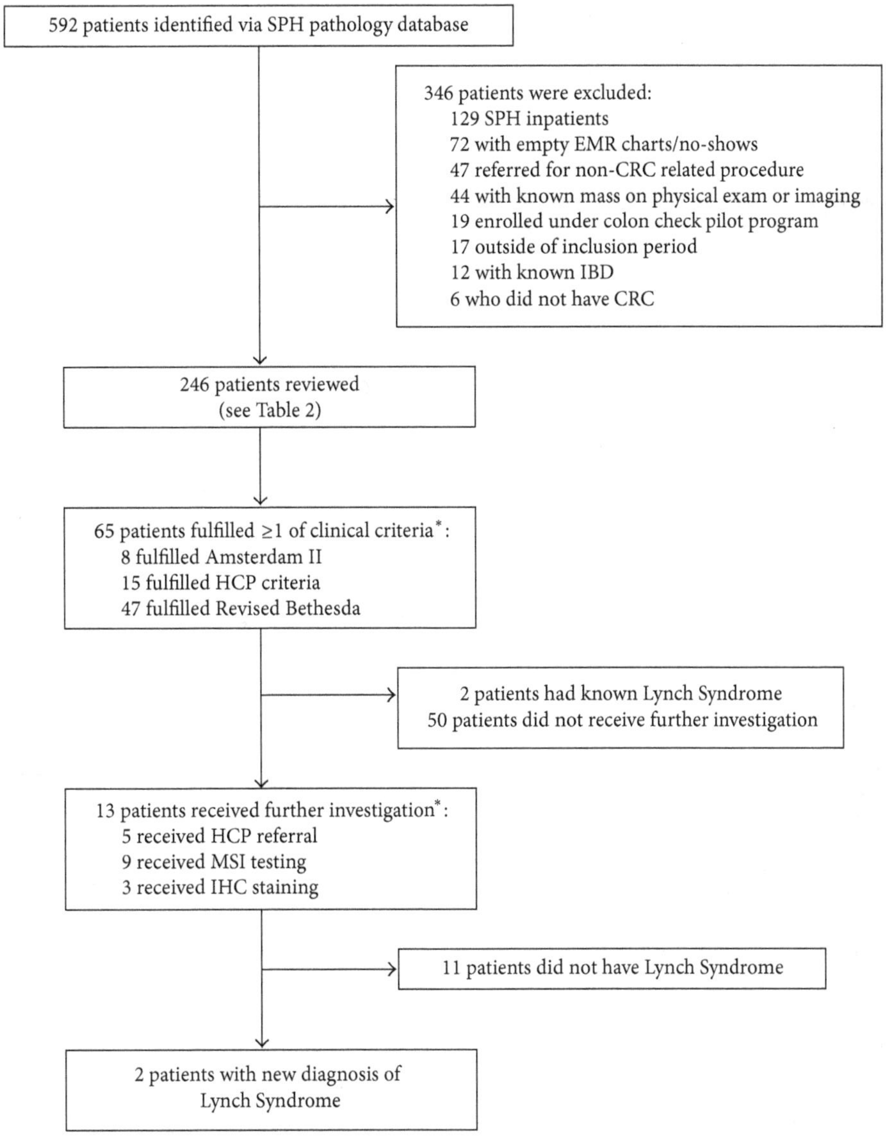

Not mutually exclusive

Figure 1: Flow chart of study and findings.

reported a positive family history for any malignancy. Of these, 76% (83 of 109 patients) were unable to recall either the specific malignancy or their respective age of diagnosis.

3.3. Completion of Family History by Physician. Of the 246 patients diagnosed with colorectal cancer, 96% (235 of 246 patients) had a family history available in their electronic chart. Of these, 46% (109 of 235 patients) had a family history of any malignancy, 35% (83 of 235 patients) had no family history of any malignancy, and 18% (43 of 235 patients) had a documentation of some equivalency of "no family history of gastrointestinal malignancy."

3.4. Pursuing of Further Investigation by Physician. 26% (65 of 246 patients) fulfilled at least one of the Amsterdam II (8 patients), Revised Bethesda (47 patients), or the HCP Criteria (15 patients). Two patients had known Lynch Syndrome. Of those without a known diagnosis, 21% (13 of 63 patients) went on to receive further investigation. Five patients were referred to the HCP, 9 received MSI testing, and 3 received IHC staining (not mutually exclusive). Patients who received further investigation had a statistically significant younger age, past medical history of malignancy, and family history of malignancy when compared to our baseline population (Table 3).

3.5. Diagnosis of Lynch Syndrome. Of the 246 patients diagnosed with colorectal cancer, 1.6% (4 patients) of these patients had a diagnosis of Lynch Syndrome. Two of these 4 patients had a previously known diagnosis of Lynch

Table 3: Characteristics of patients who received further investigation compared to all patients.

	All patients ($n = 246$)	Patients receiving further investigation ($n = 13$)	p value
History			
Average age of diagnosis	66	49	**<0.01**
Proportion of patients with past medical hx of malignancy	0.16	0.38	**0.03**
Proportion of patients with positive family hx of malignancy	0.46	0.92	**<0.01**
Pathology			
Proportion of patients with age < 60 and high risk pathology*	0.016	0.077	0.08
Colonoscopy & OR findings			
Presence of metachronous or synchronous lesion	0.057	0.15	0.132

*High risk pathology defined as any of the pathology findings fulfilling the Revised Bethesda Guidelines.

Syndrome, meaning that 0.8% (2 of 246 patients) were found to have a new diagnosis of Lynch Syndrome.

4. Discussion

Given that only 1.6% (4 of 246) of our population were diagnosed with Lynch Syndrome, our data suggests that Lynch Syndrome is indeed underrecognized when compared to the reported prevalence of 2–5% of all colorectal cancers. Our figure of 1.6% represents a population that reflects an ideal outpatient setting, where we assume that the physician (tertiary care gastroenterologist) would have the most time to complete a thorough family history and give consideration to investigating for Lynch Syndrome. Thus, our figure of 1.6% can even be considered as an overestimation of the true proportion of Lynch Syndrome amongst *all* newly diagnosed colorectal cancers at St. Paul's Hospital between 2010 and 2013. Even more concerning is the fact that St. Paul's is considered to be the major referral centre for complicated colorectal management in the Province of BC.

A number of contributing factors have emerged from this study. First, the majority of patients seem to have poor recognition of the exact type of malignancy and age of diagnosis for their family members, as 76% (83 of 109) of patients with a positive family history were unable to provide a history that was sufficient enough to be applied to any of the criteria. The exact type of malignancy can often be challenging for patients who may have difficulty discerning between various anatomical sites as well as conceptualizing primary versus metastatic disease. For example, misinterpreting a cervical cancer as an endometrial cancer can be misleading, as the latter is a Lynch Syndrome associated malignancy whereas the former is not. Another example would be a family member with metastatic disease to the liver from a colorectal cancer being misconstrued as a "liver cancer" which could mislead the physician into missing a family history of colorectal cancer. Furthermore, it is our experience that patients seem to have better recollection of their family member's age of death, as opposed to age of diagnosis. Overall, poor recollection of either the type of malignancy or its age of diagnosis inhibits the utility of the clinical criteria approach to identify patients at risk for Lynch Syndrome.

Second, our data suggests that although family history is discussed in the 96% (235 of 246 patients) of outpatient consultations, 18% (43 of 235 patients) of patients with a reportedly negative family history were only asked about a history of gastrointestinal malignancies. Given that Lynch Syndrome predisposes an individual to develop both colonic and extracolonic malignancy, a thorough family history exploring a history of any malignancy for all first-degree and second-degree relatives is warranted. It is entirely possible for a patient with unidentified Lynch Syndrome to have no family history of colorectal cancer but rather a significant history of endometrial cancer. Limiting the family history to solely gastrointestinal malignancies increases the risk of missing a diagnosis of Lynch Syndrome.

Third, only 21% (13 of 63 patients) of patients who met at least one of the criteria went on to receive further testing in the form of a HCP referral, MSI testing, or IHC staining. Our study suggests that patients with a younger age of diagnosis, past medical history of malignancy, and family history of malignancy are more likely to receive further investigation than those without. Given that this was a retrospective study, it is difficult to elicit from our data why some patients may not have received further investigation. However, we speculate that lack of recognition of the fulfillment of these criteria may be a factor. In addition, access to MSI testing or IHC staining is restricted and cannot be readily ordered by most physicians, including gastroenterologists, in British Columbia. This acts as an additional barrier to obtaining appropriate investigation for patients at high risk of Lynch Syndrome.

Overall, the underrecognition of Lynch Syndrome is multifactorial with issues at the patient, physician, and systems level. Although some factors are amenable to quality improvement intervention (e.g., encouraging physicians to ask about all malignancies in the family as opposed to just gastrointestinal related malignancy), some are not (e.g., poor patient recollection of the details of their family history). To deal with the fact that patients often have incomplete information and that physicians often do not (or cannot) obtain full family histories, the American Gastroenterology Association recommends universal MSI testing or IHC staining for all colorectal cancers [7]. Studies of molecular testing of all CRCs reveal that up to 28% of Lynch Syndrome patients could be missed with the most liberal clinical criteria, the Revised Bethesda Guidelines [8]. Furthermore, studies evaluating cost effectiveness of the various strategies have largely favoured universal testing, with initial IHC testing followed by *BRAF* mutation analysis for MLH1 absent tumours emerging as the most cost-effective approach [9].

As with any aspect in medicine, identification of these mutations must always be placed in the context of the patient and their respective wishes. A Dutch study revealed that almost half of the subjects in their cohort of family members at risk did not opt for genetic testing for LS [10]. Leenen et al. [11] further explored the motivations for the uptake or decline of genetic testing and revealed that the most important reasons for declining testing were anticipating problems with life insurance and mortgage, being content with life as is, and not experiencing any physical complaints.

Taken altogether, the present system of reliance on histories and patients to report their family histories appears to be inadequate and needs modification. A system such as that suggested by the latest AGA Guidelines where all cancers are universally tested appears to offer a cost-effective solution to these problems; however, it is essential that these results are interpreted in the perspective of the patient and the potential impact on their respective livelihood.

Acknowledgments

This manuscript was produced with the invaluable assistance of Renee Janssen who assisted with the development of our database. In addition, the authors would like to thank Cherry Galorport and Dr. Blair Walker for their assistance.

References

[1] BC Cancer Agency, "Hereditary Colorectal Cancer," 2012, http://www.screeningbc.ca/Hereditary/ForHealthProfessionals/HereditaryColorectalCancer.htm.

[2] S. Syngal, J. C. Weeks, D. Schrag, J. E. Garber, and K. M. Kuntz, "Benefits of colonoscopic surveillance and prophylactic colectomy in patients with hereditary nonpolyposis colorectal cancer mutations," *Annals of Internal Medicine*, vol. 129, no. 10, pp. 787–796, 1998.

[3] K. M. Schmeler, H. T. Lynch, L. M. Chen et al., "Prophylactic surgery to reduce the risk of gynecologic cancers in the lynch syndrome," *New England Journal of Medicine*, vol. 354, no. 3, pp. 261–269, 2006.

[4] C. M. Cremin, L. Armstrong, S. Gill, D. Huntsman, and C. Bajdik, "The identification of Lynch syndrome in British Columbia," *Canadian Journal of Gastroenterology*, vol. 23, no. 11, pp. 761–767, 2009.

[5] BC Cancer Agency, "Incident Testing for Lynch Syndrome in CRC under 50 in British Columbia," 2011, http://www.screeningbc.ca/NR/rdonlyres/F5C7A219-8D7A-457C-A2FA-D16603768EEE/62238/CRCunder51.pdf.

[6] BC Cancer Agency, "Hereditary Cancer Program Referral," 2015, http://www.screeningbc.ca/NR/rdonlyres/822D2FC7-021D-44CF-89B8-3CDFA58C7142/74062/HCPReferralFormFebruary2015.pdf.

[7] J. H. Rubenstein, R. Enns, J. Heidelbaugh, and A. Barkun, "American gastroenterological association institute guideline on the diagnosis and management of lynch syndrome," *Gastroenterology*, vol. 149, no. 3, pp. 777–782, 2015.

[8] F. M. Giardiello, J. I. Allen, J. E. Axilbund et al., "Guidelines on genetic evaluation and management of lynch syndrome: a consensus statement by the US multi-society task force on colorectal cancer," *American Journal of Gastroenterology*, vol. 109, no. 8, pp. 1159–1179, 2014.

[9] U. Ladabaum, G. Wang, J. Terdiman et al., "Strategies to identify the Lynch syndrome among patients with colorectal cancer: a cost-effectiveness analysis," *Annals of Internal Medicine*, vol. 155, no. 2, pp. 69–79, 2011.

[10] D. Ramsoekh, M. E. van Leerdam, C. M. Tops et al., "The use of genetic testing in hereditary colorectal cancer syndromes: genetic testing in HNPCC, (A)FAP and MAP," *Clinical Genetics*, vol. 72, no. 6, pp. 562–567, 2007.

[11] C. H. Leenen, M. Heijer, C. van der Meer, E. J. Kuipers, M. E. van Leerdam, and A. Wagner, "Genetic testing for Lynch syndrome: family communication and motivation," *Familial Cancer*, vol. 15, no. 1, pp. 63–73, 2016.

24

Predictive Value of Adiposity Level, Metabolic Syndrome, and Insulin Resistance for the Risk of Nonalcoholic Fatty Liver Disease Diagnosis in Obese Children

Zofia Prokopowicz, Ewa Malecka-Tendera, and Pawel Matusik

School of Medicine in Katowice, Department of Pediatrics and Pediatric Endocrinology, Medical University of Silesia, Katowice, Poland

Correspondence should be addressed to Pawel Matusik; endocrin@wp.pl

Academic Editor: Branka Filipović

Background. Nonalcoholic fatty liver disease (NAFLD) is the most common cause of chronic liver disease in obese children. Early diagnosis and treatment are essential for curing or slowing down the disease progression. The aim of the study was to assess the prevalence of NAFLD in this population and to identify anthropometrical and metabolic risk factors for NAFLD prediction and its development. *Material and Methods.* The study included 108 obese children. Anthropometric measurements, NAFLD diagnosis (based on ALT level and/or liver ultrasound), and metabolic syndrome (MS) components were assessed in all patients. Patients were divided into groups with and without NAFLD. *Results.* NAFLD was diagnosed in 49 (45%) patients with similar prevalence in boys (27; 55.10%) and girls [22 (44.9%), $p = 0.089$]. NAFLD patients had significantly greater waist circumference, WHR, and WHtR and significantly higher total cholesterol, triglyceride, and fasting insulin concentrations as well as higher glucose and insulin concentrations in 120 minutes of OGTT and higher HOMA-IR levels compared to group of patients without NAFLD. In NAFLD patients, MS was significantly more likely to be diagnosed than in group without NAFLD (40.82% versus 22.81%, $p = 0.04$), but among the MS components only hypertriglyceridemia was significantly more frequently diagnosed in the group with NAFLD ($p = 0.002$). Among analysed parameters the best independent risk factor for NAFLD was fasting insulin concentration with the cut-off point = 18,9 uIU/ml (AUC = 0.829). *Conclusions.* NAFLD is a very common disease in obese children. NAFLD predictive risk factors include increased waist circumference, elevated WHR and WHtR, and elevated total cholesterol, triglycerides, and fasting insulin as well as elevated glucose and insulin concentration in the OGTT and HOMA-IR index. NAFLD increases the risk of potential cardiovascular complications expressed by diagnosis of metabolic syndrome. The best independent predictive risk factor for diagnosing NAFLD in obese children is fasting insulin > 18.9 uIU/ml.

1. Introduction

Nonalcoholic fatty liver disease (NAFLD) is the most common cause of chronic liver disease in children [1]. Due to the growing number of obese children the prevalence of fatty liver increases, and it was assessed in around one-third of clinical population [2]. NAFLD is defined as hepatic fat infiltration > 5% of hepatocytes, assessed by liver biopsy, after exclusion of excessive alcohol intake and other liver pathologies. In children NAFLD is, usually at the time of diagnosis, a simple steatosis, which is reversible, but also can initiate further stages of disease, such as nonalcoholic steatohepatitis (NASH), fibrosis, and cirrhosis. The pathogenesis of NAFLD and its progression are complex process, called multiple-hit theory combining environmental (dietary habits, physical activity [3, 4]), molecular (lipotoxicity [5]), endoplasmic reticulum stress [6], mitochondrial dysfunction [7], organokines effect [8, 9], genetic (polymorphism involved in the onset and progression of the disease), and other factors like dysbiosis [7, 10, 11].

NAFLD not only in adults but also in children is associated with severe metabolic disorders as hypertension, dyslipidaemia, increased risk of type 2 diabetes, metabolic syndrome, and cardiovascular diseases [12, 13]. For many years, NAFLD has been perceived as a hepatic consequence of insulin resistance, but recent studies have shown that fatty liver disease can precede with type 2 diabetes and metabolic syndrome and may even be a risk factor for their development [14, 15]. Due to biopsy limitations, hepatic steatosis is also diagnosed with biochemical tests like elevated alanine transaminase, or imaging methods, especially ultrasound. Despite the limitations, ultrasonography is characterized by high sensitivity (60–94%) and specificity (84–100%) for NAFLD detection [16]. Early diagnosis in the asymptomatic period and effective therapy implementation enable curing or, at least, slow down the progression of the disease.

The aim of the study was to assess the prevalence of NAFLD, as well as identifying additional predictive anthropometrical and metabolic risk factors for NAFLD development in the obese children.

2. Materials and Methods

2.1. Study Population. The study was prospective and included 108 children aged 6 to 18, hospitalized in our department between years 2012 and 2014, whose BMI exceeded 97 pc for sex and age, after informed consent. Children with acute infectious disease, chronic hepatitis of known etiology, using hepatotoxic drugs, or consuming alcohol were excluded from the study. A general medical examination, anthropometric measurements, laboratory tests, blood pressure measurements, and abdomen ultrasound imaging were performed in all subjects.

2.2. Anthropometric Evaluation and Body Composition. All anthropometric measurements were made in the morning, with fasting with empty bladder in the upright position. Subjects were barefoot and lightly dressed. Height and weight were measured to the nearest 0,1 cm and 0,1 kg, respectively, by using calibrated scale and Harpenden stadiometer. Waist and hip circumference were measured to the nearest 0,5 cm using standard technique with nonelastic tape, at the end of normal expiration. Waist circumference (WC) was measured at a point midway between the lower border of the ribs and the iliac crest, and hip circumference was measured at the widest part of the hip. BMI, waist-hip ratio (WHR), and waist-to-height ratio (WHtR) were calculated. Standard deviations scores for height and BMI were calculated using the LMS method based on Polish reference values [17].

Body composition was evaluated by bioelectrical impedance using the Tanita MC 980 MA device-multifrequency segmental analyser. Estimates of body composition were obtained from the equipped software. Patient stand barefoot on the marked electrodes and in straightened hands held the handles equipped with electrodes. The measurement of the tissue impedance through which the six-frequency (1 kHz, 5 kHz, 50 kHz, 250 kHz, 500 kHz, and 1000 kHz) and low intensity (<90 μA) current was applied is painless and lasts for several seconds. Of the many variables, the following results were analysed: total body water in kg and % (TBW), fat mass in kg and fat%, fat-free mass in kg (FFM), muscle mass in kg, visceral fat in %, and basal metabolic rate in kJ (BMR). Moreover the following indicators were calculated: visceral fat to total body fat (visceral fat%/fat%), basal metabolic rate per kilogram body weight (BMR/kg), and standard deviations scores for fat percentage (fat%Z-score = 2 $*$ (fat% − 50 pc fat%)/(98 pc fat% − 50 pc fat%)) based on children reference values [18].

2.3. Liver Ultrasonography. Liver ultrasound examination was performed by two radiologists with Siemens Acuson Antares, convex transducer 5 MHz. Fatty liver was diagnosed on the basis of increased echogenicity of the liver parenchyma compared to the right kidney echogenicity.

2.4. Laboratory Assessment. Fasting venous blood sample was taken in the second day of hospitalization. Blood chemistry analyses, alanine transaminase (ALT), gamma glutamyltransferase (GGT), total cholesterol (Tch), high density lipoprotein (HDL), low density lipoprotein (LDL), triglycerides (TG), and bilirubin, were performed in hospital laboratory by using standard methods. Oral glucose tolerance test (OGTT; 1.75 g/kg body weight, up to 75 g) was performed in all patients. Glucose and insulin concentration were measured during fasting and in 120 minutes of the test. In this study, elevated ALT levels were identified for ALT > 35 U/l in children aged 3–11 years and ALT > 40 U/l in children aged ≥ 11 years. Hypertriglyceridemia was defined as fasting triglycerides ≥ 150 mg/dl, and low HDL cholesterol as fasting HDL < 40 mg/dl in children aged < 16 years and <40 mg/dl for boys or <50 mg/dl for girls aged > 16 years [19]. Impaired fasting glucose (IFG) was defined as fasting glucose ≥ 100 mg/dl.

2.5. Blood Pressure Measurements. Blood pressure (BP) was measured three times daily by the Korotkoff method using sphygmomanometer, on the right arm after 5–10 minutes of rest in the sitting position. The results were referred to Polish children reference values [20]. Patients with at least two measurements > 90 pc (high normal pressure) and patients with previously treated hypertension performed 24-hour ambulatory blood pressure monitoring using the Spacelabs ABP. Hypertension was diagnosed when the systolic blood pressure was above 95 pc for more than 25% of the measurements.

2.6. Insulin Resistance and Metabolic Syndrome (MS). Insulin resistance was measured by homeostasis model assessment of insulin resistance (HOMA-IR) described by Matthews et al. [21], defined as follows: HOMA-IR = fasting glucose (mg/dl) × fasting insulin (uIU/ml)/405. The outcomes were referred to Caucasian obese children reference values [22].

We used the definition of the International Diabetes Federation (IDF) for the metabolic syndrome in children and adolescents [19]. The first criterion reached in all our patients was central obesity defined as WC > 90 pc for age and sex or above adult norms (>80 cm for women and >94 cm for men). If patients reached at least 2 of the other 4 criteria (TG concentration ≥ 150 mg/dl or hypolipemic treatment; HDL levels < 40 mg/dl (for girls > 16 years, HDL < 50 mg/dl); elevated blood pressure (systolic > 130 mmHg or diastolic > 85 mm Hg) or hypertension; fasting glucose ≥ 100 mg/dl; or type 2 diabetes) then the metabolic syndrome was diagnosed.

TABLE 1: Anthropometric characteristic of studied population.

Variable	All (N = 108) Mean	All SD	Males (N = 50) Mean	Males SD	Females (N = 58) Mean	Females SD	ttest p value
BMI z-score	2.40	0.48	2.36	0.47	2.43	0.50	0.463
height z-score	0.42	1.4	0.60	1.55	0.27	1.26	0.230
WC (cm)	*103.9*	*12.9*	*108.17*	*12.06*	*100.16*	*12.49*	*0.001*
Hip circumference (cm)	108	11.3	108.12	11.47	107.90	11.29	0.922
WHR	*0.96*	*0.07*	*1.0*	*0.06*	*0.93*	*0.07*	*<0.001*
WHtR	0.63	0.06	0.64	0.06	0.62	0.06	0.073
Fat%	*39.27*	*6.79*	*37.17*	*7.36*	*41.08*	*5.71*	*0.002*
Fat% z-score	*3.06*	*1.03*	*2.84*	*0.87*	*3.31*	*1.14*	*0.017*
Visceral fat/fat%	0.46	0.45	0.44	0.45	0.48	0.45	0.769
BMR (kJ)	*7851*	*1233*	*8681*	*1056*	*7135*	*878*	*<0.001*
BMR/kg (kJ/kg)	*92*	*13.94*	*96.4*	*13.7*	*88.5*	*13.17*	*0.003*

2.7. NAFLD Diagnosis. NAFLD was diagnosed based on ultrasound examination and/or elevated ALT.

2.8. Statistical Analysis. The statistical software (Statistica v. 12.5 and Microsoft Excel) was used in data analysis. Descriptive data were expressed as median, mean values, and standard deviations (SD) for continuous variables. Patients were divided into two groups: with and without NAFLD, which were then compared for anthropometric features, biochemical parameters, and metabolic syndrome components. Mann–Whitney *U*, ANOVA Kruskal-Wallis, Spearman rank correlation tests were used to compare continuous variables. Chi-square test was used for qualitative variables. The receiver operating characteristics (ROC) analysis was used to verify the characteristics of the independent variables and to assess an appropriate cut-off. Statistical significance was set at p value less than 0.05.

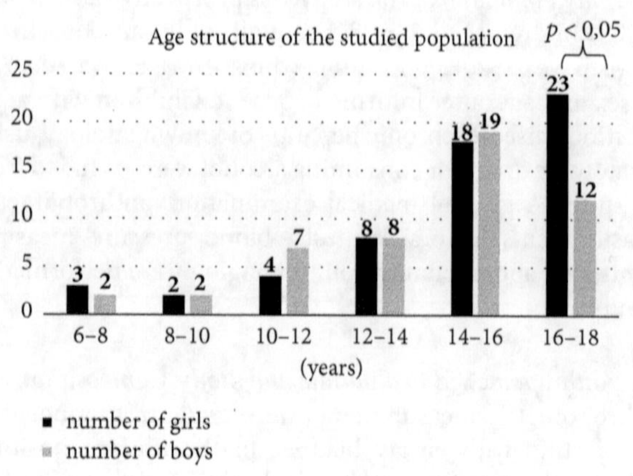

FIGURE 1: Sex distribution in particular age groups.

3. Results

The study included 108 obese children (50 boys) aged 6 years and 2 months to 17 years and 10 months. Mean age was 14.24 ± 2.73 SD. Mean age of girls was 14.75 ± 2.79 SD and of boys 13.9 ± 2.64 SD. Girls were about one year older than boys, but the difference was not statistically significant ($p = 0.074$). The age distribution of the examined group is shown in Figure 1. The only statistically significant difference was observed in the 16–18-year age group, where girls predominated. Table 1 gives the anthropometric and body composition characteristic of the study population stratified by gender. Males ($n = 50$) and females ($n = 58$) had similar BMI and height *Z*-scores while males had significantly higher mean WC and WHR. Among important anthropometrical data for obesity diagnosis, parameters of body composition males had significantly higher fat% and fat%*Z*-score; however no difference in visceral fat/fat% was observed.

3.1. NAFLD Prevalence. NAFLD was diagnosed in patients with hyperechogenic liver on ultrasound and/or elevated ALT concentration. Ultrasonographic features of fatty liver were diagnosed in 34 patients (16 girls and 18 boys) and elevated ALT in 30 patients (8 girls and 22 boys). In 15 patients (2 girls and 13 boys) both were reported. Based on proposed criteria, two groups were identified: (I) NAFLD patients ($N = 49$; 45.4%) and (II) non-NAFLD patients with normal liver and normal ALT concentration ($N = 59$; 54.6%).

NAFLD was diagnosed more often in boys than in girls; however the difference was insignificant (55.1% versus 44.9%; $p = 0.089$).

3.2. Anthropometry and Body Composition. NAFLD patients did not differ significantly from patients without NAFLD in age, height, body weight, BMI, or BMI *Z*-score, while NAFLD was associated with a significantly greater waist circumference, WHR, and WHtR. Body composition analysis did not show statistically significant differences between groups in key obesity parameters such as fat mass, fat%, fat% *Z*-score, or visceral fat%. Groups differed significantly only in fat-free mass (FFM), total body water (TBW), and basal metabolic rate (BMR); however BMR per kilogram remained similar in both groups. The comparison of the two groups in terms of basic anthropometric and body composition parameters is presented in Table 2.

TABLE 2: Anthropometry and body composition. Comparison of patients with and without NAFLD.

Variable	NAFLD ($N = 49$)			Patients without NAFLD ($N = 59$)			p value (Mann–Whitney U test)
	Mean	SD	Median	Mean	SD	Median	
Age (years)	14.40	2.49	14.83	14.17	2.94	14.92	0.828
Waist (cm)	*107.70*	*12.44*	*107.00*	*100.95*	*12.60*	*100.50*	*0.017*
Hip (cm)	108.78	11.50	109	107.53	10.97	108	0.794
WHR	*0.99*	*0.06*	*0.98*	*0.94*	*0.08*	*0.94*	*<0.001*
WHtR	*0.65*	*0.06*	*0.65*	*0.62*	*0.06*	*0.62*	*0.041*
Height (cm)	166.10	11.95	166.40	162.70	12.41	161.50	0.127
Weight (kg)	92.22	22.78	89.00	84.53	19.74	84.80	0.126
BMI (kg/m2)	32.97	5.29	32.00	31.49	4.82	31.60	0.243
BMI Z-score	2.45	0.48	2.38	2.37	0.48	2.36	0.479
Height Z-score	0.53	1.44	0.53	−0.573	0.566	−0.573	0.566
Fat%	39.40	6.34	38.90	39.15	7.23	39.60	0.897
Fat mass (kg)	36.61	11.58	36.50	33.44	10.91	34.60	0.214
FFM (kg)	*55.62*	*14.01*	*54.60*	*51.08*	*12.68*	*48.90*	*0.047*
FFM%	60.61	6.35	61.07	60.83	7.23	60.35	0.879
Muscle mass (kg)	52.40	13.72	51.80	48.57	12.13	46.60	0.094
TBW	*40.72*	*10.26*	*40.00*	*37.38*	*9.28*	*35.80*	*0.047*
TBW%	44.33	4.67	44.70	44.53	5.28	44.20	0.919
Trunk fat%	35.39	7.08	35.00	34.84	8.07	35.80	0.886
Fat% Z-score	3.15	0.99	3.04	2.98	1.07	2.92	0.577
Trunk/total	0.89	0.06	0.88	0.88	0.07	0.89	0.986
BMR	*8158*	*1293*	*7880*	*7617*	*1144*	*7512*	*0.028*
BMR/kg	90.89	12.33	86.17	92.80	14.85	88.57	0.597

TABLE 3: Biochemical analysis. Comparison of patients with and without NAFLD.

Variable	NAFLD patients ($N = 49$)			Patients without NAFLD ($N = 59$)			p value (Mann–Whitney U test)
	Mean	SD	Median	Mean	SD	Median	
Tch (mg/dl)	*185.12*	*28.64*	*185.00*	*169.02*	*30.01*	*167*	*0.004*
HDL (mg/dl)	45.34	10.26	43.90	47.77	11.38	45.85	0.298
LDL (mg/dl)	103.16	25.69	99.90	96.26	28.34	62.03	0.153
TG (mg/dl)	*183.08*	*79.69*	*173.00*	*129.15*	*62.03*	*114.00*	*<0.001*
glu 0 (mg/dl)	90.88	10.00	90.00	88.95	7.74	88.50	0.403
glu 120 (mg/dl)	*122.04*	*22.68*	*121.00*	*109.91*	*19.84*	*109.00*	*0.007*
ins 0 (μIU/ml)	*28.48*	*21.54*	*23.15*	*12.86*	*6.76*	*12.00*	*<0.001*
ins 120 (μIU/ml)	*130.38*	*98.18*	*93.80*	*81.36*	*44.03*	*70.70*	*0.004*
HOMA-IR	*6.44*	*4.83*	*4.93*	*2.86*	*1.67*	*2.58*	*<0.001*

3.3. Biochemical Analysis. Of the biochemical parameters, the serum concentration of total cholesterol, triglycerides, fasting insulin, glucose, and insulin in 120 minutes of OGTT and HOMA-IR were significantly higher in patients with NAFLD.

NAFLD was significantly more often diagnosed in patients with HOMA-IR exceeding reference values [22] than in children with the normal range of HOMA-IR (79% versus 28%, $p = 0.00$ for HOMA-IR > 90 percentile; 85% versus 15%, $p = 0.00$ for HOMA-IR > 97 percentile). A detailed summary of the biochemical parameters is presented in Table 3.

The ROC analysis was performed on variables that differentiated NAFLD patients from non-NAFLD ones. Based on the area under receiver operating curves (AUC) we established a threshold of each variable that showed the highest accuracy for identifying children at high risk of NAFLD. Figure 2 shows a comparison of the ROC curves for the evaluated parameters. The largest area under the ROC curve was obtained for fasting insulin (AUC = 0.829, 95% CI 0.746–0.911) and for HOMA-IR (AUC = 0.817; 95% CI 0,733–0,901). The optimal cut-off point of the insulin level for diagnosing NAFLD was 18,9 uIU/l with the sensitivity of 75% and specificity of 87,3%. The performance of these variables in NAFLD prediction is summarized in Table 4.

3.4. Metabolic Syndrome. In the study population 34 (31.48%) patients were diagnosed with metabolic syndrome (MS). Of the metabolic syndrome components abdominal obesity and

TABLE 4: Diagnostic value of analysed variables in NAFLD prediction.

Variable	Symbol	AUC (95% CI)	Cut point	Sensitivity	Specificity	SE
Total cholesterol	Tch	0.660 (0.557–0.764)	197 mg/dl	44.9%	80.7%	0.053
Triglycerides	TG	0.713 (0.614–0.813)	161 mg/dl	61.2%	75.4%	0.051
Glucose in 120 min of OGTT	glu 120	0.654 (0.548–0.759)	112 mg/dl	70.2%	56.4%	0.054
Fasting insulin	ins 0	0.829 (0.746–0.911)	18.9 μIU/ml	75%	87.3 %	0.042
Insulin in 120 min of OGTT	ins 120	0.666 (0.559–0.772)	129 μIU/ml	38.3%	90.9%	0.054
Insulin resistance	HOMA-IR	0.817 (0.733–0.901)	4.089	70.8%	83.6%	0.043

TABLE 5: Prevalence of metabolic factors in NAFLD and non-NAFLD group.

MS components	Total (%)	NAFLD patients (N = 49)	Patients without NAFLD (N = 59)	p
WC > 90 pc	108 (100%)	49 (100%)	59 (100%)	NS
TG > 150 mg/dl or hypolipemic treatment	49 (45.37%)	30 (61.22%)	19 (32.20%)	*0.002*
HDL < 40 mg/dl (girls > 16 years; HDL < 50 mg/dl)	39 (36.11%)	20 (40.82%)	19 (32.20%)	NS
Hypertension	21 (19.44%)	11 (22.45%)	10 (16.95%)	NS
IFG or diabetes 2	13 (12.04%)	6 (12.24%)	7 (11.86%)	NS
MS	*34 (31.48%)*	*20 (40.82%)*	*14 (23.73%)*	*0.04*

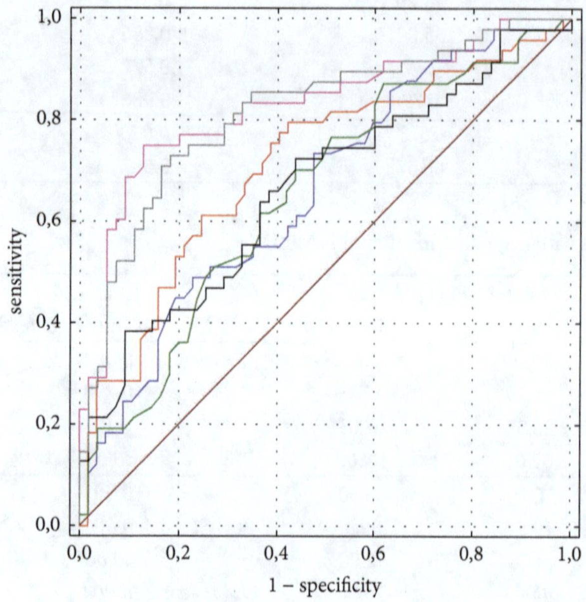

FIGURE 2: Comparison of ROC curves for parameters significantly differentiating patients with NAFLD from non-NAFLD patients.

hypertriglyceridemia were most often recognised. MS was diagnosed significantly more frequently in NAFLD group than in patients without fatty liver (40.82% versus 23.73%, p = 0.04), but of the MS components only hypertriglyceridemia was significantly more often diagnosed in NAFLD patients. The frequency of the MS and its components in the study population is presented in Table 5.

4. Discussion

We diagnosed NAFLD on the basis of elevated ALT and/or presence of steatosis on ultrasound. Both of these criteria are often used in noninvasive diagnosis of fatty liver disease. High sensitivity (60–94%) and specificity (84–100%) of ultrasonography make this examination suitable for screening [16]. Alanine aminotransferase (ALT) concentration due to wide availability and low cost is the basic marker used in liver diseases screening, including NAFLD. Interpretation difficulties are caused by different cut-off points proposed by each investigator like ALT > 52 U/L for girls and >72 U/L for boys in the Brazilian study [23], ALT > 50 U/L the in the Wiegand et al. study [24], or ALT > the laboratory standard in most authors' studies. On the other hand, we should be aware of low sensitivity of ALT at standard cut-off point (45 U/l); despite liver steatosis confirmed by imaging studies, in most pediatric patients, ALT levels remain normal. Therefore, a number of population studies suggest introducing new, sex-specific thresholds for ALT [25]: in children ALT < 25.8 IU/l for boys and ALT < 22.1 IU/l for girls in American study [26], ALT < 33 IU/l for boys and <25 IU/l for girls in Korean study [27], or ALT < 30 IU/l and <21 IU/l in Iranian study, respectively [28].

In this study we diagnosed NAFLD in 45% of patients. Such a high prevalence is caused by both group selection (obese children hospitalized for obesity) and diagnostic criteria. Fatty liver on ultrasound was reported in 34 (31.48%) patients, and elevated ALT levels were reported in 30 (27.78%) patients.

The authors of meta-analysis from 2015 [2], based on 56 clinical trials, assessed the prevalence of NAFLD in obese children on 34.2% with a prediction range from 5.2% to 83.1%. Researchers, however, emphasize significant differences in the methodology, diagnostic criteria, or accepted standards for the laboratory tests results. With the lowest frequency NAFLD was diagnosed in 2,3% patients by Brazilian researchers [23], which is caused by the inclusion criteria: abdominal obesity defined as WC > 75 pc and significantly higher ALT (52 U/L for girls and ALT > 72 U/L for boys) as well as ethnic differences (only 29% of the children were Caucasian). As much as 83.1% of patients were diagnosed with NAFLD in the American study [29]; however, the group consisted of children who were qualified to bariatric surgery. The mean prevalence of NAFLD diagnosed on ultrasound in the previously cited meta-analysis was 41%, while that diagnosed on the basis of elevated alanine aminotransferase was only 13.7% [2].

Males have higher prevalence of NAFLD than females, which is confirmed by most studies [2, 24, 30], but not in the Italian study [31] where NAFLD was similar in both sexes (58% of boys and 46% of girls, $p = 0.31$). However, in that study prepubertal population was analysed, which was significantly younger than in other studies. In our study prevalence of NAFLD was similar in males and females, which could have come from the sex distribution in age groups (there were significantly more girls in the 16–18 age group, $p < 0.05$).

In our study NAFLD patients were similar to non-NAFLD ones in age and basic anthropometric parameters such as height, weight and even BMI, and BMI Z-score. There was also no difference in the most important parameters of the body composition (fat mass, fat%, fat% Z-score, or visceral fat%). Children with NAFLD had only significantly higher fat-free mass, total body water content, and BMR (but not BMR/kg); however, these parameters, due to their weight, age, or gender dependence, have little diagnostic value.

The only anthropometric parameters discriminating NAFLD patients from non-NAFLD, in our study, are waist circumference (WC) and the indicators associated with WC, WHR and WHtR. These are important, practical pieces of information indicating that BMI, even referred to reference values, is not sufficient for obese patients, while WC, which is still not a routine medical examination, may be an effective tool for detecting patients at risk of metabolic disorders, including NAFLD. Many studies have shown that waist circumference may be used in central obesity screening, cardiovascular risk assessment in children [32], and NAFLD diagnosis [33–35].

Similar results were obtained by Italian and Taiwanese researchers who did not observe differences in BMI and body composition between the groups with and without NAFLD, but waist circumference was significantly higher in NAFLD group [31, 34]. Denzer et al. also observed significantly greater waist circumference in patients with NAFLD (mean 111 cm versus 101 cm in patients without steatosis, $p < 0.0001$) but, in contrast to our results, NAFLD patients had significantly higher BMI-Z score (mean 2, 78 versus 2.56 in non-NAFLD, $p < 0.0001$) [30].

Considering the complexity of links between NAFLD, insulin resistance (IR), and type 2 diabetes, it is extremely difficult to find out whether NAFLD is the cause or the effect of insulin resistance. For many years, NAFLD has been treated as the hepatic consequence of IR, but recent studies suggest that hepatic steatosis may precede type 2 diabetes and metabolic syndrome and may even be a risk factor for their development [14, 15].

In our survey in diagnostics of carbohydrate metabolism fasting glucose remained useless, which was confirmed in other studies [31, 36]. Significant differences between groups were observed in fasting insulin concentration and glucose and insulin concentration in 120 minutes of OGTT. In our study, the highest diagnostic value for detecting NAFLD achieved fasting insulin with AUC = 0.829, and the cut-off point of 18.9 μIU/ml with 75% sensitivity and 87.3% specificity diagnosed NAFLD. Studies in obese patients [31, 36, 37] confirm correlation of fasting insulin concentrations with NAFLD diagnosis; however there are no clear standards for this parameter, which makes it difficult to apply. In Shashaj et al. study [22] mean fasting insulin concentration in obese patients was 13.8 μIU/ml ± 9.4, while in Pacifico et al. it was 10.6 μIU/ml in obese children without steatosis and 15.6 μIU/ml in obese children with NAFLD [36]. Much higher mean concentration of fasting insulin was observed by Korean researchers, 15.1 μIU/ml ± 6.0 in obese children without NAFLD and 24.8 μIU/ml + 14.6 in children with NAFLD [37]. These results are comparable to our study (12, 86 μIU/ml ± 6.76 in children without steatosis versus 28.48 μIU/ml ± 21.53 in children with NAFLD).

NAFLD patients had significantly higher HOMA-IR values compared to non-NAFLD ones. Similar observations have been made by Denzer et al. [30] and D'Adamo et al., who confirmed that insulin resistance indexes were significantly associated with NAFLD independently of BMI [31]. In contrast Gökçe et al. concluded that neither mean HOMA-IR values nor the prevalence of insulin resistance was higher in NAFLD group [12].

It is proven that insulin resistance increases in obese patients; therefore separate standards are developed for the population of obese children [22]. Authors of this study emphasize that in obese children HOMA-IR > 75 pc is associated with an increased cardiometabolic risk defined as at least one of the following: hypercholesterolemia, hypertriglyceridemia, reduced HDL levels, and ALT > 40 U/l. They have also observed that HOMA-IR > 3.42 (AUC = 0.71) with 48.8% sensitivity and 81.3% specificity identifies cardiovascular risk in obese patients. Referring our results to the proposed standards [22] we proved that NAFLD is significantly more common in patients with increased HOMA-IR compared to obese patients with normal HOMA-IR (79% versus 28%, $p = 0.00$ for HOMA-IR > 90 pc; 85% versus 15%, $p = 0.00$ for HOMA-IR > 97 pc), and HOMA-IR > 4.089 is a good indicator of NAFLD (AUROC = 0.817, sensitivity = 70.8%, specificity = 83.6%, and 95% CI = 0.733).

Metabolic syndrome (MS) in adult patients increases the risk of cardiovascular disease. In the pediatric population such conclusions are not clear. Due to both lack of long-term follow-up of pediatric patients and different criteria for MS, some authors suggest that the prevalence of individual components of metabolic syndrome in the pediatric population would be more relevant for assessment of the cardiovascular risk than the diagnosis of metabolic syndrome [38, 39]. In the studied population, based on IDF criteria [19], 34 (31.48%) patients were diagnosed with MS, which is comparable to other studies using the same criteria (Strojny et al., 29% [40]). In contrast, Manco et al. diagnosed MS only in 10%

of children with NAFLD, which may be because only 65% of the children in the study group were obese [35]. In our study, patients with MS were more likely to have NAFLD than patients without MS (60.6% versus 39.19%, $p < 0.05$), but no correlation was found between the number of metabolic syndrome criteria and the prevalence NAFLD ($p = 0.052$), which may be caused by the fact that only fasting glucose but not the insulin resistance is considered in the IDF criteria for MS.

5. Conclusions

NAFLD is a very common disease in obese children. NAFLD risk factors include increased waist circumference, elevated WHR and WHtR, and elevated total cholesterol, triglycerides, and fasting insulin as well as glucose and insulin concentration in 120 min of OGTT and HOMA-IR index. NAFLD increases the risk of potential cardiovascular complications expressed by diagnosis of metabolic syndrome. The best independent risk factor for diagnosing NAFLD in obese children is fasting insulin concentration > 18.9 uIU/ml.

In our study, we focused on the diagnosis of obese children in the context of metabolic disorders, especially related to obesity and fatty liver disease. The prevalence of NAFLD and other metabolic disorders in the study population indicates the need to improve diagnostics in obese children already at primary health care level. Simple diagnostic methods such as waist circumference measurement and fasting plasma insulin concentration may contribute to the early identification and prediction of patients at risk of NAFLD and other metabolic complications. Appropriate therapy and lifestyle change in these patients and their families will help to prevent the negative effects of obesity in the future.

Acknowledgments

The study was financially supported by the Medical University of Silesia Grant (KNW-2-033/D/3/N), founded by Polish Ministry of Science.

References

[1] V. Giorgio, F. Prono, F. Graziano, and V. Nobili, "Pediatric non alcoholic fatty liver disease: old and new concepts on development, progression, metabolic insight and potential treatment targets," *BMC Pediatrics*, vol. 13, no. 1, article 40, 2013.

[2] E. L. Anderson, L. D. Howe, H. E. Jones, J. P. T. Higgins, D. A. Lawlor, and A. Fraser, "The prevalence of non-alcoholic fatty liver disease in children and adolescents: A systematic review and meta-analysis," *PLoS ONE*, vol. 10, no. 10, Article ID e0140908, 2015.

[3] A. A. Bremer, M. Mietus-Snyder, and R. H. Lustig, "Toward a unifying hypothesis of metabolic syndrome," *Pediatrics*, vol. 129, no. 3, pp. 557–570, 2012.

[4] M. F. Abdelmalek, A. Suzuki, C. Guy et al., "Increased fructose consumption is associated with fibrosis severity in patients with nonalcoholic fatty liver disease," *Hepatology*, vol. 51, no. 6, pp. 1961–1971, 2010.

[5] K. Cusi, "Role of obesity and lipotoxicity in the development of nonalcoholic steatohepatitis: pathophysiology and clinical implications," *Gastroenterology*, vol. 142, no. 4, pp. 711.e6–725.e6, 2012.

[6] L. Ozcan and I. Tabas, "Role of endoplasmic reticulum stress in metabolic disease and other disorders," *Annual Review of Medicine*, vol. 63, pp. 317–328, 2012.

[7] J. Yu, S. Marsh, J. Hu, W. Feng, and C. Wu, "The pathogenesis of nonalcoholic fatty liver disease: interplay between diet, gut microbiota, and genetic background," *Gastroenterology Research and Practice*, vol. 2016, Article ID 2862173, 13 pages, 2016.

[8] M. Kłusek-Oksiuta, I. Bialokoz-Kalinowska, E. Tarasów, M. Wojtkowska, I. Werpachowska, and D. M. Lebensztejn, "Chemerin as a novel non-invasive serum marker of intrahepatic lipid content in obese children," *Italian Journal of Pediatrics*, vol. 40, article 84, 2014.

[9] D. M. Lebensztejn, M. Flisiak-Jackiewicz, I. Bialokoz-Kalinowska, A. Bobrus-Chociej, and I. Kowalska, "Hepatokines and non-alcoholic fatty liver disease," *Acta Biochimica Polonica*, vol. 63, no. 3, pp. 459–467, 2016.

[10] K. Miura and H. Ohnishi, "Role of gut microbiota and Toll-like receptors in nonalcoholic fatty liver disease," *World Journal of Gastroenterology*, vol. 20, no. 23, pp. 7381–7391, 2014.

[11] E. Buzzetti, M. Pinzani, and E. A. Tsochatzis, "The multiple-hit pathogenesis of non-alcoholic fatty liver disease (NAFLD)," *Metabolism - Clinical and Experimental*, vol. 65, no. 8, pp. 1038–1048, 2016.

[12] S. Gökçe, Z. Atbinici, Z. Aycan, H. G. Çinar, and P. Zorlu, "The relationship between pediatric nonalcoholic fatty liver disease and cardiovascular risk factors and increased risk of atherosclerosis in obese children," *Pediatric Cardiology*, vol. 34, no. 2, pp. 308–315, 2013.

[13] R. Kelishadi, S. R. Cook, A. Adibi et al., "Association of the components of the metabolic syndrome with non- alcoholic fatty liver disease among normal-weight, overweight and obese children and adolescents," *Diabetology & Metabolic Syndrome*, vol. 1, no. 1, p. 29, 2009.

[14] A. Lonardo, S. Ballestri, G. Marchesini, P. Angulo, and P. Loria, "Nonalcoholic fatty liver disease: a precursor of the metabolic syndrome," *Digestive and Liver Disease*, vol. 47, no. 3, pp. 181–190, 2015.

[15] A. Kasturiratne, S. Weerasinghe, A. S. Dassanayake et al., "Influence of non-alcoholic fatty liver disease on the development of diabetes mellitus," *Journal of Gastroenterology and Hepatology*, vol. 28, no. 1, pp. 142–147, 2013.

[16] M. Koplay, M. Sivri, H. Erdogan, and A. Nayman, "Importance of imaging and recent developments in diagnosis of nonalcoholic fatty liver disease," *World Journal of Hepatology*, vol. 7, no. 5, pp. 769–776, 2015.

[17] S. K. Hourigan, S. Abrams, K. Yates et al., "Relation between vitamin D status and nonalcoholic fatty liver disease in children," *Journal of Pediatric Gastroenterology and Nutrition*, vol. 60, no. 3, pp. 396–404, 2015.

[18] H. D. McCarthy, T. J. Cole, T. Fry, S. A. Jebb, and A. M. Prentice, "Body fat reference curves for children," *International Journal of Obesity*, vol. 30, no. 4, pp. 598–602, 2006.

[19] "The IDF consensus definition of the Metabolic Syndrome in children and adolescents," International Diabetes Federation, 2007.

[20] Z. Kułaga, M. Litwin, A. Grajda, B. Gurzkowska, E. Napieralska, and K. I. Kułaga, "Rozklady wartosci cisnienia krwi w populacji referencyjnej dzieci i mlodziezy w wieku szkolnym," *Standardy Medyczne - Pediatria*, vol. 7, pp. 100–111, 2010.

[21] D. R. Matthews, J. P. Hosker, A. S. Rudenski, B. A. Naylor, D. F. Treacher, and R. C. Turner, "Homeostasis model assessment: insulin resistance and β-cell function from fasting plasma glucose and insulin concentrations in man," *Diabetologia*, vol. 28, no. 7, pp. 412–419, 1985.

[22] B. Shashaj, R. Luciano, B. Contoli et al., "Reference ranges of HOMA-IR in normal-weight and obese young Caucasians," *Acta Diabetologica*, vol. 53, no. 2, pp. 251–260, 2016.

[23] R. Rocha, H. P. Cotrim, A. G. V. Bitencourt et al., "Nonalcoholic fatty liver disease in asymptomatic Brazilian adolescents," *World Journal of Gastroenterology*, vol. 15, no. 4, pp. 473–477, 2009.

[24] S. Wiegand, K.-M. Keller, M. Röbl et al., "Obese boys at increased risk for nonalcoholic liver disease: Evaluation of 16 390 overweight or obese children and adolescents," *International Journal of Obesity*, vol. 34, no. 10, pp. 1468–1474, 2010.

[25] L. Pacifico, F. Ferraro, E. Bonci, C. Anania, S. Romaggioli, and C. Chiesa, "Upper limit of normal for alanine aminotransferase: Quo vadis?" *Clinica Chimica Acta*, vol. 422, pp. 29–39, 2013.

[26] J. B. Schwimmer, W. Dunn, G. J. Norman et al., "SAFETY study: alanine aminotransferase cutoff values are set too high for reliable detection of pediatric chronic liver disease," *Gastroenterology*, vol. 138, no. 4, pp. 1357.e2–1364.e2, 2010.

[27] S. H. Park, H. Y. Park, J. W. Kang, J. Park, and K. J. Shin, "Aminotransferase upper reference limits and the prevalence of elevated aminotransferases in the Korean adolescent population," *Journal of Pediatric Gastroenterology and Nutrition*, vol. 55, no. 6, pp. 668–672, 2012.

[28] H. Poustchi, J. George, S. Esmaili et al., "Gender differences in healthy ranges for serum alanine aminotransferase levels in adolescence," *PLoS ONE*, vol. 6, no. 6, Article ID e21178, 2011.

[29] S. Xanthakos, L. Miles, J. Bucuvalas, S. Daniels, V. Garcia, and T. Inge, "Histologic spectrum of nonalcoholic fatty liver disease in morbidly obese adolescents," *Clinical Gastroenterology and Hepatology*, vol. 4, no. 2, pp. 226–232, 2006.

[30] C. Denzer, D. Thiere, R. Muche et al., "Gender-specific prevalences of fatty liver in obese children and adolescents: roles of body fat distribution, sex steroids, and insulin resistance," *The Journal of Clinical Endocrinology & Metabolism*, vol. 94, no. 10, pp. 3872–3881, 2009.

[31] E. D'Adamo, M. Impicciatore, R. Capanna et al., "Liver steatosis in obese prepubertal children: A possible role of insulin resistance," *Obesity*, vol. 16, no. 3, pp. 677–683, 2008.

[32] K. Lo, M. Wong, P. Khalechelvam, and W. Tam, "Waist-to-height ratio, body mass index and waist circumference for screening paediatric cardio-metabolic risk factors: a meta-analysis," *Obesity Reviews*, vol. 17, no. 12, pp. 1258–1275, 2016.

[33] P. A. Monteiro, B. de Moura Mello Antunes, L. S. Silveira, D. G. D. Christofaro, R. A. Fernandes, and I. F. Freitas Junior, "Body composition variables as predictors of NAFLD by ultrasound in obese children and adolescents," *BMC Pediatrics*, vol. 14, no. 1, article no. 25, 2014.

[34] Y.-C. Lin, P.-F. Chang, S.-J. Yeh, K. Liu, and H.-C. Chen, "Risk factors for liver steatosis in obese children and adolescents," *Pediatrics and Neonatology*, vol. 51, no. 3, pp. 149–154, 2010.

[35] M. Manco, G. Bedogni, M. Marcellini et al., "Waist circumference correlates with liver fibrosis in children with non-alcoholic steatohepatitis," *Gut*, vol. 57, no. 9, pp. 1283–1287, 2008.

[36] L. Pacifico, C. Anania, F. Martino et al., "Functional and morphological vascular changes in pediatric nonalcoholic fatty liver disease," *Hepatology*, vol. 52, no. 5, pp. 1643–1651, 2010.

[37] H. R. Yang and E. J. Chang, "Insulin resistance, body composition, and fat distribution in obese children with nonalcoholic fatty liver disease," *Asia Pacific Journal of Clinical Nutrition*, vol. 25, no. 1, pp. 126–133, 2016.

[38] G. J. Paz-Filho, "Metabolic syndrome in children and teenagers: Worth assessing it, but how?" *Archives of Endocrinology and Metabolism*, vol. 61, no. 1, pp. 1–4, 2017.

[39] T. Reinehr, R. Wunsch, C. Pütter, and A. Scherag, "Relationship between carotid intima-media thickness and metabolic syndrome in adolescents," *Journal of Pediatrics*, vol. 163, no. 2, pp. 327–332, 2013.

[40] W. Strojny, D. Drozdz, K. Fijorek et al., "Looking for new diagnostic tools and biomarkers of hypertension in obese pediatric patients," *Blood Pressure Monitoring*, vol. 22, no. 3, pp. 122–130, 2017.

25

Cognitive Changes and Brain Volume Reduction in Patients with Nonalcoholic Fatty Liver Disease

Branka Filipović,[1,2] Olivera Marković,[1,3] Vesna Đurić,[4] and Branislav Filipović[1,5]

[1] *Faculty of Medicine, University of Belgrade, Dr Subotića Starijeg 8, Belgrade, Serbia*
[2] *Department of Gastroenterohepatology, Clinical and Hospital Center Bežanijska Kosa, Autoput s/n, 11080 Belgrade, Serbia*
[3] *Department of Hematology, Clinical and Hospital Center Bežanijska Kosa, Autoput s/n, 11080 Belgrade, Serbia*
[4] *Clinical and Hospital Center "Dr Dragiša Mišović-Dedinje", Belgrade, Serbia*
[5] *Institute of Anatomy "Niko Miljanić", Dr Subotića Starijeg 4/2, Belgrade, Serbia*

Correspondence should be addressed to Branka Filipović; branka.filipovic3@gmail.com

Academic Editor: Pierluigi Toniutto

Studies of psychological condition of patients suffering from nonalcoholic fatty liver disease are rather equivocal about the results: while some claim that NAFLD patients suffer from anxiety and depression more than non-NAFLD controls, others do not withstand those findings. Lower cognitive potentials have also been reported, both in patient related and in animal model-based investigations, and correlated with assessed brain tissue changes. We hypothesized that NAFLD, as a condition, affects the brain tissue and, subsequently, the cognitive state. So we compared findings in 40 NAFLD positive and 36 NAFLD negative patients and correlated their brain tissue volumes with the results of Montreal Cognitive Assessment (MoCA) test. Binomial logistic regression verified the influence of NAFLD state leading to lower cognitive potentials: odds ratio 0.096; 95% confidence interval (CI) 0.032–0.289; $p < 0.001$. Patients with NAFLD had a greater risk to suffer from the cognitive impairment and depression: RR = 3.9; 95% CI 1.815–8.381; $p = 0.0005$ and RR = 1.65; 95% CI 1.16–2.36; $p = 0.006$. NAFLD significantly influenced the cognitive deficit and tissue volume reduction and patients suffering from NAFLD had about four times higher risk of having a cognitive impairment.

1. Introduction

Psychological condition of patients with nonalcoholic fatty liver disease (NAFLD) still remains rather ambiguous. Studies related to the mentioned problem are dealing mostly with depression, but results obtained are equivocal: some studies confirmed the presence of depression in correlation with histological severity of NAFLD [1–4], while other publications denied the relationship between them [5, 6]. A systematic review by Macavei and coworkers (2016) [7] also emphasized the presence of depression and anxiety as the most frequent mood disturbances in NAFLD suffering patients. Petta and coworkers (2016) [8] outlined the relationship between decreased volume of brain white matter, lower cognitive potentials, and the type of fibrosis level in NAFLD. In both the entire cohort and NAFLD cases, only females older than 45 and with F2–F4 fibrosis level were independently associated with white matter lesions, mostly of mild grade. Some decrease in the blood oxygen concentration was revealed in female NAFLD patients and it was connected to lower cognitive performance in females affected by NAFLD [9].

The experimental investigation of NAFLD performed on Sprague-Dawley rats delineated the changes on hippocampal-related memory, but the deficit in hippocampal insulin signaling or brain-derived neurotrophic and insulin-like growth factor 1 appeared to have no influence on this [10].

We aimed to assess whether NAFLD influences the cognitive status in patients and if cognitive impairment correlates with lower volumes of various brain structures, including total brain white and gray matter volumes and volumes of the lateral ventricles in NAFLD patients.

TABLE 1: Demographic characteristics of examined cohort.

	Examined (40)	Control (36)	Difference and significance
Age (yrs., mean ± SD)	47.88 ± 6.07	47.07 ± 6.68	NS
Sex (male/female)	22/18	16/14	NS
Body mass index (BMI, kg/m^2, mean ± SD)	32.04 ± 6.67	22.18 ± 4.43	$p < 0.001$
Diabetes type 2 (yes/no)	12/28	9/27	NS
Hypertension (yes/no)	32/8	16/20	$p < 0.0001$ Spearman correlation NAFLD + and hypertension, $p < 0.0001$
HDL/LDL ratio (mean ± SE)	4.49 ± 0.23	2.94 ± 0.18	$p < 0.0001$
Status according to BMI:			
Normal	5	21	
Overweight	15	11	$p = 0.000028$
Obese	20	4	
Metabolic syndrome (yes/no)	34/6	8/28	Chi square, $p < 0.00001$
MoCA score (mean ± SD)	24.07 ± 3.18	27.17 ± 2.35	$p < 0.001$
Total brain volume (cm^3, mean ± SD)	1388 ± 127.98	1417 ± 191.83	NS
Gray matter volume (gmw in cm^3 mean ± SD)	405 ± 37.42	414 ± 56.09	NS
White matter volume (wmw, in cm^3 mean ± SD)	338 ± 31.21	344 ± 46.83	NS
Lateral ventricle volume, right/left (lvlr, lvll, in cm^3 mean ± SD)	5.97 ± 0.61 6.07 ± 0.62	5.64 ± 0.37 5.63 ± 0.37	$p = 0.009^*$ $p < 0.001^*$
AST (U/l, mean ± SE)	39.97 ± 2.61	24.03 ±3.26	$p < 0.001$
ALT (U/l mean ± SE)	39.11 ± 2.86	36.71 ± 3.5	NS
AST/ALT ratio (mean ± SE)	1.13 ± 0.11	0.7 ± 0.06	$p = 0.01$
C-reactive protein (mg/l, mean ± SE)	3.96 ± 0.45	3.52 ± 0.51	NS
Fasting glycaemia (mmol/l, l mean ± SE)	5.8 ± 0.19	3.71 ± 0.25	$p < 0.001$
Triglycerides (mmol/l, l mean ± SE)	2.87 ± 0.18	1.71 ± 0.17	$p < 0.001$

NS, not significant; SE, standard error. *Lateral ventricle volumes.

2. Material and Methods

The study group involved 89 first diagnosed, therapy naive patients, with high level of aminotransferases, out of which 40 (22 men and 18 women) aged 34–57 (mean 47.88 ± 6.07) satisfied recruiting criteria, who were treated in the Department of Gastroenterology and Hepatology, or referred to the Gastroenterology outpatients service. Control group contained 30 patients, 16 men and 14 women, aged 39–53 (mean and standard deviation = 47.07 ± 6.68) who were referred to the outpatient service for other gastroenterological problems, mostly of the functional origin (functional dyspepsia and irritable bowel syndrome), that do not involve liver nor gall bladder and gall pathways pathology, which were excluded by the abdominal ultrasonography. The demographic data are presented on Table 1.

Recruiting criteria are as follows:

(1) Older than 18

(2) No previous history of viral hepatitis of any kind, haemochromatosis, autoimmune hepatitis, cirrhosis, or other chronic liver disease

(3) No presence of severe cardiopulmonary disease

(4) Absence of obstructive sleep apnea syndrome assessed by polysomnography

(5) The absence of endocrinological disorders: hypothyroidism, hypercorticism, syndrome of the polycystic ovaria

(6) No history or clinical signs of excessive alcohol abuse (>20 g/day for males and >10 g/day for females)

(7) No psychiatric disease and/or psychiatric medication history or any other hepatotoxic drugs

(8) No visible traces of the illicit drugs abuse: negative urine multiple drug test on 10 kinds of drugs: cannabinoids, opiates, amphetamines, 3,4-methylenedioxymethamphetamine, cocaine/crack, benzodiazepines, tricyclic antidepressants, barbiturates, methadone, and buprenorphine

(9) No visible focal or diffuse changes in the gray matter of the brain on MRI

(10) Fazekas score 0 on MRI scan: Fazekas score is the estimated level of the white matter vascular changes and is the aftermath of brain vessels atherosclerotic changes

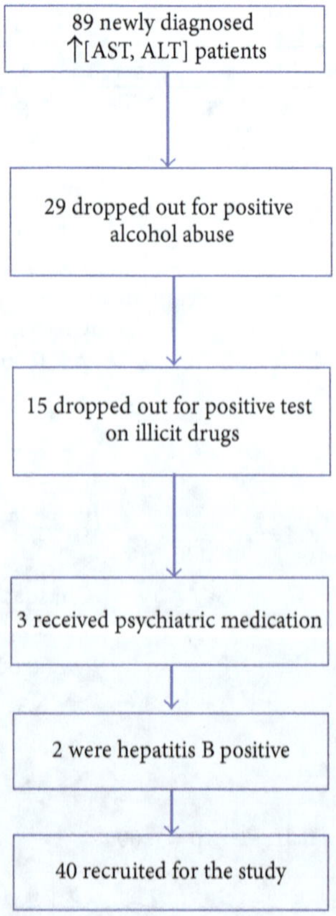

FIGURE 1: Flow diagram of patient selection from Department of Gastroenterohepatology.

(11) Absence of any rheumatological disease

(12) Patients who used antidiabetic drugs, insulin, antilipemic drugs, uricosuric drugs, steroids, and oral contraceptives were omitted from the study.

Most of the patients who were dropped out fell on the alcohol (29) and drug abuse tests (15). Flow diagram is shown on Figure 1.

Upon admittance, all the patients underwent abdominal ultrasonography and MRI brain scanning.

Abdominal ultrasound was performed using a 3.5 MHz transducer, by an experienced gastroenterologist. Both subcostal and intercostal scannings were done. Images were captured in a standard fashion with the subject in the supine position and with the right arm raised above the head. In our clinical study we measured the following ultrasonographic parameters: anterior-posterior diameter of the liver (AP), homogeneity, echogenicity of the hepatic parenchyma, and the pancreas. Normal liver parenchyma was seen as solid homogenous echo texture, which was midway between the renal cortex and pancreatic echogenicity. Fatty liver disease was diagnosed as diffusely increased echogenicity of the hepatic parenchyma compared to the kidneys, vascular blurring, and deep-echo attenuation.

Sonographic evaluation (US) of hepatic steatosis was based on five criteria: parenchymal brightness, liver to kidney contrast, deep beam attenuation, bright vessel walls, and gallbladder wall definition [11, 12]. Diffuse hepatic steatosis was graded I to III: I, increased hepatic echogenicity with visible periportal and diaphragmatic echogenicity; II, increased hepatic echogenicity with imperceptible periportal echogenicity, without obscuration of the diaphragm; and III, increased hepatic echogenicity with imperceptible periportal echogenicity and obscuration of the diaphragm.

Blood samples were collected after 12 hours of fasting. Analyses included platelet count (PC), platelet indices (MPV, PCT, and PDW), liver function tests, aspartate aminotransferase (AST), alanine aminotransferase (ALT), gamma-glutamyl transferase (GGT), alkaline phosphatase (ALP), lipid profile including triglycerides, C-reactive protein (CRP), and fasting blood glycaemia and insulin levels, by using Ilab 650 (Instrumentation Laboratory, Milano, Italy).

Volume measurements of the gray and white matter and lateral ventricles of the brain were performed on 3D T1-weighted MR images (Phillips Inc., Holland); acquisition parameters were as follows: TR = 9.8 ms; TE = 4.6 ms; fl ip angle = 8; section thickness = 1.2 mm; number of sections = 120; no section gap; whole brain coverage; FOV = 224 mm; matrix = 192; reconstruction matrix = 256. Routine T2-weighted and FLAIR images were performed to rule out a mass lesion as a contributory factor to memory loss or cognitive decline. The structures were manually outlined and compared with automatic extraction of the regions of interest in commercially available software. The software finally computed the volumes required.

After the diagnostic procedures, all the subjects underwent psychological testing for cognitive impairments using Montreal Cognitive Assessment test, Serbian version [13]. Test has several levels of testing, alternating connections (connect Figure 1 with letter A and then A to 2, to B, etc.), visuoconstructive abilities (draw a cube and a clock in 11:10 position of clock hands), memory (numbers repeated in the same and reverse order), attention (tap whenever you hear a letter A), serial subtraction of 7, starting with a hundred (100 − 7 = 93, 93 − 7 = 86, etc.), sentence repeating, and verbal fluency. Maximal score is 30, 26 being the threshold for normal cognitive functioning.

Level of the depression was tested by Hamilton's depression rating scale of 21 items. Only first 17 items were scored: equal to or lower than 7, no depression; 8–13, mild depression; 14–18, moderate; 19–22, severe; equal to or higher than 23, very severe. For all the patients with depression diagnosis, a psychiatrist was consulted, and the subsequent therapy was individually prescribed. According to the protocol, patients were controlled every three months. The protocol involved liver examination by ultrasound, laboratory parameters, and psychiatric evaluation.

Statistical testing was performed by the commercially available software. Besides the measures of central tendency (mean and standard deviation (SD), minimum, and maximum), potential differences of mean values were assessed with one way analysis of variance (ANOVA) with Bonferroni post hoc correction, Student's t-test for independent samples for parametric, and chi square test for nonparametric data. Correlation was tested with Spearman and Pierson's correlation test. Possible dependence between the nonparametric

TABLE 2: Pierson's correlation of MoCA score values and observed volumes.

Volume	B	Beta	Significance
Total brain volume	0.025	1.5	NS
latvl	−39.18	−7.48	$p = 0.005$
latvr	−38.01	−7.46	$p = 0.007$
gmw	0.019	0.279	$p = 0.015$
wmw	0.2	2.89	$p = 0.009$

Latvl: lateral ventricle volume, left hemisphere; latvr: lateral ventricle volume, right hemisphere; gmw: gray matter volume; wmw: white matter volume.

parameters was estimated by binomial logistic regression. All the testing was performed on 95% probability level.

All the participants were acquainted in detail with the study aim and design before entering the program. They all signed a written consent afterwards.

3. Results

The cognitive status, according to MoCA index, was lower in NAFLD patients (Table 1). If we observe the cutoff value (26 points) and divide both groups into normal and subnormal groups, 26 patients in NAFLD group had lower MoCA score versus 6 control members (chi square = 19.23, df = 1, and $p <$ 0,0001). Binomial logistic regression estimated significant influence of NAFLD on the reduced MoCA score: odds ratio 0.096, 95% confidence interval (CI) 0.032–0.289, and $p <$ 0.001. Patients with NAFLD had a greater risk to suffer from cognitive impairment: RR = 3.9, 95% CI 1.815–8.381, and $p =$ 0.0005, respectively.

Despite the fact that we did not evaluate differences in total brain, gray, and white volumes between the observed and control group, in NAFLD patients with lower MoCA score, the volumes of brain, gray, and white matter were significantly reduced: for brain volume, $t = 2.71$, df = 38, and $p = 0.01$, for gray matter volume, $t = 2.71$, df = 38, and $p = 0.01$ (absolutely correlated with brain volume), and for white matter, $t = 2.31$, df = 38, and $p = 0.026$. Furthermore, MoCA score values correlated with gray and white matter volumes, but not with total brain volume in NAFLD group. The increase in lateral ventricles volumes negatively correlated with total MoCA score (Table 2).

Difficulties appeared in NAFLD + group with questions that required postponed memory test to repeat the words after 5 minutes. Although no significant difference was obtained by chi square (chi = 3.5978, $p = 0.0057$), 22 examinees versus 12 controls did not solve the task. With question requiring attention, 28 examinees had more than two mistakes in tapping with pencil every time they heard the letter A, while the same mistake was revealed in controls in 9 cases (chi = 15.35, $p = 0.00009$).

Classified by Hamilton's depression score, there are more patients with moderate and severe depression in NAFLD group and this difference was verified by chi square test (Table 3). Furthermore, patients with NAFLD had a higher risk of havin depression: RR = 1.65, 95% CI 1.16–2.36, and $p = 0.006$.

TABLE 3: Depression grades in observed and control groups.

	Hamilton severity*				Total
	No depression	Mild	Moderate	Severe	
Group					
NAFLD+	7	17	14	2	40
NAFLD−	18	15	3	0	36
Total	25	32	17	2	76

*Chi square = 13.91, df = 3, and $p <$ 0,0001.

Although persons with increased body mass index (BMI), hypertension, and metabolic syndrome dominated in the NAFLD positive group, neither BMI, hypertension, nor metabolic syndrome had influence on the cognitive status. HDL/LDL ratio was not significantly related to lower MoCA index, although the risk for atherosclerosis was expressed among examinees from NAFLD positive group. Neither transaminase level nor the ratio influenced significantly the cognitive deficit.

No gender based differences were evaluated in this study.

4. Discussion

This study represents authors' effort to evaluate the cognitive status of newly recruited NAFLD patients and to correlate it to the total brain volumes, volumes of gray and white matter, and volumes of the lateral ventricles. The major finding of our study is the assessment of higher number of persons with lower cognitive abilities in NAFLD patients. Higher risk for NAFLD patients to suffer from the cognitive impairment and independent influence of NAFLD on lower cognitive scores have also been evaluated. Previous investigations also correlated the cognitive deficit with white matter changes of vascular origin [8]. Some investigations outlined the increased connection between white matter changes in menopausal and postmenopausal females [14], but, as we had not obtained statistical correlation between age and gender with any kind of volumes of interest, we did not want to involve hormonal status in our investigation. Depleted cognitive performance has been noted in NAFLD patients: increased activity of alanine (ALT) and aspartate aminotransferase (AST) correlated with poorer performance on serial digit learning test and increased activity of ALT correlated with serial digit replacement test [15]. Serial digit learning test (SDLT) is a golden standard for functional magnetic resonance memory testing and consists of three independent series of nine (sometimes eight) single digits, in which examinee must repeat correctly after maximum 12 attempts, in five to ten minutes. The other test, serial digit replacement test (SDRT), is designed for attention testing and is based on the replacement of single digit by a prescheduled sign. Obviously, NAFLD patients have a problem with memory, also found in our study, but our patients manifested less problems in postponed memory test than in attention evaluation; moreover, we found no statistically relevant correlation between transaminases activity and cognition scores. On the other side, Petta and his coworkers (2016) [8] found no difference in cognitive state in NAFLD positive patients, with and without white matter lesions. For the mentioned evaluation, they used mini mental state questionnaire, applied mostly to estimate the presence of dementia. This is not a sensitive type of questionnaire and its application is not advisable for subtle cognitive changes, as manifested in NAFLD. Reduced gray and white matter volumes, obtained in our study, combined with the increased volumes of the lateral ventricles, may be used as an explanation why total brain volume did not differ between the examinees and controls, because controls had increased volumes of gray and white matter but lower volumes of the lateral ventricles. According to VanWagner et al. (2017) [16], total brain tissue volume did not differ in groups with and without NAFLD, while gray matter perfusion was lower in NAFLD patients.

Previous reports have outlined that higher levels of adiposity including BMI, waist circumference, subcutaneous adipose tissue, and volume of adipose tissue have all been associated with lower total brain volume [17, 18]. BMI, in particular, has been associated with regional brain gray matter volume decreases, although the location and magnitude of these decreases have been inconsistent [19–22]. Some investigations reported lower gray matter volume only in those with obesity (BMI $\geq 30\,kg/m^2$) [18], although our investigation cannot confirm those findings. According to our results, BMI does not correlate with total brain, gray, or white matter volumes, nor with the depression grade.

Youssef et al. (2013) [3] published in their article that depression levels were associated with portal fibrosis grades ($p = 0.038$) and tended to be associated with hepatocyte ballooning grades ($p = 0.085$). In our study, 75% of NAFLD + examinees had depression versus 69% in cited publication [3]. Subclinical form of depression (e.g., mild + moderate) appeared in 28 out of 40 patients, while clinical form of depression (severe) was assessed in 2 patients. Our estimated risk for depression of 1.65 is related to overall NAFLD group, without difference for males and females. Gender differences in depression prevalence in NAFLD were outlined by Surdea-Blaga and Dumitraşcu (2011) [5], who stated that female NAFLD patients have higher relative risk for depression: 3.2 (95% CI = 1.6–6.7).

The previous investigation blamed insulin resistance for the predicted cognitive deficit in NAFLD + patients, indicating the prominent role of insulin resistance in Alzheimer's disease [23, 24]. Other studies, however, blamed the inflammatory process for cognitive impairment, relating it to the increased concentration of cytokines and adipokines, eventually associated with dysfunctional endothelium and oxidative stress, stating that it could be in the root of cognitive dysfunction in NAFLD patients [25–29]. Thickening of carotid arteries tunica intima, also reported in NAFLD patients and in patients with cognitive deficit as well, is the probable aftermath of the aforementioned process, which, as a definitive result, gives the volume reduction of gray and white matter and, consequently, cognitive impairment [30, 31]. Inflammatory mechanism should not be neglected as one of the causes of cognitive loss, but, according to our laboratory results, values of this inflammation marker were in the accepted range (0–10 mg/l) in both groups, without statistical difference (3.96 vs. 3.52 mg/l, examinees versus controls).

However, our study has some limitations:

(1) This is a referral, not cohort study, restricted only to the patients referred to our department and outpatient clinics.

(2) It is limited to newly diagnosed, therapy naive patients.

(3) Only noninvasive tests were used for the NAFLD estimation.

(4) The diagnosis is dependable on ultrasonographist skills and experience.

5. Conclusion

According to our results, cognitive deficit, assessed by Montreal Cognitive Assessment test, is more pronounced in persons with NAFLD. NAFLD significantly influenced the cognitive deficit and patients suffering from NAFLD had about four times higher risk to have a cognitive impairment. Depleted MoCA score correlated with the white and gray matter volume reduction. NAFLD patients are at higher risk to suffer from depression, which is, most probably, related to the revealed volume reductions as well. Nonetheless, deficit is not in a verified correlation with BMI, found to be higher in the examined group, nor with the activities of liver transaminases, although the higher concentration of AST was revealed in NAFLD patients. Future investigations should be conducted to elucidate still insufficiently known exact mechanism of cognitive deficit pathogenesis, and the therapy of NAFLD is advisable to act in such a way as to prevent it.

Acknowledgments

The investigation is partially financed by the Ministry of Education, Science and Technological Development, Government of the Republic of Serbia (Grant III41020).

References

[1] J. E. Elwing, P. J. Lustman, H. L. Wang, and R. E. Clouse, "Depression, anxiety, and nonalcoholic steatohepatitis," *Psychosomatic Medicine*, vol. 68, no. 4, pp. 563–569, 2006.

[2] A. A. Weinstein, J. Kallman Price, M. Stepanova et al., "Depression in patients with nonalcoholic fatty liver disease and chronic viral hepatitis B and C," *Psychosomatics*, vol. 52, no. 2, pp. 127–132, 2011.

[3] N. A. Youssef, M. F. Abdelmalek, M. Binks et al., "Associations of depression, anxiety and antidepressants with histological

severity of nonalcoholic fatty liver disease," *Liver International*, vol. 33, no. 7, pp. 1062–1070, 2013.

[4] W. Tomeno, K. Kawashima, M. Yoneda et al., "Non-alcoholic fatty liver disease comorbid with major depressive disorder: The pathological features and poor therapeutic efficacy," *Journal of Gastroenterology and Hepatology*, vol. 30, no. 6, pp. 1009–1014, 2015.

[5] T. Surdea-Blaga and D. L. Dumitraşcu, "Depression and anxiety in nonalcoholic steatohepatitis: is there any association?" *Romanian Journal of Internal Medicine*, vol. 49, pp. 273–280, 2011.

[6] K. Lee, M. Otgonsuren, Z. Younoszai, H. M. Mir, and Z. M. Younossi, "Association of chronic liver disease with depression: a population-based study," *Psychosomatics*, vol. 54, no. 1, pp. 52–59, 2013.

[7] B. Macavei, A. Baban, and D. L. Dumitrascu, "Psychological factors associated with NAFLD/NASH: a systematic review," *European Review for Medical and Pharmacological Sciences*, vol. 20, pp. 5081–5097, 2016.

[8] S. Petta, A. Tuttolomondo, C. Gagliardo et al., "The presence of white matter lesions is associated with the fibrosis severity of nonalcoholic fatty liver disease," *Medicine*, vol. 95, no. 16, Article ID e3446, 2016.

[9] A. Takahashi, S. Kono, A. Wada et al., "Reduced brain activity in female patients with non-alcoholic fatty liver disease as measured by near-infrared spectroscopy," *PLoS ONE*, vol. 12, no. 4, Article ID e0174169, 2017.

[10] A. P. Ross, E. C. Bruggeman, A. W. Kasumu, J. G. Mielke, and M. B. Parent, "Non-alcoholic fatty liver disease impairs hippocampal-dependent memory in male rats," *Physiology & Behavior*, vol. 106, no. 2, pp. 133–141, 2012.

[11] S. Kahl, K. Straßburger, and B. Nowotny, "Comparison of liver fat indices for the diagnosis of hepatic steatosis and insulin resistance," *PLoS ONE*, vol. 9, no. 4, Article ID A1453, 2014.

[12] D. Singh, C. J. Das, and M. P. Baruah, "Imaging of non alcoholic fatty liver disease: a road less travelled," *Indian Journal of Endocrinology and Metabolism*, vol. 17, no. 6, pp. 990–995, 2013.

[13] V. Kljajevic, *Aktuelnosti u neurologiji i psihijatriji*, vol. 17, 2009.

[14] T. S. Mikkola, P. Tuomikoski, H. Lyytinen et al., "Estradiol-based postmenopausal hormone therapy and risk of cardiovascular and all-cause mortality," *Menopause*, vol. 22, no. 9, pp. 976–983, 2015.

[15] S. W. Seo, R. F. Gottesman, J. M. Clark et al., "Nonalcoholic fatty liver disease is associated with cognitive function in adults," *Neurology*, vol. 86, no. 12, pp. 1136–1142, 2016.

[16] L. B. VanWagner, J. G. Terry, L. S. Chow et al., "Nonalcoholic fatty liver disease and measures of early brain health in middle-aged adults: the CARDIA study," *Obesity*, vol. 25, no. 3, pp. 642–651, 2017.

[17] S. Debette, A. Beiser, U. Hoffmann et al., "Visceral fat is associated with lower brain volume in healthy middle-aged adults," *Annals of Neurology*, vol. 68, no. 2, pp. 136–144, 2010.

[18] J. Gunstad, R. H. Paul, R. A. Cohen et al., "Relationship between body mass index and brain volume in healthy adults," *International Journal of Neuroscience*, vol. 118, no. 11, pp. 1582–1593, 2008.

[19] C. A. Raji, A. J. Ho, N. N. Parikshak, JT. Becker, O. L. Lopez, L. H. Kuller et al., "Brain structure and obesity," *Human Brain Mapping*, vol. 31, no. 3, pp. 353–364, 2010.

[20] Y. Taki, S. Kinomura, K. Sato et al., "Relationship between body mass index and gray matter volume in 1,428 healthy individuals," *Obesity*, vol. 16, no. 1, pp. 119–124, 2008.

[21] N. Pannacciulli, A. Del Parigi, K. Chen, D. S. N. T. Le, E. M. Reiman, and P. A. Tataranni, "Brain abnormalities in human obesity: a voxel-based morphometric study," *NeuroImage*, vol. 31, no. 4, pp. 1419–1425, 2006.

[22] E. Albanese, B. Davis, P. V. Jonsson et al., "Overweight and obesity in midlife and brain structure and dementia 26 years later," *American Journal of Epidemiology*, vol. 181, no. 9, pp. 672–679, 2015.

[23] S. Craft, "Insulin resistance and Alzheimer's disease pathogenesis: potential mechanisms and implications for treatment," *Current Alzheimer Research*, vol. 4, no. 2, pp. 147–152, 2007.

[24] M. Tong, A. Neusner, L. Longato, M. Lawton, J. R. Wands, and S. M. De La Monte, "Nitrosamine exposure causes insulin resistance diseases: relevance to type 2 diabetes mellitus, non-alcoholic steatohepatitis, and alzheimer's disease," *Journal of Alzheimer's Disease*, vol. 17, no. 4, pp. 827–844, 2009.

[25] N. Villanova, S. Moscatiello, S. Ramilli et al., "Endothelial dysfunction and cardiovascular risk profile in nonalcoholic fatty liver disease," *Hepatology*, vol. 42, no. 2, pp. 473–480, 2005.

[26] L. F. Van Gaal, I. L. Mertens, and C. E. De Block, "Mechanisms linking obesity with cardiovascular disease," *Nature*, vol. 444, no. 7121, pp. 875–880, 2006.

[27] G. Targher, F. Marra, and G. Marchesini, "Increased risk of cardiovascular disease in non-alcoholic fatty liver disease: causal effect or epiphenomenon?" *Diabetologia*, vol. 51, no. 11, pp. 1947–1953, 2008.

[28] G. A. Rosenberg, M. Bjerke, and A. Wallin, "Multimodal markers of inflammation in the subcortical ischemic vascular disease type of vascular cognitive impairment," *Stroke*, vol. 45, no. 5, pp. 1531–1538, 2014.

[29] S. Takeda, N. Sato, and R. Morishita, "Systemic inflammation, blood-brain barrier vulnerability and cognitive/non-cognitive symptoms in Alzheimer disease: relevance to pathogenesis and therapy," *Frontiers in Aging Neuroscience*, vol. 6, article 171, 2014.

[30] S. A. E.-K. El-Sayed, R. F. El-Folly, and A. M. Ahmed, "Assessment of the co-incidence between non alcoholic fatty liver disease and carotid atherosclerosis," *Journal of the Egyptian Society of Parasitology*, vol. 44, no. 1, pp. 187–195, 2014.

[31] C. R. Wendell, A. B. Zonderman, E. J. Metter, S. S. Najjar, and S. R. Waldstein, "Carotid intimal medial thickness predicts cognitive decline among adults without clinical vascular disease.," *Stroke*, vol. 40, no. 10, pp. 3180–3185, 2009.

26

Characteristics and Changes over Time of Alcohol-Related Chronic Liver Diseases in Italy

Tommaso Stroffolini,[1] Evangelista Sagnelli,[2] Caterina Sagnelli,[2] Filomena Morisco,[3] Sergio Babudieri,[4] Caterina Furlan,[1] Mario Pirisi,[5] Maurizio Russello,[6] Antonina Smedile,[7] Mariantonietta Pisaturo,[8] and Piero Luigi Almasio[9]

[1] *Department of Tropical and Infectious Diseases, Policlinico Umberto I, Rome, Italy*
[2] *Department of Mental Health and Public Medicine, Campania University Luigi Vanvitelli, Naples, Italy*
[3] *Department of Clinical Medicine and Surgery, Gastroenterology Unit, University of Naples "Federico II", Naples, Italy*
[4] *Clinic of Infectious Diseases, University of Sassari, Sassari, Italy*
[5] *Department of Translational Medicine, Università del Piemonte Orientale, Novara, Italy*
[6] *Liver Unit, Hospital "G. Garibaldi" Catania, Catania, Italy*
[7] *Department of Medical Sciences, University of Turin, Turin, Italy*
[8] *Unit of Infectious Diseases, S. Anna and S. Sebastian Hospital, Caserta, Italy*
[9] *Biomedical Department of Internal Medicine e Specialities (Di.Bi.M.I.S.), University of Palermo, Palermo, Italy*

Correspondence should be addressed to Piero Luigi Almasio; piero.almasio@unipa.it

Academic Editor: Peter Jarčuška

Introduction. To evaluate the characteristics of alcohol-related chronic liver disease (CLD) in Italy and their potential changes over time. *Patients and Methods*. Subjects with CLD were enrolled in two national surveys performed in 2001 and in 2014 in Italy. The two surveys prospectively recruited patients aged ≥ 18 years referring to more than 80 Italian liver units scattered all over the country using similar clinical approach, analytical methods, and threshold of risky alcohol intake definition (≥ 3 units/day in men and ≥ 2 units/day in women). *Results*. Out of 12,256 enrolled subjects, 2,717 (22.2%) reported a risky alcohol intake. Of them, anti-HCV positive was observed in 48.3% of subjects. The overall sex ratio (M/F) was 3.1, decreasing from 3.8 in 2001 to 1.3 in 2014. Women were significantly older than men (58.9 versus 53.1 years; $p < 0.01$) and an increasing ageing over time was observed in both sexes. The proportion of subjects with liver cirrhosis increased over time in both sexes, and decompensated stage (Child B or C) was detected in 55.9% of cases in 2001 and 46.0% in 2014. *Conclusions*. Risky alcohol intake plays a role in more than one-fifth of CLD in Italy, with a shift over time towards an older age and a more severe liver disease stage. These data put alcohol back in the spotlight with an important role in CLD in the years to come in Italy.

1. Introduction

Alcohol consumption is a major cause of chronic liver disease, particularly in Western and Eastern Europe, where the highest worldwide per capita intake of alcohol is reported [1, 2]. In the United Kingdom there was a 5-fold increase in cirrhosis mortality among men and a 4-fold increase among women from 1950 through 2000, which parallels the doubled alcohol consumption recorded in these countries over the same period [3]. However, only about 35% of heavy drinkers develop the disease [4], suggesting that, beyond alcohol abuse, other factors are involved in the development of liver cirrhosis [5]. In Italy, a significant decrease in the proportion of risky alcohol consumers has been over time observed, from 21.3% in 2007 to 15.7% in 2015. This downtrend was greater in men (from 30.6% to 23.0%) than in women (from 12.6% to 9.0%) [6].

The wealth on information on hepatitis viruses has decreased the attention paid to the role of alcohol intake in the development of chronic liver disease (CLD) and progression to cirrhosis, so that information on alcoholic liver diseases in Italy is scanty and fragmentary.

Pooling the cases recruited in two Italian national surveys performed in 2001 [7] and in 2014 [8, 9] on the characteristics of subjects with chronic liver diseases (CLD) referring more than 80 liver units, we have evaluated the main aspects of alcohol-related CLD and their potential changes over time.

2. Patients and Methods

The two national surveys have been previously described [7–9]. The first one enrolled 9,997 persons with CLD consecutively referring to 79 hospital liver units for a six months' period in 2001. The second one recruited 2,557 CLD cases consecutively referring to 15 hospital liver units in 2014. Subjects enrolled in 2014 were different from those in the 2001 survey. Criteria of enrolment were aged over 18 years and either altered hepatic biochemistry, presence of etiologic markers of liver damage, or history of symptoms consistent with CLD. Both inpatients and outpatients were recruited. In both studies, the enrolling liver units were scattered all over the country. Most of the 15 hospitals participating in the second study had also taken part in the first one. The liver units participating to the two surveys collected the data prospectively had comparable access procedures and used similar approach and similar analytical methods.

Personal data were collected in full compliance with the Italian law on personal data protection, and each patient gave his/her informed consent to participate. All procedures applied in the two studies were in accordance with the international guidelines, with the standards of human experimentation of the local Ethics Committees and with the Helsinki Declaration of 1975, revised in 1983. At the time of the first observation, each patient signed their informed consent for the collection of personal data. Patients who agreed to undergo liver biopsy signed an appropriate informed consent before biopsy was performed. Patients were enrolled only once at their first observation. For each patient, a precoded questionnaire containing demographic, epidemiological, and clinical data was filled out. No patient refused to participate in the studies.

2.1. Diagnostic Criteria. In both surveys, the presence of serum hepatitis B surface antigen (HBsAg) identified hepatitis B virus (HBV) aetiology and that of antibody to hepatitis C virus (anti-HCV), an HCV aetiology. Autoimmune chronic hepatitis and primary biliary cholangitis, hereditary hemochromatosis, and Wilson's disease were diagnosed according to standardized international criteria [10–13].

An alcohol intake > 40 g/day for males (≥ 3 drinks a day) and > 30 g/day for females (≥ 2 drinks a day) for at least 5 years was considered an etiologic factor for alcoholic liver disease [14, 15].

Nonalcoholic fatty liver disease (NAFLD/NASH) was diagnosed based on abnormal serum values of alanine aminotransferase (ALT) associated with hepatic steatosis identified by liver histology and/or ultrasound (US), in the absence of other known causes of liver disease [16]. CLD was considered cryptogenic in the absence of any viral, autoimmune, or metabolic aetiology.

Chronic hepatitis was diagnosed based on liver histology, when available, or on the persistence (>6 months) of abnormal ALT in the absence of clinical, biochemical, and US evidence of liver cirrhosis [17]. Liver cirrhosis was diagnosed by liver biopsy (LB) or, in the absence, on the presence of characteristic clinical, biochemical, and ultrasound signs [17]. The diagnosis of hepatocellular carcinoma (HCC) was based on histological and/or imaging findings and alfa-1-fetoprotein serum levels [18].

Percutaneous LB was performed, if requested by the physician in care for diagnostic purposes, under US guidance using a disposable modified Menghini's needle. In each liver unit, a skilled pathologist unaware of the clinical and laboratory data evaluated liver histology. Liver necro-inflammation and fibrosis were assessed by the Ishak [19] or Metavir scoring system [20] and standardized criteria were used to convert the Ishak score to a Metavir scores [21]. Liver biopsy slices were read by local of central pathologist.

2.2. Serologic Assays. Serum HBsAg and antibody to HCV were sought using commercial immunoenzymatic assays. Routine tests were applied to seek the etiologic markers of autoimmune hepatitis, primary biliary cholangitis, iron and copper overload, and liver functions.

2.3. Statistical Analysis. The data were collected in a preestablished electronic CRF database (web-based data collection, e-CRF provided by Air-Tel®, Airon Telematica, Milan, Italy). Differences in means and in proportion were evaluated by Student's t-test and chi square test or Fisher's exact test, respectively. A p value < 0.05 was considered to be significant. All p values were two-tailed.

3. Results

Out of the 12,754 enrolled subjects with CLD (9,997 in 2001 and 2,557 in 2014), 2,717 (22.2%) reported a risky alcohol intake. The mean age was 54.2 years with a sex ratio (M/F) of 3.2. The mean Body Mass Index (BMI) resulted in 25.6. A nearly similar proportion of cases was observed in northern/central areas (47.7%) and in southern/islands (49.8%). Nearly one-third (35.5%) of subjects had liver cirrhosis without (30.7%) or with (4.5%) HCC. Of these 2,717 patients, 1,313 (48.3%) were also anti-HCV positive, while 1,163 (42.7 %) reported a risky alcohol intake as the only etiologic agent of CLD. The comparison of the two studies shows an over time statistically significant older mean age (53.2 years versus 60.2 years, $p < 0.001$), a decreasing M/F sex ratio (from 3.8 to 1.3, $p < 0.001$), an increasing proportion of cases from northern/central areas ($p < 0.001$), an increase in the proportion of subjects declaring alcohol abuse with a decrease in the proportion of those having alcoholism plus anti-HCV positivity ($p < 0.02$), and, finally, an increase of subjects with liver cirrhosis without or with HCC (39.9% versus 43.4%, $p < 0.01$) (Table 1).

TABLE 1: Baseline characteristics of 2,717 enrolled subjects with chronic liver disease alcohol related in Italy, by year of recruitment.

Characteristic	Overall (n=2,717)	Study 2001 (n=2,342)	Study 2014 (n=375)	p-value
Age, years, mean ± SD	54.2 ± 12.8	53.2 ± 14.8	60.2 ± 13.4	<0.001
Sex Ratio (M/F)	3.1	3.8	1.3	<0.001
BMI, mean ± SD	25.6 ± 3.8	25.5 ± 3.8	23.0 ± 4.3	0.015
Area of birth				
(i) Northern/Central Italy	1,295 (47.7%)	1,099 (46.9%)	196 (52.3%)	<0.001
(ii) Southern Italy/Islands	1,354 (49.8%)	1,192 (50.9%)	159 (42.4%)	
(iii) Born abroad	71 (2.6%)	51 (2.2%)	20 (5.3%)	
Risk factors				
(i) Alcohol intake alone	1,163 (42.8%)	983 (42.0%)	179 (47.7%)	0.02
(ii) Alcohol intake/HBsAg positive	172 (6.3%)	140 (6.0%)	32 (8.5%)	
(iii) Alcohol intake/anti-HCV positivity	1,313 (48.3%)	1,157 (49.4%)	154 (41.1%)	
(iv) Alcohol intake/HBsAg positive/anti-HCV positive	72 (6.3%)	62 (2.6%)	10 (2.7%)	
Diagnosis				
(i) Chronic hepatitis	1,762 (64.8%)	1,550 (66.1%)	212 (56.5%)	<0.001
(ii) Liver cirrhosis without HCC	834 (30.7%)	697 (29.8%)	137 (36.5%)	
(iii) Liver cirrhosis with HCC	121 (4.5%)	95 (4.1%)	26 (6.9%)	

BMI: body mass index. HCC: hepatocellular carcinoma.

TABLE 2: Characteristics of 2,717 enrolled subjects with chronic liver disease alcohol related in Italy, by sex.

Characteristics	Males (n=2,059)	Females (n=658)	Sex Ratio (M/F)	p-value
Age, years, mean ± SD	53.0 ± 14.7	58.0 ± 14.5	-	<0.001
BMI, mean ± SD	25.7 ± 3.7	25.1 ± 4.4	-	0.001
Area of birth				
(i) Northern/Central Italy	943 (45.8%)	352 (53.5%)	2.7	<0.001
(ii) Southern Italy/Islands	1,069 (51.9%)	282 (42.9%)	3.8	
(iii) Born abroad	47 (2.3%)	24 (3.6%)	2.0	
Risk factors				
(i) Alcohol intake alone	810 (39.3%)	352 (53.5%)	2.3	<0.001
(ii) Alcohol intake/HBsAg positive	147 (7.1%)	25 (3.8%)	5.9	
(iii) Alcohol intake/anti-HCV positivity	1,040 (50.5%)	271 (41.2%)	3.8	
(iv) Alcohol intake/HBsAg positive/anti-HCV positive	62 (3.0%)	10 (1.5%)	6.2	
Diagnosis				
(i) Chronic hepatitis	1,348 (65.5%)	414 (62.9%)	3.3	0.15
(ii) Liver cirrhosis without HCC	614 (29.8%)	220 (33.4%)	2.8	
(iii) Liver cirrhosis with HCC	97 (4.7%)	24 (3.6%)	4.0	

BMI: body mass index. HCC: hepatocellular carcinoma.

As compared to males, females were over time more likely older (58.0 years versus 53.0 years, $p < 0.01$), were born in northern/central areas (53.5% versus 45.7%, $p < 0.01$), and more frequently declared alcohol abuse (53.5% versus 39.3%, $p < 0.01$). No significant difference by gender was observed according to diagnosis (Table 2).

Statistically significant intragender over time differences were observed in males, with an ageing age, an increasing proportion of cases related to alcohol abuse alone, and an increasing proportion of cirrhotic patients with or without HCC (Table 3). Intragender differences over time were observed even in females with an ageing age, a higher proportion of cases with liver cirrhosis, and a decreasing proportion of subjects with alcohol abuse alone (Table 4).

Characteristics of liver cirrhosis cases are reported in Table 5. The most relevant findings are the over time decrease of both the M/F sex ratio ($p < 0.001$) and the rate of cases (55.9% to 46.8%; $p < 0.05$) with in a decompensated stage (Child B/C).

4. Discussion

The present work is a careful subanalysis of data only generically stated in an earlier publication [8], focusing

TABLE 3: Characteristics of chronic liver diseases alcohol related in male sex over time in Italy.

Characteristics	2001 Study (n°=1,852)	2014 Study (n°=207)	p-value
Age (years), mean ± SD	52.4 ± 14.7	58.0 ± 13.9	<0.001
BMI (kg/m^2), mean ± SD	25.6 ± 3.6	26.4 ± 4.1	<0.05
Area of origin			
(i) Northern/Central Italy	888 (45.8%)	95 (45.9%)	0.03
(ii) Southern Italy/Islands	967 (52.2%)	102 (49.3%)	
(iii) Born abroad	37 (2.0%)	10 (4.8%)	
Risk factors			
(i) Alcohol intake alone	710 (38.3%)	100 (48.3%)	0.015
(ii) Alcohol intake/HBsAg positive	129 (7.0%)	18 (8.7%)	
(iii) Alcohol intake/anti-HCV positivity	957 (51.7%)	83 (40.1%)	
(iv) Alcohol intake/HBsAg positive/anti-HCV positive	56 (3.0%)	6 (2.9%)	
Diagnosis			
(i) Chronic hepatitis	1,231 (66.5%)	117 (56.5%)	0.004
(ii) Liver cirrhosis without HCC	541 (29.2%)	73 (35.3%)	
(iii) Liver cirrhosis with HCC	80 (4.3%)	17 (8.2%)	

BMI: body mass index. HCC: hepatocellular carcinoma.

TABLE 4: Characteristics of chronic liver diseases alcohol related in female sex over time, in Italy.

Characteristics	2001 Study (n°=490)	2014 Study (n°=168)	p-value
Age (years), mean ± SD	56.3 ± 14.8	63.0 ± 12.3	<0.001
BMI (kg/m^2), mean ± SD	24.9 ± 4.3	25.6 ± 4.4	0.1
Area of origin			
(i) Northern/Central Italy	251 (51.2%)	101 (60.1%)	0.009
(ii) Southern Italy/Islands	225 (45.9%)	57 (33.9%)	
(iii) Born abroad	14 (2.9%)	10 (6.0%)	
Risk factors			
(i) Alcohol intake alone	273 (55.7%)	79 (47.0%)	0.002
(ii) Alcohol intake/HBsAg positive	11 (2.2%)	14 (8.3%)	
(iii) Alcohol intake/anti-HCV positivity	200 (40.8%)	71 (42.3%)	
(iv) Alcohol intake/HBsAg positive/anti-HCV positive	6 (1.2%)	4 (2.4%)	
Diagnosis			
(i) Chronic hepatitis	319 (65.1%)	95 (56.5%)	0.09
(ii) Liver cirrhosis without HCC	156 (31.8%)	64 (38.1%)	
(iii) Liver cirrhosis with HCC	15 (3.1%)	9 (5.4%)	

BMI: body mass index. HCC: hepatocellular carcinoma.

exclusively on alcohol-related CLD. The 2001 and the 2014 nationwide prevalence surveys were structurally similar. Both studies were cross-sectional and prospectively enrolled for a given time inpatients and outpatients aged 18 or more with CLD of any aetiology referring for altered hepatic biochemistry or positivity of hepatitis virus serum markers to one of the participating liver units located all over the country. The same clinical approach, analytical methods, and facilities to access the participating liver units, operating in district general or academic hospitals, have been adopted. In addition, several of these liver units have participated to both 2001 and 2014 surveys. Finally, the same threshold of a risky alcohol intake was adopted in both surveys [14, 15]. Consequently, the pooling and the comparison of the two studies may be no matter of concern. The most striking findings of this large series of subjects with CLD alcohol-related are a male preponderance, an older mean age of women, an increasing ageing over time in both sexes, a high proportion of subjects with a history of alcohol abuse and anti-HCV positive, and the majority of liver cirrhosis cases presenting at a decompensated stage.

The greater vulnerability of women and lower safe limits for alcohol consumption have been long recognized [22]. Women have a higher risk of alcoholic cirrhosis compared to men for a given level of alcohol intake [22, 23]. Some factors may explain this sex difference: lower production

TABLE 5: Characteristics of 955 subjects with alcohol-related liver cirrhosis in Italy, by year of recruitment.

Characteristics	Overall (n°=955)	Study 2001 (n°=792)	Study 2014 (n°=163)	p-value
Age (years), mean ± SD	60.0 ± 12.3	59.8 ± 12.1	60.7 ± 13.4	0.4
Sex Ratio (M/F)	2.9	3.6	1.3	<0.001
BMI, mean ± SD	25.8 ± 4.1	25.7 ± 4.0	25.7 ± 4.0	0.3
Area of origin				
(i) Northern/Central Italy	423 (44.2%)	349 (44.1%)	74 (45.4%)	0.005
(ii) Southern Italy/Islands	510 (53.3%)	429 (54.2%)	79 (48.5%)	
(iii) Born abroad	24 (2.5%)	14 (1.8%)	10 (6.1%)	
Risk factors				
(i) Alcohol intake alone	459 (48.0%)	374 (47.2%)	85 (52.1%)	0.7
(ii) Alcohol intake/HBsAg positive	63 (6.6%)	54 (6.8%)	9 (5.5%)	
(iii) Alcohol intake/anti-HCV positivity	407 (42.5%)	340 (42.9%)	65 (39.9%)	
(iv) Alcohol intake/HBsAg positive/anti-HCV positive	28 (2.9%)	24 (3.0%)	4 (2.5%)	
Diagnosis				
(i) Liver cirrhosis without HCC	836 (87.4%)	697 (88.0%)	137 (84.0%)	0.2
(ii) Liver cirrhosis with HCC	121 (12.6%)	95 (12.0%)	26 (16.0%)	
Child-Pugh class				
(i) A	381 (45.6%)	307 (44.1%)	74 (54.0%)	0.04
(ii) B/C	455 (54.4%)	390 (55.9%)	63 (46.0%)	

BMI: body mass index. HCC: hepatocellular carcinoma.

of gastric alcohol dehydrogenase and smaller volume of alcohol distribution. In addition, it has been suggested that female hormones increase alcohol mediated liver injury in an unknown fashion [24]. However, males account worldwide for 67% of liver cirrhosis deaths due to alcohol, and worldwide reports (enclosed the present study) have indicated a higher prevalence of alcoholic liver disease in men [2]. This could be because men typically drink more frequently than women do and, more frequently, they are heavy drinkers and alcoholics, regardless of geographic locations [25].

The great decrease of sex ratio from 2001 to 2014 parallels the consistent linear reduction of alcohol intake in the last decade in Italy, particularly among men [6], likely due to both Italian Sanitary Authorities' campaign to prevent alcohol abuse and to economic crisis, which reduces the likelihood of purchase alcohol beverages for money restriction.

The statistically significant younger age of male subjects suggests an earlier in the life exposure to alcohol in this sex. However, the cross-sectional structure of the two studies may have generated a potential survival bias; i.e., men might have died for other diseases more likely than women might do. On the other hand, the biphasic course of liver disease progression in women [26], with a more rapid increase of liver fibrosis in the late menopause than in the reproductive/premenopausal/early menopausal status [27], should be also considered. These explanations are not mutually exclusive, but all may have played a role in the observed different age pattern by sex. In any case, the observed ageing over time in both sexes may suggest an improvement of CLD managing over the past 13 years.

The high proportion of alcoholic and anti-HCV positive subjects reflects both the wide spread of HCV infection occurring in Italy after the world war II and the likelihood of behaviours at higher risk of exposure to this infection in these subjects.

A large case-control study showed that two-thirds of decompensated liver cirrhosis in Italy were attributable to alcohol abuse [28]. This figure, even if overestimated for having the authors inaccurately used the proportion of risky alcohol consumers in the hospital controls instead of in the general population for calculating the Population Attributable Risk [29], reflects the tendency of alcoholics to seek medical care only once symptoms are disclosed.

We acknowledge some potential limitations of the present study. Firstly, the history of alcohol intake was retrospectively recorded so that findings may be influenced by a recall bias and by the tendency of alcoholics to minimize or deny alcohol abuse at the time of observation to avoid the negative stigmata associated with alcoholism.

Secondly, some concern for a potential referral bias exists, since about 50% of patients with alcohol abuse were also anti-HCV positive (this condition that may have favoured the enrolment) and the remaining 50% anti-HCV negative often showed a severe liver disease (i.e., liver cirrhosis), a clinical condition that may have favoured the request for medical assistance and the enrolment in the study. This limitation, however, affects any study focusing on alcoholic CLD, as alcoholics tend to refer to hospitals only once severe symptoms have developed.

Thirdly, the definition of risky alcohol intake used in the present study does not capture the pattern of binge drinking, i.e., the consumption of 5 or more drinks in males or 4 or more drinks in women in about two hours [30], a phenomenon poorly investigated even in other published studies although continuously increasing in western countries [31]. Finally, type of beverage has not been assessed; the abuse in drinking wine has been recently shown to be associated with a lower risk of severe liver disease than the abuse in drinking beer and liquor [32].

In conclusion, this survey evidences that risky alcohol intake plays a role in more than one-fifth of CLD in Italy, with a shift over time towards an older age and a more severe disease stage. Considering the decreasing role of chronic HCV [33] and HBV [34] infections in Italy, these data put alcohol back in the spotlight with an important role in CLD in the years to come.

Abbreviations

HCV: Hepatitis C virus
HCC: Hepatocellular carcinoma
anti-HCV: Antibody to HCV
HCV RNA: Hepatitis C virus ribonucleic acid
HBV: Hepatitis B virus
HbsAg: Hepatitis B surface antigen
CLD: Chronic liver disease
PCR: Polymerase chain reaction
ALT: Alanine aminotransferase
US: Ultrasound.

Authors' Contributions

All authors contributed equally to this work, designed the study, and wrote the manuscript.

Acknowledgments

The authors acknowledge the contribution to data collection of the following coauthors: Sergio Babudieri, Bruno Cacopardo, Guido Colloredo, Massimo De Luca, Anna Licata, Mario Pirisi, Mariantonietta Pisaturo, Floriano Rosina, Maurizio Russello, and Teresa Santantonio.

References

[1] J. Rehm, A. V. Samokhvalov, and K. D. Shield, "Global burden of alcoholic liver diseases," *Journal of Hepatology*, vol. 59, no. 1, pp. 160–168, 2013.

[2] S. Liangpunsakul, P. Haber, and G. W. McCaughan, "Alcoholic Liver Disease in Asia, Europe, and North America," *Gastroenterology*, vol. 150, no. 8, pp. 1786–1797, 2016.

[3] D. A. Leon and J. McCambridge, "Liver cirrhosis mortality rates in Britain from 1950 to 2002: An analysis of routine data," *The Lancet*, vol. 367, no. 9504, pp. 52–56, 2006.

[4] European Association for the Study of Liver, "EASL Clinical Practical Guidelines: Management of Alcoholic Liver Disease," *Journal of Hepatology*, vol. 57, no. 2, pp. 399–420, 2012.

[5] M. K. Dam, T. Flensborg-Madsen, M. Eliasen, U. Becker, and J. S. Tolstrup, "Smoking and risk of liver cirrhosis: A population-based cohort study," *Scandinavian Journal of Gastroenterology*, vol. 48, no. 5, pp. 585–591, 2013.

[6] E. Scafato, "Sistema Italiano Monitoraggio Alcol (SISMA) on line," 2015, http://www.epicentro.iss.it/alcol/aggiornamenti.asp.

[7] E. Sagnelli, T. Stroffolini, A. Mele et al., "The importance of HCV on the burden of chronic liver disease in Italy: A multicenter prevalence study of 9,997 cases," *Journal of Medical Virology*, vol. 75, no. 4, pp. 522–527, 2005.

[8] E. Sagnelli, T. Stroffolini, C. Sagnelli et al., "Epidemiological and clinical scenario of chronic liver diseases in Italy: Data from a multicenter nationwide survey," *Digestive and Liver Disease*, vol. 48, no. 9, pp. 1066–1071, 2016.

[9] E. Sagnelli, T. Stroffolini, C. Sagnelli et al., "Gender differences in chronic liver diseases in two cohorts of 2001 and 2014 in Italy," *Infection*, vol. 46, no. 1, pp. 93–101, 2018.

[10] F. Alvarez, P. A. Berg, F. B. Bianchi et al., "International autoimmune hepatitis group report: review of criteria for diagnosis of autoimmune hepatitis," *Journal of Hepatology*, vol. 31, no. 5, pp. 929–938, 1999.

[11] B. G. Taal, S. W. Schalm, F. W. J. Ten Kate, J. Hermans, R. G. Geertzen, and B. E. Feltkamp, "Clinical diagnosis of primary biliary cirrhosis: A classification based on major and minor criteria," *Hepato-Gastroenterology*, vol. 30, no. 5, pp. 178–182, 1983.

[12] P. C. Adams and S. Chakrabarti, "Genotypic/phenotypic correlations in genetic hemochromatosis: Evolution of diagnostic criteria," *Gastroenterology*, vol. 114, no. 2, pp. 319–323, 1998.

[13] P. Ferenci, K. Caca, G. Loudianos et al., "Diagnosis and phenotypic classification of Wilson disease," *Liver International*, vol. 23, no. 3, pp. 139–142, 2003.

[14] U. Becker, A. Deis, and T. I. A. Sorensen, "Prediction of risk of liver disease by alcohol intake, sex, and age: A prospective population study," *Hepatology*, vol. 23, no. 5, pp. 1025–1029, 1996.

[15] A. McCullough and J. F. Barry O' Connor, "Alcoholic liver disease: proposed recommendations for the American College of Gastroenterology," *American Journal of Gastroenterology*, vol. 93, no. 11, pp. 2022–2036.

[16] P. Angulo and K. D. Lindor, "Non-alcoholic fatty liver disease," *Journal of Gastroenterology and Hepatology*, vol. 17, supplement sl, pp. S186–S190, 2002.

[17] S. Gaiani, L. Gramantieri, N. Venturoli et al., "What is the criterion for differentiating chronic hepatitis from compensated cirrhosis? A prospective study comparing ultrasonography and percutaneous liver biopsy," *Journal of Hepatology*, vol. 27, no. 6, pp. 979–985, 1997.

[18] J. Bruix, M. Sherman, J. M. Llovet et al., "Clinical management of hepatocellular carcinoma, conclusions of the barcelona-2000 EASL conference," *Journal of Hepatology*, vol. 35, no. 3, pp. 421–430, 2001.

[19] K. Ishak, A. Baptista, L. Bianchi et al., "Histological grading and staging of chronic hepatitis," *Journal of Hepatology*, vol. 22, no. 6, pp. 696–699, 1995.

[20] P. Bedossa and T. Poynard, "An algorithm for the grading of activity in chronic hepatitis C," *Hepatology*, vol. 24, no. 2, pp. 289–293, 1996.

[21] S. Gamal and Z. Khaled, *Ishak versus METAVIR: Terminology, Convertibility and Correlation with Laboratory Changes in*

Chronic Hepatitis C, Liver Biopsy, Takahashi, H., InTech, 2011, http://www.intechopen.com/books/liver-biopsy/ishak-versus-metavir-terminology-convertibility-and-correlation-with-laboratory-changes-in-chronic-h.

[22] J. Rehm, B. Taylor, S. Mohapatra et al., "Alcohol as a risk factor for liver cirrhosis: a systematic review and meta-analysis," *Drug and Alcohol Review*, vol. 29, no. 4, pp. 437–445, 2010.

[23] M. Kamper-Jørgensen, M. Grønbæk, J. Tolstrup, and U. Becker, "Alcohol and cirrhosis: Dose-response or threshold effect?" *Journal of Hepatology*, vol. 41, no. 1, pp. 25–30, 2004.

[24] P. K. Eagon, "Alcoholic liver injury: Influence of gender and hormones," *World Journal of Gastroenterology*, vol. 16, no. 11, pp. 1377–1384, 2010.

[25] R. E. Mann, R. G. Smart, and R. Govoni, "The epidemiology of alcoholic liver disease," *Alcohol Research & Health*, vol. 27, pp. 209–219, 2003.

[26] T. Poynard, P. Bedossa, and P. Opolon, "Natural history of liver fibrosis progression in patients with chronic hepatitis C," *The Lancet*, vol. 349, no. 9055, pp. 825–832, 1997.

[27] E. Villa, R. Vukotic, C. Cammà et al., "Reproductive status is associated with the severity of fibrosis in women with hepatitis C," *PLoS ONE*, vol. 7, no. 9, Article ID e44624, 2012.

[28] G. Corrao, A. Zambon, P. Torchio, S. Aricò, C. La Vecchia, and F. Di Orio, "Attributable risk for symptomatic liver cirrhosis in Italy," *Journal of Hepatology*, vol. 28, no. 4, pp. 608–614, 1998.

[29] T. Stroffolini, "Alcohol, HCV infection, and liver cirrhosis: Is the cup half full or half empty?" *Journal of Hepatology*, vol. 28, no. 4, pp. 728–730, 1998.

[30] S. Zakhari and T.-K. Li, "Determinants of alcohol use and abuse: impact of quantity and frequency patterns on liver disease," *Hepatology*, vol. 46, no. 6, pp. 2032–2039, 2007.

[31] P. Mathurin and R. Bataller, "Trends in the management and burden of alcoholic liver disease," *Journal of Hepatology*, vol. 62, no. 1, supplement, pp. S38–S46, 2015.

[32] G. Askgaard, M. Grønbæk, M. S. Kjær, A. Tjønneland, and J. S. Tolstrup, "Alcohol drinking pattern and risk of alcoholic liver cirrhosis: A prospective cohort study," *Journal of Hepatology*, vol. 62, no. 5, pp. 1061–1067, 2015.

[33] T. Stroffolini, E. Sagnelli, P. L. Almasio et al., "Etiological factors of chronic hepatitis in Italy," *European Journal of Gastroenterology & Hepatology*, vol. 29, no. 9, pp. 994–997, 2017.

[34] E. Sagnelli, T. Stroffolini, C. Sagnelli et al., "Influence of universal HBV vaccination on chronic HBV infection in Italy: Results of a cross-sectional multicenter study," *Journal of Medical Virology*, vol. 89, no. 12, pp. 2138–2143, 2017.

27

Urinary Elimination of Bile Acid Glucuronides under Severe Cholestatic Situations: Contribution of Hepatic and Renal Glucuronidation Reactions

Martin Perreault,[1] Ewa Wunsch,[2] Andrzej Białek,[2] Jocelyn Trottier,[1] Mélanie Verreault,[1] Patrick Caron,[1] Guy G. Poirier,[3] Piotr Milkiewicz,[4] and Olivier Barbier[1]

[1]*Laboratory of Molecular Pharmacology, CHU-Québec Research Centre and the Faculty of Pharmacy, Laval University, Quebec City, QC, Canada*
[2]*Translation Medicine Group, Pomeranian Medical University, Szczecin, Poland*
[3]*Proteomics Platform, Québec Genomic Center, CHU-Québec Research Centre and Faculty of Medicine, Laval University, Quebec City, QC, Canada*
[4]*Liver and Internal Medicine, Medical University of Warsaw, Warsaw, Poland*

Correspondence should be addressed to Olivier Barbier; olivier.barbier@crchudequebec.ulaval.ca

Academic Editor: Pascal Lapierre

Biliary obstruction, a severe cholestatic complication, causes accumulation of toxic bile acids (BAs) in liver cells. Glucuronidation, catalyzed by UDP-glucuronosyltransferase (UGT) enzymes, detoxifies cholestatic BAs. Using liquid chromatography coupled to tandem mass spectrometry, 11 BA glucuronide (-G) species were quantified in prebiliary and postbiliary stenting serum and urine samples from 17 patients with biliary obstruction. Stenting caused glucuronide- and fluid-specific changes in BA-G levels and BA-G/BA metabolic ratios. *In vitro* glucuronidation assays with human liver and kidney microsomes revealed that even if renal enzymes generally displayed lower K_M values, the two tissues shared similar glucuronidation capacities for BAs. By contrast, major differences between the two tissues were observed when four human BA-conjugating UGTs 1A3, 1A4, 2B4, and 2B7 were analyzed for mRNA and protein levels. Notably, the BA-24G producing UGT1A3 enzyme, abundant in the liver, was not detected in kidney microsomes. In conclusion, the circulating and urinary BA-G profiles are hugely impacted under severe cholestasis. The similar BA-glucuronidating abilities of hepatic and renal extracts suggest that both the liver and kidney may contribute to the urine BA-G pool.

1. Introduction

Bile acids (BAs) play a major role in cholesterol homeostasis. In the liver, cholesterol is efficiently converted into the primary cholic (CA) and chenodeoxycholic (CDCA) acids for subsequent secretion into intestine via the bile [1]. In the duodenum, these acids act as natural detergents to facilitate the absorption of dietary lipids, liposoluble vitamins, and cholesterol [2]. Significant proportions of CDCA and CA are then converted in the respective secondary lithocholic acid (LCA) and deoxycholic acid (DCA) by resident bacteria [2]. Both primary and secondary acids are reabsorbed and return to the liver via the portal circulation. Back in the liver, LCA and CDCA sustain additional biotransformations into the 6α-hydroxylated hyodeoxycholic acid (HDCA) and hyocholic acid (HCA), respectively [2, 3].

BAs are cytotoxic at elevated concentrations [4], and their accumulation in liver cells favors oxidative stress, inflammation, apoptosis, and subsequent damage to the liver parenchyma [2]. Such features are characteristic of cholestatic situations, where a reduction of the bile flow limits BA elimination from hepatocytes [5]. A reduction of BA hepatic levels is therefore an important goal for anticholestatic strategies [5].

Glucuronidation, catalyzed by members of the UDP-glucuronosyltransferase (UGT) family, is a major elimination mechanism for a variety of exogenous and endogenous molecules [6]. This enzymatic reaction consists in the transfer of the glucuronosyl group from uridine 5′-diphosphoglucuronic acid (UDPGA) to acceptor substrates. In humans, 19 functional UGTs have been categorized into three major UGT subfamilies, UGT1A, UGT2A, and UGT2B [7]. Among these enzymes, hepatic UGT1A3, 1A4, 2B4, and 2B7 isoforms have a remarkable capacity to convert BAs into glucuronide *in vitro* [8–12]. Bile acid glucuronidation involves either the 3/6-hydroxyl or 24-carboxyl groups of the BA steroid nucleus for the respective formation of ether 3/6G or acyl/ester 24G [8, 9, 11, 12]. UGT1A3 is the major enzyme for hepatic production of BA-24G, while UGT1A4, 2B4, and 2B7 are the main producers of ether glucuronides [8, 9, 11, 12].

An important consequence of glucuronidation is the introduction of an additional negative charge to the BA molecule, which allows BA-G transport by conjugate-transporters such as the multidrug resistance related proteins (MRPs) 3 and 4 that are present at the basolateral membrane of hepatocytes [4]. These transporters facilitate BA-G secretion into the blood, followed by enhanced urinary excretion. While increased BA-G urinary elimination has been reported in patients with acute cholestasis, the profile of these conjugates in both the circulation and urine has only been partially resolved [13–17]. On the other hand, the dogma that liver is the major site for glucuronidation has been challenged by the recent evidences that human kidney also has significant drug glucuronidation capacity [18]. Until now, only few investigations were performed to determine the contribution of renal UGTs to BA glucuronidation during cholestasis [19]. In the present study, 11 BA-G species have been quantified in serum and urine samples from patients with biliary obstruction obtained before and after biliary stenting. In parallel experiments, the BA-conjugating activities of microsomal extracts from human liver and kidney were compared.

2. Materials and Methods

2.1. Ethics Statement. All work has been conducted in accordance with the declaration of Helsinki (1964). This study was approved by the appropriate clinical study review boards at the CHU-Québec Research Centre, Laval University (*"Comité d'éthique de la recherche Clinique du CHUL,"* Québec City, QC, Canada: Projects #95.05.14 and #97.05.14) and Pomeranian Medical University (Bioethics Commission, Pomeranian Medical University in Szczecin, Poland: Resolution number BN-001/43/06). Experiments were conducted with the human subjects' understanding and consent. All patients had signed a written consent form before each procedure.

2.2. Materials. Bile acid glucuronides were obtained as described [11, 21]. Commercially available microsomes from human liver (pool of 26 men and 24 women, *#HO620*) and kidney (pool of 4 female and 4 male donors, *#H0610.R*) were purchased from Xenotech (Walkersville, MD). Human liver samples were from kidney donors as previously described (livers 2 to 8) [10, 12, 22]. Total RNA from individual human liver and kidney tissues was purchased from Ambion (Streetsville, Canada) (liver 1 and kidney 1) and Stratagene (Santa Clara, CA) (kidney 2). Total RNA from a pool of 5 human kidney donors was purchased from Ambion (Abingdon, UK). The Tri Reagent® was from Molecular Research Center Inc. (Cincinnati, OH). Protein assay reagents were obtained from Bio-Rad Laboratories Inc. (Marnes-la-Coquette, France). UGT antibodies were as previously described [10, 23, 24]. The secondary anti-rabbit IgG horse antibody was from Amersham (Oakville, Canada).

2.3. Patients with Biliary Obstruction. Seventeen patients (8 men and 9 women; mean age: 64 ± 10 years) with clinical and biochemical features of cholestasis were recruited as previously reported [20] (Supplementary Material 1). Diagnosis, biliary tree dilatation evidences, and biliary stenting procedures were extensively described in a previous report [20]. Stored urine was available from only 12 of these patients (6 men and 6 women) for BA-G measurement. Informed consent was obtained from each patient.

2.4. Bile Acid Glucuronides Measurement. Bile acid-glucuronide concentrations were determined from serum and urine samples (100 μL) using liquid chromatography coupled to tandem mass spectrometry (LC-MS/MS) with an electrospray interface, as previously reported [11, 12, 21]. The chromatographic system consisted of an Alliance 2690 HPLC apparatus (Waters, Milford, MA), and the tandem mass spectrometry system was an API3200 mass spectrometer (Applied Biosystems, Concord, Canada).

2.5. Glucuronidation Assays. All glucuronidation assays were performed for 2 hours in the presence of 10 μg microsomal proteins in a previously reported assay buffer [11, 12]. Kinetic parameters were assessed in liver and kidney samples using substrate concentrations ranging from 1 to 350 μM. The enzyme kinetic model was selected as recommended [25], using the Sigma Plot 11.2 assisted by Enzyme Kinetics 1.3 program (SSI, San Jose, CA).

2.6. RNA Extraction, Reverse Transcription, and Real-Time PCR Analyses. Total RNA was isolated according to the Tri Reagent acid: phenol protocol as specified by the supplier (Molecular Research Center Inc.). The reverse transcription (RT) and quantitative PCR reactions were performed as previously described [11, 26]. The real-time PCR amplifications were performed using an ABI Prism 7500FAST instrument from Applied Biosystems (Foster City, CA). For each reaction, the final volume of 20 μL comprised 10 μL of SYBR Green PCR Mix, 2 μL (4 μM) of each previously reported primer [11], and 6 μL of the indicated dilution of RT products. For each gene in each tissue, the amplification efficiency was tested using 2 to 5 log of cDNA produced from liver- or kidney-purified RNA and sequential dilutions of UGT cDNA constructs (0.0001 to 10 pg/μl). The difference between standard curve and sample efficiency was below 10%, as recommended [27]. The amount of target genes was derived from linear regression with standard curves of these UGT constructs according to reported protocols [28].

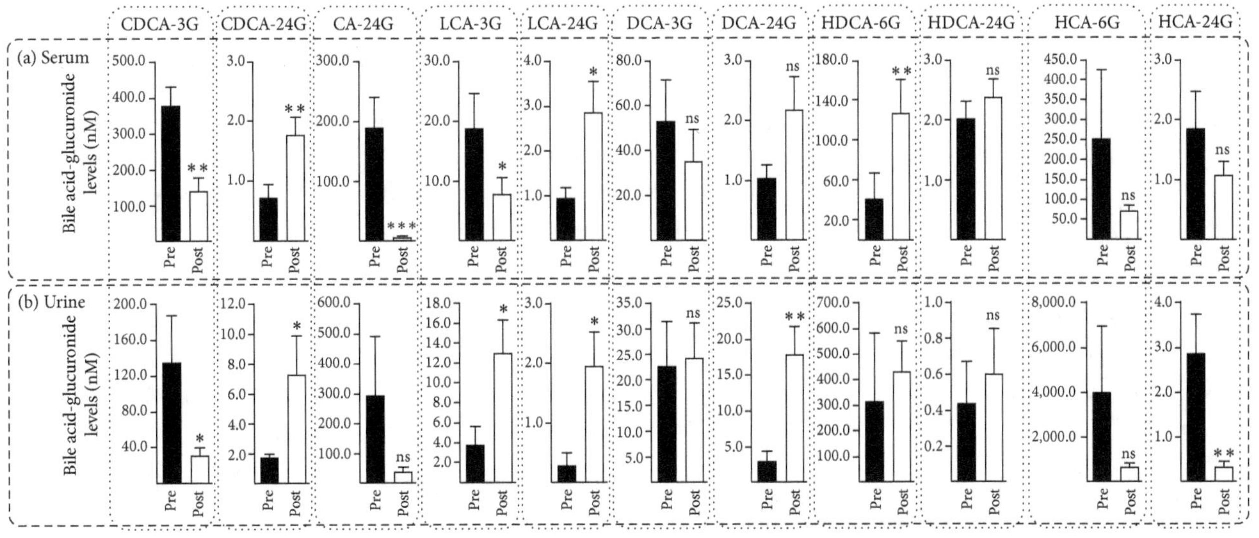

FIGURE 1: *Endoscopic stenting of the bile duct differentially affects the serum (a) and urine (b) bile acid-glucuronide profiles in patients suffering from biliary obstruction.* Serum ((a); $n = 17$) and urine ((b); $n = 12$) samples drawn before *(pre)* and after *(post)* endoscopic biliary stenting from patients with stenosed bile ducts were analyzed for their concentrations in 11 bile acid-glucuronide species using LC-MS/MS. Results represent the mean concentration ± SEM and are expressed as nM. p values were determined by the Wilcoxon matched-pairs signed-rank test. $^{*}p < 0.05$; $^{**}p < 0.01$; $^{***}p < 0.001$. ns: not significant.

Messenger RNA levels were calculated using the average molecular weight of one base-paired nucleotide (660 g/mol) and Avogadro's constant (6.022×10^{23} mol^{-1}).

2.7. UGT Protein Determination. For Western blotting, microsomes (5 μg) were size-separated by 10% SDS-polyacrylamide gels and transferred onto nitrocellulose membranes. All antibodies were used at 1:2,000 dilutions [10, 23, 24]. The housekeeping protein β-actin was used to ensure the equal protein loading in each lane. An anti-rabbit IgG horse antibody (1:10,000) conjugated with peroxidase (Amersham) was used as the second antibody, and the resulting immunocomplexes were visualized as described [12, 26].

Determination of UGT1A3 protein levels was also achieved using LC-MS/MS quantification according to the previously reported analytical strategy [10].

2.8. Data Analyses. Bile acid-glucuronide levels were calculated as mean ± standard error of the mean (SEM). BA-G concentrations did not satisfy the normal distribution according to the Shapiro-Wilk test; thus the Wilcoxon matched-pairs signed-rank test was used for statistical analyses of the response to treatment. Correlations were assessed by Spearman's rank correlation coefficient using the JMP Statistical Discovery V7.0.1 program (SAS Institute, Cary, NC).

3. Results

3.1. Biliary Stenting Modulates Circulating and Urinary BA-G Levels in Patients with Biliary Obstruction. The circulating and urinary BA-G profiles in prestenting and poststenting samples from biliary stenosed patients are illustrated in Figure 1. In sera, the species distribution was CDCA-3G > HCA-6G > CA-24G > DCA-3G = HDCA-6G > LCA-3G ≫ HDCA-24G = HCA-24G > DCA-24G = LCA-24G ≥ CDCA-24G. In urine, the most abundant species was HCA-6G > HDCA-6G = CA-24G > CDCA-3G > DCA-3G. As in serum, other species were minor components. Bile flow restoration caused significant reduction in serum CDCA-3G (2.7-fold), CA-24G (25-fold), and LCA-3G (2.4-fold) contents (Figure 1(a)). By contrast, CDCA-24G (2.4-fold), LCA-24G (3.0-fold), and HDCA-6G (3.0-fold) concentrations were significantly increased in poststenting versus prestenting sera (Figure 1(a)). Other changes failed to reach the statistical significance. As we previously reported [11], serum levels of BA-G in noncholestatic volunteers varied from 0.7 ± 0.1 nM for HDCA-24G to 63.5 ± 8.6 nM for HCA-6G. As observed in the present study, the most abundant species were HCA-6G, CDCA-3G, DCA-3G, and HDCA-6G. Biliary stenting also changed urine BA-G levels (Figure 1(b)): CDCA-24G (4.1-fold), LCA-3G (3.5-fold), LCA-24G (6.5-fold), and DCA-24G (5.9-fold) were increased; and CDCA-3G (4.3-fold) and HCA-24G (8.3-fold) were reduced.

3.2. Biliary Stenting Differentially Affects the BA-G versus BA Metabolic Ratios in Serum and Urine from Biliary Stenosed Patients. The serum and urine samples were previously analyzed for their content in the 6 unconjugated precursors of the glucuronide derivatives analyzed here [20]. These concentrations were used to calculate the metabolic ratio (i.e., BA-G/BA) for each glucuronide (Figure 2 and Supplementary Material 2). This parameter translates the glucuronide production capability from the available pool of unconjugated precursor, thus ensuring that changes in blood or urine levels of BA-G species do not only reflect changes in their precursors [11]. In serum samples, only the 6.5-, 20.6-, and 17.2-fold reductions in the respective

Metabolic ratios	Serum		Urine	
	Before stenting	After stenting	Before stenting	After stenting
CDCA-3G/CDCA	25.2 ± 4.3	3.9 ± 2.8***	6.9 ± 1.2	4.2 ± 0.8
CDCA-24G/CDCA	0.1 ± 0.1	0.1 ± 0.1	0.2 ± 0.1	1.1 ± 0.3
CA-24G/CA	10.2 ± 3.3	0.5 ± 0.2**	4.4 ± 1.2	0.8 ± 0.3**
LCA-3G/LCA	1.4 ± 0.8	0.3 ± 0.1	NA	NA
LCA-24G/LCA	0.2 ± 0.1	0.1 ± 0.1	NA	NA
DCA-3G/DCA	6.4 ± 2.8	0.4 ± 0.2**	4.3 ± 2.8	2.1 ± 0.5
DCA-24G/DCA	0.2 ± 0.1	0.1 ± 0.0	0.7 ± 0.6	1.7 ± 0.2
HDCA-6G/HDCA	4.1 ± 4.0	4.9 ± 1.5	5.0 ± 2.5	41.4 ± 11.3
HDCA-24G/HDCA	0.1 ± 0.1	0.1 ± 0.1	0.0 ± 0.0	0.0 ± 0.0
HCA-6G/HCA	15.5 ± 5.6	19.8 ± 3.5	4,159.1 ± 3,745.9	295.4 ± 235.3
HCA-24G/HCA	0.3 ± 0.1	0.3 ± 0.1	1.5 ± 0.7	0.1 ± 0.1

(a)

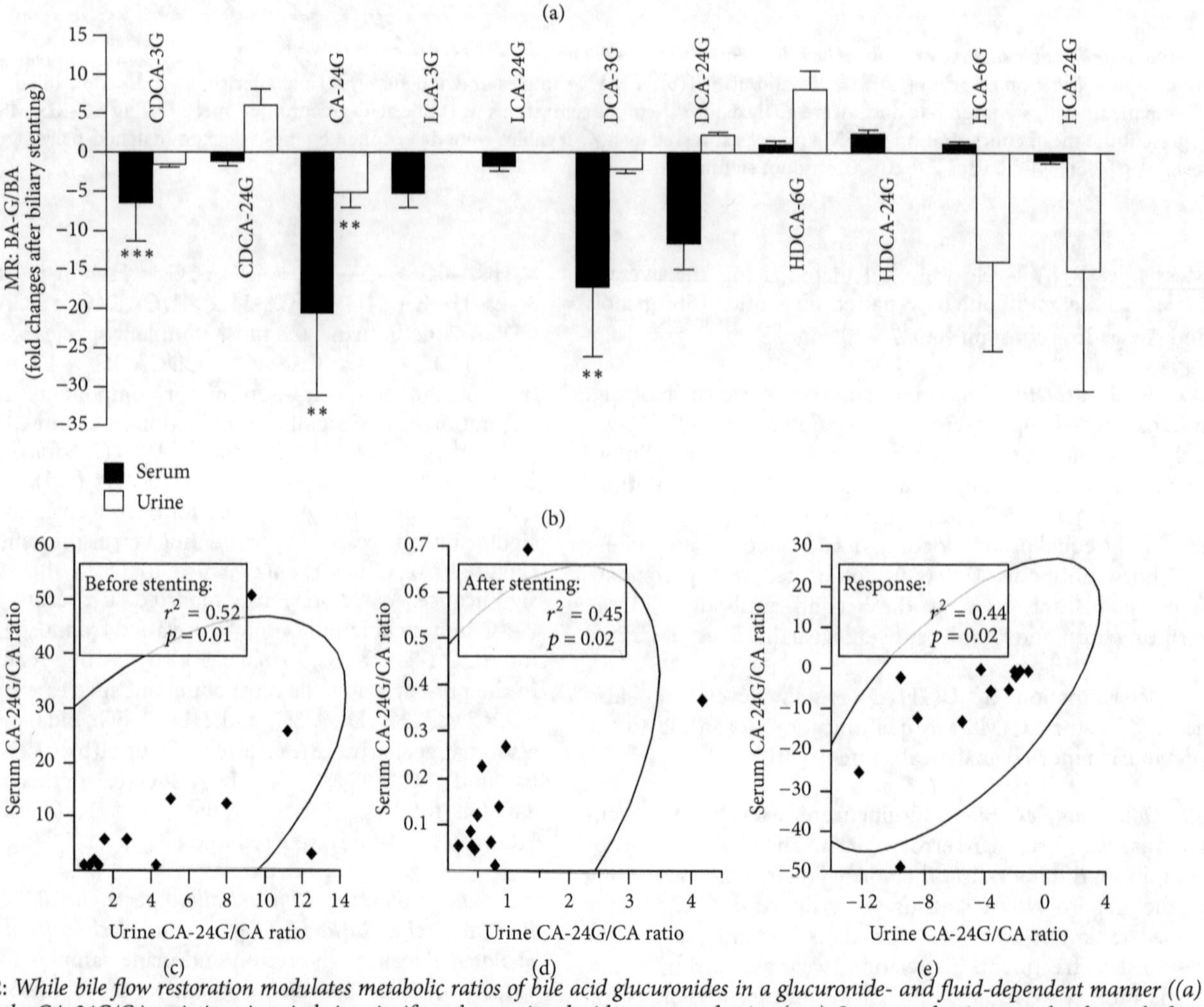

FIGURE 2: *While bile flow restoration modulates metabolic ratios of bile acid glucuronides in a glucuronide- and fluid-dependent manner ((a) and (b)), the CA-24G/CA ratio is unique in being significantly associated with serum and urine (c–e).* Serum and urine samples drawn before and after endoscopic biliary stenting from patients with stenosed bile ducts were analyzed for their concentrations in 11 bile acid-glucuronide species using LC-MS/MS. Concentrations of unconjugated acids were determined as reported [20], and the metabolic ratio for each species (a) was calculated as the ratio of glucuronide versus unconjugated precursor. (b) Black (serum; $n = 17$) and white (urine; $n = 12$) bars represent the mean ± SEM of fold changes (posttreatment values divided by pretreatment values) in MRs. Statistically significant differences between prestenting versus poststenting samples were determined using the Wilcoxon matched-pairs signed-rank test: $^{**}P < 0.01$; $^{***}P < 0.001$. Other changes failed to reach statistical significance. The absence of unconjugated LCA in urine impaired such analysis for LCA-3 and -24G [20], while urine HDCA-24G/HDCA was null. (c–e) Correlation analyses of paired ($n = 12$) prestenting (c) and poststenting (d) serum and urine CA-24G/CA values or response to stenting determined as the difference between post- and pretreatment levels (e) were performed using the Spearman rank-order correlation (r^2), and p values for comparisons are indicated.

TABLE 1: Summary of the correlation studies between serum and urine bile acid-glucuronide profiles.

Urine levels	Before stenting (r^2; p value)	After stenting (r^2; p value)	Response (r^2; p value)
CDCA-3G	0.10; 0.30	0.02; 0.67	0.25; 0.10
CDCA-24G	0.01; 0.69	0.05; 0.50	0.02; 0.63
CA-24G	0.32; 0.05	***0.51; 0.01***	0.07; 0.42
LCA-3G	0.00; 0.97	0.19; 0.15	0.01; 0.81
LCA-24G	0.14; 0.22	***0.47; 0.01***	***0.42; 0.02***
DCA-3G	***0.82; <0.0001***	0.14; 0.23	0.01; 0.71
DCA-24G	0.06; 0.43	0.16; 0.19	***0.58; 0.004***
HDCA-6G	0.29; 0.07	0.31; 0.06	***0.35; 0.04***
HDCA-24G	0.00; 1.00	0.05; 0.47	0.03; 0.59
HCA-6G	0.29; 0.07	0.15; 0.20	***0.67; 0.001***
HCA-24G	0.00; 0.83	0.27; 0.08	0.04; 0.54

Correlation analyses were performed using the Spearman rank-order correlation (r^2), and p values for comparisons are indicated. Response is calculated as the difference between post- and prestenting values. CA: cholic acid; CDCA: chenodeoxycholic acid; DCA: deoxycholic acid; HCA: hyocholic acid; HDCA: hyodeoxycholic acid; LCA: lithocholic acid; G: glucuronide.

CDCA-3G/CDCA, CA-24G/CA, and DCA-3G/DCA ratios were statistically significant (Figures 2(a) and 2(b)). Other changes, even the reduction in DCA-24G/DCA (11.7-fold) and LCA-3G/LCA (5.3-fold) or the 2.5-fold increase of the HDCA-24G/HDCA ratio, failed to reach statistical significance (Figure 2(b)). In urine (Supplementary Material 2), the unique significant change corresponded to the 5.2-fold reduction of the CA-24G/CA ratio (Figure 2(b)), while the 14- and 15-fold reductions in HCA-6 and -24G MRs also failed to reach statistical significance.

3.3. Serum and Urine BA-G Profiles Are Only Feebly Associated. Correlation studies of circulating and urinary BA-G levels in paired samples identified only few significant associations (Table 1). In prestenting samples, only the serum DCA-3G was significantly and positively correlated ($r^2 = 0.82$) to its urinary concentration, while in poststenting fluids, no correlation for this conjugate was detected. Serum and urine CA-24G ($r^2 = 0.51$) and LCA-24G ($r^2 = 0.47$) levels were significantly correlated but only in samples obtained after bile flow restoration (Table 1). When the response to stenting (determined as the difference between post- and prestenting values) was analyzed, only changes for LCA-24G ($r^2 = 0.42$), DCA-24G ($r^2 = 0.58$), HDCA-6G ($r^2 = 0.35$), and HCA-6G ($r^2 = 0.67$) were positively and significantly associated (Table 1). Finally, when similar analyses were performed for MRs, the unique significant association in prestenting ($r^2 = 0.52$) and poststenting ($r^2 = 0.45$) levels and response ($r^2 = 0.44$) was obtained with the ratio CA-24G/CA (Figures 2(c)–2(e)).

3.4. Bile Acid Glucuronidation by Human Liver and Kidney Extracts. The limited associations between circulating and urinary profiles observed above suggest a potential extra-hepatic origin for urinary levels of BA-G. To test such a hypothesis, we sought to compare the kinetic parameters of BA glucuronidation by human liver (pool of 50 donors) and kidney (pool of 8 donors) microsomes (Figures 3–5). No differences in kinetic models were observed, with the BA-specific glucuronidation reactions being distributed among 3 models:

(i) The sigmoidal pattern for CA-24G and CDCA-24 and -3G (Figure 3), DCA-3 and -24G (Figures 4(c) and 4(d)), and HDCA-6 and -24G (Figures 5(a) and 5(b)) production

(ii) The Michaelis-Menten model for the formation of LCA-24G (Figure 4(b)) and HCA-6 and -24G (Figures 5(c) and 5(d))

(iii) The substrate-inhibition model for LCA-3G with respective K_I values of 240.3 ± 53.5 and 255.4 ± 69.9 μM for liver and kidney extracts (Figure 4(a)).

With the exception of CA-24G, HDCA-24G, and HCA-24G, kidney UGTs generally displayed lower K_M values. For example, kidney microsomes exhibited a 6-fold lower K_M value than liver ones for LCA-3G production (Figure 4(a)). Another notable difference between liver and kidney microsomes relates to the 10-fold higher V_{max} value of HDCA-24G production obtained with the hepatic microsomal preparation (Figure 5(b)). Nevertheless, the most efficient reactions were obtained with the conversion of HDCA and HCA into 6G derivatives that occurred at high velocities (i.e., V_{max}) with both liver and kidney microsomes (Figures 5(a) and 5(c)). In both tissue extracts, the 6α-hydroxylated acids were more actively converted into 6-glucuronide when compared to their 24-glucuronide counterparts (Figure 5). Interestingly, the opposite was observed for CDCA (Figures 3(a) and 3(b)) and LCA (Figures 4(a) and 4(b)). The V_{max} values for DCA-3 and -24G formation were, however, similar (Figures 4(c) and 4(d)).

3.5. Differential BA-Conjugating UGT Expression in the Human Liver and Kidney. Results from kinetic experiments indicate that the human kidney possesses an efficient BA-conjugating UGT system. We next investigated whether the BA-conjugating UGTs 1A3, 1A4, 2B4, and 2B7 [8–11] are differentially expressed in human liver and kidney

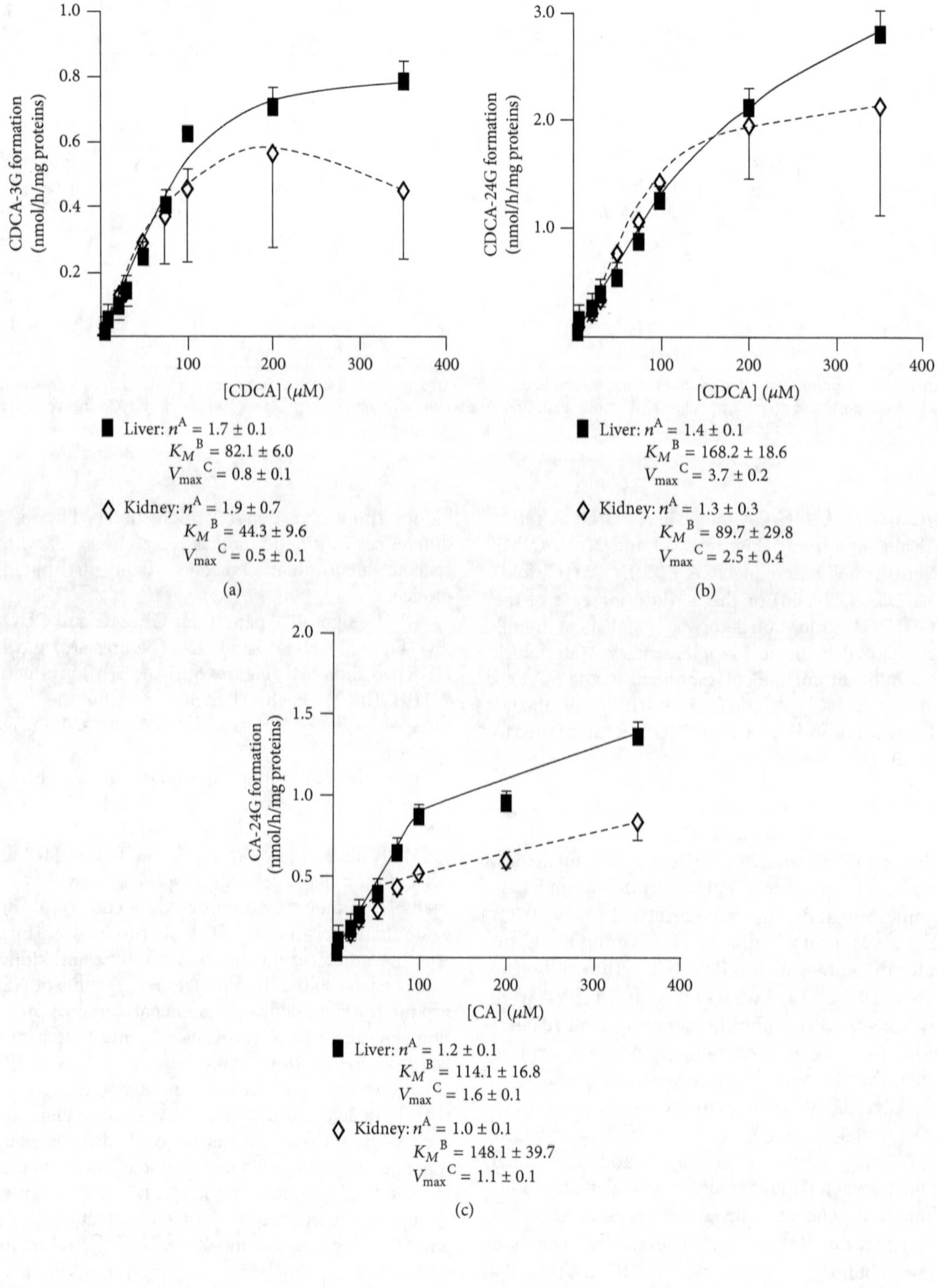

FIGURE 3: *Kinetic analyses of CDCA-3G (a), CDCA-24G (b), and CA-24G (c) formation by microsomes from human liver and kidney.* Human liver (black squares, pool of 50 donors) and kidney (white diamonds; pool of 8 donors) microsomes (10 μg) were incubated in the presence of increasing concentrations (1 to 350 μM) of chenodeoxycholic acid (CDCA, (a) and (b)) or cholic acid (CA, (c)) for 2 hours at 37°C. The formation of CDCA-3G (a), CDCA-24G (b), and CA-24G (c) was analyzed by LC-MS/MS. For each panel, graphs represent the rate of product formation (y-axis) versus substrate concentration (x-axis) of two experiments performed in triplicate. The listed kinetic parameters were determined as indicated in "Materials and Methods." $^A n$: Hill coefficient; $^B K_M$: calculated Michaelis constant expressed as μM; $^C V_{max}$: calculated maximal velocity expressed as nmol/h/mg proteins.

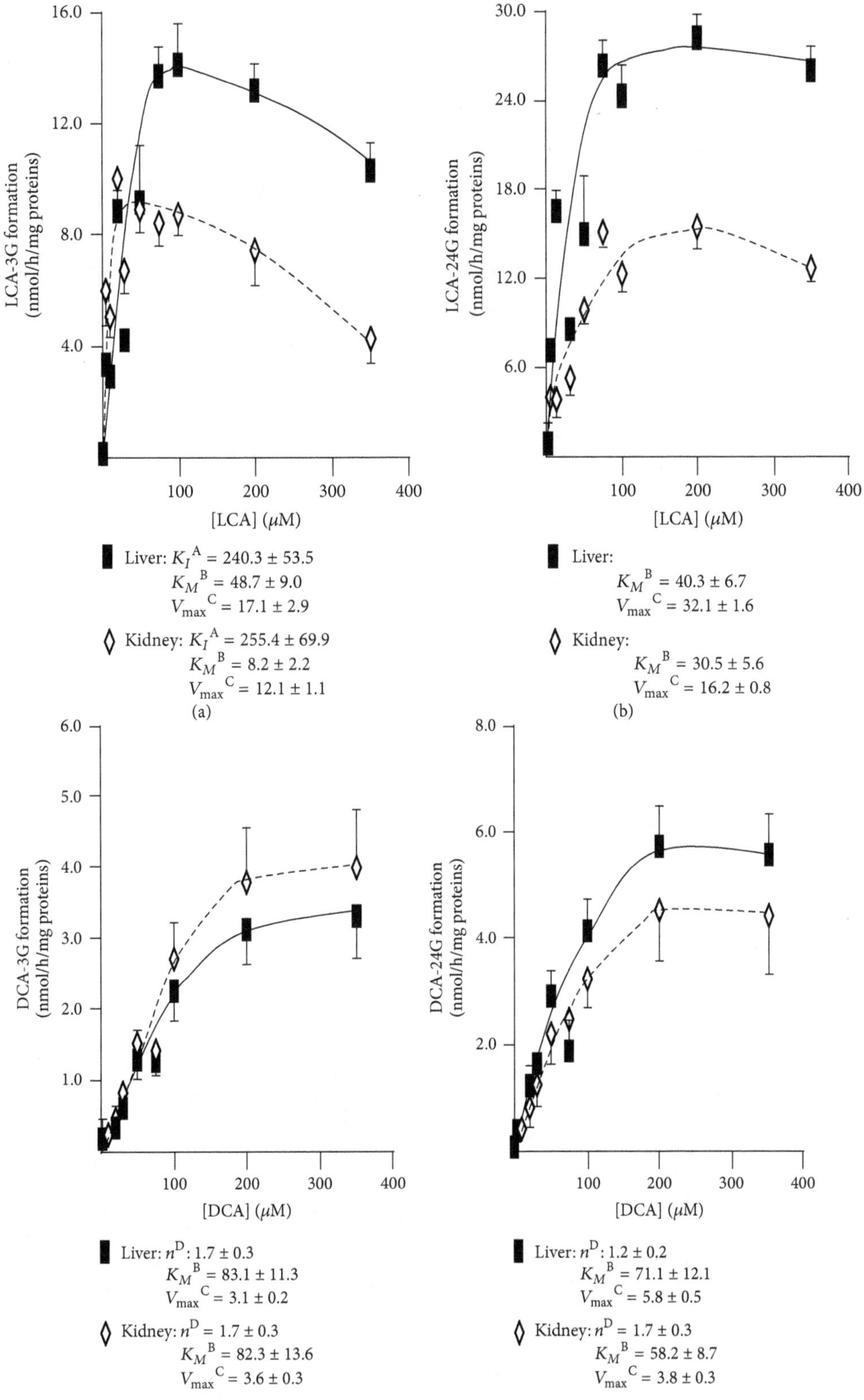

FIGURE 4: *Kinetic analyses of LCA-3G (a), LCA-24G (b), DCA-3G (c), and DCA-24G (d) formation by microsomes from human liver and kidney.* Human liver (black squares, pool of 50 donors) and kidney (white diamonds; pool of 8 donors) microsomes (10 μg) were incubated in the presence of increasing concentrations (1 to 350 μM) of lithocholic acid (LCA, (a) and (b)) or deoxycholic acid (DCA, (c) and (d)) for 2 hours at 37°C. The formation of LCA-3G (a), LCA-24G (b), DCA-3G (c), and DCA-24G (d) was analyzed by LC-MS/MS. For each panel, graphs represent the rate of product formation (y-axis) versus substrate concentration (x-axis) of two experiments performed in triplicate. The listed kinetic parameters were determined as indicated in "Materials and Methods." $^{A}K_I$: constant of inhibition expressed as μM; $^{B}K_M$: calculated Michaelis constant expressed as μM; $^{C}V_{max}$: calculated maximal velocity expressed as nmol/h/mg proteins; ^{D}n: Hill coefficient.

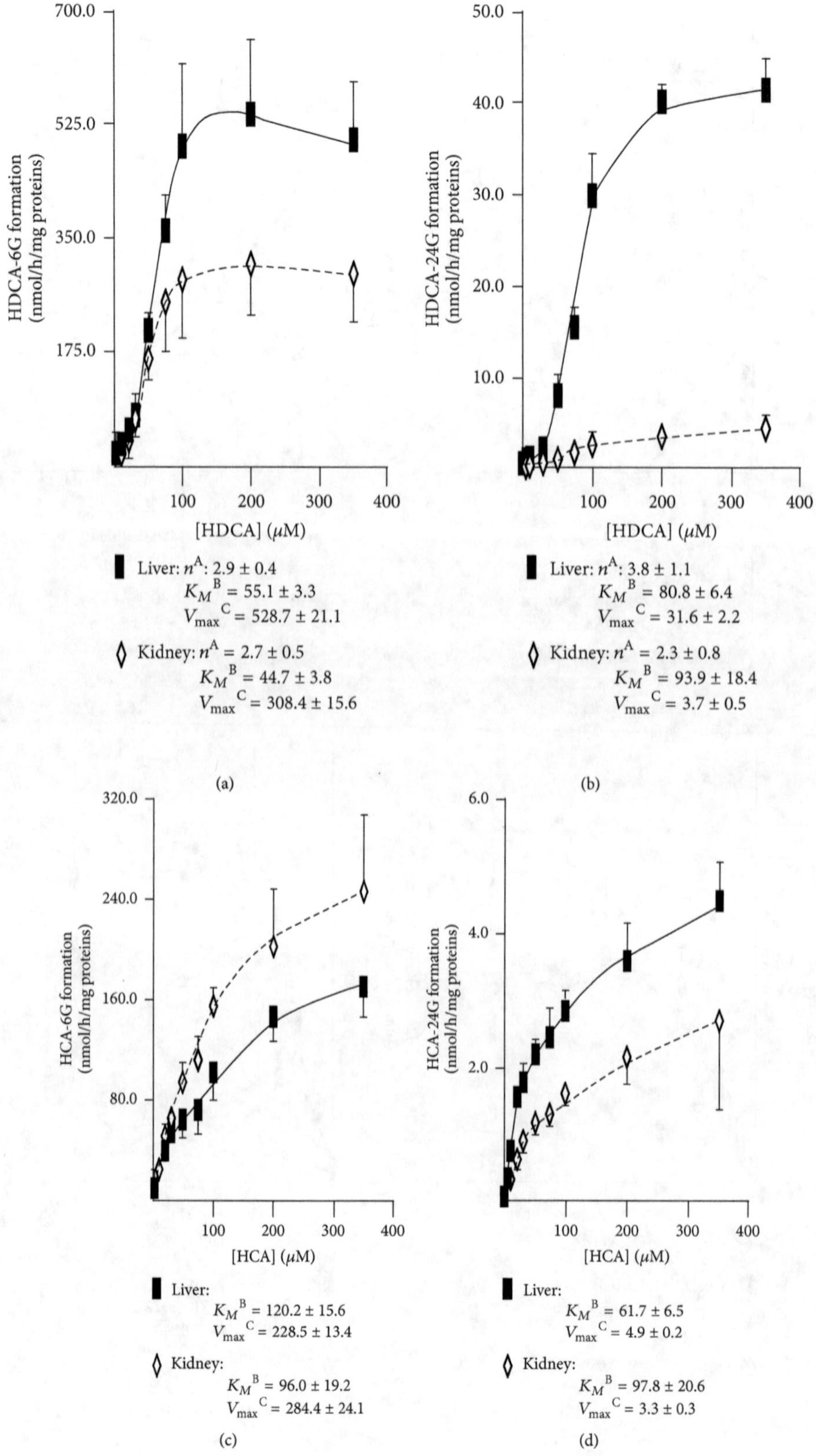

FIGURE 5: *Kinetic analyses of HDCA-6G (a), HDCA-24G (b), HCA-6G (c), and HCA-24G (d) formation by microsomes from human liver and kidney.* Human liver (black squares, pool of 50 donors) and kidney (white diamonds; pool of 8 donors) microsomes (10 μg) were incubated in the presence of increasing concentrations (1 to 350 μM) of hyodeoxycholic acid (HDCA, (a) and (b)) or hyocholic acid (HCA, (c) and (d)) for 2 hours at 37°C. The formation of HDCA-6G (a), HDCA-24G (b), HCA-6G (c), and HCA-24G (d) was analyzed by LC-MS/MS. For each panel, graphs represent the rate of product formation (y-axis) versus substrate concentration (x-axis) of two experiments performed in triplicate. The listed kinetic parameters were determined as indicated in "Materials and Methods." $^A n$: Hill coefficient; $^B K_M$: calculated Michaelis constant expressed as μM; $^C V_{max}$: calculated maximal velocity expressed as nmol/h/mg proteins.

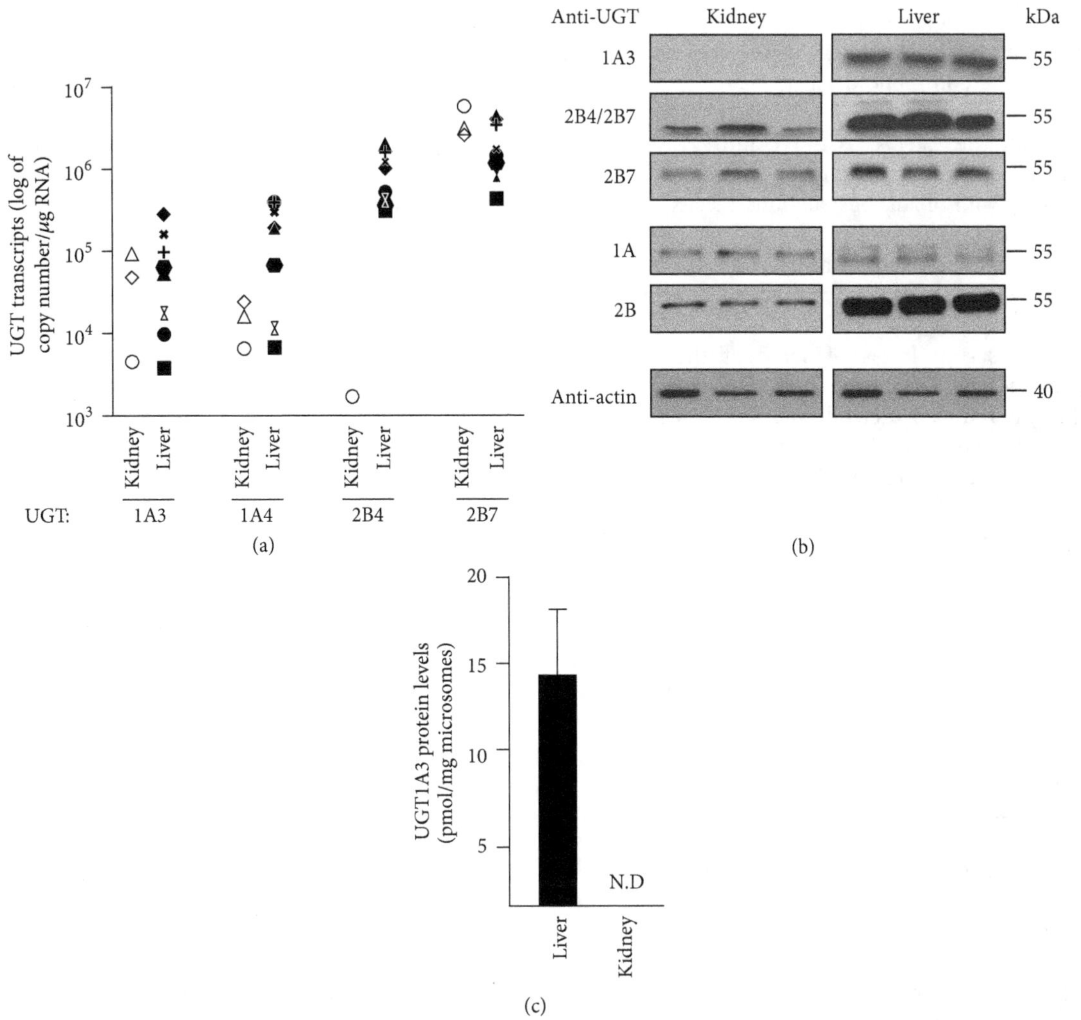

FIGURE 6: *Differential expression of the bile acid-conjugating UGT enzymes in the human liver and kidney.* (a) UGTs 1A3, 1A4, 2B4, and 2B7 mRNA levels in total RNA samples from human kidney (1 pool of 5 donors and 2 individual donors) and liver (8 individual donors) were determined through qRT-PCR analyses as described in "Materials and Methods." Results are expressed as $\log_{10}$ of mRNA copy number per μg of total RNA. Each symbol represents 1 donor, with the exception of the white triangle that corresponds to a pool of the 5 kidney donors. (b) The UGT protein contents in microsomal preparations (5 μg) from human kidney (pool of 4 female and 4 male donors) and liver (pool of 26 male and 24 female donors) were determined after size separation on SDS-PAGE and hybridization with the anti-UGT1A3, anti-UGT2B4/7, anti-UGT2B7, anti-UGT1A, and anti-UGT2B antibodies (1 : 2,000 dilution). The housekeeping protein β-actin was used to ensure the equal protein loading in each lane. Data presented are representative of two experiments. (c) The UGT1A3 protein content in human liver and kidney microsomes was determined using LC-MS/MS analyses as previously described [10]. Data represent the mean ± SD of two different experiments performed in triplicate. N.D: not detected.

(Figure 6). With the exception of UGT2B4 transcripts that were detected only in 1 kidney mRNA sample, other UGT messengers were detected in all kidney and liver preparations (Figure 6(a)). As expected [28, 29], their mRNA levels sustained a strong interindividual variability. Western blot analyses evidenced, however, major differences between liver and kidney (Figure 6(b)). A clear UGT1A3 immunoreactive complex was obtained with liver extracts, while this UGT protein was not detected in microsomal proteins from kidney (Figure 6(b)). While the UGT2B7 protein was found at similar levels in both tissues, the use of an anti-UGT2B4/2B7 antibody indicated that the UGT2B4 protein may be more abundant in liver than in kidney extracts (Figure 6(b)). The lack of an accurate and specific anti-UGT1A4 antibody impaired the quantification of this BA-conjugating UGT; however, we were able to further confirm the absence of the UGT1A3 protein in kidney microsomes through the use of our previously established LC-MS/MS-based proteomic method (Figure 6(c)) [10].

4. Discussion

Urinary and circulating levels of BA-Gs detected in the present study are similar to previous findings in terms of both glucuronide concentrations and species distribution [13, 14, 16]. However, an important improvement of the present investigations resides in our ability to discriminate between ether and ester glucuronides of a single BA. For example, while glucuronide conjugates of CDCA, CA, and DCA were previously identified as accumulating metabolites in sera from patients undergoing bile drainage [20], the nature of these glucuronides has not been resolved until now. Our results point out the ester CDCA-3G and DCA-3G and the acyl CA-24G as the most abundant glucuronide species found in patients with biliary obstruction. Because acyl, but not ester, glucuronides can be potentially toxic molecules (reviewed in [30]), such information may be critical in anticipating the consequences of their accumulation during cholestasis.

Interestingly, serum levels of some of the bile acid glucuronides, such as CDCA-3G, CA-24G, and LCA-3G, were significantly reduced after biliary stenting, while some others, like CDCA-24G, LCA-24G, and HDCA-6G, were significantly increased. While additional investigations are warranted to decipher the mechanisms beyond such a glucuronide species-dependent responsiveness, one can speculate that these changes may actually reflect the differential manner in which the UGT enzymes and/or the BA-G transporters may be altered upon biliary obstruction and after stenting. Therefore, it would have been of interest to compare how these proteins behave in tissues (i.e., liver and kidney) from cholestatic donors to validate such a hypothesis. Actually, one limitation of the current study is that the liver and kidney microsomes used are not from donors with biliary obstruction. When compared to other glucuronide conjugates, CA-24G presented a unique behavior: (1) in contrast to other acyl BA-Gs that are only minor components of the urine and serum glucuronide pools, CA-24G is the 3rd most abundant glucuronidated acid in prestenting samples; (2) this species is the most spectacularly affected when poststenting versus prestenting sera profiles are compared; (3) the serum CA-24G/CA ratio sustains the stronger reduction after biliary stenting; (4) this MR is also unique in being significantly reduced in posttreatment urines; and (5) only the CA-24G/CA ratio exhibits positive serum/urine association in terms of prestenting and poststenting distribution, as well as treatment response. These last observations support a hepatic origin for the formation of CA-24G and the strong CA-24G accumulation in prestenting fluids, and its spectacular reduction after bile flow restoration suggests that, under noncholestatic situations, this compound, formed in liver cells, is normally secreted in bile. This hypothesis is further supported by previous investigations, in which the intravenous injections of cholate glucuronide to rats resulted in a rapid and efficient secretion in bile of the unchanged glucuronide conjugate [31]. By contrast, when the same procedure was applied to bile duct ligated animals, 95% of the radioactivity was recovered in urine [31]. The present study indicates that similar rerouting of CA-24G elimination to urine may also occur in cholestatic patients, since circulating levels detected in prestenting cholestatic donors were almost 50-fold higher than those previously quantified in samples from noncholestatic volunteers (~2 nM, [11]). Privileging secretion from liver cells into the blood for subsequent urinary elimination may actually protect the liver against the accumulation of such abundant and potentially toxic glucuronide species during cholestasis. In the same vein, the improved formation of other conjugates such as CDCA-3G and DCA-3G, which we recently identified as nontoxic BAs [32], may also participate in the hepatic detoxification of their unconjugated CDCA and DCA precursors. Consistent with the above stated hypothesis, circulating MRs for these 2 conjugates (i.e., 25.2 and 6.4 for CDCA-3G and DCA-3G, resp.) are spectacularly increased when compared to those previously found in noncholestatic donors (0.6 and 0.1) [11]. However, the fact that circulating and urinary MRs for these species were not associated and the fact that biliary stenting exerted only minor effects on these ratios in urine are also indicative of an extrahepatic origin for urine CDCA- and DCA-3G species, at least after bile flow restoration.

We next compared the human liver and kidney in terms of bile acid glucuronidation activity and BA-conjugating UGT expression. With 2 exceptions (i.e., the 6- and 10-fold difference in K_M and $V_{\max}$ values for LCA-3G and HDCA-24G formations, resp.), these experiments reveal the remarkable similarity of renal and hepatic bile acid glucuronidation processes and the clear preference of both tissues in producing HDCA-6 and HCA-6G. Such preference may actually explain the predominance of these conjugates in various human fluids as previously described [11]. However, the most intriguing observation issuing from these analyses relates to the UGT1A3 enzyme. Indeed, not only was this enzyme detected in kidney extracts only at the mRNA (but not protein) level, but also the absence of such an active enzyme, previously identified as the main isoform for acyl BA glucuronidation [8–10, 12], is inconsistent with the elevated acyl glucuronide production capability of kidney microsomes. A plausible explanation for the conflicting observation on UGT1A3 mRNA and protein expression in kidney samples relates to the fact that protein and RNA extracts were from different sources and thus were not paired. It is therefore possible that only donors for mRNA express these isoforms in the kidney. Meanwhile, unlikely, such a possibility is supported by the controversial nature of the UGT1A3 expression in the human kidney [29, 33–35]. Additional investigations are therefore warranted to clarify whether this BA-conjugating protein is found or not in the human kidney.

Nevertheless, the present study clearly establishes the major contributions that liver and kidney play in glucuronidating bile acid during cholestasis. Interestingly, Zhou and colleagues reported that intestinal glucuronidation also plays an important role in controlling the local bile acid homeostasis and the pathological development of colitis [36]. These authors elegantly demonstrated that, in the intestine, bile acids glucuronidation leads to reduced intracellular levels of ligands for the nuclear receptor FXR. Reduced FXR activation limits the secretion of FGF15/19 in the portal circulation, which in turns leads to an increase of de novo formation of bile acid in the liver [36]. Thus, in contrast to the liver and kidney, where glucuronidation is thought to facilitate the removal of bile acids, the intestinal glucuronidation seems to increase the delivery of bile acids. However, it should be noted that, during obstructive cholestasis, the delivery of hepatic bile acids to the intestine is compromised, and thus only minor intestinal glucuronidation may occur.

5. Conclusion

In conclusion, the present study evidences the major impact that bile flow restoration exerts on the circulating and urinary bile acid-glucuronide profiles and demonstrates the elevated capability of the human kidney to glucuronidate these endogenous compounds. Future investigations are required to clarify the mechanism allowing kidney extracts to convert bile acids into acyl glucuronides in the absence of the UGT1A3 protein.

Abbreviations

BA:	Bile acid
BO:	Biliary obstruction
CA:	Cholic acid
CDCA:	Chenodeoxycholic acid
DCA:	Deoxycholic acid
FXR:	Farnesoid X receptor
G:	Glucuronide
HDCA:	Hyodeoxycholic acid
HCA:	Hyocholic acid
LCA:	Lithocholic acid
LC-MS/MS:	Liquid chromatography-tandem mass spectrometry
UDPGA:	UDP-glucuronic acid
UGT:	UDP-glucuronosyltransferase
MRPs:	Multidrug resistance related proteins.

Acknowledgments

The authors wish to thank Dr. Virginie Bocher for critical reading of the manuscript. This study was supported by grants from the Canadian Institute of Health Research (CIHR #119331), the Canadian Liver Foundation, the Natural Sciences and Engineering Research Council of Canada (NSERC #402213-2012), and the Canadian Foundation for Innovation (CFI #25712). Martin Perreault is holder of a scholarship from the "Fonds pour la Recherche en Santé du Québec" (FRSQ #23444). Olivier Barbier is holder of a salary grant from CIHR (New Investigator #MSH95330). Piotr Milkiewicz was supported by Grants #DEC-2011/01/B/NZ5/04216 and 2011/02/A/NZ5/00321 from the National Science Centre in Poland.

References

[1] D. W. Russell, "The enzymes, regulation, and genetics of bile acid synthesis," *Annual Review of Biochemistry*, vol. 72, pp. 137–174, 2003.

[2] M. J. Monte, J. J. G. Marin, A. Antelo, and J. Vazquez-Tato, "Bile acids: Chemistry, physiology, and pathophysiology," *World Journal of Gastroenterology*, vol. 15, no. 7, pp. 804–816, 2009.

[3] A. F. Hofmann, "Detoxification of lithocholic acid, a toxic bile-acid: relevance to drug hepatotoxicity," *Drug Metabolism Reviews*, vol. 36, no. 3-4, pp. 703–722, 2004.

[4] C. Pauli-Magnus, B. Stieger, Y. Meier, G. A. Kullak-Ublick, and P. J. Meier, "Enterohepatic transport of bile salts and genetics of cholestasis," *Journal of Hepatology*, vol. 43, no. 2, pp. 342–357, 2005.

[5] G. Paumgartner, "Pharmacotherapy of cholestatic liver diseases," *Journal of Digestive Diseases*, vol. 11, no. 3, pp. 119–125, 2010.

[6] M. Verreault, J. Kaeding, P. Caron et al., "Regulation of endobiotics glucuronidation by ligand-activated transcription factors: Physiological function and therapeutic potential," *Drug Metabolism Reviews*, vol. 42, no. 1, pp. 106–118, 2010.

[7] P. I. Mackenzie, K. W. Bock, B. Burchell et al., "Nomenclature update for the mammalian UDP glycosyltransferase (UGT) gene superfamily," *Pharmacogenetics and Genomics*, vol. 15, no. 10, pp. 677–685, 2005.

[8] M. H. Court, S. Hazarika, S. Krishnaswamy, M. Finel, and J. A. Williams, "Novel polymorphic human UDP-glucuronosyltransferase 2A3: Cloning, functional characterization of enzyme variants, comparative tissue expression, and gene induction," *Molecular Pharmacology*, vol. 74, no. 3, pp. 744–754, 2008.

[9] W. E. Gall, G. Zawada, B. Mojarrabi et al., "Differential glucuronidation of bile acids, androgens and estrogens by human UGT1A3 and 2B7," *The Journal of Steroid Biochemistry and Molecular Biology*, vol. 70, no. 1–3, pp. 101–108, 1999.

[10] J. Trottier, D. El Husseini, M. Perreault et al., "The human UGT1A3 enzyme conjugates norursodeoxycholic acid into a C23-ester glucuronide in the liver," *The Journal of Biological Chemistry*, vol. 285, no. 2, pp. 1113–1121, 2010.

[11] J. Trottier, M. Perreault, I. Rudkowska et al., "Profiling serum bile acid glucuronides in humans: Gender divergences, genetic determinants, and response to fenofibrate," *Clinical Pharmacology & Therapeutics*, vol. 94, no. 4, pp. 533–543, 2013.

[12] P. Caron, J. Trottier, M. Verreault, J. Bélanger, J. Kaeding, and O. Barbier, "Enzymatic production of bile acid glucuronides used as analytical standards for liquid chromatography-mass spectrometry analyses," *Molecular Pharmaceutics*, vol. 3, no. 3, pp. 293–302, 2006.

[13] B. Alme and J. Sjovall, "Analysis of bile acid glucuronides in urine. identification of $3\alpha,6\alpha,12\alpha$-trihydroxy-5β-cholanoic acid," *The Journal of Steroid Biochemistry and Molecular Biology*, vol. 13, no. 8, pp. 907–916, 1980.

[14] A. Stiehl, R. Raedsch, G. Rudolph, P. Czygan, and S. Walker, "Analysis of bile acid glucuronides in urine: group separation on a lipophilic anion exchanger," *Clinica Chimica Acta*, vol. 123, no. 3, pp. 275–285, 1982.

[15] A. Stiehl, R. Raedsch, G. Rudolph, U. Gundert-Remy, and M. Senn, "Biliary and urinary excretion of sulfated, glucuronidated and tetrahydroxylated bile acids in cirrhotic patients," *Hepatology*, vol. 5, no. 3, pp. 492–495, 1985.

[16] H. Takikawa, T. Beppu, and Y. Seyama, "Urinary concentrations of bile acid glucuronides and sulfates in hepatobiliary diseases," *Gastroenterologia Japonica*, vol. 19, no. 2, pp. 104–109, 1984.

[17] H. Wietholtz, H. Marschall, R. Reuschenbach, H. Matern, and S. Matern, "Urinary excretion of bile acid glucosides and glucuronides in extrahepatic cholestasis," *Hepatology*, vol. 13, no. 4, pp. 656–662, 1991.

[18] K. M. Knights, A. Rowland, and J. O. Miners, "Renal drug metabolism in humans: The potential for drug-endobiotic interactions involving cytochrome P450 (CYP) and UDP-glucuronosyltransferase (UGT)," *British Journal of Clinical Pharmacology*, vol. 76, no. 4, pp. 587–602, 2013.

[19] S. Matern, H. Matern, E. H. Farthmann, and W. Gerok, "Hepatic and extrahepatic glucuronidation of bile acids in man. Characterization of bile acid uridine 5'-diphosphate-glucuronosyltransferase in hepatic, renal, and intestinal microsomes," *The Journal of Clinical Investigation*, vol. 74, no. 2, pp. 402–410, 1984.

[20] J. Trottier, A. Białek, P. Caron, R. J. Straka, P. Milkiewicz, and O. Barbier, "Profiling circulating and urinary bile acids in patients with biliary obstruction before and after biliary stenting," *PLoS ONE*, vol. 6, no. 7, Article ID e22094, 2011.

[21] M. Perreault, L. Gauthier-Landry, J. Trottier et al., "The human UDP-glucuronosyltransferase UGT2A1 and UGT2A2 enzymes are highly active in bile acid glucuronidation," *Drug Metabolism and Disposition*, vol. 41, no. 9, pp. 1616–1620, 2013.

[22] M. E. Campbell, D. M. Grant, T. Inaba, and W. Kalow, "Biotransformation of caffeine, paraxanthine, theophylline, and theobromine by polycyclic aromatic hydrocarbon-inducible cytochrome(s) P-450 in human liver microsomes," *Drug Metabolism and Disposition*, vol. 15, no. 2, pp. 237–249, 1987.

[23] J. Lépine, O. Bernard, M. Plante et al., "Specificity and regioselectivity of the conjugation of estradiol, estrone, and their catecholestrogen and methoxyestrogen metabolites by human uridine diphospho-glucuronosyltransferases expressed in endometrium," *The Journal of Clinical Endocrinology & Metabolism*, vol. 89, no. 10, pp. 5222–5232, 2004.

[24] J. Thibaudeau, J. Lépine, J. Tojcic et al., "Characterization of common UGT1A8, UGT1A9, and UGT2B7 variants with different capacities to inactivate mutagenic 4-hydroxylated metabolites of estradiol and estrone," *Cancer Research*, vol. 66, no. 1, pp. 125–133, 2006.

[25] J. O. Miners, P. I. MacKenzie, and K. M. Knights, "The prediction of drug-glucuronidation parameters in humans: UDP-glucuronosyltransferase enzyme-selective substrate and inhibitor probes for reaction phenotyping and in vitroin vivo extrapolation of drug clearance and drug-drug interaction potential," *Drug Metabolism Reviews*, vol. 42, no. 1, pp. 189–201, 2010.

[26] M. Verreault, K. Senekeo-Effenberger, J. Trottier et al., "The liver X-receptor alpha controls hepatic expression of the human bile acid-glucuronidating UGT1A3 enzyme in human cells and transgenic mice," *Hepatology*, vol. 44, no. 2, pp. 368–378, 2006.

[27] R. G. Rutledge, "Mathematics of quantitative kinetic PCR and the application of standard curves," *Nucleic Acids Research*, vol. 31, no. 16, pp. 93e–93, 2003.

[28] T. Izukawa, M. Nakajima, R. Fujiwara et al., "Quantitative analysis of UDP-glucuronosyltransferase (UGT) 1A and UGT2B expression levels in human livers," *Drug Metabolism and Disposition*, vol. 37, no. 8, pp. 1759–1768, 2009.

[29] S. Ohno and S. Nakajin, "Determination of mRNA expression of human UDP-glucuronosyltransferases and application for localization in various human tissues by real-time reverse transcriptase-polymerase chain reaction," *Drug Metabolism and Disposition*, vol. 37, no. 1, pp. 32–40, 2009.

[30] S. L. Regan, J. L. Maggs, T. G. Hammond, C. Lambert, D. P. Williams, and B. K. Park, "Acyl glucuronides: The good, the bad and the ugly," *Biopharmaceutics & Drug Disposition*, vol. 31, no. 7, pp. 367–395, 2010.

[31] J. M. Little, M. V. Chari, and R. Lester, "Excretion of cholate glucuronide," *Journal of Lipid Research*, vol. 26, no. 5, pp. 583–592, 1985.

[32] M. Perreault, A. Białek, J. Trottier et al., "Role of glucuronidation for hepatic detoxification and urinary elimination of toxic bile acids during biliary obstruction," *PLoS ONE*, vol. 8, no. 11, Article ID e80994, 2013.

[33] H. Girard, E. Lévesque, J. Bellemare, K. Journault, B. Caillier, and C. Guillemette, "Genetic diversity at the UGT1 locus is amplified by a novel 3′ alternative splicing mechanism leading to nine additional UGT1A proteins that act as regulators of glucuronidation activity," *Pharmacogenetics and Genomics*, vol. 17, no. 12, pp. 1077–1089, 2007.

[34] A. Nakamura, M. Nakajima, H. Yamanaka, R. Fujiwara, and T. Yokoi, "Expression of UGT1A and UGT2B mRNA in human normal tissues and various cell lines," *Drug Metabolism and Disposition*, vol. 36, no. 8, pp. 1461–1464, 2008.

[35] D. E. Harbourt, J. K. Fallon, S. Ito et al., "Quantification of human uridine-diphosphate glucuronosyl transferase 1A isoforms in liver, intestine, and kidney using nanobore liquid chromatography-tandem mass spectrometry," *Analytical Chemistry*, vol. 84, no. 1, pp. 98–105, 2012.

[36] X. Zhou, L. Cao, C. Jiang et al., "PPARα-UGT axis activation represses intestinal FXR-FGF15 feedback signalling and exacerbates experimental colitis," *Nature Communications*, vol. 5, 2014.

28

MicroRNAs as Immunotherapy Targets for Treating Gastroenterological Cancers

Yixin Yang,[1] Christopher Alderman,[2] Ayoub Sehlaoui,[3] Yuan Xiao,[3] and Wei Wang[4]

[1]*College of Natural, Applied and Health Sciences, Kean University, 100 Morris Avenue, Union, NJ 07083, USA*
[2]*School of Medicine, University of Colorado, 13001 E 17th Pl, Aurora, CO 80045, USA*
[3]*Department of Biological Sciences, Emporia State University, 1 Kellogg Circle, Emporia, KS 66801, USA*
[4]*Department of Thoracic Surgery III, Cancer Hospital of China Medical University, No. 44 Xiaoheyan Road, Dadong District, Shenyang, Liaoning 110042, China*

Correspondence should be addressed to Yixin Yang; yyang@kean.edu and Wei Wang; wangwei_9111@hotmail.com

Academic Editor: Fernand Pierre Gendron

Gastroenterological cancers are the most common cancers categorized by systems and are estimated to comprise 18.4% of all cancers in the United States in 2017. Gastroenterological cancers are estimated to contribute 26.2% of cancer-related death in 2017. Gastroenterological cancers are characterized by late diagnosis, metastasis, high recurrence, and being refractory to current therapies. Since the current targeted therapies provide limited benefit to the overall response and survival, there is an urgent need for developing novel therapeutic strategy to improve the outcome of gastroenterological cancers. Immunotherapy has been developed and underwent clinical trials, but displayed limited therapeutic benefit. Since aberrant expressions of miRNAs are found in gastroenterological cancers and miRNAs have been shown to regulate antitumor immunity, the combination therapy combining the traditional antibody-based immunotherapy and novel miRNA-based immunotherapy is promising for achieving clinical success. This review summarizes the current knowledge about the miRNAs and long noncoding RNAs that exhibit immunoregulatory roles in gastroenterological cancers and precancerous diseases of digestive system, as well as the miRNA-based clinical trials for gastroenterological cancers. This review also analyzes the ongoing challenge of identifying appropriate therapy candidates for complex and dynamic tumor microenvironment, ensuring efficient and targeted delivery to specific cancer tissues, and developing strategy for avoiding off-target effect.

1. Introduction

Gastroenterological cancers are most common cancers categorized by systems and are estimated to comprise 18.4% of all cancers in the United States in 2017 [1]. Gastroenterological cancers constitute a leading cause of cancer-related deaths, contributing 26.2% of estimated cancer death in 2017. Colorectal cancer, liver and intrahepatic bile carcinoma, and pancreatic cancer continue to be ranked as three of the top 10 cancers with the largest number of new cases and deaths [1]. Most gastroenterological cancers, especially hepatocellular carcinoma and pancreatic cancer, are characterized by latent disease course, metastasis, high recurrence, and being refractory to current therapies. Therefore, gastroenterological cancers are often associated with poor prognosis.

With better understanding of molecular mechanisms of carcinogenesis, cell self-renewal and uncontrolled growth, metastasis, and other landmarks of cancer, progress has been made in developing and obtaining FDA approval of biological therapies targeting oncogenic signaling driver molecules including vascular-endothelial growth factor (VEGF) and its receptor VEGF-R [2], epidermal growth factor receptor (EGFR) [3], and human epidermal growth factor receptor-2 (HER2/Neu) [4]. The monoclonal antibodies antagonizing these cell growth driver molecules have achieved improved response rate (RR), progression-free survival (PFS), and overall survival (OS), demonstrating varying levels of success in colorectal and gastroesophageal cancers. However, the response is not durable and resistance is almost inevitably developed due to both innate and acquired mechanisms [5]. Gemcitabine, a standard treatment choice for advanced pancreatic cancer, produces only modest effect on survival (5.65 months versus 4.41 months) [6]. The very limited clinical efficacy is attributed to poor cell uptake of the drug, dense fibrous tumor stroma, and the development of gemcitabine resistance [7]. Sorafenib, a multikinase inhibitor, is the only FDA-approved drug for metastasized HCC, improving overall survival by only 2.8 months [8]. Since the current therapies provide limited benefit to the overall response and survival and are susceptible to resistance development, there is pressing need for developing novel therapeutic strategies to improve the outcome of gastroenterological cancers.

The aberrant expressions of genetically or epigenetically altered proteins in cancers produce cancer specific antigens. Since the cancer specific antigens were discovered in melanoma in 1990s, cancer immunotherapy has become a promising treatment strategy that deliberately uses the activated innate immunity and cancer specific adaptive immunity to reject tumors and prevent metastasis and reoccurrence [9]. Cancer immunotherapy employing cancer peptide vaccine [10], adaptive T cell therapies [11], and antibodies modulating regulatory T cells and achieving immunity checkpoint blockage [12] has been extensively studied in both basic research and clinical trials. Immunotherapy aims to induce strong, specific, and persistent anticancer immune response in tumor microenvironment.

It is well understood that tumors develop sophisticated mechanisms to disarm the immune system and evade the immune surveillance. Many cancers can produce or induce the immune cells in tumor stroma to produce an array of immunosuppressive cytokines including transforming growth factor (TGF-β) and IL-10, which inhibit the recruitment and activation of antitumor T lymphocytes [12]. In addition, IL-6 suppresses antigen presentation ability of dendritic cells through activation of signal transducer and transcription activator 3 (STAT3) and attenuates $CD4^+$ T cell-mediated immune responses [13, 14]. Furthermore, immunosuppressive cells including $Foxp3^+$ $CD4^+$ regulatory T cells (Tregs) and myeloid-derived suppressor cells (MDSC) in tumor microenvironments play significant roles in suppressing anticancer immunity [15, 16]. Therefore, immunotherapy using monoclonal antibody antagonizing the immunosuppressive cytokines or inactivating immunosuppressive cells can enhance anticancer immunity and inhibit tumor growth [17].

Immunotherapy that has achieved acclaimed clinical success primarily targets on two immune checkpoint molecules: PD-1/PD-L1 and CTLA4. Programmed cell death 1 (PD-1, *pdcd1*) is a type I transmembrane glycoprotein belonging to the CD28/CTLA-4 family. PD-1 is expressed on T cells in thymus and on peripheral B and T cells [18]. PD-L1 and PD-L2 are type I transmembrane glycoprotein and serve as the ligands of PD-1. PD-L1 and -L2, especially PD-L1, are extensively expressed in both lymphoid and nonlymphoid tissues [19, 20], suggesting that PD-1-PD-L1 pathway regulates the immune response in lymphoid tissues as well as in target organs. Upon binding to either PD-L1 or PD-L2, PD-1 negatively regulates the antigen receptor signaling and immune activation by recruiting protein tyrosine phosphatase to dephosphorylate the downstream molecules involved in B cell receptor mediated signaling [21] and T cell activation [22]. PD-1-PD-L1 pathway plays integral role in developing central and peripheral immune tolerance by inhibiting proliferation and maturation of T lymphocytes [23, 24]. PD-1 is highly expressed in tumors and a large portion of Tumor-Infiltrating Lymphocytes (TILs), consisting of both $CD4^+$ T_{reg} cells and $CD8^+$ cells with resulting decreased production of cytokines [25]. The expression of PD-L1 is elevated, often responding to IFN-γ [26], in a variety of malignancies including gastroenterological cancers. PD-1-PD-L1 axis is exploited by tumors to inhibit tumor antigen-specific immunity and achieve tumor immunity escape [27–34]. Higher expression of PD-L1 in cancers is usually correlated to poorer prognosis [35–37]. In gastroenterological cancers, expression of PD-L1 is linked to higher α-fetoprotein level, blood vessel invasion, and overall poor prognosis of hepatocellular carcinoma [32, 35]. In addition, PD-L1 status is associated with visceral metastasis and more $FOXP3^+$ T_{reg} cell infiltration in gastric cancers [27]. Similarly, in cholangiocarcinoma, PD-L1 expression is found in up to 30% patients and is linked to worse prognosis [30, 31]. Therefore, PD-L1 blockade can relieve tumor suppression, enhance tumor antigen-specific immunity, and improve prognosis. The antitumor activity of PD-1 blockade has been confirmed in both animal experiment [38] and clinical trials [39], where the tumor regression in response to PD-1 antibody treatment was observed in refractory solid cancers including colon, renal, and lung cancers and melanoma. It was observed that 22% of patients with PD-L1 positive metastatic adenocarcinoma of gastric or gastroesophageal junction showed overall response to Pembrolizumab, the humanized antibody to PD-1 receptor [40]. Cytotoxic T Lymphocyte Associated Antigen 4 (CTLA-4) is a coinhibitory molecule stored in intracellular vesicles of the naïve $CD4^+$ and $CD8^+$ T cells located in the lymph nodes, and it can be transported to the membrane of T cells and inhibit the activation of naïve T cells in the priming phase upon binding to its ligand B7 expressed on antigen-presenting cells (APC) [41]. CTLA4 expression is elevated by T cell activation status and an inflammatory environment for exerting brake on immune response [42]. Ipilimumab, a monoclonal antibody antagonizing CTLA-4, was approved by US Food and Drug Administration in 2011 to treat melanoma. Ipilimumab is undergoing clinical trials for other cancers including lung, bladder, and hormone-refractory prostate cancers.

Besides immune checkpoint blockade and immunosuppressive cytokine inactivation, therapeutic strategies targeting on enhancing activation of nature killer cells and macrophages, reversing the immune tolerogenic profile of tumor microenvironment, and ablating the immunosuppressive tumor-associated macrophages (TAMs) have been developed and evaluated. In addition, the low expression of the tumor antigen-derived peptide presented on major histocompatibility complex class I (MHC I) is a major reason for the limited clinical benefit of antigen-specific cancer immunotherapy [43]. Peptide intratumor injection has been shown to enhance tumor cell antigenicity for specific cytotoxic T lymphocyte activity and be effective in inhibiting tumor growth and prolonging survival time [44].

MicroRNAs (miRNAs) are a group of short (~ 22 nt), evolutionally conserved, single stranded noncoding RNA molecules that regulate expression of target genes by either cleaving mRNAs or destabilizing the translational system through interacting with sites of imperfect complementarity at 3' untranslated region (UTR) of target mRNAs [45]. With over a thousand of miRNAs present in higher eukaryotes and with each miRNA targeting on several genes, miRNAs can regulate the expressions of about 60% human protein-encoding genes [46]. miRNAs are involved in various biological processes including embryonic development [47], DNA repair [48], cell proliferation and senescence [49], differentiation [50], and apoptosis [51]. Dysregulation of miRNAs is associated with various diseases including Schizophrenia, obesity, alcoholism, and heart disease [52–54]. Notably, dysregulation of miRNA expression profiles is common in most malignancies, and the deregulation of miRNAs may lead to creation of favorable environment for the development of hallmarks of cancer [55]. The regulatory roles of miRNAs in metabolic and cellular pathways, especially those controlling cell proliferation, differentiation, apoptosis, and survival, are crucial to tumor initiation and progression.

Since miRNAs modulate the differentiation, activation, and mobilization of diverse immune cells and the complex cytokine network, miRNAs play vital roles in both innate and adaptive immunity. miRNAs regulates innate immune system by modulating the functions of its major players including natural killer cells (NK), microphage, and $\gamma\delta$ T cells, as well as the production of inflammatory cytokines and chemokines [56]. NK cells achieve immune surveillance by cytotoxicity and type I Interferon-α (INF-α) activation. miR-27a has been demonstrated to negatively regulate NK cells by repressing the genes PRF1 and GZMB [57]. Also, miR-30c-1 is known to affect the activation of NK cells by regulating the expression of tumor necrosis factor α (TNF-α) and HMBOX1 [58]. For regulatory roles for macrophage, it was reported that miR-511-3p modulated the inflammatory activity of tumor-associated macrophage [59]. In addition, miR-125b has been shown to regulate the expression of inflammatory cytokines by repressing the expression of TNF-α in macrophage [60]. miR-19 was also reported to modulate NF-κB mediated inflammation [61]. Adaptive immunity is characterized by specificity and memory of the immune response produced by the orchestrated interplay among T cell, B cell, dendritic cells, and complex network of inflammatory cytokines. miRNAs have been found to be involved in differentiation of B cells and the activation of T cells and dendritic cells [62]. miR-150 and miR-34 were found to inhibit B cells from developing from Pro-B to Pre-B stage through the downregulating c-MYB [63] and FOXP1 [64], respectively. Also, the expression of miR-155 was elevated in B cell precursors of lymphoblast leukemia, suggesting that miR-155 may cause development stalk and accumulation of pre-B cells by downregulating SHIP and C/EBPβ [65]. In addition, miRNAs have been demonstrated to be involved in the regulation of T lymphocyte activation and the antigen-presenting ability of dendritic cells, which engage all other immune cells in the immune response. miR-135b was shown to negatively regulate Th2 lymphocyte regulator genes STAT6 and GATA3 [66]. Also, miR-140-5p, miR-409-3p, and miR-433-3p can regulate the tumor antigen recognition and cytotoxicity of $CD8^+$ T lymphocytes and NK cells by regulating the expression of ULBP1, which is a ligand of NKG2D, an immunoreceptor found on T cells and NK cells [67]. Furthermore, Zheng et al. reported that the differentiation of $FOXP3^+CD4^+$ T regulatory cells and the tolerogenic property of dendritic cells could be enhanced by miR-23b through repressing the expression of NOTCH1 and the NF-κB [67] (21406206). Moreover, microRNAs also regulate the immune checkpoint activity. For example, miR-155 overexpression in $CD4^+$ T cells leads to decreased CTLA-4 levels and the subsequent activation of T cell immune response [68].

Since microRNAs are intricately involved in the modulation of activation of innate and adaptive immunity, in the regulation of inflammatory response and cytokine signaling, and in the molecular trafficking and cytokine crosstalk between the tumor and its microenvironment, miRNAs are promising targets for developing immunotherapy against gastroenterological cancers, for which the current targeted chemotherapy has not provided significant clinical benefit for overall response and survival. This review will focus on the regulatory roles of miRNAs on the immunity of digestive system and the antitumor immunity against gastroenterological cancers. For each type of cancers, miRNAs possessing the following functions will be featured: (1) directly modulating the activation of immune cells (macrophages, CD^+4 or CD^+8 T cells, T_{regs}, NK cells, dendritic cells, etc.) and subsequently affecting growth and metastasis of cancers; (2) presenting a cytokine profile that shapes the immunosuppressive microenvironment of cancers; (3) directly impacting the cellular components of tumor microenvironment niche including the cells lodging in the tumor stroma that contributes to cancer immune evasion; (4) being implicated in the development of preneoplastic conditions (e.g., hepatitis B and C, liver lipid metabolism disorder, and steatohepatitis for liver cancers; Crohn's disease, ulcerative colitis, and other colonic inflammation for colorectal cancer); (5) being targeted by transcriptional factors (such as STAT3) that are involved in immunity and cancer immune evasion; (6) sensitizing the cytotoxicity of immunotherapeutic agents.

2. MicroRNAs' Immunoregulatory Ability in Hepatocellular Carcinoma (HCC)

The incidence of liver and intrahepatic bile duct cancers has been increasing in the past decade, with estimated 40,710 new cases and 28,920 deaths in 2017 in the United States [1]. Liver and intrahepatic bile duct cancers have been the fifth deadliest cancers in men and account for 4.8% of overall cancer-related cancers in both sexes [1]. Due to the increasing hepatic virus infections of both hepatitis B and C viruses and rising incidence of both alcoholic and nonalcoholic fatty liver disease (NAFLD), hepatocellular carcinoma has been the 5th most common cancer and the third leading cause of cancer-related deaths worldwide [69]. It is predicted that liver cancers would surpass breast, prostate, and colorectal cancers to become the third leading cause of cancer-related deaths worldwide by 2030 [70]. The low survival rate is attributed to the latent disease course, late diagnosis, metastasis, and recurrence. Sorafenib, the only FDA-approved drug for advanced HCC, improves overall survival by only 2.8 months [8]. Recent phase 3 clinical trials have shown that sorafenib did not improve the median recurrence-free survival as an adjuvant therapy after resection or ablation of HCC [71]. Therefore, it is imperative to develop novel treatment strategies employing therapeutic molecules that boost antitumor immunity for combating HCC.

2.1. MicroRNA Removes Immune Checkpoint Blockade Imposed by PD-1/PD-L1 Pathway. Immune checkpoint blockade using antibody antagonizing PD-1 achieved overall response for some gastroenterological cancers. However, due to intrinsically poor immunogenicity and suppressive desmoplastic tumor microenvironment, anti-PD-1/PD-L1 monotherapy had not shown significant therapeutic benefit [34, 39]. Therefore, the new strategy that combines anti-PD-1 antibody and PD-L1 expression knockout would further remove the immune blockage imposed by PD-1/PD-L1 pathway. Targeting PD-1 or PD-L1 genes, a number of microRNAs have been found to inhibit tumor growth, initiate PD-1 specific T lymphocyte apoptosis, and reverse chemoresistance by blocking PD-1 immune checkpoint [72, 73].

miR-34a has become a rising star of microRNA-based therapy since it targets on over 30 oncogenic genes across distinct cellular pathways, modulates immune response, and prevents cancer cells from achieving immune evasion. In addition to activating dendritic cell mediated innate immune response by repressing DAPK2/SP1 pathway in gastric cancer [74], miR-34a also increases tumor-infiltrating CD8 expression T lymphocytes and decreases CD8/PD1 expression T lymphocyte by directly targeting PD-L1 3'-untranslated region [75]. Clinical delivery of MRX34, a liposome formulated mimic of miR-34a and the first-in-human clinical trial of microRNA therapy, has been evaluated for treating advanced solid tumors including unresectable liver cancers and metastatic tumors with liver involvement. Some patients achieved prolonged confirmed partial response (PR) per Response Evaluation in Solid Tumors (REIST) or stable disease (SD).

2.2. MicroRNA Alters Immunosuppressive Cytokine Profile by Serving as an Effector of STAT3. Signal transducer and activator of transcription 3 (STAT3) is an important transcriptional factor for cell differentiation, proliferation, and death and is implicated in tumor induced immune suppression in hepatocellular carcinoma (HCC) [76]. STAT3 can inhibit antitumor activity of NK cells against HCC cells by suppressing the expression of NKG2D ligands and type 1 interferon (IFN) [76]. In addition, STAT3 signaling has been found to regulate both innate and adaptive immunity by increasing the expressions of growth factors and cytokines including TGF-β, VEGF, interleukin 6 (IL-6), and IL-10 [76–78], which collectively repress the host immune response and facilitate tumor immune evasion. Therefore, understanding the molecular mechanisms through which the effectors of STAT3 network contribute to STAT3-mediated immune suppression is valuable for developing therapeutic strategy for HCC. miR-146a has been shown to be a direct target of STAT3 and its expression is activated by binding of STAT3 to the promoter of miR-146a gene [76]. Inactivation of STAT3 leads to downregulation of miR-146a, which subsequently alters aforementioned STAT3-associated immunosuppressive cytokines profile and restores the function of NK cells and antitumor lymphocytes.

2.3. MicroRNAs Affect the Cytotoxicity of NK Cells. A number of microRNAs can quench the tumor response by suppressing the MHC class 1-related chain molecule A and B (MICA and MICB), which are expressed on tumor cells and are ligands of the natural killer (NK) cell activating receptor NKG2D [79]. Suppression of MICA and MICB decreases the susceptibility of tumor cells to the cytotoxicity of NK cells [80]. miR-20a, miR-93, and miR-106b are MICA/B-targeting microRNAs and are encoded by host genes miR-17-92 cluster and maintenance complex component 7 (MCM7) [79]. These MICA/B-targeting miRNAs have been found to contribute to immune response evasion, and the epigenetic downregulation of MICA/B-targeting miRNAs by histone deacetylase inhibitor sensitizes HCC cells to the cytolytic effect of NK cells [81].

2.4. MicroRNAs Regulate the Activation of Tumor-Associated Macrophages. Tumor-associated macrophages (TAMs) are infiltrating macrophage subpopulation differentiated from circulating monocytes induced by cytokines produced by type 2 T helper cells (Th2). Dual-specificity phosphatase (DUSP1) is a negative regulator of MAPKs and thus inhibits the production of cytokines including TNF-α, TGF-β, IL-1, and IL-6. miR-101 directly targets on DUSP1 and increases HCC growth and metastasis by suppressing the expression of DUSP1 and the resulting increase in proinflammatory cytokines [82].

miR-26a has been identified as a tumor suppressor that inhibits tumor growth and metastasis by downregulating its oncogenic targets [83]. For HCC, overexpression of miR-26a reduced the expression of macrophage colony-stimulating factor (M-CSF), decreased expression of chemokine (C-C motif) ligand (CCL)22, CCL17, and IL-10, and inhibited the macrophage infiltration in tumors [84].

2.5. MicroRNAs Are Implicated in Hepatitis B and C Infections, High Risk Factors of HCC. Hepatitis B and C can produce prolonged chronic inflammatory status and subsequent liver cirrhosis and eventually HCC. Since chronic infection of hepatitis B or C virus (HBV or HCV) is a high risk factor of HCC [85], microRNAs that affect the life cycle and infection of HBV or HCV also have profound effects on the tumorigenesis and progression of HCC.

miR-122 has been discovered to assist replication of hepatitis C virus RNA [86]. Based on this finding, a miR-122 inhibitor miravirsen was developed and achieved prolonged dramatically reduced viremia without dose-related toxicity in a phase 2a trial in HCV type I patients [87]. Even though anti-miR-122 drug has shown satisfactory clinical outcome without emergency of viral resistance, due to the integral roles of miR-122 in liver homeostasis and maintenance of hepatocytic phenotype, the long-term inhibition of miR-122 in patients with underlying liver pathological conditions needs more thorough clinical evaluations. In contrast, miR-122 expression has been found to be reduced in patients with HBV infection and negatively correlate to the virus load and necroinflammation of liver [88]. Transfection of miR-122 mimics inhibited virus production. miR-122 inhibits HBV replication by suppressing the expression of cyclin G_1, which can negatively regulate p53-mediated inhibition of HBV transcription [88]. In addition, miR-122 has been found to suppress the interferon-stimulated response element (ISRE) mediated gene expression by enhancing methylation at gene promoter of suppressor of cytokine signaling 3 (SOCS3) and subsequently increasing expression of SOCS3 in liver cells [89]. Therefore, silencing miR-122 can improve response of liver cells to interferon-α in treatment against hepatic B or C, which are major causes of liver cirrhosis and cancer.

Besides miR-122, miR-185 interferes with the HCV life cycle by targeting several genes encoding critical proteins for entry, replication, and assembly of HCV infection. In addition, through inhibiting the lipid accumulation and other immunometabolic modulation, miR-130b and miR-185 inhibit the infection of hepatitis C virus by reinforcing the antiviral activity of 25-hydroxycholesterol (25-HC), an oxysterol secreted by interferon-stimulated macrophages and dendritic cells [91].

2.6. miR-122 Is a Liver-Specific MicroRNA That Plays Vital Roles in Liver Homeostasis and Immunity. The implication of miR-122 in the infection of HBV and HCV discussed above provides an example of how miR-122 is involved in liver disease. miR-122 is the most abundant liver-specific microRNA, constituting about 70% of overall microRNAs in liver. It is conserved in all vertebrates, indicating its crucial roles in the liver [115, 116]. miR-122 plays important roles in lipid metabolism, iron homeostasis, and maintenance of hepatocyte differentiation by regulating a large number of genes involved in various hepatic functions and repressing nonhepatic genes [117, 118]. The expression of miR-122 is downregulated in human HCC patients [119], and the deletion of miR-122 in hepatocytes leads to progressive development of stages of liver cancer: steatohepatitis, inflammation, hepatocyte regeneration, fibrosis, cirrhosis, and primary and metastatic HCC [120]. The loss of miR-122 has been associated with metastasis and poor prognosis of HCCs [121], whereas the restoration of ectopic miR-122 suppresses cell replication and invasion, inhibits angiogenesis, and sensitizes the liver cancer cells to sorafenib. miR-122 has been found to contribute to the liver disease outcome by modulating both innate and adaptive immunity. Mice with miR-122 knockout develops chronic inflammation that progresses to HCC since miR-122 deletion leads to upregulation of chemokine (C-C motif) ligand 2 (CCL2) in liver [90]. CCL2 recruits $CCR2^+CD11b^{high}Gr1^+$ immune cells to the liver, where these cells produce proinflammatory cytokines and subsequently cause hepatitis and progressively HCC [122].

In addition, miR-122 is significantly downregulated in primary biliary cirrhosis (PBC), which is an autoimmune disease that causes destruction and cirrhosis of intrahepatic bile duct [123]. The deregulation of miR-122 in PBC suggests that miR-122 either mediates the intrahepatic bile duct cell damage or modulates the autoimmune reaction process.

3. The Implications of MicroRNAs in Immunotherapy for Pancreatic Cancer

It is estimated that there will be 53,670 new pancreatic cancer cases and 43,096 death cases in the United States in 2017 [1]; both will be higher than the cases in 2016. Although pancreatic cancer is the eleventh most cancer among men and ninth most cancer among women, it is the fourth leading cause of cancer death of both sexes, accounting for 7% of overall death caused by cancers [1]. Limited progress has been made for improving the outcome of pancreatic cancer, with its 5-year survival rate modestly increased from 2.5% in 1975-1977 to 8.5% in 2006-2012 [124]. Due to the rapid development of therapies for other cancers, pancreatic cancer is projected to become the second leading cause of cancer death by 2030 [70]. The early systemic metastasis is the primary reason for the grooming prognosis of this disease.

3.1. MicroRNAs Transferred by Tumor-Derived Exosomes Engage in Immune Regulation. Tumor-derived exosome, a secreted membrane vesicle produced from inward budding of endosomal membrane, is generally considered as a promising source of tumor vaccine since it contains abundant immune regulatory proteins including MHCI [125], MHCII [126], and heat shock protein 70 [127] and various tumor rejection antigens including gp96, Her2, and tyrosinase related protein (TRP) [128]. Tumor-derived exosome presents tumor specific antigens to dendritic cells and induced potent $CD8^+$-dependent antitumor [128]. Due to the antitumor immune activation capacity, nanoscale size (30-100nM), and chemical stability, exosome has been targeted and exploited to develop novel cancer immunotherapeutic vaccine, which progressed to the clinical trials [129]. Since tumor-derived exosome contains various cytosolic components of donor cells, it can profoundly modify the biological behaviors including immune responses of recipient immune cells (macrophage, dendritic cells, NK cells, T lymphocyte, etc.) in proximity as well as at distance sites by transferring signaling molecules, receptors, enzymes, and gene expression regulatory molecules including microRNAs. Exosome was found to mediate the microRNA transfer and thus the exosome was proposed to be a novel mechanism of gene transfer between cells [130]. Since exosomes can be secreted by a myriad of tumors and immune cells including dendritic cells, macrophage, B cells, cytotoxic T lymphocytes, fibroblasts, platelets, mastocytes, and tumor cells [128, 131], microRNAs transferred via exosome can effectively affect the tumor antigen-specific immune response of the immune cells and facilitate the immune tolerance of tumor cells. It was reported that miR-203 was present in pancreatic cancer cell derived exosomes, and miR-203 suppressed the expression of toll-like receptor 4 (TLR4) resulting in the decreased levels of tumor necrosis factor-α (TNF-α) and interleukin-12 (IL-12) in pancreatic cancer cell line Panc-1 [92]. Since TNF-α and IL-12 both play critical roles in maturation of immune cells, enhancing antigen presentation of APCs, and augmenting cell immunity, miR-203 may modulate TLR-mediated immune response and facilitate immune escape of pancreatic cancer cells. The engagement of microRNAs in the immune regulation of pancreatic cancer was further consolidated by the discovery that the pancreatic cancer derived exosome with depleted microRNAs by ultrafiltration displayed stronger potency of activating dendritic cells and cytokine induced killer cells to exert cytotoxicity against pancreatic cancer cells [132].

3.2. MicroRNAs Disarm PD-1/PD-L1 Immune Blockade Pathway. Like in HCC, microRNAs targeting PD-1/PD-L1 pathway can suppress pancreatic cancer progression by activating anticancer immunity. Among these microRNAs, miR-142-5p was found to downregulate the expression of PD-L1 by directly binding 3' UTR of PD-L1 mRNA, and the overexpression of miR-142-5p increases CD4+ and CD8+ T lymphocytes and concomitantly decreases PD-1+ T lymphocytes [93]. Therefore, miR-142-5p is promising in developing microRNA-based therapy targeting PD-1/PD-L pathway.

3.3. MicroRNAs Regulate the Functions of Immune Cells and Lymphatic Vessel Formation. MicroRNAs have been found to directly regulate the maturation, recruitment, and activation of macrophages and NK cells in the microenvironment of pancreatic cancers. miR-454 directly targets and downregulates stromal cell derived factor-1 (SDF-1), which is a target of hypoxia-induced factor-1 (HIF-1). Since macrophages are recruited to tumor tissues by its expression of CXCR4 in response to SDF-1, miR-454 was found to inhibit the recruitment of bone marrow-derived macrophages to pancreatic ductal adenocarcinoma (PDAC) cells by downregulating SDF-1 [94]. In addition, miR-146a expression level is elevated in dendritic cells treated by conditioned medium of pancreatic cancer cells, which leads to impaired differentiation and antigen presentation function of dendritic cells [133]. Therefore, miR-146a is implicated in the maturation and antigen presentation of dendritic cells in response to the invasion of pancreatic cancer cells.

miR-206 has been identified as a negative regulator of proinflammatory factors including the chemokines (C-X-C motif) ligand 1 and (C-C motif) ligand 2, Interleukin-8, and the granulocyte macrophage colony-stimulating factor in pancreatic adenocarcinoma. It also abolishes the expression of prolymphangiogenic factor, vascular-endothelial growth factor C, thus inhibiting blood and lymphatic vessel formation and suppressing tumor progression [95].

3.4. MicroRNAs Regulate the Inflammation of Pancreatitis, a High Risk Factor of Pancreatic Cancer. Acute pancreatitis (AP) is a sterile inflammation in pancreas with severity ranging from mild to high mortality despite aggressive medical intervention. AP is a risk factor of pancreatic cancer. MicroRNAs were aberrantly expressed in acute pancreatitis and can serve as biomarkers for diagnosis and prognosis [134, 135]. miR-9, produced by bone marrow-derived mesenchymal stem cells (BMSCs), negatively regulates the inflammatory response induced by lipopolysaccharide (LPS). It was reported that miR-9-modified BMSCs (pri-miR-9-BMSCs) significantly decreased release of inflammatory factors and reduced pancreatic injury, indicating that miR-9 may play an anti-inflammatory role in the pathogenesis of AP and a promising candidate target for microRNA-based treatment of AP [96].

miR-216a is a highly expressed miRNA in pancreas. miR-216a is found to repress the expression of PTEN, Smad7, pAkt, and TGF-β receptor 1 and, thus, it is implicated in the pathogenesis of AP. Inhibition of miR-216a expression by TGF-β inhibitor significantly decreased serum amylase, TNF-α, IL6, and TGF- β and alleviated histopathological changes of pancreas [97].

Chronic pancreatitis (CP) is defined as "a pathologic fibro-inflammatory syndrome of the pancreas in individuals who develop persistent pathologic responses to parenchymal injury or stress." [136]. CP is characterized by chronic inflammation of the pancreas and the resulting progressive pancreatic endocrine and exocrine dysfunction [137] and widely accepted to be a strong risk factor of pancreatic cancer [138]. The microRNA that is known to be involved in CP is miR-146a, which suppressed the production of proinflammatory factors including IL-1β, IL-6, and TNF-α and is involved in innate immunity and inflammatory response pathways [98]. A common G/C SNP polymorphism rs2910164, which is located in the crucial seed sequence of the mir-146a, is found to affect the expression of mature miR-146a and is correlated to the increased chronic pancreatitis risk [139].

4. Immunoregulatory Roles of miRNAs in Colorectal Cancer (CRC)

The estimated number of new cases for colorectal cancers in 2017 for the United States is 135,430. The only cancers with higher rates of new cases are lung and bronchus, breast, and prostate. In fact, it is estimated that 50,260 people will die from CRC in the United States in 2017, which is only behind lung and bronchus cancers [1].

4.1. miRNAs Regulate the Regulatory T Lymphocytes. In order to display the relevance that microRNA has in CRC, Cobb et al. performed a Dicer KO in Treg cells. This study displayed that Dicer was a requirement for Treg cell development. Without Dicer, Treg cell numbers are diminished [140]. Moreover, a previous Dicer KO study has shown that cytotoxic T lymphocytes (CTLs) have increased ability to lyse CRC cells [99, 101]. This is thought to occur through the inactivation of miR-222/339, which typically downregulates ICAM-I [99]. However, due to the essential role of Dicer in RNA regulation, targeting it in patients would lead to unwanted side effects. Therefore, future studies should look at using anti-miRs to directly knock down miR-222/339.

Another method for regulating T cells with microRNAs in CRC is with miR-21. According to a recent study by Mima et al., miR-21 is inversely associated with $CD3^+$ and $CD45RO^+$ T cells. The proposed mechanism for this is by targeting PDCD4, which is a known IL10 repressor [100]. The correlation was determined by looking at a cohort of 538 cases of CRC. This is significant because it shows the ability for miR-21 therapy to improve the immunity against CRC. Specifically, $CD3^+$ cells are known for their ability to activate $CD3^+$ and $CD8^+$ cells, which will increase the likelihood of antitumor activities in these cell types [141]. In addition, $CD45RO^+$ T cells are a population that has been associated with increased TNM stage but still needs further investigation [142].

4.2. miRNAs Modulate the Function of MDSCs. Cancer cells and their co-opted microenvironments often take a multi-pronged approach to evade immune responses. For this reason, it is important for scientists to also look at multipronged approaches in order to improve immune responses. Myeloid-derived (immune) suppressor cells (MDSCs) are often a key player in creating the microenvironment. These cells are able to control CRC and immune cell development. Typically, MDSCs inhibit the growth of antigen-specific $CD4^+$ and $CD8^+$ cells [143]. However, we are able to modify the function of MDSCs with microRNA. The miR-17-92 cluster contains miR-17-5p and miR-20a. These microRNAs are both beneficial and harmful to CRC development. Unfortunately, they are found to promote CRC development by decreasing the burden of reactive oxygen species [101]. However, they are also able to inhibit the immunosuppressive action of MDSCs [102]. Thus, their usefulness for treating cancer still needs further exploration. Another mechanism that modulates MDSC action is with miR-494. miR-494 expression inhibits PTEN while simultaneously activating AKT. This leads to an increased number of procancer MDSCs [144].

4.3. miRNAs Modulate the Pathogenesis of Inflammatory Diseases of Colon. The role of miRs in chronic inflammatory disorders is also of key importance due to the ability of these disorders to induce CRC [101]. Some of the strongest associations have been with ulcerative colitis, Crohn's disease, and inflammatory bowel disease [145]. In ulcerative colitis, overexpression of STAT3 is common and leads to progression from ulcerative colitis to CRC. miR-124 targets STAT3 and is downregulated in these patients [103]. miR replacement therapy could be a viable option for these patients to decrease the risk of developing CRC. In patients with Crohn's disease, miR-19b has been identified as an anti-inflammatory molecule that has potential to decrease the tumor-promoting capability of Crohn's disease. miR-19b does this by modulating the expression of cytokine suppressors [146]. Moreover, miR-210 has a similar ability to decrease inflammation in inflammatory bowel disease by targeting HIF-alpha [104]. In addition, miR-511-3p, carried on the gene of the macrophage mannose receptor CD206 (mrc-1), is expressed by macrophage and dendritic cells. miR-511-3p targets toll-like receptor 4 (tlr-4) and reduces the production of proinflammatory cytokines in response to microbial stimulus. Therefore, miR-511-3p regulates the intestinal inflammation by regulating toll-like receptor 4 [147].

4.4. miRNAs Regulate the Recruitment and Activation of Macrophage and Neutrophils. miR-484 has been found to inhibit CD137L and thus have significant anticancer properties. CD137L has two characteristics that make it a procancer protein. First, CD137L induces cell viability via the PI3K and mTOR cell pathways. Secondly, CD137L induces IL-8 production which is used to recruit macrophages and neutrophils into the procancer microenvironment. If this is successful, the procancer macrophages and neutrophils then assist with tumor invasiveness. In microsatellite instable CRC, miR-484 plays a key role in regulating IL-8 secretion [105]. IL-8 is dangerous for the tumor microenvironment because of its proliferative effects and ability to promote tumor-associated immune cells such as macrophages and neutrophils into the microenvironment [148].

Procancer neutrophil function has been elucidated more in recent years. Although not all neutrophilic functions promote cancer, one example of cancer induction is shown by their ability to inhibit the immune system [149]. Along with other functions they have also been found to help tumors induce angiogenesis [150]. The role of tumor-associated macrophages in cancer has been more clearly elucidated, stimulating malignancy via metastasis, angiogenesis, and immunosuppression [151]. Fortunately, miR-484 and miR-19a have been found to inhibit CD137L and thereby improve the cancer microenvironment [152, 153].

4.5. miRNAs Regulate the Expression of PD-L1. MicroRNAs are also able to improve the immune response to CRC through targeting PD-L1. PD-L1 has been popularized recently due to its ability to reduce the viability of T cells [154]. It has also been discovered that miR-142-5p targets PD-L1 [93]. Moreover, miR-20b, 21, and -130b are overexpressed in CRC and target phosphatase and tensin homolog (PTEN), leading to PD-L1 overexpression [101, 106]. These events in turn block the PD-L1/PD-1 signaling pathway, allowing T cells to survive in the tumor microenvironment, thus improving anticancer immunity.

5. Immunoregulatory Roles of MicroRNAs in Gastric Cancer (GC)

Although the rate of gastric cancer has been decreasing, there are still around 22,220 patients diagnosed annually in the United States with approximately 10,990 annual deaths [155]. Moreover, the rate of noncardia gastric cancer for whites aged 25 to 39 in the United States increased between 1977 and 2006, showing that it is still a disease that needs to be studied further [156]. MicroRNA has also been discovered to modulate the anticancer immune response in GC, although in a somewhat convoluted manner. It is understood that the downregulation of E2F-1 in dendritic cells successfully inhibits the immune response. E2F-1 controls the activity of P53 and also regulates cell activity including proliferation [157]. Moreover, death-associated protein kinase 2 (DAPK2) along with the transcription factor specificity 1 (SP1) is able to inhibit the activity of E2F-1. This also leads to an inhibition in the activity of dendritic cells in the immune response. However, we can counteract this procancer activity by inhibiting the expression of DAPK2/SP1 using miR-34a [74].

6. MicroRNAs' Immunoregulatory Ability in Gallbladder Cancer

Gallbladder cancer (GBC) is a difficult to diagnose gastroenterological cancer. Detection in early stages is limited due to a poor understanding of the mechanisms involved in the development of cancerous hyperplasias [158]. The diagnosis of GBC is typically seen in advanced and late stage development. Unfortunately, this accounts for a 5-year survival rate of only 20-40% [159]. The available literature on GBC investigates methodologies that would potentially allow for more progressive detection. Abnormalities in cytokine profiles in the cellular microenvironment have long been a known contributor to oncogenesis. Current advancements and continued research allow for advanced genetic screening capabilities. With the capacity to screen for a range of miRNA and lncRNA, early diagnosis seems more promising.

The gallbladder is the bile producing organ of the body. These biliary secretions are channeled through ducts from the gallbladder to the liver. In a pancreaticobiliary maljunction (PBM) the bile ducts themselves are conjoined in such a way that allows for reflux of biliary secretions [107]. The presence of a PBM presents an increased risk factor for the development of GBC. This abnormal buildup of bile causes lecithin to convert endogenously to lysolecithin, which has been shown to induce chronic inflammation of the biliary epithelial cells [160]. The inflammatory response to lysolecithin disrupts the extracellular microenvironment causing an influx in inflammatory cytokines [161].

6.1. Cytokines and GBC. Cytokine expression profiles of healthy gallbladder cells in mice were shown to express mRNA for TNF-α along with RANTES and macrophage inflammatory protein 2 (MIP-20). Once these cells were treated with lipopolysaccharides, the expression profiles changed to exhibit an increase in mRNA for monocyte chemoattractant protein-1 (MCP-1), Interleukin-6 (IL-6), and IL-1b [162]. With immunotherapeutic treatments these abnormal cytokines could be used to aggregate genetically enhanced immune cells to the site of carcinoma. However, such an inflammatory response can thus lead to mutations and overexpression of cell-cycle associated proteins such as p53 and MUCI [163]. The implications of p53 mutations has been shown to potentiate atypical hyperplasia, thus resulting in lesions and subsequent malignancy [163]. MUCl is a mucin class glycoprotein produced by epithelial cells and involved in cell signaling and adhesion. Left unchecked, this overexpression thus potentiates the formation of cancerous cells in the lining of the biliary tract. This protein has been found in increased, lowered, and erratic expression in tumor cells related to GBC [163]. Expression profiles of MUCI and MUC5AC showed predictable patterns which accounted for metastasis of tumor cells. H. Kono et al. demonstrated that, along with P53, K-ras mutations have also been studied as biomarkers in GBC with PBM [160], with K-ras being a well understood and studied prooncogene [164]. In addition, miR-133a-3p was reported to inhibit the gallbladder carcinoma by directly targeting on recombination signal-binding protein Jκ (RBPJ) [109]. RBPJ is a key downstream transcription factor in the Notch signaling pathway that regulates the differentiation of T cell lineage from common lymphoid precursor.

6.2. miRNA and lncRNA in GBC Prognosis. Other potential biomarkers associated with GBC include a range of miRNA and lncRNA (long noncoding RNA). lncRNA CCAT1 (colon cancer-associated transcript-1) has been shown to promote GBC development through downregulation of miRNA 218-5p. This regulatory ability is associated with the direct binding of miRNA 218-5p to CCAT1 [107]. This class of lncRNA is categorized as ceRNA (competitive endogenous RNA) which acts as molecular 'sponges' through endogenous miRNA binding sites. This mechanism could be a factor in the down-regulation of tumor suppressing miRNA seen in miRNA profiles in GBC [158]. Alternately, overexpression of miRNA 155 has also been shown to increase the malignancy of late neoplastic conditions in GBC. This miRNA shows promise as a potential for detection in patients with symptoms associated with GBC. miRNA 155 elevation was also associated with an increase in metastasis to the lymph node [160]. In a miRNA study performed by P. Letelier et al. in human GBC cell lines, it was determined that miR-1 and miR-145 possess antitumor properties. These miRNAs along with miR-143 and miR-133 directly targeted signaling pathways associated with cell motility and adhesion, thus having implications in malignancy and carcinoma [110].

7. Immunoregulatory Ability of miRNAs in Esophageal Cancer (EC)

In esophageal cancer (EC), there can be several differing morphologies characterized by the cells that are affected. In ESCC the epithelial tissue lining the esophageal tract becomes cancerous [165]. Another manifestation of esophageal carcinoma is known as esophageal adenocarcinoma (EAC) which effects the glandular epithelium [166]. The manifestation of these carcinomas has been shown to increase with the prominence of a condition known as Barrett's esophagus (BE) where the cells of the squamous epithelium are replaced by glandular epithelium [165]. When analysis of both transcriptomes was performed, notable differences arose between the two subtypes of esophageal cancers. Esophageal squamous cell carcinoma (ESCC) is a high risk and difficult to detect carcinoma. Not accounting for the western world, ESCC is the one of the most diagnosed cancers [167]. Tobacco smoking and chronic alcohol consumption have been shown as risk factors for ESCC, with a high prevalence in Asian countries [165]. With a 5-year survival rate of 4.5%, early detection and prognosis are prudent for successful remission. Nonetheless, recurrence of ESCC is common and met with low rates of survival. Given these grim statistics, development of alternative detection and therapeutic methods is crucial.

7.1. lncRNA in EC. W. Wu et al. set out to characterize potential noncoding DNA and its implications on EAC. Through hypomethylation of DNA overexpression of otherwise noncoding regions can occur. This lack of methylation could induce genomic instability and downstream activation of oncogenes [14]. In EAC it was found that the lncRNA AFAP1-AS1 was subsequently overexpressed due to hypomethylated DNA regions in the transcriptome of EAC cells. The overexpression of AFAP1-AS1 was shown in vitro to induce cell proliferation and tumorigenic growth in EAC cell lines [166]. This invasiveness and tumorigenic growth was reversed with treatment using AFAP1-AS1-specific siRNA, showing promise for siRNA-targeted therapies. The researchers also postulated that AFAP1-AS1 is a potential biomarker for the detection of EAC. The exact function of AFAP1-AS1 is unknown and further studies must be performed. lncRNA MALAT1 has also been shown to induce and promote tumorigenesis in ESCC. In a study to elucidate the potential for MALAT1 miRNA therapies X. Wang et al. demonstrated in vivo suppression of ESCC growth by using miR-101 and miR-217. These mi-RNAs were shown to target MALAT1 consequentially silencing its tumor-promoting action [167].

7.2. miRNA in EC. Potential for noncoding RNA biomarkers for esophageal cancer (EC) includes a wide range of dysregulated miRNAs. A study performed by Shang-guo Liu et al. set out to establish a baseline of miRNA expression profiles in human EC. To achieve this, researchers took EC patient cells and analyzed them using miRNA chip technology; these results were then further verified using RT-qPCR methods for comparison to noncancerous cells. This research identified 59 upregulated miRNAs along with 9 downregulated miRNAs [168]. According to R. B. Koumangoye et al., miR-31 was shown to suppress tumor oncogenesis when SOX4, EZH2, and HDAC3 genes are downregulated. However, in ESCC these genes are typically expressed and were shown to cooperatively downregulate the effectiveness of miR-31 *in vitro* [169]. Measuring levels of miR-31 could provide a potential biomarker in GSCC detection. More notably, miR-31 directly regulates Stk40 and activates the STK40-NF-κB-controlled inflammatory pathway in esophageal cancer. Therefore, the anti-miR-31 can repress inflammation and neoplasm of esophageal cancer [111]. Invasion and metastasis is controlled by a host of proteins responsible for motility and cytoskeletal construction and distribution. FSCN1 and MMP14 are proteins that facilitate tumor progression and formation of a suitable tumor microenvironment. N. Akanuma et al. performed a study correlating the anticancer effects of miR-133a through its direct modulation of these two proteins [170]. This shows promise for miR-133a as a tumor suppressor in ESCC. Further studies have identified a host of well-defined miRNAs that elicit a notable and prominent promotion of migration and invasiveness of GC cells. miR-92 was found to be highly expressed in ESCC and to modulate the migration and invasion of ESCC cells through repressing the tumor suppressor CDH1 gene [171]. Y. Tian et al. studied the effects of miRNA-10b along with elucidating its target gene KLF4. This study showed that with overexpression of miR-10b came a direct underexpression of the tumor suppressor KLF-4. Along with this study, the researchers also performed a literature review showing miR-10b expression being downregulated in 95% of human EC tissues [172]. This direct correlation of miR-10b and tumorigenesis suggests potential as a generalized biomarker for EC detection. ESCC senescence and apoptosis have also been shown to be mediated by the expression of miRNA. miR-34a was shown to act as a p53-dependant tumor suppressor [173]. The expression of miR-34a was shown to be affected by DNA damaging agents traditionally used in chemotherapy. This expression was notably downregulated by the mutant p53 variant. Through the patient specific regulation of the wild type p53/p21 pathway miR-34a can be used as a diagnostic marker for therapeutic effectiveness in p53 mutant ESCC. In addition, miR-34a expression can be elevated by NF-κB, a central regulator of inflammation [112].

7.3. The Implication of Exosomes Transporting miRNAs in EC. Secretion of exosomes is a well-known method of cellular communication and excretion. Small noncoding RNA molecules such as miRNA can also be secreted in exosomes and circulate in the blood or other extracellular matrix [114]. Exosome secretion adds to the plethora of intercellular communicatory systems that play a large role in mediating the cellular microenvironment. Through the use of Transmission Electron Microscopy and western blot analysis, the exosomal protein CD63 was confirmed in serum exosome isolate purified by Y. Tanaka et al. showing a reliable analysis of serum exosomes. Exosomal miR-21 was confirmed using a bioanalyzer in serum samples [114]. This research showed that the transmission of extracellular miRNA was indeed possible and could be transmitted intercellularly. This study also elucidated miR-21 as a potential cancer promoting miRNA which was determined through previous studies to increase proliferation and oncogenesis in vitro [174].

7.4. Immunosuppression in GSCC. CD4 and CD25 regulatory T cell (Treg) expression has been shown to increase in association with both gastric and esophageal cancer (EC) progression. Treg cells, which have been shown to inhibit immune responses otherwise mediated by T cells, have been noted in higher abundance with proximity to cancerous lesions. K. Kono et al. looked at the prevalence of Treg cells in PBMCs (Peripheral Blood Mononuclear Cells) in patients with ranging progression of both gastric and esophageal cancers. Through flow cytometry, RT-PCR and intracellular cytokine assays, the researchers were successful in separating Treg cells by unique markers such as CD45RO and CTLA-4 [175]. The proportional analysis also revealed a correlation between cancer stage and Treg prevalence. A speculative outlook on why this happens could be explained by the expression of chemokine CCL20, secreted by macrophages at the site of tumorigenesis. This chemokine has been shown to facilitate Treg migration [176]. Otherwise, the exact mechanism of action that allows for such an increase in Treg cells is currently unknown. Response to traditional inflammatory

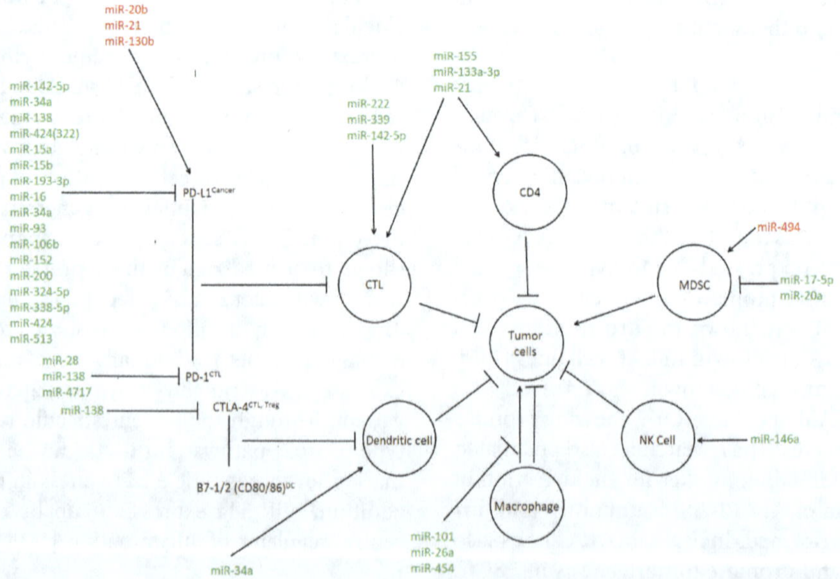

FIGURE 1: The miRNA modulation of cellular immunity in gastrointestinal cancers. Red denotes procancer miRNA interactions while green denotes anticancer interactions.

factors could also play a large role. A well-documented and studied protein pathway for inflammation induced cancer is NF-κB and STAT3 [165]. These proteins have been shown to be expressed when induction of an inflammatory response occurs. Once induced, these proteins potentiate downstream cascades, activating a spectrum of oncogenes such as miR-21 and IL-6 [165].

Along the same lines of intracellular immunosuppression, myeloid-derived suppressor cells (MDSCs) have also been studied as a potential antagonist in immunotherapy. In a study performed on EC patients' PBMCs, R. F. Gabitass et al. demonstrated that elevated numbers of MDSCs were also associated with an increase of Treg cells in EC [177]. MDSCs impose immunosuppression through impairment of T cell differentiation. This overexpression was strongly correlated with elevated levels of the Th2 cytokine IL-13. By utilizing IL-13, Treg, and MDSC detection this study sheds light on these potential prognostic biomarkers EC detection. From an immunotherapeutic perspective, the abundance of MDSC and Treg cells presents a challenge in therapies which rely on the successful implantation of genetically altered T cells [177].

8. Immune Checkpoint Blockade and miRNA Therapy

With the known antioncogenic and microenvironment altering properties of miRNA, the potential positive effects on the immune mediated response are of great interest. A critical adaptation of cancerous cells is their ability to imitate otherwise healthy cells and avoid immune detection [178]. In current literature, immune checkpoint blockade in cancer cells has been shown to elicit antitumor effects in late stage cancer development [179]. The widely studied and targeted immune checkpoint proteins are CTLA-4, PD-1, and PD-L1 [73, 180, 181]. PD-1 and PD-L1, also known as programmed death receptor and ligand, are of particular interest as the PD-L1 ligand is expressed on tumor cells, thus evading the imminent immune response [182]. The modulation of CTLA-4 is not as researched as the PD pathways; however miR-138 was shown to elicit an effect [183]. A major setback that has been seen when immune checkpoint antibodies are used in combinatorial therapy on multiple checkpoint pathways is risk of toxicity [183]. This is due to the nature of the immune checkpoint receptors being present on most cells. However, the use of miRNA to induce immune checkpoint blockade by selectively upregulating or downregulating miRNA expression for specific immune checkpoint proteins could prove to be a useful tool in our antioncogenic arsenal. Figure 1 presents possible miRNA targets that are involved in the modulation of PD-L1, PD-1, and CTLA-4; this figure is modified and adapted from Q. Wang et al. [182].

9. Challenges and Future Study

Gastroenterological cancers have been considered to be poorly immunogenic, and, along with enhanced immune checkpoint inhibition, cancer cells can escape from the recognition and clearance of immune system. Pembrolizumab, a monoclonal antibody antagonizing PD-1 receptor, and Ipilimumab, the monoclonal antibody binding CTLA-4, have achieved some clinical success [40, 42]. However, due to poor immunogenicity and desmoplastic tumor microenvironment, mono-immunotherapy using antibody for achieving immune checkpoint blockade has not shown therapeutic benefit. The combination therapy combining traditional monoclonal antibody-based immunotherapy and the novel miRNA-based immunotherapy is expected to achieve more effective and sustained therapeutic effect. Liposome formulated mimic of miR-34a entered the first-in-human clinical trial of microRNA therapy and obtained favorable clinical results with prolonged partial response. In addition, since STAT3 has been found to play crucial roles in magnitude of tumor mediated immunosuppression and immune escape in tumor microenvironment [76, 78], miRNA-based immunotherapy targeting on STAT3 should be aggressively pursued.

The extensive involvement of miRNAs in modulation of tumor-associated immune cells, immune checkpoint blockage, and maintenance of immunosuppressive status of tumor microenvironment presents miRNAs as promising therapeutic agents or molecular targets for developing novel immunotherapy for awakening or augmenting antitumor immunity. The miRNAs, the target genes, and the immunoregulatory roles of these miRNAs in some gastroenterological cancers are summarized in Table 1. However, since a miRNA can regulate a number of target genes that may have fundamentally different and even contradictory effects on regulating immune response to tumors and the gene expression regulatory capacity of miRNAs and the biological roles of their target genes may be vastly different in various tissues and pathophysiological status, the actual net immunoregulatory effect of a miRNA has to be evaluated within a holistic and evolving immunomodulation network. Some microRNAs are known to positively regulate the functions of immune cells and enhance antitumor activity; however, augmenting immune response alone does not warrant the tumor suppressing effect of the microRNAs. The roles of miR-155 in antitumor immunity present a good example. miR-155 expression in T cells is required for maintaining the number of IFNγ-expressing $CD4^+$ and $CD8^+$ T cells and suppressing tumor growth [108, 184]. miR-155 also modulates the innate immunity by regulating IFNγ production in NK cells [185]. In addition, miR-155 in liver macrophage Kupffer cells plays an important role for normal antigen-presenting function and SOCS1/JAK/STAT inflammatory pathways of Kupffer cells [113]. Therefore, miR-155 can serve as a regulator of tumor immunity that enhances the tumor antigen recognition, surveillance, and clearance. However, miR-155 is highly expressed in multiple solid tumors and is commonly associated with more aggressive phenotype. miR-155 was reported to promote invasiveness of pancreatic cancer cells, through regulating suppressor of cytokine signaling 1 (SOCS1) and P-signal transducer and activator of transcription-3 (STAT3) [186], and promote the hepatocellular carcinoma progression by targeting PTEN [187]. In addition, expression of miR-155 in tumor tissue at a high level is positively correlated with lymph node metastasis, as well as poorer overall and disease-free survival in colorectal cancer patients [188]. Similarly, miR-155 expression is a biomarker indicating poor prognosis for gallbladder cancer [189]. Therefore, the precise delivery of microRNA mimics or inhibitors to specific cell types in tumor tissues or immune system is the key to the success of microRNA-based immunotherapy.

Differential expression level of the same miRNA in different tissues and cell types further complicates the prediction of the role of the miRNA in antitumor immunity. In addition, it is known that he expression of miRNAs is deregulated in tumors compared with that in normal tissues. However, the normal baseline level of miRNAs varies dramatically in different individuals. It is not uncommon that literature reports inconsistent or even conflicting discoveries regarding the expression level of miRNAs. Therefore, a challenge for better understanding the immunoregulatory roles of miRNAs and developing miRNAs-based immunotherapy is establishing a set of endogenous miRNA controls for normalization.

Another challenge lies in the difficulty of identifying miRNA candidates for treating a tumor due to the heterogeneity of miRNAs in tumor tissues. Inflammation and hypoxia in tumor microenvironment cause complex and dynamic heterogeneity in miRNA expression profile [190, 191]; therefore, multiple-point biopsy and temporal monitoring of expression of mRNAs are critical to the constructing of a more meaningful regulatory network of miRNAs and the identifying of miRNA candidate (usually the common regulatory miRNA) for developing immunotherapy for that particular cancer.

Safe, efficient, stable, and specific delivery of miRNAs to tumor neoplasm and microenvironment has been a major challenge for any RNA-based therapy [192]. Cationic polymers or viral vectors are efficient delivery vehicles; however, the systemic toxicity and immunogenicity cause significant side effects and limit the transition from bench to bedside. Recently, the delivery system that loads miRNA mimics or anti-miRNAs to nanoparticles conjugated with targeting antibodies/peptides displayed efficient targeting and achieved high cellular uptake and bioavailability [193].

Off-target effect is another challenge for developing miRNA-based immunotherapy. Since many miRNAs belonging to the same family have very conserved seed sequence and most anti-miRs contain perfect complementary sequences to the seed sequence, anti-miRs are not able to distinguish the miRNAs of the same family and may produce off-target effect [192]. A novel strategy addressing off-target effect targets on miRNAs at their precursor stage. Since the precursors of miRNAs contain secondary structure that is required for recruiting enzymes and the miRNA precursors contain sequences that are not found in seed sequences, anti-miRs can be designed to specifically bind to nonseed sequences on the miRNA precursors, which may disrupt the hairpin and affect the RNA processing by Drosha-DGCR8 complex [192]. Therefore, targeting secondary structure scaffold sequence but not seed sequence may help avoid off-target effects. Continued effort on assessing the effectiveness and off-target effect of this novel strategy is important for developing a safe miRNA-based immunotherapy with least side effects.

Authors' Contributions

Christopher Alderman and Ayoub Sehlaoui equally contributed to this work. Yixin Yang and Wei Wang contributed equally to this work.

TABLE 1: miRNAs involved in immunity and immunotherapy for gastroenterological cancers.

Cancer types/cell type	MicroRNAs	Target genes	Immunological component/process	References
Hepatocellular Carcinoma	miR-34a	DAPK2/SP1 pathway	Dendritic cell activation	[74]
	miR-34a	PD-L1	PD-1/PD-L1 immune checkpoint blockade	[75]
	miR-146a	Effector of STAT3	NK cells and anti-tumor lymphocytes	[76]
	miR-20a, miR-93 and miR-106b	MICA/B	Antigen presentation and immune evasion	[79]
	miR-101	DUSP1	Proinflammatory factors and tumor-associated macrophages	[82]
	miR-26a	Macrophage colony-stimulating factor (M-CSF)	Chemokine ligand (CCL) 22, IL10 and macrophage infiltration	[84]
	miR-122	HCV genome	Assisting replication of HCV	[86]
	miR-122	Cyclin G_1	Inhibiting transcription of HBV	[88]
	miR-122	Suppressor of cytokine signaling 3 (SOCS3)	Interferon production	[89]
	miR-122	Chemokine (C-C motif) ligand 2 (CCL2)	$CCR2^+CD11b^{high}Gr1^+$ immune cells recruitment, proinflammatory cytokine production	[90]
	miR-185	LDLR, SCD1, SCARB1 and SREBP2	HCV replication	[91]
	miR-130b	LDLR, lipid metabolism pathway	HCV replication; reinforcing the antiviral activity of 25-hydroxycholesterol (25-HC),	[91]
Pancreatic Cancer	miR-203	Toll-Like Receptor 4	Modulating TLR-mediated immune response and facilitate immune escape	[92]
	miR-142-5p	PD-L1	PD-1/PD-L1 immune checkpoint blockade	[93]
	miR-454	Stromal cell derived factor-1	Macrophage recruitment and dendritic cell maturation	[94]
	miR-206	Chemokines (C-X-C motif) ligand 1 and (C-C motif) ligand 2, Interleukin-8 and the granulocyte macrophage colony-stimulating factor	Inhibiting inflammation and immune reaction	[95]
	miR-206	Vascular endothelial growth factor C	Inhibiting blood and lymphatic vessel formation	[95]
	miR-9	unknown	Inflammation of acute pancreatitis	[96]
	miR-216a	PTEN, Smad7, pAkt and TGF-β receptor 1	Inflammation of acute pancreatitis	[97]
	miR-146a	IL-1b, IL-6 and TNF-a	Inflammation of chronic pancreatitis	[98]

Table 1: Continued.

Cancer types/cell type	MicroRNAs	Target genes	Immunological component/process	References
Colorectal Cancer	miR-222 and -339	ICAM-1	Promotes cytotoxicity of CTL's	[99]
	miR-21	PDCD4	IL-10 transcription and $CD3^+$ and $CD45RO^+$ cell selection	[100]
	miR-17-5p and -20a	STAT3	Decreased burden from reactive oxygen species and inhibition of MDSC immunosuppression	[101, 102]
	miR-124	STAT3	Decreased progression of ulcerative colitis	[103]
	miR-19b	HIF-alpha	Anti-inflammatory in Crohn's disease	[104]
	miR-494	PTEN	Increased number of pro-cancer MDSC's	
	miR-484 and -19a	CD137L	Decreased PI3K/mTOR signaling and IL-8 production	[105]
	miR-142-5p	PD-L1	Increased viability of CTL's	[93]
	miR-20b, -21, and -130b	PTEN	PD-L1 overexpression and CRC proliferation	[101, 106]
Gastric Cancer	miR-34a	DAPK2/SP1	Increased dendritic cell immune response	[74]
Gallbladder Cancer	miR-218-5p	Downregulated by lncRNA CCAT1	Modulation of the tumor micro-environment	[107]
	miR-155	IFNγ	Activation and proliferation of $CD4^+$ and $CD8^+$ T cells	[108]
	miR-133a-3p	Recombination signal-binding protein Jκ	Differentiation of T cell lineage from common lymphoid precursor.	[109]
	miR-1, miR-133, miR-143 and miR-145	VEGF-A, ErbB3, AXL	Modulation of the tumor micro-environment	[110]
Esophageal Cancer	miR-31	STK40	Inflammatory signaling	[111]
	miR-34a	Upregulated by NF-kappaB	Inflammation signaling	[112]
	miR-155	SOCS1/JAK/STAT pathway	Normal function of Kupffer cells	[113]
	miR-21	Exosomal miRNA	T cells and macrophages activation	[114]

Acknowledgments

The authors are grateful for the institutional support provided by Kean University.

References

[1] R. L. Siegel, K. D. Miller, and A. Jemal, "Cancer statistics, 2017," *CA: A Cancer Journal for Clinicians*, vol. 67, no. 1, pp. 7–30, 2017.

[2] H. Hurwitz, "Integrating the anti-VEGF - A humanized monoclonal antibody bevacizumab with chemotherapy in advanced colorectal cancer," *Clinical Colorectal Cancer*, vol. 4, no. 2, pp. S62–S68, 2004.

[3] S. J. Dutton, D. R. Ferry, J. M. Blazeby et al., "Gefitinib for oesophageal cancer progressing after chemotherapy (COG): a phase 3, multicentre, double-blind, placebo-controlled randomised trial," *The Lancet Oncology*, vol. 15, no. 8, pp. 894–904, 2014.

[4] Y.-J. Bang, E. Van Cutsem, and A. Feyereislova, "Trastuzumab in combination with chemotherapy versus chemotherapy alone for treatment of HER2- positive advanced gastric or gastro-oesophageal junction cancer (ToGA): a phase 3, open-label, randomised controlled trial," *The Lancet*, vol. 376, no. 9742, pp. 687–697, 2010.

[5] S. J. Lubner, N. V. Uboha, and D. A. Deming, "Primary and acquired resistance to biologic therapies in gastrointestinal cancers," *Journal of Gastrointestinal Oncology*, vol. 8, no. 3, pp. 499–512, 2017.

[6] H. A. Burris III, M. J. Moore, J. Andersen et al., "Improvements in survival and clinical benefit with gemcitabine as first-line therapy for patients with advanced pancreas cancer: a randomized trial," *Journal of Clinical Oncology*, vol. 15, no. 6, pp. 2403–2413, 1997.

[7] M. Amrutkar and I. P. Gladhaug, "Pancreatic cancer chemoresistance to gemcitabine," *Cancers*, vol. 9, no. 11, article no. 157, 2017.

[8] J. M. Llovet, S. Ricci, and V. Mazzaferro, "Sorafenib in Advanced Hepatocellular Carcinoma," *The New England Journal of Medicine*, vol. 359, no. 23, pp. 2497–2499, 2008.

[9] P. van der Bruggen, C. Traversari, P. Chomez et al., "A gene encoding an antigen recognized by cytolytic T lymphocytes on a human melanoma," *Science*, vol. 254, no. 5038, pp. 1643–1647, 1991.

[10] T. Kumai, "Peptide vaccines in cancer-old concept revisited," *Current Opinion in Immunology*, vol. 45, pp. 1–7, 2017.

[11] J. C. Yang and S. A. Rosenberg, "Adoptive T-Cell Therapy for Cancer," *Advances in Immunology*, vol. 130, pp. 279–294, 2016.

[12] Y. Takeuchi and H. Nishikawa, "Roles of regulatory T cells in cancer immunity," *International Immunology*, vol. 28, no. 8, pp. 401–409, 2016.

[13] S. J. Park, T. Nakagawa, H. Kitamura et al., "IL-6 regulates in vivo dendritic cell differentiation through STAT3 activation," *The Journal of Immunology*, vol. 173, no. 6, pp. 3844–3854, 2004.

[14] H. Kitamura, Y. Ohno, Y. Toyoshima et al., "Interleukin-6/STAT3 signaling as a promising target to improve the efficacy of cancer immunotherapy," *Cancer Science*, vol. 108, no. 10, pp. 1947–1952, 2017.

[15] A. Tanaka and S. Sakaguchi, "Regulatory T cells in cancer immunotherapy," *Cell Research*, vol. 27, no. 1, pp. 109–118, 2017.

[16] V. Bronte, S. Brandau, S.-H. Chen et al., "Recommendations for myeloid-derived suppressor cell nomenclature and characterization standards," *Nature Communications*, vol. 7, Article ID 12150, 2016.

[17] K. Sumida, D. Wakita, Y. Narita et al., "Anti-IL-6 receptor mAb eliminates myeloid-derived suppressor cells and inhibits tumor growth by enhancing T-cell responses," *European Journal of Immunology*, vol. 42, no. 8, pp. 2060–2072, 2012.

[18] Y. Agata, A. Kawasaki, H. Nishimura et al., "Expression of the PD-1 antigen on the surface of stimulated mouse T and B lymphocytes," *International Immunology*, vol. 8, no. 5, pp. 765–772, 1996.

[19] G. J. Freeman, A. J. Long, Y. Iwai et al., "Engagement of the PD-1 immunoinhibitory receptor by a novel B7 family member leads to negative regulation of lymphocyte activation," *The Journal of Experimental Medicine*, vol. 192, no. 7, pp. 1027–1034, 2000.

[20] Y. Latchman, C. R. Wood, T. Chernova et al., "PD-L2 is a second ligand for PD-1 and inhibits T cell activation," *Nature Immunology*, vol. 2, no. 3, pp. 261–268, 2001.

[21] T. Okazaki, A. Maeda, H. Nishimura, T. Kurosaki, and T. Honjo, "PD-1 immunoreceptor inhibits B cell receptor-mediated signaling by recruiting src homology 2-domain-containing tyrosine phosphatase 2 to phosphotyrosine," *Proceedings of the National Academy of Sciences of the United States of America*, vol. 98, no. 24, pp. 13866–13871, 2001.

[22] R. V. Parry, J. M. Chemnitz, K. A. Frauwirth et al., "CTLA-4 and PD-1 receptors inhibit T-cell activation by distinct mechanisms," *Molecular and Cellular Biology*, vol. 25, no. 21, pp. 9543–9553, 2005.

[23] H. Nishimura, T. Honjo, and N. Minato, "Facilitation of β selection and modification of positive selection in the thymus of PD-1-deficient mice," *The Journal of Experimental Medicine*, vol. 191, no. 5, pp. 891–897, 2000.

[24] H. C. Probst, K. McCoy, T. Okazaki, T. Honjo, and M. van den Broek, "Resting dendritic cells induce peripheral $CD8^+$ T cell tolerance through PD-1 and CTLA-4," *Nature Immunology*, vol. 6, no. 3, pp. 280–286, 2005.

[25] M. Ahmadzadeh, "OR.93. Tumor Antigen-specific CD8 T Cells Infiltrating the Tumor Express High Levels of PD-1 and are Functionally Impaired," *Clinical Immunology*, vol. 131, p. S38, 2009.

[26] S. Lee, S. Seo, B. Kim et al., "Corrigendum to "IFN-gamma regulates the expression of B7-H1 in dermal fibroblast cells" [J. Dermatol. Sci. 40 (2005) 95–103]," *Journal of Dermatological Science*, vol. 42, no. 3, p. 273, 2006.

[27] C. Wu, Y. Zhu, J. Jiang, J. Zhao, X.-G. Zhang, and N. Xu, "Immunohistochemical localization of programmed death-1 ligand-1 (PD-L1) in gastric carcinoma and its clinical significance," *Acta Histochemica*, vol. 108, no. 1, pp. 19–24, 2006.

[28] J. Hou, Z. Yu, R. Xiang et al., "Correlation between infiltration of FOXP3+ regulatory T cells and expression of B7-H1 in the tumor tissues of gastric cancer," *Experimental and Molecular Pathology*, vol. 96, no. 3, pp. 284–291, 2014.

[29] D. T. Le, J. N. Uram, H. Wang et al., "PD-1 Blockade in Tumors with Mismatch-Repair Deficiency," *The New England Journal of Medicine*, vol. 372, no. 26, pp. 2509-20, 2015.

[30] F. Sabbatino, V. Villani, J. H. Yearley et al., "PD-L1 and HLA class i antigen expression and clinical course of the disease in intrahepatic cholangiocarcinoma," *Clinical Cancer Research*, vol. 22, no. 2, pp. 470–478, 2016.

[31] D. Walter, E. Herrmann, A. A. Schnitzbauer et al., "PD-L1 expression in extrahepatic cholangiocarcinoma," *Histopathology*, vol. 71, no. 3, pp. 383–392, 2017.

[32] J. Calderaro, B. Rousseau, G. Amaddeo et al., "Programmed death ligand 1 expression in hepatocellular carcinoma: Relationship With clinical and pathological features," *Hepatology*, vol. 64, no. 6, pp. 2038–2046, 2016.

[33] L. Wang, Q. Ma, X. Chen, K. Guo, J. Li, and M. Zhang, "Clinical significance of B7-H1 and B7-1 expressions in pancreatic carcinoma," *World Journal of Surgery*, vol. 34, no. 5, pp. 1059–1065, 2010.

[34] P. Zheng and Z. Zhou, "Human Cancer Immunotherapy with PD-1/PD-L1 Blockade," *Biomarkers in Cancer*, vol. 7s2, p. BIC.S29325, 2015.

[35] F. Finkelmeier, Ö. Canli, A. Tal et al., "High levels of the soluble programmed death-ligand (sPD-L1) identify hepatocellular carcinoma patients with a poor prognosis," *European Journal of Cancer*, vol. 59, pp. 152–159, 2016.

[36] R. H. Thompson et al., "Costimulatory B7-H1 in renal cell carcinoma patients: Indicator of tumor aggressiveness and potential therapeutic target," *Proceedings of the National Academy of Sciences of the United States*, vol. 101, no. 49, p. 17174, 2004.

[37] J. Hamanishi et al., "Programmed cell death 1 ligand 1 and tumor-infiltrating CD8+ T lymphocytes are prognostic factors of human ovarian cancer," *Proceedings of the National Academy of Sciences of the United States*, vol. 104, no. 9, p. 3360, 2007.

[38] Y. Iwai, M. Ishida, Y. Tanaka, T. Okazaki, T. Honjo, and N. Minato, "Involvement of PD-L1 on tumor cells in the escape from host immune system and tumor immunotherapy by PD-L1 blockade," *Proceedings of the National Acadamy of Sciences of the United States of America*, vol. 99, no. 19, pp. 12293–12297, 2002.

[39] J. R. Brahmer, C. G. Drake, I. Wollner et al., "Phase I study of single-agent anti-programmed death-1 (MDX-1106) in refractory solid tumors: safety, clinical activity, pharmacodynamics, and immunologic correlates," *Journal of Clinical Oncology*, vol. 28, no. 19, pp. 3167–3175, 2010.

[40] K. Muro, H. C. Chung, V. Shankaran et al., "Pembrolizumab for patients with PD-L1-positive advanced gastric cancer (KEYNOTE-012): a multicentre, open-label, phase 1b trial," *The Lancet Oncology*, vol. 17, no. 6, pp. 717–726, 2016.

[41] E. I. Buchbinder and A. Desai, "CTLA-4 and PD-1 pathways: similarities, differences, and implications of their inhibition," *American Journal of Clinical Oncology*, 2015.

[42] J. D. Wolchok and Y. Saenger, "The mechanism of anti-CTLA-4 activity and the negative regulation of T-cell activation.," *The Oncologist*, vol. 13, pp. 2–9, 2008.

[43] C.-C. Chang, M. Campoli, and S. Ferrone, "HLA class I antigen expression in malignant cells: Why does it not always correlate with CTL-mediated lysis?" *Current Opinion in Immunology*, vol. 16, no. 5, pp. 644–650, 2004.

[44] D. Nobuoka, T. Yoshikawa, T. Fujiwara, and T. Nakatsura, "Peptide intra-tumor injection for cancer immunotherapy: Enhancement of tumor cell antigenicity is a novel and attractive strategy," *Human Vaccines & Immunotherapeutics*, vol. 9, no. 6, pp. 1234–1236, 2013.

[45] T. A. Farazi, S. A. Juranek, and T. Tuschl, "The growing catalog of small RNAs and their association with distinct Argonaute/Piwi family members," *Development*, vol. 135, no. 7, pp. 1201–1214, 2008.

[46] R. C. Friedman, K. K. Farh, C. B. Burge, and D. P. Bartel, "Most mammalian mRNAs are conserved targets of microRNAs," *Genome Research*, vol. 19, no. 1, pp. 92–105, 2009.

[47] E. Wienholds, W. P. Kloosterman, E. Miska et al., "MicroRNA expression in zebrafish embryonic development," *Science*, vol. 309, no. 5732, pp. 310-311, 2005.

[48] G. Wan, R. Mathur, X. Hu, X. Zhang, and X. Lu, "miRNA response to DNA damage," *Trends in Biochemical Sciences*, vol. 36, no. 9, pp. 478–484, 2011.

[49] G. Liu, Y. Sun, and P. Ji, "MiR-506 suppresses proliferation and induces senescence by directly targeting the CDK4/6-FOXM1 axis in ovarian cancer," *The Journal of Pathology*, vol. 233, no. 3, pp. 308–318, 2014.

[50] C. Chen, L. Li, H. F. Lodish, and D. P. Bartel, "MicroRNAs modulate hematopoietic lineage differentiation," *Science*, vol. 303, no. 5654, pp. 83–86, 2004.

[51] E. H. Baehrecke, "miRNAs: Micro managers of programmed cell death," *Current Biology*, vol. 13, no. 12, pp. R473–R475, 2003.

[52] L. G. Hommers, K. Domschke, and J. Deckert, "Heterogeneity and Individuality: microRNAs in Mental Disorders," *Journal of Neural Transmission*, vol. 122, no. 1, pp. 79–97, 2015.

[53] J. M. Lewohl, Y. O. Nunez, P. R. Dodd, G. R. Tiwari, R. A. Harris, and R. D. Mayfield, "Up-regulation of microRNAs in brain of human alcoholics," *Alcoholism: Clinical and Experimental Research*, vol. 35, no. 11, pp. 1928–1937, 2011.

[54] R. J. A. Frost and E. N. Olson, "Control of glucose homeostasis and insulin sensitivity by the Let-7 family of microRNAs," *Proceedings of the National Acadamy of Sciences of the United States of America*, vol. 108, no. 52, pp. 21075–21080, 2011.

[55] R. Garzon, M. Fabbri, A. Cimmino, G. A. Calin, and C. M. Croce, "MicroRNA expression and function in cancer," *Trends in Molecular Medicine*, vol. 12, no. 12, pp. 580–587, 2006.

[56] R. Zhou, S. P. O'Hara, and X.-M. Chen, "MicroRNA regulation of innate immune responses in epithelial cells," *Cellular & Molecular Immunology*, vol. 8, no. 5, pp. 371–379, 2011.

[57] T.-D. Kim, S. U. Lee, S. Yun et al., "Human microRNA-27a*targets Prf1 and GzmB expression to regulate NK-cell cytotoxicity," *Blood*, vol. 118, no. 20, pp. 5476–5486, 2011.

[58] J. Gong, R. Liu, R. Zhuang et al., "MiR-30c-1* promotes natural killer cell cytotoxicity against human hepatoma cells by targeting the transcription factor HMBOX1," *Cancer Science*, vol. 103, no. 4, pp. 645–652, 2012.

[59] M. L. Squadrito, F. Pucci, L. Magri et al., "MiR-511-3p modulates genetic programs of tumor-associated macrophages," *Cell Reports*, vol. 1, no. 2, pp. 141–154, 2012.

[60] E. Tili, J. J. Michaille, A. Cimino et al., "Modulation of miR-155 and miR-125b levels following lipopolysaccharide/TNF-α stimulation and their possible roles in regulating the response to endotoxin shock," *The Journal of Immunology*, vol. 179, no. 8, pp. 5082–5089, 2007.

[61] S.-Y. Hwang, H.-Y. Sun, K.-H. Lee et al., "5′-Triphosphate-RNA-independent activation of RIG-I via RNA aptamer with enhanced antiviral activity," *Nucleic Acids Research*, vol. 40, no. 6, pp. 2724–2733, 2012.

[62] K. P. Hoefig and V. Heissmeyer, "MicroRNAs grow up in the immune system," *Current Opinion in Immunology*, vol. 20, no. 3, pp. 281–287, 2008.

[63] Y.-C. Lin, M.-W. Kuo, J. Yu et al., "c-Myb is an evolutionary conserved miR-150 target and miR-150/c-Myb interaction is important for embryonic development," *Molecular Biology and Evolution*, vol. 25, no. 10, pp. 2189–2198, 2008.

[64] D. S. Rao, R. M. O'Connell, A. A. Chaudhuri, Y. Garcia-Flores, T. L. Geiger, and D. Baltimore, "MicroRNA-34a perturbs B lymphocyte development by repressing the forkhead box transcription factor Foxp1," *Immunity*, vol. 33, no. 1, pp. 48–59, 2010.

[65] S. Costinean, S. K. Sandhu, and I. M. Pedersen, "Src homology 2 domain-containing inositol-5-phosphatase and CCAAT enhancer-binding protein β are targeted by miR-155 in B cells of Eμ-*MiR*-155 transgenic mice," *Blood*, vol. 114, no. 7, pp. 1374–1382, 2009.

[66] H. Matsuyama, H. I. Suzuki, H. Nishimori et al., "miR-135b mediates NPM-ALK-driven oncogenicity and renders IL-17-producing immunophenotype to anaplastic large cell lymphoma," *Blood*, vol. 118, no. 26, pp. 6881–6892, 2011.

[67] H. Himmelreich, A. Mathys, A. Wodnar-Filipowicz, and C. P. Kalberer, "Post-transcriptional regulation of ULBP1 ligand for the activating immunoreceptor NKG2D involves 3' untranslated region," *Human Immunology*, vol. 72, no. 6, pp. 470–478, 2011.

[68] Y. Zhang, E. Sun, X. Li et al., "miR-155 contributes to Df1-induced asthma by increasing the proliferative response of Th cells via CTLA-4 downregulation," *Cellular Immunology*, vol. 314, pp. 1–9, 2017.

[69] H. B. El-Serag and K. L. Rudolph, "Hepatocellular carcinoma: epidemiology and molecular carcinogenesis," *Gastroenterology*, vol. 132, no. 7, pp. 2557–2576, 2007.

[70] L. Rahib, B. D. Smith, R. Aizenberg, A. B. Rosenzweig, J. M. Fleshman, and L. M. Matrisian, "Projecting cancer incidence and deaths to 2030: the unexpected burden of thyroid, liver, and pancreas cancers in the United States," *Cancer Research*, vol. 74, no. 11, pp. 2913–2921, 2014.

[71] J. Bruix, T. Takayama, V. Mazzaferro et al., "Adjuvant sorafenib for hepatocellular carcinoma after resection or ablation (STORM): A phase 3, randomised, double-blind, placebo-controlled trial," *The Lancet Oncology*, vol. 16, no. 13, pp. 1344–1354, 2015.

[72] X. Wang, J. Li, K. Dong et al., "Tumor suppressor miR-34a targets PD-L1 and functions as a potential immunotherapeutic target in acute myeloid leukemia," *Cellular Signalling*, vol. 27, no. 3, pp. 443–452, 2015.

[73] S. Xu, Z. Tao, B. Hai et al., "miR-424(322) reverses chemoresistance via T-cell immune response activation by blocking the PD-L1 immune checkpoint," *Nature Communications*, vol. 7, Article ID 11406, 2016.

[74] L.-H. Yan, Z.-N. Chen, L. Li et al., "E2F-1 promotes DAPK2-induced anti-tumor immunity of gastric cancer cells by targeting miR-34a," *Tumor Biology*, vol. 37, no. 12, pp. 15925–15936, 2016.

[75] M. A. Cortez, "PDL1 Regulation by p53 via miR-34," *Journal of the National Cancer Institute*, vol. 108, 2016.

[76] X. Sun, Q. Sui, C. Zhang, Z. Tian, and J. Zhang, "Targeting blockage of stat3 in hepatocellular carcinoma cells augments nk cell functions via reverse hepatocellular carcinoma-induced immune suppression," *Molecular Cancer Therapeutics*, vol. 12, no. 12, pp. 2885–2896, 2013.

[77] T. Wang, G. Niu, M. Kortylewski et al., "Regulation of the innate and adaptive immune responses by Stat-3 signaling in tumor cells," *Nature Medicine*, vol. 10, no. 1, pp. 48–54, 2004.

[78] H. Yu, D. Pardoll, and R. Jove, "STATs in cancer inflammation and immunity: a leading role for STAT3," *Nature Reviews Cancer*, vol. 9, no. 11, pp. 798–809, 2009.

[79] N. Stern-Ginossar, C. Gur, M. Biton et al., "Human microRNAs regulate stress-induced immune responses mediated by the receptor NKG2D," *Nature Immunology*, vol. 9, no. 9, pp. 1065–1073, 2008.

[80] S. Armeanu, M. Bitzer, U. M. Lauer et al., "Natural killer cell-mediated lysis of hepatoma cells via specific induction of NKG2D ligands by the histone deacetylase inhibitor sodium valproate," *Cancer Research*, vol. 65, no. 14, pp. 6321–6329, 2005.

[81] H. Yang, P. Lan, Z. Hou et al., "Histone deacetylase inhibitor SAHA epigenetically regulates miR-17-92 cluster and MCM7 to upregulate MICA expression in hepatoma," *British Journal of Cancer*, vol. 112, no. 1, pp. 112–121, 2015.

[82] X. Wei, C. Tang, X. Lu et al., "MiR-101 targets DUSP1 to regulate the TGF-ß secretion in sorafenib inhibits macrophage-induced growth of hepatocarcinoma," *Oncotarget* , vol. 6, no. 21, pp. 18389–18405, 2015.

[83] H. Qian, C. Yang, and Y. Yang, "MicroRNA-26a inhibits the growth and invasiveness of malignant melanoma and directly targets on MITF gene," *Cell Death Discovery*, vol. 3, p. 17028, 2017.

[84] Z.-T. Chai, X.-D. Zhu, J.-Y. Ao et al., "MicroRNA-26a suppresses recruitment of macrophages by down-regulating macrophage colony-stimulating factor expression through the PI3K/Akt pathway in hepatocellular carcinoma," *Journal of Hematology & Oncology*, vol. 8, no. 1, article no. 56, 2015.

[85] H. B. El-Serag, "Epidemiology of viral hepatitis and hepatocellular carcinoma," *Gastroenterology*, vol. 142, no. 6, pp. 1264–1273, 2012.

[86] C. L. Jopling, M. Yi, A. M. Lancaster, S. M. Lemon, and P. Sarnow, "Molecular biology: modulation of hepatitis C virus RNA abundance by a liver-specific MicroRNA," *Science*, vol. 309, no. 5740, pp. 1577–1581, 2005.

[87] H. L. A. Janssen, H. W. Reesink, E. J. Lawitz et al., "Treatment of HCV infection by targeting microRNA," *The New England Journal of Medicine*, vol. 368, no. 18, pp. 1685–1694, 2013.

[88] S. Wang, L. Qiu, X. Yan et al., "Loss of microRNA 122 expression in patients with hepatitis B enhances hepatitis B virus replication through cyclin G 1-modulated P53 activity," *Hepatology*, vol. 55, no. 3, pp. 730–741, 2012.

[89] T. Yoshikawa, A. Takata, M. Otsuka et al., "Silencing of microRNA-122 enhances interferon-α signaling in the liver through regulating SOCS3 promoter methylation," *Scientific Reports*, vol. 2, no. 1, 2012.

[90] C. Li, M. Deng, J. Hu et al., "Chronic inflammation contributes to the development of hepatocellular carcinoma by decreasing miR-122 levels," *Oncotarget* , vol. 7, no. 13, pp. 17021–17034, 2016.

[91] R. Singaravelu, S. O'Hara, D. M. Jones et al., "MicroRNAs regulate the immunometabolic response to viral infection in the liver," *Nature Chemical Biology*, vol. 11, no. 12, pp. 988–993, 2015.

[92] M. Zhou, J. Chen, L. Zhou, W. Chen, G. Ding, and L. Cao, "Pancreatic cancer derived exosomes regulate the expression of TLR4 in dendritic cells via miR-203," *Cellular Immunology*, vol. 292, no. 1-2, pp. 65–69, 2014.

[93] L. Jia, Q. Xi, H. Wang et al., "miR-142-5p regulates tumor cell PD-L1 expression and enhances anti-tumor immunity," *Biochemical and Biophysical Research Communications*, vol. 488, no. 2, pp. 425–431, 2017.

[94] Y. Fan, C. Shi, T. Li, and T. Kuang, "microRNA-454 shows anti-angiogenic and anti-metastatic activity in pancreatic ductal adenocarcinoma by targeting LRP6," *American Journal of Cancer Research*, vol. 7, no. 1, pp. 139–147, 2017.

[95] I. Keklikoglou, K. Hosaka, C. Bender et al., "MicroRNA-206 functions as a pleiotropic modulator of cell proliferation, invasion and lymphangiogenesis in pancreatic adenocarcinoma by targeting ANXA2 and KRAS genes," *Oncogene*, vol. 34, no. 37, pp. 4867–4878, 2015.

[96] D. Qian, G. Wei, C. Xu et al., "Bone marrow-derived mesenchymal stem cells (BMSCs) repair acute necrotized pancreatitis by secreting microRNA-9 to target the NF-κB1/p50 gene in rats," *Scientific Reports*, vol. 7, no. 1, 2017.

[97] J. Zhang, X. Ning, W. Cui, M. Bi, D. Zhang, and J. Zhang, "Transforming Growth Factor (TGF)-β-Induced MicroRNA-216a Promotes Acute Pancreatitis Via Akt and TGF-β Pathway in Mice," *Digestive Diseases and Sciences*, vol. 60, no. 1, pp. 127–135, 2015.

[98] M. El Gazzar, A. Church, T. F. Liu, and C. E. McCall, "MicroRNA-146a regulates both transcription silencing and translation disruption of TNF-α during TLR4-induced gene reprogramming," *Journal of Leukocyte Biology*, vol. 90, no. 3, pp. 509–519, 2011.

[99] R. Ueda, G. Kohanbash, K. Sasaki et al., "Dicer-regulated microRNAs 222 and 339 promote resistance of cancer cells to cytotoxic T-lymphocytes by down-regulation of ICAM-1," *Proceedings of the National Acadamy of Sciences of the United States of America*, vol. 106, no. 26, pp. 10746–10751, 2009.

[100] K. Mima, R. Nishihara, Z. Qian, H. Baba, and S. Ogino, "173PD MicroRNA MIR21, T cells, and PTGS2 expression in Colorectal Cancer," *Annals of Oncology*, vol. 27, no. suppl_9, 2016.

[101] X. Li, J. Nie, Q. Mei, and W.-D. Han, "MicroRNAs: novel immunotherapeutic targets in colorectal carcinoma," *World Journal of Gastroenterology*, vol. 22, no. 23, pp. 5317–5331, 2016.

[102] M. Zhang, Q. Liu, S. Mi et al., "Both miR-17-5p and miR-20a alleviate suppressive potential of myeloid-derived suppressor cells by modulating STAT3 expression," *The Journal of Immunology*, vol. 186, no. 8, pp. 4716–4724, 2011.

[103] G. Koukos, C. Polytarchou, J. L. Kaplan et al., "MicroRNA-124 regulates STAT3 expression and is down-regulated in colon tissues of pediatric patients with ulcerative colitis," *Gastroenterology*, vol. 145, no. 4, pp. 842.e2–852.e2, 2013.

[104] H. Wang, H. Flach, M. Onizawa, L. Wei, M. T. Mcmanus, and A. Weiss, "Negative regulation of Hif1a expression and TH17 differentiation by the hypoxia-regulated microRNA miR-210," *Nature Immunology*, vol. 15, no. 4, pp. 393–401, 2014.

[105] H. W. H. Yu, D. M. Y. Sze, and W. C. S. Cho, "MicroRNAs involved in anti-tumour immunity," *International Journal of Molecular Sciences*, vol. 14, no. 3, pp. 5587–5607, 2013.

[106] J. Zhu, L. Chen, L. Zou et al., "MiR-20b, -21, and -130b inhibit PTEN expression resulting in B7-H1 over-expression in advanced colorectal cancer," *Human Immunology*, vol. 75, no. 4, pp. 348–353, 2014.

[107] M.-Z. Ma, B.-F. Chu, Y. Zhang et al., "Long non-coding RNA CCAT1 promotes gallbladder cancer development via negative modulation of miRNA-218-5p," *Cell Death & Disease*, vol. 6, no. 1, Article ID e1583, 2015.

[108] T. B. Huffaker, S.-H. Lee, W. W. Tang et al., "Antitumor immunity is defective in T cell-specific microRNA-155- deficient mice and is rescued by immune checkpoint blockade," *The Journal of Biological Chemistry*, vol. 292, no. 45, pp. 18530–18541, 2017.

[109] Y. Huang, Y. Wu, J. Dong, D. Han, S. Yang, and L. Jiang, "MicroRNA-133a-3p exerts inhibitory effects on gallbladder carcinoma via targeting RBPJ," *American Journal of Cancer Research*, vol. 6, no. 11, pp. 2448–2462, 2016.

[110] P. Letelier, "miR-1 and miR-145 act as tumor suppressor microRNAs in gallbladder cancer," *International Journal of Clinical and Experimental Pathology*, vol. 7, no. 5, p. 67, 1849.

[111] C. Taccioli, M. Garofalo, H. Chen et al., "Repression of esophageal neoplasia and inflammatory signaling by anti-MIR-31 delivery in vivo," *Journal of the National Cancer Institute*, vol. 107, no. 11, Article ID djv220, 2015.

[112] J. Li, K. Wang, X. Chen et al., "Transcriptional activation of microRNA-34a by NF-kappaB in human esophageal cancer cells," *BMC Molecular Biology*, vol. 13, article 4, 2012.

[113] J. Li, J. Gong, P. Li et al., "Knockdown of MicroRNA-155 in kupffer cells results in immunosuppressive effects and prolongs survival of mouse liver allografts," *Transplantation*, vol. 97, no. 6, pp. 626–635, 2014.

[114] Y. Tanaka, H. Kamohara, K. Kinoshita et al., "Clinical impact of serum exosomal microRNA-21 as a clinical biomarker in human esophageal squamous cell carcinoma," *Cancer*, vol. 119, no. 6, pp. 1159–1167, 2013.

[115] J. Chang, E. Nicolas, D. Marks et al., "miR-122, a mammalian liver-specific microRNA, is processed from hcr mRNA and may downregulate the high affinity cationic amino acid transporter CAT-1," *RNA Biology*, vol. 1, no. 2, pp. 106–113, 2004.

[116] P. Landgraf, *A mammalian microRNA expression atlas based on small RNA library sequencing*, vol. 129, Cell, 2007.

[117] C. L. Jopling, "Liver-specific microRNA-122: biogenesis and function," *RNA Biology*, vol. 9, no. 2, pp. 137–142, 2012.

[118] G. Szabo and S. Bala, "MicroRNAs in liver disease," *Nature Reviews Gastroenterology & Hepatology*, vol. 10, no. 11, pp. 542–552, 2013.

[119] H. Kutay, S. Bai, J. Datta et al., "Downregulation of miR-122 in the rodent and human hepatocellular carcinomas," *Journal of Cellular Biochemistry*, vol. 99, no. 3, pp. 671–678, 2006.

[120] W.-C. Tsai, S.-D. Hsu, C.-S. Hsu et al., "MicroRNA-122 plays a critical role in liver homeostasis and hepatocarcinogenesis," *The Journal of Clinical Investigation*, vol. 122, no. 8, pp. 2884–2897, 2012.

[121] C. Coulouarn, V. M. Factor, J. B. Andersen, M. E. Durkin, and S. S. Thorgeirsson, "Loss of miR-122 expression in liver cancer correlates with suppression of the hepatic phenotype and gain of metastatic properties," *Oncogene*, vol. 28, no. 40, pp. 3526–3536, 2009.

[122] S.-H. Hsu, B. Wang, J. Kota et al., "Essential metabolic, anti-inflammatory, and anti-tumorigenic functions of miR-122 in liver," *The Journal of Clinical Investigation*, vol. 122, no. 8, pp. 2871–2883, 2012.

[123] K. A. Padgett, R. Y. Lan, P. C. Leung et al., "Primary biliary cirrhosis is associated with altered hepatic microRNA expression," *Journal of Autoimmunity*, vol. 32, no. 3-4, pp. 246–253, 2009.

[124] A. Jemal, E. M. Ward, C. J. Johnson et al., "Annual Report to the Nation on the Status of Cancer, 1975-2014, Featuring Survival," *Journal of the National Cancer Institute*, vol. 109, no. 9, Article ID djx030, 2017.

[125] C. Admyre, S. M. Johansson, S. Paulie, and S. Gabrielsson, "Direct exosome stimulation of peripheral human T cells detected by ELISPOT," *European Journal of Immunology*, vol. 36, no. 7, pp. 1772–1781, 2006.

[126] G. Raposo, H. W. Nijman, W. Stoorvogel et al., "B lymphocytes secrete antigen-presenting vesicles," *The Journal of Experimental Medicine*, vol. 183, no. 3, pp. 1161–1172, 1996.

[127] C. Théry, A. Regnault, J. Garin et al., "Molecular characterization of dendritic cell-derived exosomes. Selective accumulation of the heat shock protein hsc73," *The Journal of Cell Biology*, vol. 147, no. 3, pp. 599–610, 1999.

[128] J. Wolfers, A. Lozier, G. Raposo et al., "Tumor-derived exosomes are a source of shared tumor rejection antigens for CTL cross-priming," *Nature Medicine*, vol. 7, no. 3, pp. 297–303, 2001.

[129] A. Tan, H. de la Peña, and A. M. Seifalian, "The application of exosomes as a nanoscale cancer vaccine," *International Journal of Nanomedicine*, vol. 5, no. 1, pp. 889–900, 2010.

[130] H. Valadi, K. Ekström, A. Bossios, M. Sjöstrand, J. J. Lee, and J. O. Lötvall, "Exosome-mediated transfer of mRNAs and microRNAs is a novel mechanism of genetic exchange between cells," *Nature Cell Biology*, vol. 9, no. 6, pp. 654–659, 2007.

[131] C. Théry, M. Ostrowski, and E. Segura, "Membrane vesicles as conveyors of immune responses," *Nature Reviews Immunology*, vol. 9, no. 8, pp. 581–593, 2009.

[132] R.-S. Que, C. Lin, G.-P. Ding, Z.-R. Wu, and L.-P. Cao, "Increasing the immune activity of exosomes: the effect of miRNA-depleted exosome proteins on activating dendritic cell/cytokine-induced killer cells against pancreatic cancer," *Journal of Zhejiang University SCIENCE B*, vol. 17, no. 5, pp. 352–360, 2016.

[133] J. Du, J. Wang, G. Tan et al., "Aberrant elevated microRNA-146a in dendritic cells (DC) induced by human pancreatic cancer cell line BxPC-3-conditioned medium inhibits DC maturation and activation," *Medical Oncology*, vol. 29, no. 4, pp. 2814–2823, 2012.

[134] S. Meng, H. Wang, D. Xue, and W. Zhang, "Screening and validation of differentially expressed extracellular miRNAs in acute pancreatitis," *Molecular Medicine Reports*, vol. 16, no. 5, pp. 6412–6418, 2017.

[135] X.-X. Zhang, L.-H. Deng, W.-W. Chen et al., "Circulating microRNA 216 as a Marker for the Early Identification of Severe Acute Pancreatitis," *The American Journal of the Medical Sciences*, vol. 353, no. 2, pp. 178–186, 2017.

[136] D. C. Whitcomb, L. Frulloni, P. Garg et al., "Chronic pancreatitis: An international draft consensus proposal for a new mechanistic definition," *Pancreatology*, vol. 16, no. 2, pp. 218–224, 2016.

[137] J. Kleeff, D. C. Whitcomb, T. Shimosegawa et al., "Chronic pancreatitis," *Nature Reviews Disease Primers*, vol. 3, p. 17061, 2017.

[138] U. C. Bang, T. Benfield, L. Hyldstrup, F. Bendtsen, and J.-E. Beck Jensen, "Mortality, cancer, and comorbidities associated with chronic pancreatitis: A Danish nationwide matched-cohort study," *Gastroenterology*, vol. 146, no. 4, pp. 989–994, 2014.

[139] Z. Wang, D. Li, J. Jin, Q. Wang, S. Zhao, and Y. Bai, "Association between microRNA polymorphisms and chronic pancreatitis," *Pancreatology*, vol. 16, no. 2, pp. 244–248, 2016.

[140] B. S. Cobb, A. Hertweck, J. Smith et al., "A role for Dicer in immune regulation," *The Journal of Experimental Medicine*, vol. 203, no. 11, pp. 2519–2527, 2006.

[141] J. E. de Vries, H. Yssel, and H. Spits, "Interplay between the TCR/CD3 Complex and CD4 or CD8 in the Activation of Cytotoxic T Lymphocytes," *Immunological Reviews*, vol. 109, no. 1, pp. 119–142, 1989.

[142] K. Hotta, M. Sho, K. Fujimoto et al., "Prognostic significance of CD45RO memory T cells in renal cell carcinoma," *British Journal of Cancer*, vol. 105, no. 8, pp. 1191–1196, 2011.

[143] M. K. Srivastava, P. Sinha, V. K. Clements, P. Rodriguez, and S. Ostrand-Rosenberg, "Myeloid-derived suppressor cells inhibit T-cell activation by depleting cystine and cysteine," *Cancer Research*, vol. 70, no. 1, pp. 68–77, 2010.

[144] Y. Liu, L. Lai, Q. Chen et al., "MicroRNA-494 is required for the accumulation and functions of tumor-expanded myeloid-derived suppressor cells via targeting of PTEN," *The Journal of Immunology*, vol. 188, no. 11, pp. 5500–5510, 2012.

[145] S. I. Grivennikov, "Inflammation and colorectal cancer: colitis-associated neoplasia," *Seminars in Immunopathology*, vol. 35, no. 2, pp. 229–244, 2013.

[146] X. Cheng, X. Zhang, J. Su et al., "MiR-19b downregulates intestinal SOCS3 to reduce intestinal inflammation in Crohn's disease," *Scientific Reports*, vol. 5, Article ID 10397, 2015.

[147] S. E. M. Heinsbroek, M. L. Squadrito, R. Schilderink et al., "MiR-511-3p, embedded in the macrophage mannose receptor gene, contributes to intestinal inflammation," *Mucosal Immunology*, vol. 9, no. 4, pp. 960–973, 2016.

[148] S. B. Coffelt, M. D. Wellenstein, and K. E. De Visser, "Neutrophils in cancer: Neutral no more," *Nature Reviews Cancer*, vol. 16, no. 7, pp. 431–446, 2016.

[149] D. I. Gabrilovich, S. Ostrand-Rosenberg, and V. Bronte, "Coordinated regulation of myeloid cells by tumours," *Nature Reviews Immunology*, vol. 12, no. 4, pp. 253–268, 2012.

[150] S. Tazzyman, H. Niaz, and C. Murdoch, "Neutrophil-mediated tumour angiogenesis: Subversion of immune responses to promote tumour growth," *Seminars in Cancer Biology*, vol. 23, no. 3, pp. 149–158, 2013.

[151] R. Noy and J. W. Pollard, "Tumor-associated macrophages: from mechanisms to therapy," *Immunity*, vol. 41, no. 1, pp. 49–61, 2014.

[152] Q. Mei, G. Xue, X. Li et al., "Methylation-induced loss of miR-484 in microsatellite-unstable colorectal cancer promotes both viability and IL-8 production via CD137L," *The Journal of Pathology*, vol. 236, no. 2, pp. 165–174, 2015.

[153] B. Chen, "Role of miR-19a targeting TNF-alpha in mediating ulcerative colitis," *Scandinavian Journal of Gastroenterology*, vol. 48, no. 7, pp. 815-24, 2013.

[154] S. P. Patel and R. Kurzrock, "PD-L1 expression as a predictive biomarker in cancer immunotherapy," *Molecular Cancer Therapeutics*, vol. 14, no. 4, pp. 847–856, 2015.

[155] R. Siegel, J. Ma, Z. Zou, and A. Jemal, "Cancer statistics, 2014," *CA: A Cancer Journal for Clinicians*, vol. 64, no. 1, pp. 9–29, 2014.

[156] W. F. Anderson, M. C. Camargo, J. F. Fraumeni Jr., P. Correa, P. S. Rosenberg, and C. S. Rabkin, "Age-specific trends in incidence of noncardia gastric cancer in US adults," *Journal of the American Medical Association*, vol. 303, no. 17, pp. 1723–1728, 2010.

[157] D. Ginsberg, "E2F1 pathways to apoptosis," *FEBS Letters*, vol. 529, no. 1, pp. 122–125, 2002.

[158] Z. Li, X. Yu, J. Shen, P. T. Y. Law, M. T. V. Chan, and W. K. K. Wu, "MicroRNA expression and its implications for diagnosis and therapy of gallbladder cancer," *Oncotarget* , vol. 6, no. 16, pp. 13914–13924, 2015.

[159] B. C. Chapman, T. Jones, M. C. McManus, R. Shah, and C. Gajdos, "Metastatic papillary gallbladder carcinoma with a unique presentation and clinical course," *JOP*, vol. 15, no. 5, pp. 515–519, 2014.

[160] H. Kono, M. Nakamura, T. Ohtsuka et al., "High expression of microRNA-155 is associated with the aggressive malignant behavior of gallbladder carcinoma," *Oncology Reports*, vol. 30, no. 1, pp. 17–24, 2013.

[161] Y. Li, J. Zhang, and H. Ma, "Chronic inflammation and gallbladder cancer," *Cancer Letters*, vol. 345, no. 2, pp. 242–248, 2014.

[162] C. E. Savard, T. A. Blinman, H. Choi, S. Lee, S. J. Pandol, and S. P. Lee, "Expression of cytokine and chemokine mRNA and secretion of tumor necrosis factor-α by gallbladder epithelial cells: Response to bacterial lipopolysaccharides," *BMC Gastroenterology*, vol. 2, no. 1, 2002.

[163] L. Xiong, Z. Yang, L. Yang, J. Liu, and X. Miao, "Expressive levels of MUC1 and MUC5AC and their clinicopathologic significances in the benign and malignant lesions of gallbladder," *Journal of Surgical Oncology*, vol. 105, no. 1, pp. 97–103, 2012.

[164] N. Tsuchida, T. Ryder, and E. Ohtsubo, "Nucleotide sequence of the oncogene encoding the p21 transforming protein of Kirsten murine sarcoma virus," *Science*, vol. 217, no. 4563, pp. 937–939, 1982.

[165] G. M. Sundaram and P. V. Bramhachari, "Molecular interplay of pro-inflammatory transcription factors and non-coding RNAs in esophageal squamous cell carcinoma," *Tumor Biology*, vol. 39, no. 6, 2017.

[166] W. Wu, T. D. Bhagat, X. Yang et al., "Hypomethylation of noncoding DNA regions and overexpression of the long noncoding RNA, AFAP1-AS1, in Barrett's esophagus and esophageal adenocarcinoma," *Gastroenterology*, vol. 144, no. 5, pp. 956.e4–966.e4, 2013.

[167] X. Wang, M. Li, Z. Wang et al., "Silencing of long noncoding rna malat1 by mir-101 and mir-217 inhibits proliferation, migration, and invasion of esophageal squamous cell carcinoma cells," *The Journal of Biological Chemistry*, vol. 290, no. 7, pp. 3925–3935, 2015.

[168] S. G. Liu, X. G. Qin, B. S. Zhao et al., "Differential expression of miRNAs in esophageal cancer tissue," *Oncology Letters*, vol. 5, no. 5, pp. 1639–1642, 2013.

[169] R. B. Koumangoye, T. Andl, K. J. Taubenslag et al., "SOX4 interacts with EZH2 and HDAC3 to suppress microRNA-31 in invasive esophageal cancer cells," *Molecular Cancer*, vol. 14, no. 1, article no. 24, 2015.

[170] N. Akanuma, I. Hoshino, Y. Akutsu et al., "MicroRNA-133a regulates the mRNAs of two invadopodia-related proteins, FSCN1 and MMP14, in esophageal cancer," *British Journal of Cancer*, vol. 110, no. 1, pp. 189–198, 2014.

[171] Z.-L. Chen, X.-H. Zhao, and J.-W. Wang, "microRNA-92a promotes lymph node metastasis of human esophageal squamous cell carcinoma via E-cadherin," *The Journal of Biological Chemistry*, vol. 286, no. 12, pp. 10725–10734, 2011.

[172] Y. Tian, A. Luo, and Y. Cai, "MicroRNA-10b promotes migration and invasion through KLF4 in human esophageal cancer cell lines," *The Journal of Biological Chemistry*, vol. 285, no. 11, pp. 7986–7994, 2010.

[173] Z. Ye, J. Fang, S. Dai et al., "MicroRNA-34a induces a senescence-like change via the down-regulation of SIRT1 and up-regulation of p53 protein in human esophageal squamous cancer cells with a wild-type p53 gene background," *Cancer Letters*, vol. 370, no. 2, pp. 216–221, 2016.

[174] Y. Hiyoshi, H. Kamohara, R. Karashima et al., "MicroRNA-21 regulates the proliferation and invasion in esophageal squamous cell carcinoma," *Clinical Cancer Research*, vol. 15, no. 6, pp. 1915–1922, 2009.

[175] K. Kono, H. Kawaida, A. Takahashi et al., "CD4(+)CD25^{high} regulatory T cells increase with tumor stage in patients with gastric and esophageal cancers," *Cancer Immunology, Immunotherapy*, vol. 55, no. 9, pp. 1064–1071, 2006.

[176] T. J. Curiel, G. Coukos, L. Zou et al., "Specific recruitment of regulatory T cells in ovarian carcinoma fosters immune privilege and predicts reduced survival," *Nature Medicine*, vol. 10, no. 9, p. 942, 2004.

[177] R. F. Gabitass, N. E. Annels, D. D. Stocken, H. A. Pandha, and G. W. Middleton, "Elevated myeloid-derived suppressor cells in pancreatic, esophageal and gastric cancer are an independent prognostic factor and are associated with significant elevation of the Th2 cytokine interleukin-13," *Cancer Immunology, Immunotherapy*, vol. 60, no. 10, pp. 1419–1430, 2011.

[178] S. Topalian, C. Drake, and D. Pardoll, "Immune checkpoint blockade: a common denominator approach to cancer therapy," *Cancer Cell*, vol. 27, no. 4, pp. 450–461, 2015.

[179] P. A. Ott, F. S. Hodi, and C. Robert, "CTLA-4 and PD-1/PD-L1 blockade: New immunotherapeutic modalities with durable clinical benefit in melanoma patients," *Clinical Cancer Research*, vol. 19, no. 19, pp. 5300–5309, 2013.

[180] M. A. Postow, M. K. Callahan, and J. D. Wolchok, "Immune checkpoint blockade in cancer therapy," *Journal of Clinical Oncology*, vol. 33, no. 17, pp. 1974–1982, 2015.

[181] D. M. Pardoll, "The blockade of immune checkpoints in cancer immunotherapy," *Nature Reviews Cancer*, vol. 12, no. 4, pp. 252–264, 2012.

[182] Q. Wang, W. Lin, X. Tang et al., "The roles of microRNAs in regulating the expression of PD-1/PD-l1 immune checkpoint," *International Journal of Molecular Sciences*, vol. 18, no. 12, article no. 2540, 2017.

[183] D. A. Mitchell, "MicroRNAs provide a novel pathway toward combinatorial immune checkpoint blockade," *Neuro-Oncology*, vol. 18, no. 5, pp. 601-602, 2016.

[184] J. C. Dudda, B. Salaun, Y. Ji et al., "MicroRNA-155 is required for effector cd8+ t cell responses to virus infection and cancer," *Immunity*, vol. 38, no. 4, pp. 742–753, 2013.

[185] R. Trotta, L. Chen, D. Ciarlariello et al., "miR-155 regulates IFN-γ production in natural killer cells," *Blood*, vol. 119, no. 15, pp. 3478–3485, 2012.

[186] C. Huang, H. Li, W. Wu, T. Jiang, and Z. Qiu, "Regulation of miR-155 affects pancreatic cancer cell invasiveness and migration by modulating the STAT3 signaling pathway through SOCS1," *Oncology Reports*, vol. 30, no. 3, pp. 1223–1230, 2013.

[187] X. Fu, H. Wen, L. Jing et al., "MicroRNA-155-5p promotes hepatocellular carcinoma progression by suppressing PTEN through the PI3K/Akt pathway," *Cancer Science*, vol. 108, no. 4, pp. 620–631, 2017.

[188] H. Shibuya, H. Iinuma, R. Shimada, A. Horiuchi, and T. Watanabe, "Clinicopathological and prognostic value of microRNA-21 and microRNA-155 in colorectal cancer," *Oncology*, vol. 79, no. 3-4, pp. 313–320, 2011.

[189] X. L. Zhang, J. H. Chen, and C. K. Qin, "MicroRNA-155 expression as a prognostic factor in patients with gallbladder carcinoma after surgical resection," *International Journal of Clinical and Experimental Medicine*, vol. 8, no. 11, p. 21241, 2015.

[190] E. Tili, J.-J. Michaille, and C. M. Croce, "MicroRNAs play a central role in molecular dysfunctions linking inflammation with cancer," *Immunological Reviews*, vol. 253, no. 1, pp. 167–184, 2013.

[191] R. Rupaimoole, S. Y. Wu, and S. Pradeep, "Hypoxia-mediated downregulation of miRNA biogenesis promotes tumour progression," *Nature Communications*, vol. 5, article 5202, 2014.

Permissions

All chapters in this book were first published in CJGH, by Hindawi Publishing Corporation; hereby published with permission under the Creative Commons Attribution License or equivalent. Every chapter published in this book has been scrutinized by our experts. Their significance has been extensively debated. The topics covered herein carry significant findings which will fuel the growth of the discipline. They may even be implemented as practical applications or may be referred to as a beginning point for another development.

The contributors of this book come from diverse backgrounds, making this book a truly international effort. This book will bring forth new frontiers with its revolutionizing research information and detailed analysis of the nascent developments around the world.

We would like to thank all the contributing authors for lending their expertise to make the book truly unique. They have played a crucial role in the development of this book. Without their invaluable contributions this book wouldn't have been possible. They have made vital efforts to compile up to date information on the varied aspects of this subject to make this book a valuable addition to the collection of many professionals and students.

This book was conceptualized with the vision of imparting up-to-date information and advanced data in this field. To ensure the same, a matchless editorial board was set up. Every individual on the board went through rigorous rounds of assessment to prove their worth. After which they invested a large part of their time researching and compiling the most relevant data for our readers.

The editorial board has been involved in producing this book since its inception. They have spent rigorous hours researching and exploring the diverse topics which have resulted in the successful publishing of this book. They have passed on their knowledge of decades through this book. To expedite this challenging task, the publisher supported the team at every step. A small team of assistant editors was also appointed to further simplify the editing procedure and attain best results for the readers.

Apart from the editorial board, the designing team has also invested a significant amount of their time in understanding the subject and creating the most relevant covers. They scrutinized every image to scout for the most suitable representation of the subject and create an appropriate cover for the book.

The publishing team has been an ardent support to the editorial, designing and production team. Their endless efforts to recruit the best for this project, has resulted in the accomplishment of this book. They are a veteran in the field of academics and their pool of knowledge is as vast as their experience in printing. Their expertise and guidance has proved useful at every step. Their uncompromising quality standards have made this book an exceptional effort. Their encouragement from time to time has been an inspiration for everyone.

The publisher and the editorial board hope that this book will prove to be a valuable piece of knowledge for researchers, students, practitioners and scholars across the globe.

List of Contributors

Cheryl Kluthe, Matthew Carroll, Eytan Wine and Hien Quoc Huynh
Edmonton Pediatric IBD Clinic (EPIC), Edmonton, AB, Canada

Jenkin Tsui
University of Edinburgh, Edinburgh, UK

Donald Spady
Division of Pediatric GI Nutrition, Stollery Children's Hospital, University of Alberta, Edmonton, AB, Canada

Peyda Korhan, Yeliz Yılmaz, Ezgi Bağırsakçı, Ayşim Güneş, Hande Topel, Brian I. Carr and Neşe Atabey
Izmir Biomedicine and Genome Center, 35340, Turkey

Yeliz Ylimaz and Hande Topel
Medical Biology and Genetics, Heath Sciences Institute, Dokuz Eylul University, 35340, Turkey
Ezgi Bağırsakçı
Izmir International Biomedicine and Genome Institute, Dokuz Eylul University, 35340, Turkey

Malgorzata Sidorkiewicz, Martyna Grek-Kowalinska and Anna Piekarska
Medical University of Lodz, Poland

Seogsong Jeong, Ying Tong, Lei Xia, Ning Xu, Meng Sha, Jianjun Zhang, Xiaoni Kong, Jinyang Gu and Qiang Xia
Department of Liver Surgery, Renji Hospital, School of Medicine, Shanghai Jiao Tong University, Shanghai 200127, China

Lei Gao
Institute of Liver Diseases, 81st Hospital of People's Liberation Army, Nanjing 210002, China

Seogsong Jeong, Ying Tong, Lei Xia, Ning Xu, Meng Sha, Jianjun Zhang, Xiaoni Kong, Jinyang Gu and Qiang Xia
Department of Liver Surgery, Renji Hospital, School of Medicine, Shanghai Jiao Tong University, Shanghai 200127, China

Lei Gao
Institute of Liver Diseases, 81st Hospital of People's Liberation Army, Nanjing 210002, China

Nikhil R. Kalva, Vishwas Vanar and Srinivas Reddy Puli
Internal Medicine, University of Illinois College of Medicine at Peoria, Peoria, IL, USA

David Forcione
Interventional Endoscopy Services, Gastrointestinal Unit, Massachusetts General Hospital, Harvard Medical School, Boston, MA, USA

Matthew L. Bechtold
Division of Gastroenterology and Hepatology, University of Missouri-Columbia, Columbia, MO, USA

Wandong Hong and Suhan Lin
Department of Gastroenterology and Hepatology, The First Affiliated Hospital of Wenzhou Medical University, Wenzhou, Zhejiang, China

Maddalena Zippi
Unit of Gastroenterology and Digestive Endoscopy, Sandro Pertini Hospital, Rome, Italy

Wujun Geng
Department of Anesthesiology, The First Affiliated Hospital ofWenzhou Medical University, Wenzhou, Zhejiang, China

Simon Stock
Department of Surgery, World Mate Emergency Hospital, Battambang, Cambodia

Zarrin Basharat
Microbiology and Biotechnology Research Lab, Department of Environmental Sciences, Fatima JinnahWomen University, Rawalpindi 46000, Pakistan

Bicheng Cheng
Zhejiang Provincial Top Key Discipline in Surgery, Wenzhou Key Laboratory of Surgery, Department of Surgery, The First Affiliated Hospital, Wenzhou Medical University, Wenzhou, Zhejiang, China

Jingye Pan
Intensive Care Unit, The First Affiliated Hospital ofWenzhou Medical University, Wenzhou, Zhejiang, China

Mengtao Zhou
Department of Surgery, The First Affiliated Hospital of Wenzhou Medical University, Wenzhou, Zhejiang, China

Feiyue Zhang, Tong Liu and Pan Gao
Department of Gastroenterology, Xuzhou Medical University, Xuzhou, Jiangsu 221000, China

Sujuan Fei
Department of Gastroenterology, The Affiliated Hospital of XuzhouMedical University, Xuzhou, Jiangsu 221000, China

Xi-Zhen Chen, Wei Kevin Zhang, He-Bin Tang, Xiao-Jun Li and Yu-Sang Li
Department of Pharmacology, School of Pharmaceutical Sciences, South-Central University for Nationalities, Wuhan, China

Gui-Hua Tian and Hong-Cai Shang
Key Laboratory of Chinese Internal Medicine of MOE, Beijing Dongzhimen Hospital, Beijing University of Chinese Medicine, Beijing, China

Min Woo Lee, Hyo Keun Lim, Hyunchul Rhim, Dong Ik Cha, Tae Wook Kang, Kyoung Doo Song and Ji Hye Min
Department of Radiology and Center for Imaging Science, Samsung Medical Center, Sungkyunkwan University School of Medicine, Seoul 06351, Republic of Korea

Min Woo Lee, Hyo Keun Lim and Hyunchul Rhim
Department of Health Sciences and Technology, SAIHST, Sungkyunkwan University, Seoul 06351, Republic of Korea

Geum-Youn Gwak
Department of Medicine, Samsung Medical Center, Sungkyunkwan University School of Medicine, Seoul 06351, Republic of Korea

Seonwoo Kim
Statistics and Data Center, Samsung Medical Center, Seoul 06351, Republic of Korea

David S. K. Lu
Department of Radiological Sciences, David Geffen School ofMedicine at UCLA, 757Westwood Plaza, Los Angeles, CA 90095, USA

Jiaxin Xu, Tianyin Chen, Meidong Xu, Yunshi Zhong, Yiqun Zhang, Weifeng Chen, Wenzheng Qin, Mingyan Cai and Pinghong Zhou
Endoscopy Centre and Endoscopy Research Institute, Zhongshan Hospital, Fudan University, Shanghai, China

Shaimaa Elkholy
Internal Medicine Department, Gastroenterology Division, Faculty of Medicine, Cairo University, Egypt

Yuanji Ma, Yan Xu, Fang Chen, Ying Wang, Lang Bai and Hong Tang
Center of Infectious Diseases, West China Hospital of Sichuan University, Chengdu 610041, China
Division of Infectious Diseases, State Key Laboratory of Biotherapy, Sichuan University, Chengdu 610041, China

Preya J. Patel, Leigh U. Horsfall, Katherine A. Stuart and Elizabeth E. Powell
Department of Gastroenterology and Hepatology, Princess Alexandra Hospital, Brisbane, QLD, Australia

Preya J. Patel, Leigh U. Horsfall, Kelly L. Hayward, Andrew D. Clouston, Katharine M. Irvine, Patricia C. Valery and Elizabeth E. Powell
Centre for Liver Disease Research, Translational Research Institute, School of Medicine, The University of Queensland, Brisbane, QLD, Australia

David Smith
QIMR Berghofer Medical Research Institute, Brisbane, QLD, Australia

Jason P. Connor
Discipline of Psychiatry, The University of Queensland, Brisbane, QLD, Australia

Fabrina Hossain, Suzanne Williams and Tracey Johnson
Inala Primary Care, Brisbane, QLD, Australia

Nigel N. Brown
Pathology Queensland, Brisbane, QLD, Australia

Nivene Saad
Department of Radiology, Princess Alexandra Hospital, Brisbane, QLD, Australia

Katharine M. Irvine
Mater Research, Translational Research Institute, University of Queensland, Brisbane, QLD, Australia

Anthony W. Russell and Patricia C. Valery
School of Clinical Medicine, The University of Queensland, Brisbane, QLD, Australia

Anthony W. Russell
Department of Diabetes and Endocrinology, Princess Alexandra Hospital, Brisbane, QLD, Australia

Glynis Byrne
Department of Medicine, University of British Columbia, Vancouver, BC, Canada

Greg Rosenfeld, Yvette Leung and Brian Bressler
Department of Medicine, Division of Gastroenterology, University of British Columbia, Vancouver, BC, Canada

Hong Qian
Centre for Health Evaluation and Outcome Sciences, University of British Columbia, St. Paul's Hospital, Vancouver, BC, Canada

Julia Raudzus and Carlos Nunez
Department of Psychiatry, University of British Columbia, Vancouver, BC, Canada

Lumir Kunovsky, Pavla Tesarikova, Radek Kroupa, Jiri Dolina and Jan Trna
Department of Gastroenterology, University Hospital Brno Bohunice, Faculty of Medicine, Masaryk University, Czech Republic

Lumir Kunovsky, Zdenek Kala and Petr Kysela
Department of Surgery, University Hospital Brno Bohunice, Faculty of Medicine, Masaryk University, Czech Republic

Pavla Tesarikova and Jan Trna
Department of Internal Medicine, Hospital Boskovice, Czech Republic

Umberto Vespasiani-Gentilucci, Chiara Dell'Unto, Antonio De Vincentis, Giovanni Galati, Paolo Gallo, Francesco Valentini, Raffaele Antonelli-Incalzi and Antonio Picardi
Internal Medicine, Geriatrics, and Hepatology Unit, University Campus Bio-Medico, Rome, Italy

Andrea Baiocchini and Franca Del Nonno
Laboratory of Pathology of The National Institute for Infectious Diseases, Lazzaro Spallanzani, Rome, Italy

Marco Delle Monache and Roberto Cecere
Hepatology Outpatient Clinic, Colleferro Hospital, Rome, Italy

Adriano Maria Pellicelli and Valerio Giannelli
Liver Disease Unit, San Camillo-Forlanini Hospital, Rome, Italy

Simone Carotti and Sergio Morini
Laboratory of Microscopic and Ultrastructural Anatomy, CIR, University Campus Bio-Medico, Rome, Italy

Davide Rosati
University La Sapienza of Rome, Rome, Italy

Konstantinos Argyriou, Andreas Kapsoritakis, Konstantinos Oikonomou, Anastassios Manolakis, Eirini Tsakiridou, and Spyridon Potamianos
Department of Gastroenterology, University Hospital of Larissa, Mezourlo 1, 41110 Larissa, Greece

Yangjie Dang and Xingxing Shi
Department of Anesthesiology, Xi'an Children's Hospital, Xi'an, Shaanxi 710032, China

William Xu
Department of Anesthesiology, Carver College of Medicine, University of Iowa, Iowa City, IA 52246, USA

Mingzhang Zuo
Department of Anesthesiology, Beijing Hospital, National Center of Gerontology, No. 1 Dahua Road, Dongdan, Beijing 100730, China

Suhan Lin, Wandong Hong and Qipin Wang
Department of Gastroenterology and Hepatology, The First Affiliated Hospital ofWenzhou Medical University, Wenzhou, Zhejiang, China

Suhan Lin and Qipin Wang
School of the First Clinical Medical Sciences, Wenzhou Medical University, Wenzhou, Zhejiang, China

Zarrin Basharat and Wandong Hong
Microbiology and Biotechnology Research Lab, Department of Environmental Sciences, Fatima Jinnah Women University, Rawalpindi 46000, Pakistan

Jingye Pan and Qipin Wang
Intensive Care Unit, The First Affiliated Hospital of Wenzhou Medical University, Wenzhou, Zhejiang, China

Mengtao Zhou
Department of Surgery, The First Affiliated Hospital of Wenzhou Medical University, Wenzhou, Zhejiang, China

Xiaoping Wang
Laboratory of Molecular Biology and Pathology, Shaanxi University of Chinese Medicine, Xianyang, Shaanxi 712046, China

Qiaoxia Wang
Department of Infectious Diseases, Xi'an Central Hospital, Xi'an, Shaanxi 710000, China

Irene S. Yu
University of British Columbia, Vancouver, Canada

Winson Y. Cheung
University of Calgary, Calgary, Canada

Xuefeng Luo, Wanqin Wang, Xiaoli Fan, Ying Zhao, Xiaoze Wang, Jinlin Yang and Li Yang
Department of Gastroenterology and Hepatology, West China Hospital, Sichuan University, Chengdu, China

Gonca Handan Ustundag and Yasemin Dilek Soysal
Faculty of Medicine, Department of Pediatric Gastroenterology, Hepatology and Nutrition, Bulent Ecevit University, Zonguldak, Turkey

Halime Altuntas
Faculty of Medicine, Department of Pediatrics, Bulent Ecevit University, Zonguldak, Turkey

Furuzan Kokturk
Faculty of Medicine, Department of Biostatistics, Bulent Ecevit University, Zonguldak, Turkey

Steven Pi
Department of Medicine, University of British Columbia Faculty of Medicine, Vancouver, BC, Canada

Estello Nap-Hill
Pacific Gastroenterology Associates, Vancouver, BC, Canada

Jennifer Telford and Robert Enns
Department of Gastroenterology, Division of Gastroenterology, St. Paul's Hospital, Vancouver, BC, Canada

Zofia Prokopowicz, Ewa Malecka-Tendera and Pawel Matusik
School of Medicine in Katowice, Department of Pediatrics and Pediatric Endocrinology, Medical University of Silesia, Katowice, Poland

Branka Filipović and Olivera Marković
Faculty of Medicine, University of Belgrade, Dr Subotíca Starijeg 8, Belgrade, Serbia

Branka Filipović
Department of Gastroenterohepatology, Clinical and Hospital Center Bežanijska Kosa, Autoput s/n, 11080 Belgrade, Serbia

Olivera Marković
Department of Hematology, Clinical and Hospital Center Bežanijska Kosa, Autoput s/n, 11080 Belgrade, Serbia

Vesna Đurić
Clinical and Hospital Center "Dr Dragiša Mišović-Dedinje", Belgrade, Serbia

Branislav Filipović
Institute of Anatomy "Niko Miljani´c", Dr Subotića Starijeg 4/2, Belgrade, Serbia

Tommaso Stroffolini and Caterina Furlan
Department of Tropical and Infectious Diseases, Policlinico Umberto I, Rome, Italy

Evangelista Sagnelli and Caterina Sagnelli
Department of Mental Health and Public Medicine, Campania University Luigi Vanvitelli, Naples, Italy

Iomena Morisco
Department of Clinical Medicine and Surgery, Gastroenterology Unit, University of Naples "Federico II", Naples, Italy

Sergio Babudieri
Clinic of Infectious Diseases, University of Sassari, Sassari, Italy

Mario Pirisi
Department of Translational Medicine, Universit`a del Piemonte Orientale, Novara, Italy

Maurizio Russello
Liver Unit, Hospital "G. Garibaldi" Catania, Catania, Italy

Antonina Smedile
Department of Medical Sciences, University of Turin, Turin, Italy

Mariantonietta Pisaturo
Unit of Infectious Diseases, S. Anna and S. Sebastian Hospital, Caserta, Italy

Piero Luigi Almasio
Biomedical Department of Internal Medicine e Specialities (Di.Bi.M.I.S.), University of Palermo, Palermo, Italy

Martin Perreault, Jocelyn Trottier, Mélanie Verreault, Patrick Caron and Olivier Barbier
Laboratory of Molecular Pharmacology, CHU-Qúebec Research Centre and the Faculty of Pharmacy, Laval University, Quebec City, QC, Canada

Ewa Wunsch and Andrzej Białek
Translation Medicine Group, Pomeranian Medical University, Szczecin, Poland

Guy G. Poirier
Proteomics Platform, Qúebec Genomic Center, CHU-Qúebec Research Centre and Faculty of Medicine, Laval University, Quebec City, QC, Canada

Piotr Milkiewicz
Liver and Internal Medicine, Medical University ofWarsaw, Warsaw, Poland

Yixin Yang
College of Natural, Applied and Health Sciences, Kean University, 100Morris Avenue, Union, NJ 07083, USA

Christopher Alderman
School of Medicine, University of Colorado, 13001 E 17th Pl, Aurora, CO 80045, USA

Ayoub Sehlaoui and Yuan Xiao
Department of Biological Sciences, Emporia State University, 1 Kellogg Circle, Emporia, KS 66801, USA

Wei Wang
Department ofThoracic Surgery III, Cancer Hospital of China Medical University, No. 44 Xiaoheyan Road, Dadong District, Shenyang, Liaoning 110042, China

Index